Geriatric Emergencies

Current Topics in Emergency Medicine

Series editor-in-chief, Peter L. Rosen
Associate series editor-in-chief, Shamai A. Grossman

Geriatric Emergencies

A discussion-based review

Edited by

Amal Mattu
University of Maryland School of Medicine, Department of Emergency Medicine, USA

Shamai A. Grossman
Harvard Medical School, USA
Beth Israel Deaconess Medical Center, Boston Massachusetts, USA

Peter L. Rosen
Harvard Medical School, USA
Beth Israel Deaconess Medical Center, Boston Massachusetts, USA

Associate Editors

Robert Anderson, MD
Christopher Carpenter, MD, MSC
Andrew Chang, MD, MS
Jon Mark Hirshon, MD, MPH, PhD
Ula Hwang, MD, MPH
Maura Kennedy, MD, MPH
Don Melady, MD, MSC(Ed)
Vaishal Tolia, MD, MPH
Scott Wilber, MD, MPH

WILEY Blackwell

Contents

List of Contributors

Nissa J. Ali, MD
Beth Israel Deaconess Medical Center
Harvard Affiliated Emergency Medicine Residency
Department of Emergency Medicine
West Campus Clinical Center
Boston, MA, USA

Robert S. Anderson, Jr., MD
Assistant Professor
Tufts University School of Medicine
Departments of Emergency Medicine and Internal
    Medicine and Division of Geriatric Medicine
Maine Medical Center
Portland, ME, USA

Kevin Biese, MD, MAT
Vice Chair of Academic Affairs
Department of Emergency Medicine
University of North Carolina at Chapel Hill Chapel
Hill, NC, USA

Michael C. Bond, MD
Associate Professor, Residency Program Director
Department of Emergency Medicine
University of Maryland School of Medicine
Baltimore, MD, USA

Alexander Bromfield, MD
Clinical Instructor, Department of Emergency
    Medicine
University of California San Diego Health System
San Diego, CA, USA

Kenneth H. Butler, DO
Associate Professor, Associate Residency Program
    Director
Department of Emergency Medicine
University of Maryland School of Medicine
Baltimore, MD, USA

Colleen Campbell, MD
Associate Clinical Professor
Department of Emergency Medicine
Division of Emergency Ultrasound
University of California
    San Diego Health System
San Diego, CA, USA

Alessandro Cancelliere, MD PhD
Assistant Professor
Department of Emergency Medicine
University of Massachusetts Medical School
Worcester, MA, USA

Christopher R. Carpenter, MD, MSC
Associate Professor
Division of Emergency Medicine
Washington University in St. Louis School of
    Medicine
St. Louis, MO, USA

Andrew K. Chang, MD, MS
Vincent P. Verdile Vice Chair for Research and
    Academic Affairs
Professor of Emergency Medicine
Albany Medical College
Attending Physician
Albany Medical Center
Albany, New York

Eric A. Coleman, MD, MPH
Professor of Medicine and Head, Division of Health
    Care Policy and Research
Director
Care Transitions Program University of Colorado
    Denver
Anschutz Medical Campus
Aurora, CO, USA

Elizabeth Couser, MSW
Gerontology PhD Candidate
Doctoral Program in Gerontology
University of Maryland
Baltimore, MD, USA

Susanne DeMeester, MD
Attending Physician and Director Emergency
    Observation Center
St Joseph Mercy Hospital
Ann Arbor, MI, USA

Jonathan Edlow, MD
Vice-Chair, Department of Emergency Medicine
Beth Israel Deaconess Medical Center
Professor of Medicine and Emergency Medicine
Harvard Medical School
Boston, MA, USA

Benjamin W. Friedman, MD, MS
Associate Professor of Emergency Medicine
Albert Einstein College of Medicine
Montefiore Medical Center
Bronx, NY, USA

Shamai A. Grossman, MD
Associate Professor of Medicine and Emergency
    Medicine
Harvard Medical School
Vice Chair for Health Care Quality
Director
Observation Medicine
Department of Emergency Medicine
Beth Israel Deaconess Medical Center
Boston, MA, USA

Kama Guluma, MD
Clinical Professor
Department of Emergency Medicine
University of California San Diego Health System
San Diego, CA, USA

Marianne Haughey, MD
Associate Professor of Emergency Medicine
Albert Einstein College of Medicine
Jacobi Medical Center
Bronx, New York, NY, USA

Bryan Hayes, PharmD
Clinical Associate Professor
Department of Emergency Medicine
University of Maryland School of Medicine
    Baltimore, MD, USA

Jon Mark Hirshon, MD, MPH, PhD
Professor
Departments of Emergency Medicine and of
    Epidemiology and Public Health
University of Maryland School of Medicine
Baltimore, MD, USA

Teresita M. Hogan, MD
Director of Geriatric Emergency Medicine
Department of Medicine
Sections of Emergency Medicine and Geriatrics &
    Palliative Care
The University of Chicago
Chicago, IL, USA

Ula Hwang, MD, MPH
Associate Professor
Department of Emergency Medicine
Brookdale Department of Geriatrics and Palliative
    Medicine
Icahn School of Medicine at Mount Sinai
New York, NY
Geriatric Research, Education and Clinical Center
James J. Peters VAMC
Bronx, NY, USA

Joshua W. Joseph, MD
Fellow in Clinical Informatics
Department of Emergency Medicine
Beth Israel Deaconess Medical Center
Clinical Fellow in Emergency Medicine
Harvard Medical School, Boston, MA, USA

Maura Kennedy, MD, MPH
Associate Director for Emergency
    Medicine Research
Department of Emergency Medicine
Beth Israel Deaconess Medical Center
Assistant Professor of Emergency Medicine
Harvard Medical School
Boston, MA, USA

Phillip D. Magidson, MD, MPH
Departments of Emergency Medicine and Medicine
University of Maryland Medical Center
Baltimore, MD, USA

Amal Mattu, MD
Professor of Emergency Medicine and Vice Chair
Department of Emergency Medicine
University of Maryland School of Medicine
Baltimore, MD, USA

Colleen M. McQuown, MD
Associate Professor, Northeast Ohio Medical
   University
Rootstown, OH, USA
Associate Research Director
Department of Emergency Medicine
Summa Akron City Hospital
Akron, OH, USA

Don Melady, MD, MSC(Ed)
Schwartz/Reisman Emergency Centre
Mount Sinai Hospital
Assistant Professor, Faculty of Medicine
University of Toronto
Toronto, ON, Canada

Siamak Moayedi, MD
Assistant Professor
Department of Emergency Medicine
University of Maryland School of Medicine
Baltimore, MD, USA

Barbara Morano, MPH, LCSW
Program Manager
Department of Geriatrics
Icahn School of Medicine at Mount Sinai
New York, NY, USA

Carmen Morano, PhD, LCSW
Associate Professor
Silberman School of Social Work at Hunter College
Director
Silberman Aging: A Hartford Center of Excellence in
   Diverse Aging
Managing Editor
Journal of Gerontological Social Work
New York, NY, USA

Denise Nassisi, MD
Director of the Geriatric Emergency Department
Mount Sinai Medical Center
Associate Professor Departments of Emergency
   Medicine & Medicine Icahn School of Medicine at
   Mount Sinai
New York, NY, USA

Rebecca Nerenberg, MD
Assistant Professor of Clinical Emergency Medicine
Department of Emergency Medicine
Montefiore Medical Center
Albert Einstein College of Medicine
Bronx, NY, USA

Charles W. O'Connell, MD
Clinical Instructor
Department of Emergency Medicine
Division of Medical Toxicology
University of California San Diego Health System
San Diego, CA, USA

Ruben E. Olmedo, MD
Director
Division of Toxicology
Department of Emergency Medicine
Mount Sinai Medical Center
Assistant Professor
Icahn School of Medicine at Mount Sinai
New York, NY, USA

Jason Ondrejka, DO
Summa Akron City Hospital
Department of Emergency Medicine
Akron, OH, USA

Leslie C. Oyama, MD
Associate Clinical Professor
Associate Residency Director
University of California San Diego Health System
San Diego, CA, USA

Timothy C. Peck, MD
Beth Israel Deaconess Medical Center
Harvard Affiliated Emergency Medicine Residency
Department of Emergency Medicine
West Campus Clinical Center
Boston, MA, USA

Peter L. Rosen, MD
Senior Lecturer Emergency Medicine
Harvard Medical School
Attending Emergency Physician Beth
  Israel/Deaconess Medical Center
Visiting Clinical Professor of Emergency Medicine
University of Arizona School of Medicine Tucson
Emeritus Professor of Emergency Medicine
University of California
San Diego, CA, USA

Roxanna Sadri, MD
Department of Emergency Medicine
University of California San Diego Health System
San Diego, CA, USA

Nicholas Santavicca, MD
Fellow, Emergency Medicine/Internal
  Medicine/Critical Care Program
University of Maryland Medical Center
Baltimore, MD, USA

Davut Savaser, MD
Clinical Instructor
Department of Emergency Medicine
Division of Hyperbaric and Undersea Medicine
University of California San Diego Health System
San Diego, CA, USA

John G. Schumacher, PhD
Graduate Program Director, Associate Professor
Department of Sociology and Anthropology
University of Maryland
Baltimore County (UMBC),
  Baltimore, MD, USA

Kirk A. Stiffler, MD, MPH
Department of Emergency Medicine,
  Summa Akron City Hospital
Associate Professor of Emergency Medicine
Northeast Ohio Medical University
Akron, OH, USA

Tania D. Strout, PhD, RN, MS
Associate Professor
Tufts University School of Medicine
Director of Research
Department of Emergency Medicine
Maine Medical Center
Portland, ME, USA

Alison Southern, MD
Associate Program Director, Department of
  Emergency Medicine
Summa Health System
Associate Professor of Emergency Medicine
Northeast Ohio Medical University
Akron, OH, USA

Vaishal Tolia, MD, MPH
Associate Clinical Professor
Emergency & Internal Medicine
Medical Director & Director of Observation
  Medicine
Department of Emergency Medicine
UCSD Health System
San Diego, CA

Mercedes Torres, MD
Clinical Assistant Professor
Department of Emergency Medicine
University of Maryland School of Medicine
Baltimore, MD, USA

Julie Watkins-Torrey, MD
Resident Physician
Department of Emergency Medicine
University of California San Diego Health System
San Diego, CA, USA

Katren Tyler, M.B.B.S.
Associate Professor and Associate Program
  Director, Geriatric Emergency
  Medicine Fellowship Director,
  Vice Chair for Faculty Development,
  Wellness and Outreach
Department of Emergency Medicine
University of California, Davis
Sacramento, CA, USA

Gabriel Wardi, MD
Department of Emergency Medicine, Fellow,
  Division of Pulmonary and Critical Care Medicine,
  University of California San Diego Health System
San Diego, CA, USA

Scott Wilber, MD, MPH
Chair, Department of Emergency Medicine
Summa Health System
Professor of Emergency Medicine
Northeast Ohio Medical University
Akron, Ohio, USA

Michael Winters, MD
Associate Professor of Emergency Medicine and
  Medicine
Departments of Emergency Medicine and Medicine
University of Maryland School of Medicine
Baltimore, MD, USA

Richard E. Wolfe, MD
Chief of Emergency Medicine
Beth Israel Deaconess Medical Center
Boston, MA, USA

Alexandra Wong, BA
Research Associate
Department of Medicine
Section of Geriatrics and Palliative Care
The University of Chicago
Chicago, IL, USA

Kate D. Zimmerman, DO
Assistant Professor
Tufts University School of Medicine, Associate
  Director of Medical Student Education
Department of Emergency Medicine
Maine Medical Center
Portland, ME, USA

1

General assessment of the elderly patient

Alison Southern & Scott Wilber

Department of Emergency Medicine, Summa Akron City Hospital, Northeast Ohio Medical University, Akron, OH, USA

Section I: Case presentation

The patient is a 96-year-old man who presented with a chief complaint of slurred speech and generalized weakness. A history was obtained from the paramedic run sheet and family, who arrived in the emergency department (ED) 15 min after the patient. His symptoms have been waxing and waning over the last few days. Today, he had slurred speech and left-sided weakness, which has now resolved.

The patient's daughter reported that since his wife died 3 months ago, he has had a 20 lb weight loss. He has decreased appetite, decreased activity, and decreased function, which has waxed and waned. For the last 2 days, he has required wheelchair transport to the cafeteria for meals and assistance with transfer. The family stated that he has not had a recent change in his confusion.

The past medical history was significant for dementia, gastroesophageal reflux disease, hypertension, aortic stenosis, and benign prostatic hypertrophy. His social history notes that he currently lives in an assisted living facility. His daughter visits daily and assists with instrumental activities of daily living (ADLs).

On examination, the vital signs were normal. Head, eyes, ears, nose, and throat examinations were normal. Results of cardiopulmonary, abdomen, and extremity examinations were normal. On neurologic examination, he was oriented to year and person. He was not oriented to day or month. He had 0/3 items on 3 item recall. The Six-Item Screener (SIS)

score was 1. The modified Richmond Agitation and Sedation Scale (RASS) score was 0. The NIH Stroke Scale was 1 for confusion. The skin examination revealed a Stage 2 sacral decubitus ulcer.

The laboratory studies revealed an albumin of 2.3 and a hemoglobin of 9.

The family felt that the patient had been declining since his wife died and requested hospice evaluation, as a hospice had been beneficial for the patient's wife.

Section II: Case discussion

Dr Peter Rosen (PR): I would like to remind everyone what we tell our interns when we first get a presentation like this. We should have our exact vital signs instead of just saying normal, because normal may not be normal at this age. I think one of the critical assessment points of the older patient is to understand what are the normal changes in physiology as you age, so that you aren't fooled by them. Just as when you look at an infant, a resting heart rate of 120 doesn't bother you, which it would if the child were 10 years old. That's number one. Number two: it's impossible not to be that age without taking 42 different medications, so we really need to know what they are. Without those, it's really hard to get to the root of any geriatric problem. What are some of the physiologic changes you would expect in this age group?

Dr Amal Mattu (AM): You mentioned the vital signs, so we can start with that. To reiterate, vital signs can be unreliable. Elderly patients can have a resting bradycardia as opposed to the infants you mentioned who might have a resting tachycardia. In addition, if they're on beta-blockers, calcium channel blockers, or digoxin, any of these can produce a further reduction in the heart rate so that even in the presence of overwhelming sepsis they may not mount a tachycardia; or if they are bleeding out, they may not mount a tachycardia we've all been led to expect from those ATLS charts. Elderly patients often will have isolated systolic hypertension and may walk around with a systolic pressure of 180 or 190 torr. Thus, when they come in with a systolic pressure of 120 torr, it appears to be a normal pressure, but they may actually be in shock. These are the two vital signs that are the most misleading. Elderly patients tend to take longer to mount a fever as well. If they have an infection, they may also be more likely to develop a hypothermic response to the infection.

PR: Furthermore, not knowing what medications the patient is on prevents us from knowing what vital sign responses we can expect. Even though we are supposed to take temperatures on all patients, we frequently don't. It's just prudent to get used to having to ask for a temperature, if we don't see it right away. Can you think of any other physiologic changes to this age group that we should be aware of, such as vital capacity or respiratory rate or something to do with the neurologic system?

Dr Scott Wilber (SW): Dr Mattu mentioned the lack of tachycardia even in the case of overwhelming sepsis. One of the things we also see is that frequently tachypnea is a better indication of serious illness such as hemorrhage or infection, and you will frequently see a patient with only tachypnea as the manifestation of serious illness.

PR: The issues in this case are both medical and ethical. It seems to me that we rarely need to start ethical evaluations before we finish our medical evaluations, but here's a difference in the management of the geriatric patient. I think that unless you're willing to answer the ethical question of how much workup is this patient going to profit from, then you really can't do a good medical evaluation. This case seems to be a perfect example of that. Here's a patient with declining status, he can't take care of himself. Even from an already observed level of dementia, his family

has noticed a decline. I think a good ethical question is at what point do workup and treatment become futile and an unnecessary expense rather than trying to reach the medical endpoint that we might try to achieve in someone, who was say 30 years younger leading a normal life.

AM: I agree managing expectations is going to be very important. I think we were very fortunate that in this case, the family is actually present, and we can have that discussion with them. Moreover, the patient is somewhat stable. We can query the family about what their expectations may be for the patient's care. Also, we need to determine whether the patient had been to other facilities or his primary care physician to see if any aggressive changes might have been made to the medication regimen that might have led to the today's ED presentation. Then, we can ask that question: how much should we be doing? Other providers may not have done that, and that could actually explain why that person is here.

Dr Shamai Grossman (SG): I think the problem we are raising reflects some of the limitations of emergency medicine. We rarely have all the information about the patient, and often this is the first time we are seeing this patient. If you just read this case, you would realize we're missing vital parts of the history. You know the patient has had decreasing function since his wife died. Is that depression? Is it a physiologic process going on? The problem is we're seeing this patient fresh in the ED, and we're not his primary care doctor. In an ideal world, all these things would have been worked out by the primary care physician. At best, we will have only a brief discussion with the family members, and making these decisions is going to be very challenging. I think approaching older adults in the ED, given all these limitations that we have, requires a different method. I think a major responsibility is determining the goals of care that the patient or by proxy, the family or the caregivers would like. It's new for emergency physicians to be thinking in terms like this. Then, when we understand the immediate care goals, we can begin to find out about intermediate, and then long-term goals.

PR: I think that's a very strong point, which can also affect decision-making in terms of how aggressively you manage that patient. In any patient, you need to discover why they are there, and I think it can be useful to ask what are the expectations from the emergency care that this family wishes to derive. If he's having a stroke, do they want us to treat that stroke? If he's just declining, then why did they bring them to the ED? Often, the primary care physician may have the answers, but they frequently don't share them with the ED. What would you suggest in terms of the workup for what sounds to be a transient ischemic attack (TIA)?

AM: I would again start with trying to find out what the family's goals are in terms of the short-term and long-term outcomes. If this were a younger patient who had fewer medical problems and many years ahead of him, then you would probably get a head CT scan, and have neurology come and do the full workup that we usually perform for TIA and stroke. On the other hand, if this is a patient for whom the family just wants to make the patient comfortable, then we do not need to do much of anything. The family requested a hospice, which certainly suggests comfort care, and may preclude doing anything but giving that comfort care.

SW: I think oftentimes it does take a few minutes of conversation with the family to explain to them the different kinds of evaluations we can do in the ED. For instance, in this situation, the family may say they do not want a stroke aggressively treated, they may not want surgery to evacuate a subdural hematoma, but if the patient had a urinary tract infection (UTI) and needed antibiotics, they might consent to that. Or, if the patient were hyponatremic, and needed some IV fluids for a day, they might consent to that. I therefore might spend time with the family just to explain the kind of testing we can do, and what that would lead to. In this particular situation, a CT scan often may lead to more aggressive treatment than checking the patient's electrolytes or checking a urinalysis.

SG: I might add one more thing. We are concentrating on the wishes of the family, but what we need to be sure of is that these also are the patient's wishes. If the patient can't articulate what he really thought, we are obliged to make sure that the person you're talking to is really the healthcare proxy and make sure that when you talk to the family that they're actually communicating the patient's best wishes and not the family

member's vested interests, and that they're not trying to make someone who potentially has some viability into a hospice patient. I think it's an ethical imperative that when we talk about patient autonomy, it's not solely the family's autonomy. When the patient is decisionally incapacitated, then you have to do the next best thing, which is to try to figure out what the patient would want.

SW: The ethical terms we use are using substituted judgment rather than best interest. Whenever possible, we want to substitute for our judgment what the patients would want, rather than just acting in their best interest. When we have no ability to ascertain what the patient would have wanted, then we act using the patient's best interest, but whenever possible, we use substituted judgment.

PR: A number of EDs have benefited from having a pharmacologist available in the department to help in the evaluation of complex drug interactions. I think that's particularly useful in the geriatric population because they have so many different medications that none of us can keep all the interactions in our head. We need to be cautious because the patient may have been taking inappropriate and just wrong medications, which somehow became the patient's ordered therapy at the nursing home. Diabetic medications are one of the most common sources of increasing confusion in the elderly patient, and it would be useful to check the patient's glucose level. Do you have any solutions for how we can ensure the quality of this patient's medications?

AM: In terms of a simple solution, I don't know that there is one. ED pharmacists can be very helpful here as they can focus on scrutinizing the medications these patients are taking and look for drug interactions and potential adverse effects, especially if you are planning on adding a new drug to the regimen. There is probably not as great a need for them or for us to scrutinize medications in young patients, but in older patients the effort is very important. Sometimes, 5 min of study of past records or computer drug records will identify the single cause of the patient's presentation, the patient's delirium, or whatever else it is that brings them into the hospital.

PR: Most of us are not familiar with all of these scores that are mentioned here and are not likely to learn them. Do you have any suggestions for how

3

the emergency physician can make a quick mental status assessment that might identify an acute organic brain syndrome (delirium), as opposed to declining dementia?

SW: So I think it's important that we try to be objective when we do a mental status examination. Frequently, I will have residents present to me that a patient is alert and oriented times three (A&Ox3). I generally think that means that the patient was awake and interactive and that they didn't specifically ask the patients the questions to determine their orientation. So I think it's important to be objective about that. In this case, we used something called a SIS. A very quick test where we just ask the patient to remember three items (apple, table, and penny) and then to tell us the day, the month, and the year, and then to repeat back the objects we asked. And a score of 4 or less out of 6 is equivalent of a mini mental status examination (MMSE) of approximately 23 or less. Now none of us are going to do a full MMSE on a patient that might take 15 min, but the SIS might be incorporated into your examination without increasing your time with the patient significantly. The RASS score is something that a lot of residents are probably familiar with right now, but those of us who are older may not be. The reason the residents are familiar with this is that often it is used in the ICU to titrate sedation. Basically, a RASS of 0 means the patient is awake, alert, and interactive. Scores that are negative mean that the patient is more lethargic and may be aroused only to verbal and painful stimuli; scores that are positive indicate a patient who is more agitated. Whether they use this scale or a descriptive scale, it is important to determine if the patient is alert and attentive. A patient who is unable to pay attention to you while you are doing a history and is obsessed with the beeping monitor and with things going on outside of the room may be exhibiting the first signs of delirium, that is, lack of attention. So I think those are the two ways to evaluate the two parts of their consciousness: the content of their consciousness, or how confused they are, and their level of consciousness, or how awake they are.

PR: We used to use the clock as a quick delirium screen in younger patients. Can the patient draw a time that you give them on a clock face? It's a very quick assessment of someone who may from time to time appear to be normal and alert, but who is actually confused. We used to use the "string sign" for withdrawing alcoholics, where you ask "Do you see the string?" and you of course hold no string. If the patient reports seeing a string, then the patient is confabulating and has an acute organic brain syndrome (delirium). I think that the point being that many of these patients are acutely altered as opposed to being at baseline demented. If they were normal before they have the drug interactions, it's useful to know that this is a form of dementia that you can reverse. Amal, we also know that the patient has a history of prostatic hypertrophy. While we know that UTIs are more common in the elderly and are one of the more common causes of acute organic brain syndromes, would you do any special kind of workup for this man's prostate? That is, would you do a bladder evaluation to see if this man's emptying, or if what the patient would benefit from would be an indwelling Foley as we are again unlikely to recommend surgery?

AM: I've seen a couple of patients who have developed delirium simply from significant urinary retention. Checking the urine and confirming that the patient is able to void and is not retaining is simple and should be probably done. With ready access to ultrasound, everywhere it's easy to take a look at the bladder and see if it's significantly distended. If it is, then putting a catheter in to decompress the bladder would be useful as would sending a urinalysis. If the bladder does not appear to be distended, my preference would be to not put the catheter in because it would be a portal of entry for bacteria.

SG: I would also remember to do a rectal exam as prostatitis is an often-missed cause of elderly UTIs, who bounce back to the ED with recurrent or worsened infections after their antibiotics are completed, but their infection has yet to be adequately treated.

PR: In reading the case, it sounds like the family's desire is to change the focus of his care from nursing home to hospice. I'm not personally aware of any of the hospice restrictions although I thought that death had to be imminent – 30 days or less, to get into a hospice, and I don't know how I'd be able to make that argument in this patient. Maybe you could help us in terms of whether or not this patient is even a candidate for hospice.

SW: Most hospices require that two physicians certify that the patient has a projected prognosis of 6 months or less. It is really not imminent death but a best guess of 6 months or less. The estimate can be extended if the patient doesn't die within 6 months, and the patient can be recertified for an additional 6 months. There are different categories for hospice qualification. There are criteria for failure to thrive, stroke, chronic renal disease, chronic liver disease, and dementia. The general indicators that I keep in mind are that if someone is having functional decline and problems with nutrition, they may be appropriate for hospice. For failure to thrive, they have to have increasing symptoms, progression of disease, or frequent ED visits plus impaired nutritional status and failure to thrive. We see that this patient had an albumin of 2.3 showing impaired nutritional status, and also a decubitus ulcer suggesting impaired nutritional status as well. Thus, we do have a documented functional decline. Functional decline and impaired nutritional status with weight loss and low albumin are two things to indicate to an emergency physician that the patient may qualify for hospice.

Dr Ula Hwang (UH): There are two things I would bring up in terms of approaching the family's wishes. We've discussed a lot about the potential medical evaluation, but another thing that may also be of benefit for this patient is a quick evaluation for depression. I know that the patient has significant dementia; it sounds like he hasn't varied much from his baseline, but the history does include the fact that his wife died 3 months ago, and we saw this significant weight loss, perhaps he has had some functional decline, decreased appetite. Some of this may also contribute to the big picture of what's going on. It's probably not the only cause, but that may also be part of the family's decision-making in terms of palliative care evaluation and end-of-life discussions with the family. The physician can think not necessarily in terms of imminent death, but rather withdrawal of active treatment. If he is not undergoing active treatment, he could and should be evaluated by palliative medicine, if not for hospice, then at least for comfort measures that may be useful for him.

PR: Perhaps you could tell us the outcome of this case and what precisely ended up being the cause of this patient coming to the hospital that day.

SW: I had a discussion with the family. We did agree to evaluate for potentially reversible conditions such as a UTI, which they would have wanted to have treated, and we did decide to do a CT scan of the head, which was done more for prognosis than for treatment. They felt that if the patient had a significant abnormality on CT scan, it would have made them more likely to want to have the patient in hospice. The CT scan of the head did not show anything acute. He did not have any evidence of infection. His medications were reviewed, and there was nothing obvious that was a medication interaction or a new medication added. In fact, he had been evaluated for depression and had been on antidepressant since his wife had gotten sick several months ago; so, it was not thought that new depression was the cause of his functional decline and symptoms. The patient was admitted to the hospital and evaluated by the palliative care team on the acute palliative care unit and was found eligible for hospice. He lived for several more months under hospice care before he died.

PR: I would like to discuss one more idea brought up by this case. We went through most of the responsibilities of the emergency physician. What we did not discuss are some of the painful life realities. That is, patients like this are very difficult to admit. Most medical services do not feel that they have anything to offer the patient and do not want to admit patients for whom there is no easy outcome that they can see. When I was a young physician, we had a service at the hospital where I trained that would admit patients like this. They were basically sociologic admissions or administrative admissions, where you had to put patients in the hospital before you could get them into a nursing home, and it was more custodial care rather than diagnostic or therapeutic care. I wonder if we shouldn't be developing more services like that as we have populations that age, and more patients who are developing these kinds of problems. It is especially frustrating with all the crowding problems we have now and the increasing focus as to whether patients qualify for admission in terms of reimbursement. It is certainly getting tougher for all of us to get these patients admitted. I don't have a simple solution except to remind all the readers that our job is to be advocates for the patients. We have to remember why we went into medicine, which is to take care of people and not just to focus on reimbursement, and

5

to be an advocate for the patient as much as possible. Sometimes, advocating for patients doesn't involve giving drugs or IV fluids but merely doing the best thing for the patient. This may involve a fight to get them admitted just to protect them in some way, or to facilitate their transit to a nursing home or hospice.

SW: I think that this case illustrates a new kind of approach that we need to take with older patients in the ED. We need to look at the whole patient. We do not always need to offer aggressive medical treatment, and sometimes the best thing we can offer is palliative treatment or hospice care. These patients are complex, but we went into emergency medicine for the challenge, and I think that these patients do challenge us. We can end up with good outcomes, and I think this patient had a good outcome.

UH: I would add that the approach to older patients and their assessment in the ED does incorporate different and new approaches with regard to assessment. The vitals must be interpreted differently. We must think about cognitive and functional status. We must make a diligent attempt to ascertain what the goals of care would be for the patient and for the family members.

AM: I was just thinking that when I was in medical school, the medical professors used to talk about this holistic approach to patients and a biopsychosocial model of medical care. It was a bit soft or too theoretical for many of us. We went into emergency medicine because we wanted to do focused evaluations. Fast, quick, "treat 'em and street 'em" approaches. Yet, now I think we're realizing that as the population is aging, and we're seeing more and more patients who have more than just isolated medical issues, the focused approach is very short-sighted and inappropriate to successfully caring for these patients. The reality is that emergency medicine needs to become a more holistic, at least in our approach to older patients. We need to consider not only the medical issues but also the psychosocial aspects of patient care as well. More and more I'm realizing that when you take the time to do that, it turns out to be a very good investment in the medical care of these patients. It does result in fewer bounce backs. The population is changing, and our practice needs to change as well. A case like this is a really good demonstration of that.

Section III: Concepts

Background

A key concept that is evident from this case presentation and discussion is that the general assessment of the elderly patient in the ED is complex and different from practice upon younger patients, and this patient population requires special attention. These patients often have complex past medical histories and interrelated psychosocial issues contributing to their current presentation. Although the hallmark of the initial stabilization of the elderly patient remains airway, breathing, and circulation, the remainder of the assessment becomes a biopsychosocial evaluation. It is essential that the emergency physician be able to see the whole picture, with the ultimate goal of care to manage the elderly patient as the patient would wish. This presents many challenges including accurate history taking and gathering, diagnosing medical problems within the context of physiologic changes related to age, treating complex medical problems along with polypharmacy, assessing cognitive and functional status, and determining end-of-life decisions and goals of care.

In most cases, the assessment of the older patient in the ED should be comprised of four specific areas of focus: (1) medical evaluation, (2) cognitive evaluation, (3) functional evaluation, and (4) social evaluation [1].

Medical evaluation

The medical evaluation comprises the standard approach to ED patients. It should include a thorough history and physical examination. At times, given the circumstances of the patient and ED, these may not proceed in the ordered manner one was taught in medical school, but both should be performed.

History
The initial history, including a review of the chief complaint, and a history of present illness should be reviewed in all patients. Some older patients may not be able to provide adequate history due to cognitive impairment, hearing impairment, or acuity of illness; in these patients, alternative sources of history should be obtained and documented. Serious conditions often present atypically in the older ED patients, and

vague presenting complaints such as "weakness" may be indicative of serious disease [2].

The patient's past medical history should be elicited and the medications reviewed. This would include the current medication list and dosages, paying close attention to any new or recently removed medications. Older patients are often prescribed multiple medications for chronic illnesses; this may lead to increased adverse effects and drug–drug interactions. The number of medications taken by older patients is increasing. In 2002, the Sloan Survey collected data on drug usage from a random sample of US patients. This survey showed that of patients ≥65 years of age, 23% of women and 19% of men took at least five medications and 12% of both women and men took >10 medications [3].

It is estimated that 5–10% of admissions to the hospital for older patients are due to adverse drug reactions [4]. According to data from estimates of the 58 nonpediatric hospitals that participate in the National Electronic Injury Surveillance System– Cooperative Adverse Drug Event Surveillance (NEISS–CADES) project, drug interactions result in an estimated 99,628 emergency hospitalizations each year among older adults. Warfarin is implicated in approximately one third of these adverse events; insulin, oral anti-platelet agents, and oral hypoglycemic agents account for approximately another third [5].

In 2012, the American Geriatric Society updated the Beers criteria for potentially inappropriate medication use in older adults. This was accomplished through an extensive literature search and expert panel. The Beers criteria are used as an educational tool and a quality measure; the goal of these criteria is to improve older patients' care by reducing their exposure to potentially inappropriate medications. Fifty-three medications or medication classes make up the updated 2012 AGS Beers Criteria, which are divided into three categories. The first category is the potentially inappropriate medications and classes to avoid in older adults. The next category summarizes potentially inappropriate medications and classes to avoid in older adults with certain diseases and syndromes that the drugs listed can exacerbate. The third group, medications that should be used with caution, was added with the 2012 update [6]. The Beers Criteria help in the review of a patient's medication list for potential medications causing side effects. It also aids physician's decision making when new medications are needed.

Vital signs

All too often, a quick review of the vital signs in an elderly patient leads to the conclusion that he/she is "normal," as in the case presentation above. However, in this age group, subtle changes in vital signs may be easily overlooked and lead physicians in the wrong direction. Each vital sign can give objective information in a patient whose history is already most likely limited. Therefore, a thorough review of a complete set of vital signs is crucial.

Blood pressure can be misleading in the elderly population. A blood pressure that may appear normal may be markedly abnormal compared to the patient's baseline blood pressure. Due to physiologic changes of aging, there is a loss of elastic fibers, causing vessels to be more rigid and less compliant. This hardening of the major vessels leads to systolic hypertension, increased peripheral resistance, and ventricular hypertrophy [7]. Ventricular hypertrophy can lead to diastolic dysfunction with decreased cardiac filling [8]. In a patient with systolic hypertension, it is important to know the patient's baseline systolic blood pressure as "normal" blood pressures may actually be a sign of shock.

Older patients are also subject to orthostatic hypotension, or the inability of the body to adjust the blood pressure during postural changes, resulting in hypotension. Orthostatic hypotension is estimated to occur in 20–30% of community-dwelling older patients and 50% of nursing home residents. Orthostatic hypotension is associated with falls, syncope, dizziness, and confusion in older patients [9].

Another cardiovascular physiologic change of aging is a reduction in the number of atrial pacemaker cells. This leads to a decreased intrinsic heart rate. There is also a decreased responsiveness to beta adrenergic receptor stimulation that leads to a decreased heart rate response to exercise and stress [10]. Older patients are more likely to have a resting bradycardia, sick sinus syndrome, and atrial dysrhythmias [11]. This can add additional risk to a patient who is already at risk for falls and syncope. A patient's medication may also mask problems normally evident by abnormal vital signs [12]. For example, a patient with severe sepsis or hemorrhagic shock may be unable to mount a tachycardia due to beta-blockers, calcium channel blockers, or digoxin. This lends further importance to a thorough review of the patient's medication list.

Aging results in many changes in the respiratory system. There is a loss of elastic lung recoil, leading to an increasing number of alveoli that do not participate in gas exchange. The chest wall loses ability to expand, and the lungs lose defense mechanisms, such as mucociliary reflex [13]. Kyphosis can reduce chest wall compliance and diaphragm function. These changes can increase the work of breathing and decrease functional reserve [14].

The respiratory rate may be a subtle sign of distress in older patients and may be the only vital sign that appears abnormal on initial evaluation. As it requires some time to obtain an adequate respiratory rate, and it may be poorly recorded, it may be prudent for the physician to verify the respiratory rate personally. Tachypnea is associated with cardiac arrest in admitted patients, transfer to higher level of care within 24 h of ED admission, and 30-day mortality in ED patients [15, 16]. Tachypnea can be a sign of impending respiratory distress or failure, infection, cardiac disease, or shock. In patients with sepsis, tachypnea is independently associated with in-hospital mortality [17]. There is also an association with mortality and tachypnea in older patients with suspected infection [18].

Accurate testing of pulse oximetry is also important as many geriatric patients have underlying chronic lung diseases as well as peripheral vascular disease, which may make an accurate pulse oximeter reading more difficult to obtain [19].

Older patients have limitations in body temperature regulation resulting in a lower core body temperature [20]. They may not mount a febrile response to infection and are apt to be hypothermic as a result of infection [21]. The cutoff defining a fever may need to be adjusted in older patients in order to improve the detection of serious infections. For example, with older nursing home patients in the ED, a temperature of 99°F (37.2°C) has a sensitivity of 83% and a specificity of 89% for significant bacterial infections [22]. As baseline temperatures may be lower in older patients, a change from baseline temperature of at least 1.3°C or 2.4°F may be an important indicator of infection [23].

Physical examination

After initial stabilization and review of the vital signs, it is important to perform a full physical examination when assessing the elderly patient. Oftentimes, history may be limited secondary to chronic dementia or a newly altered mental status. These patients may not be able to relate that they have a sore on their back or a neglect of their right side. Therefore, a complete head-to-toe examination including skin examination and neurologic assessment is essential. When assessing the patient's skin, it is important to remove clothes including socks to assess whether there is skin breakdown. This is especially important in the evaluation of potential infections. It may be necessary to roll immobile patients to examine their buttocks, sacrum, and back.

Laboratory studies

There are a number of laboratory studies whose normal values do not change with aging. These include electrolytes, blood urea nitrogen, hemoglobin, platelet count, and white blood cell count. In these situations, comparison to a baseline value is helpful to evaluate whether abnormal values are an acute or chronic change [24]. There are other laboratory parameters whose normal ranges do change with age. For instance, the erythrocyte sedimentation rate upper limit of normal should be age adjusted (age/2 for men and (age + 10)/2 for women) [25]. Since creatinine values are related to lean body mass, normal creatinine values decline with aging. In this situation, "normal" values may indicate reduced glomerular filtration rate [26]. In addition, D-dimer values may need adjustment with aging, a series of recent studies suggest that a value of (age × 10) mg/l may be a reasonable cutoff for excluding pulmonary embolism [27].

Cognitive assessment

Cognitive impairment is common in the elderly patient population and the emergency physician should be able to utilize tools available to aid in recognition of this impairment. Commonly physicians will document that the patient is "A&Ox3." This likely reflects that the patient was able to carry on a conversation and answer historical questions. More formal testing should be used to avoid an inadequate and incomplete assessment. The Geriatric Emergency Medicine Task

Force recommends a mental status evaluation of all elderly patients presenting to the ED [28].

As it is often difficult to discern worsening dementia from acute delirium in confused ED patients, additional information from paramedics, family, primary care providers, and caretakers should be sought. The emergency physician should not assume that confusion or altered mental status is the patient's baseline status without verification.

The classic cognitive screening test is the MMSE. This test is difficult to perform in the ED as it is time-consuming and scoring is complex. Alternatives include screening tests that are sensitive, quick, and easy for the physician to remember and score. The SIS and Ottawa 3DY (O3DY) meet these criteria [29].

The SIS consists of item recall plus orientation. The SIS takes approximately 1 min to complete. It begins by asking the patient to repeat three items such as apple, table, and penny. The patient is asked to recall these items in a few minutes. They are then asked year, month, and day. Finally, they are asked to recall the initial three items. It is scored as a sum of the correct answers with 6 being the highest score. A score of 4 or less suggests cognitive impairment. A cutoff of 3 or more errors has a similar sensitivity and specificity for a diagnosis of dementia *as does* a cutoff score of 23 on the MMSE [30]. In a study of 352 subjects with 111 cognitively impaired by MMSE, the SIS is 63% sensitive and 81% specific in detecting cognitive impairment. The sensitivity in this study is lower than reported in prior studies [31].

The O3DY consists of asking the patient to spell "world" backward (Dlrow), the day, the date, and the year. This tests for orientation and verbal fluency. The O3DY was derived from the Canadian Study of Health and Aging (CSHA-1). The test was meant to be extremely brief, yet sensitive at the expense of specificity. It is 95% sensitive and 51% specific for cognitive impairment [32].

Differentiating dementia from delirium is a challenge for the emergency physician. Many patients who present with delirium also have an underlying dementia. The Confusion Assessment Method may be used quickly and easily and has a high specificity (100%) and sensitivity (86%) for the diagnosis of delirium [33]. This tool features four items and requires the presence of an acute change from baseline and either inattention or fluctuation of behavior, along with either disorganized thinking or altered level of consciousness.

In assessing level of consciousness, the modified RASS score can be used quickly and has the benefit of reproducibility. A modified RASS of 0 means the patient is awake and interactive. A negative score means the patient is more lethargic and a positive score means the patient is more agitated. A positive score may lead the emergency physician down the path to the diagnosis of acute delirium, recognizing that one of the first signs of delirium is inattention. A prospective cohort study was performed in a tertiary VA hospital in New England. As a single screen, the modified RASS has a sensitivity of 64% and specificity of 93% for delirium. When serial scores were used the sensitivity increased to 85%. The modified RASS score should therefore be considered for daily screening for delirium [34].

After assessing both cognition and level of consciousness, if both are found to be normal, the physician can then document "normal mental status." If the patient has impairment of either cognition or level of consciousness, further evaluation should follow. Determining onset of symptoms should be attempted with all sources available, including family, friends, caretakers, and primary providers [35].

Functional assessment

The functional assessment of the elderly patient includes things such as ADLs, mobility, continence, and hearing and vision impairment. A complex geriatric assessment may be necessary but is not practical in the ED. Simplified tools have been developed to aid the emergency physician in quickly identifying functional impairments.

The ability to perform ADLs is pertinent to the overall assessment of the elderly patient and determining goals of care. Examples of basic self-care ADLs include dressing, using the toilet, and walking. Instrumental ADLs evaluate executive function, the higher level ADLs necessary for function within the community. Examples include driving, shopping, and paying bills [36]. Some ADLs from both basic and instrumental scales can contribute to ED visits. Declines in mobility-related ADLs such as ability to dress, transfer, walk (basic ADLs) and transportation, shopping, meal preparation, and housework (instrumental ADLs) have been shown to contribute to ED visits in older patients [37]. When impairments in ability to perform ADLs are identified, these patients are at higher risk for falls and are more likely to require skilled nursing facility placement [38].

Mobility is determined by gait, balance, ability to transfer, and joint function [39]. The "Get Up and Go" Test is a practical approach to gait assessment in the elderly. This involves instructing the patient to get up, stand still, walk forward, turn around, walk back to chair, and sit down. There is no score associated with this test; the test is considered abnormal if the patient appears at risk of falling at any time during the test [40].

Vision and hearing impairment are associated with a substantial increased risk of falls [41]. Progressive loss of vision and hearing can lead to impairment of the ability to perform basic and advanced ADLs. Although generally beyond the scope of ED practice, in select circumstances patients should be screened for difficulty with vision and hearing in the ED and referred for specialty testing when indicated.

The geriatric syndrome of frailty is related to functional decline and is characterized by weight loss, fatigue, reduced muscle strength, reduced physical activity, and reduced walking speed [42]. Frailty is associated with increased risk of ED visits, hospitalization, disability, and death [43].

Social assessment

The social assessment of a patient is important for making disposition decisions. Obtaining important information early can make the emergency physician more efficient by avoiding inappropriate discharges and addressing concerns proactively. Important questions include the following: Does the patient have friends or family nearby who could provide support with ADLs? Would these people be available occasionally, daily, or 24/7? Does the patient use any assistive devices, such as a walker or a cane? Is it mandatory to use steps in the home, or are the bedroom, bathroom, and kitchen all on one floor? If the patient is sent home with a walker, are the hallways wide enough for the walker?

Posing these types of questions to the patient and family will help determine if the home environment is appropriate and may uncover potential difficulties that the patient or family had not previously considered. In a trial conducted to study the effectiveness of distributing fall prevention information to patients 65 years or older, it is suggested that even minimum discussion of fall prevention may lead to home modification [44].

A large part of the case discussion for this chapter involved establishing goals of care and managing expectations. This can be a time-consuming and challenging aspect of the management of elderly patients, but this can also be a beneficial and rewarding aspect as well. If these difficult discussions are possible early on in the patient's visit, goals of care for the patient can be established, and in many cases, the patient may avoid unnecessary testing, financial burden, and inappropriate admissions.

It is necessary to determine whether the patient has decision-making capacity, and if not, identify a surrogate decision-maker. State laws vary in this regard. When using a surrogate decision-maker, the emergency physician and the surrogate decision-maker act using substituted judgment. In other words, the surrogate decision-maker should make decisions based on what the patient would have wanted, not what they themselves would want. Only when the patient's wishes are unknown, should the decision-maker decide what would be in the patient's best interest [45]. The emergency physician can assist the surrogate decision-maker in using substituted judgment rather than best interest by phrasing questions as "What would the patient want us to do in this situation" rather than "What would you like us to do."

Section IV: Decision-making

- The general assessment of the elderly patient in the ED is unique and requires special attention.
- Each older patient should have an assessment of the medical condition, cognition, function, and social situation.
- A thorough review of a complete set of vital signs is crucial.
- Pay close attention to the patient's medication list, and recognize any new or recently removed medications.
- The Geriatric Emergency Medicine Task Force recommends a mental status evaluation of all elderly patients presenting to the ED.
- The SIS and O3DY are screening tests that are sensitive, quick, and easy for the physician to remember and score.

- The functional assessment of the elderly patient should include things such as ADLs, mobility, continence, and hearing and vision impairment.
- The ultimate goal of care is to manage the elderly patient, using substituted judgement, or as the patient would wish.

References

1 Siebens, H. (2005) The domain management model – a tool for teaching and management of older adults in emergency departments. *Acad. Emerg. Med.*, **12** (2), 162–168.

2 Sanders, A.B. and Force S for AEM (U S) GEMT (1996) *Emergency Care of the Elder Person*, Beverly Cracom Publications, 328 p.

3 Kaufman, D.W., Kelly, J.P., Rosenberg, L. *et al.* (2002) Recent patterns of medication use in the ambulatory adult population of the United States: the Slone survey. *J. Am. Med. Assoc.*, **287** (3), 337–344.

4 Halter, J., Ouslander, J., Tinetti, M. *et al.* (2009) *Hazzard's Geriatric Medicine and Gerontology*, 6th end edn, McGraw-Hill Professional, New York, 1760 p.

5 Budnitz, D.S., Lovegrove, M.C., Shehab, N., and Richards, C.L. (2011) Emergency hospitalizations for adverse drug events in older Americans. *N. Engl. J. Med.*, **365** (21), 2002–2012.

6 American Geriatrics Society 2012 Beers Criteria Update Expert Panel (2012) American Geriatrics Society updated Beers Criteria for potentially inappropriate medication use in older adults. *J. Am. Geriatr. Soc.*, **60** (4), 616–631.

7 Narang, A.T. and Sikka, R. (2006) Resuscitation of the elderly. *Emerg. Med. Clin. North Am.*, **24** (2), 261–272, v.

8 Chester, J.G. and Rudolph, J.L. (2011) Vital signs in older patients: age-related changes. *J. Am. Med. Dir. Assoc.*, **12** (5), 337–343.

9 Gupta, V. and Lipsitz, L.A. (2007) Orthostatic hypotension in the elderly: diagnosis and treatment. *Am. J. Med.*, **120** (10), 841–847.

10 Cheitlin, M.D. (2003) Cardiovascular physiology-changes with aging. *Am. J. Geriatr. Cardiol.*, **12** (1), 9–13.

11 Pavri, B.B. and Ho, R.T. (2003) Syncope. Identifying cardiac causes in older patients. *Geriatrics*, **58** (5), 26–31; quiz 32.

12 Douglas, G., Nicol, E.F., and Robertson, C. (2013) *Macleod's Clinical Examination*, Churchill Livingstone Elsevier, Edinburgh.

13 American College of Emergency Medicine (2004) *Geriatric Emergency Medicine*, 1st edn (eds S. Meldon, O.J. Ma, and R. Woolard), McGraw-Hill, Health Professions Division, New York, 585 p.

14 Pedone, C., Bellia, V., Sorino, C. *et al.* (2010) Prognostic significance of surrogate measures for forced vital capacity in an elderly population. *J. Am. Med. Dir. Assoc.*, **11** (8), 598–604.

15 Farley, H., Zubrow, M.T., Gies, J. *et al.* (2010) Emergency department tachypnea predicts transfer to a higher level of care in the first 24 hours after ED admission. *Acad. Emerg. Med.*, **17** (7), 718–722.

16 Fieselmann, J.F., Hendryx, M.S., Helms, C.M., and Wakefield, D.S. (1993) Respiratory rate predicts cardiopulmonary arrest for internal medicine inpatients. *J. Gen. Intern. Med.*, **8** (7), 354–360.

17 Shapiro, N.I., Wolfe, R.E., Moore, R.B. *et al.* (2003) Mortality in Emergency Department Sepsis (MEDS) score: a prospectively derived and validated clinical prediction rule. *Crit. Care Med.*, **31** (3), 670–675.

18 Caterino, J.M., Kulchycki, L.K., Fischer, C.M. *et al.* (2009) Risk factors for death in elderly emergency department patients with suspected infection. *J. Am. Geriatr. Soc.*, **57** (7), 1184–1190.

19 Valdez-Lowe, C., Ghareeb, S.A., and Artinian, N.T. (2009) Pulse oximetry in adults. *Am. J. Nurs.*, **109** (6), 52–59; quiz 60.

20 Gomolin, I.H., Lester, P., and Pollack, S. (2007) Older is colder: observations on body temperature among nursing home subjects. *J. Am. Med. Dir. Assoc.*, **8** (5), 335–337.

21 Ball, J. (2015) *Seidel's Guide to Physical Examination*, 8th edn, Elsevier/Mosby, St. Louis, MO.

22 Castle, S.C., Norman, D.C., Yeh, M. *et al.* (1991) Fever response in elderly nursing home residents: are the older truly colder? *J. Am. Geriatr. Soc.*, **39** (9), 853–857.

23 Castle, S.C. (2000) Clinical relevance of age-related immune dysfunction. *Clin. Infect. Dis.*, **31** (2), 578–585.

24 Kane, R.L., Ouslander, J.G., and Abrass, I.B. (1999) *Essentials of Clinical Geriatrics*, McGraw-Hill, Health Professions Division, New York.

25 Miller, A., Green, M., and Robinson, D. (1983) Simple rule for calculating normal erythrocyte sedimentation rate. *Br. Med. J. (Clin. Res. Ed)*, **286** (6361), 266.

26 Levey, A.S., Stevens, L.A., Schmid, C.H. *et al.* (2009) A new equation to estimate glomerular filtration rate. *Ann. Intern. Med.*, **150** (9), 604–612.

27 Righini, M., Van Es, J., Den Exter, P.L. *et al.* (2014) Age-adjusted D-dimer cutoff levels to rule out pulmonary embolism: the ADJUST-PE study. *J. Am. Med. Assoc.*, **311** (11), 1117–1124.

28 Samaras, N., Chevalley, T., Samaras, D., and Gold, G. (2010) Older patients in the emergency department: a review. *Ann. Emerg. Med.*, **56** (3), 261–269.

29 Wilber, S.T., Lofgren, S.D., Mager, T.G. *et al.* (2005) An evaluation of two screening tools for cognitive impairment in older emergency department patients. *Acad. Emerg. Med.*, **12** (7), 612–616.

30 Callahan, C.M., Unverzagt, F.W., Hui, S.L. *et al.* (2002) Six-item screener to identify cognitive impairment among potential subjects for clinical research. *Med. Care*, **40** (9), 771–781.

31 Wilber, S.T., Carpenter, C.R., and Hustey, F.M. (2008) The Six-Item Screener to detect cognitive impairment in older emergency department patients. *Acad. Emerg. Med.*, **15** (7), 613–616.

32 Carpenter, C.R., Bassett, E.R., Fischer, G.M. *et al.* (2011) Four sensitive screening tools to detect cognitive dysfunction in geriatric emergency department patients: brief Alzheimer's Screen, Short Blessed Test, Ottawa 3DY, and the caregiver-completed AD8. *Acad. Emerg. Med.*, **18** (4), 374–384.

33 Monette, J., Galbaud du Fort, G., Fung, S.H. *et al.* (2001) Evaluation of the Confusion Assessment Method (CAM) as a screening tool for delirium in the emergency room. *Gen. Hosp. Psychiatry.*, **23** (1), 20–25.

34 Chester, J.G., Beth Harrington, M., Rudolph, J.L., and VA Delirium Working Group (2012) Serial administration of a modified Richmond Agitation and Sedation Scale for delirium screening. *J. Hosp. Med.*, **7** (5), 450–453.

35 Wilber, S.T. (2006) Altered mental status in older emergency department patients. *Emerg. Med. Clin. North Am.*, **24** (2), 299–316, vi.

36 Lawton, M.P. and Brody, E.M. (1969) Assessment of older people: self-maintaining and instrumental activities of daily living. *Gerontologist*, **9** (3), 179–186.

37 Wilber, S.T., Frey, J.A., Poland, S.A. *et al.* (2012) Muscle strength, muscle mass, and muscle fatigue and their relationship with mobility-related activities of daily living in older emergency department patients. *Ann. Emerg. Med.*, **60** (4), S29–S30.

38 Robbins, A.S., Rubenstein, L.Z., Josephson, K.R. *et al.* (1989) Predictors of falls among elderly people. Results of two population-based studies. *Arch. Intern. Med.*, **149** (7), 1628–1633.

39 Tinetti, M.E. and Ginter, S.F. (1988) Identifying mobility dysfunctions in elderly patients. Standard neuromuscular examination or direct assessment? *J. Am. Med. Assoc.*, **259** (8), 1190–1193.

40 Mathias, S., Nayak, U.S., and Isaacs, B. (1986) Balance in elderly patients: the "get-up and go" test. *Arch. Phys. Med. Rehabil.*, **67** (6), 387–389.

41 Tinetti, M.E., Inouye, S.K., Gill, T.M., and Doucette, J.T. (1995) Shared risk factors for falls, incontinence, and functional dependence. Unifying the approach to geriatric syndromes. *J. Am. Med. Assoc.*, **273** (17), 1348–1353.

42 Robertson, D.A., Savva, G.M., and Kenny, R.A. (2013) Frailty and cognitive impairment – a review of the evidence and causal mechanisms. *Ageing Res. Rev.*, **12** (4), 840–851.

43 Stiffler, K.A., Finley, A., Midha, S., and Wilber, S.T. (2013) Frailty assessment in the emergency department. *J. Emerg. Med.*, **45** (2), 291–298.

44 Gerson, L.W., Camargo, C.A., and Wilber, S.T. (2005) Home modification to prevent falls by older ED patients. *Am. J. Emerg. Med.*, **23** (3), 295–298.

45 Combs, M.P., Rasinski, K.A., Yoon, J.D., and Curlin, F.A. (2013) Substituted judgment in principle and practice: a national physician survey. *Mayo Clin. Proc.*, **88** (7), 666–673.

2

Physiologic changes with aging

Kate D. Zimmerman[1] *& Robert S. Anderson, Jr.*[2]

[1]*Department of Emergency Medicine, Maine Medical Center, Portland, ME, USA*
[2]*Departments of Emergency Medicine and Internal Medicine and Division of Geriatric Medicine, Tufts University School of Medicine, Maine Medical Center, Portland, ME, USA*

Section I: Case presentation

This was an 85 year old woman with progressive dementia who presented from home with family with non-specific complaints of functional decline over the prior week. She was normally ambulatory with minor assistance. She was usually attentive and conversant. Family noted that over the prior week, she had required an increasing level of ambulatory support, was sleeping more, was not as conversant, and had been eating less. The family denied cough, abdominal pain, chest pain, diarrhea, falls, or rash. They reported an oral temperature of 37.2 degrees Centigrade (99.0 degrees Fahrenheit) on the day prior to presentation.

The past medical history was notable for hypertension and hyperlipidemia. Given her age and dementia, a decision was made to scale back on medications 6 months prior. Her current medications were aspirin and as needed colace.

On examination, her oral temperature was 37.3 C (99.1 degrees Fahrenheit), supine blood pressure was 105/60 mm/hg and pulse of 80 beats/min. With standing her blood pressure was 95/50 mm/hg and pulse 110 beats/min. Her respiratory rate was 22 breaths/min. with a pulse oximetry of 93% on ambient air. She was able to follow commands and was attentive. She was unable to stand without assistance. Pulmonary, cardiac, and abdominal examinations were unremarkable. She had dry axillae, poor skin turgor, and dry mucous membranes.

Laboratory studies included CBC, CMP, and UA. They were notable for lack of leukocytosis, an elevated BUN and creatinine, urine specific gravity of 1.030, positive leukocyte esterase and nitrite, and occasional bacteria in the urine. Given the pulse oximetry reading, low grade fever, and elevated respiratory rate a chest radiograph was ordered that showed a right middle lobe infiltrate.

Section II: Case discussion

Peter Rosen: Rob, this is a fascinating case in regards to the diligence of the family that has managed this elderly patient at home a lot longer than most families seem to be able to do. Rather than a physiology of aging issue, I'm wondering if this isn't more of an ethical case because the reality is we have a demented patient who has not been stable in her dementia who is beginning to fail. I think the family has already addressed some of the issues of how much medical support to give her. But clearly they haven't come to terms with her getting worse. I find it yet, once again, interesting that the presentation of the patient is to the emergency department (ED) as opposed to a family primary care physician. Perhaps you could comment on the why they came to the ED, and also some of the ethical issues of how do you define futility in a demented patient.

Rob Anderson: Peter, your perspective is interesting because the case was intended to paint a picture of a woman with dementia who was usually attentive and interactive with her family. She was a woman whose life has a value to her and her family, and for whom treating an acute infectious process makes

Geriatric Emergencies: A Discussion-Based Review, First Edition.
Edited by Amal Mattu, Shamai A. Grossman and Peter L. Rosen.

a lot of sense. This is in contrast to people who have very endstage dementia, who are no longer communicative, who are no longer mobile, and for whom the treatment of an infectious process might be debated.

PR: You have to gauge your decisions about futility to some degree on what you're starting from, and that unfortunately leads to subjective errors. Qualities of life that we don't particularly want for ourselves we presume someone else doesn't want, and yet, as you've pointed out, here is a family who gets some sort of positive interaction with this patient, and wants to preserve it. Therefore, the decisions for futility are going to be made on an individual family construct as opposed to necessarily the patient alone.

Also, would you comment on, do you think it provides some degree of comfort care to always treat infections?

RA: That's a very complicated question as well, I'm not sure I have the answer. Some folks feel antibiotics are can be palliative for treatment of urinary tract infections. The decision to use or not use antibiotics is addressed on the Physician Orders for Life Sustaining Treatment order form, or the POLST form. In the correct setting, it would be ideal to have started the discussion with family prior to the acute issue. I think the decision should be made on a case-by-case basis.

Amal Mattu: I would just add on to that, first of all, I agree with what you said that it is a case-by-case decision. What is the patient's baseline in terms of where you hope to get them back to, and it also makes a difference what type of infection you're treating. If the patient had a reasonable quality of life, which of course if very subjective, but the family was content with that, and you think this is an infection that is going to be reasonable to treat, then I would think that you're going to go full force. On the other hand, if the patient has an overwhelming infection, and you think that the chances of getting the patient back to baseline are very low, then you probably want to treat anyway, but I think you're going to focus more on keeping the patient as comfortable as possible. In this particular case, it looks like the patient has what appears to be a unilobar pneumonia and the patient doesn't appear to be toxic in appearance. We can talk about some of the pitfalls associated with these relatively normal-looking vital signs, nevertheless, the patient doesn't appear to be toxic.

PR: Maura, pneumonia has been called the old person's friend. I think that even in severe cases of dementia, urinary tract infection and pneumonia are worth treating because they clearly worsen the mental status. How do you feel about those issues?

Maura Kennedy: I absolutely agree. I would concur with both Amal and Rob about the spectrum of dementia. This patient at baseline is ambulatory with minor assistance, so it sounds like she has a higher degree of function than many patients at the farther end of the spectrum. Her vital signs indicate that she's tachypneic and hypoxic. I would presume that she's uncomfortable in the setting of this infection, and I think it would be entirely appropriate to treat this patient with antibiotics to try to improve her symptomatically and hopefully return her back to her level of functioning. Though currently she is attentive, so possibly not yet delirious, delaying treatment could result in her becoming delirious, and certainly that can further impair her quality of life.

PR: Rob, this is a patient who I initially would not be inclined to admit to an ICU, and I guess most ICUs would not take her even though she's probably the patient who would most benefit from aggressive care of this infection before she deteriorates. Would you consider treating a patient like this at home to try to avoid some of the negative effects of hospitalization such as delirium?

RA: I think that's an excellent question and discussion point because and we should always be asking ourselves "what is the best thing for this person?" She might come into the hospital and get delirious to go home and then potentially decompensate. I think that it also based on the resources that you have at hand, family preference, and the ability to follow up with the PCP. We have a very robust home health visiting nurses program in Maine, so this kind of person could have a visiting nurse be at the house the very next day to check her pulse oximetry and see how she's doing. Discussion with family is paramount and should guide final decision.

PR: Maura, you've made very useful points in past case discussions about the sociology of the old patient at home. Would you comment a little bit on at what point you think someone like this would perhaps do better not to be with the family, but needs to be placed in assisted living? The family has done a terrific job with her, and I don't know the construct here whether there's somebody who's capable of being at home with her, but at what point to do you think both the patient and the family would benefit from an assisted living program assuming its available and finances permit?

MK: Outside of the acute illness or with respect to the acute illness we're dealing with?

PR: Well maybe triggered by the acute illness, but I was thinking more in spite of or after the acute illness has been taken care of.

MK: I think some of the things that need to go into that consideration is "what function do the patients have at home?" Are they able to do things such as make meals and eat unassisted? Are they able to go out and do food shopping? Do they need assistance with bathing? Also, what sort of social interactions they're getting, and is that adequate for this individual? While many of these things can be done in a private home with aids and visiting nursing, if there needs to be assistance with delivery of medication, sometimes it's easier to coordinate that in an assisted living facility where there are the opportunities to attend meals and set social events that enable the person to participate with others. One must also think about, this particular person walks with minor assistance, but if someone is in a wheelchair or requires a walker, being in a living situation that doesn't require lots of stairs would be another consideration. I would probably look both at their ambulatory status and their ability to do their activities of daily living.

PR: I think those are really excruciatingly difficult points to meet in many cases, and, as we've mentioned before, the financial resources for the elderly become more diminished all the time. One of the things I've been struck by is the older patient who lives alone, perhaps because of divorce, perhaps because of the demise of the spouse, but there seems to be a rapid decline in function for people who live alone. Rob, do you think that that almost by itself is an indication for assisted living?

RA: No, I think again it's a case-by-case situation. In fact I just came from a house call where I visited a man who really should not be alone anymore. He is really not doing well and his family is quite worried about him. He did very poorly on my cognitive testing. He doesn't understand his medications. He's taking high risk medications such as warfarin and oxycodone and a fentanyl patch. But he is adamant that he will stay home, and he does not want to leave. And he's still driving. So there's a whole host of issues that come up that we have to face and help families face. How we respect a person's autonomy and also do the safe thing for them is a very complicated issue.

AM: The interesting thing in the United States is that personal liberties are such a tremendous emphasis and focus in our laws, and just in terms of our culture that it's very, very difficult to make decisions like that. I would imagine that even the court systems would have a tough time taking the keys away from someone, and taking away their personal liberties. Moreover, driving is considered a tremendous personal liberty in the United States. I would guess that in other countries they don't worry as much about taking away personal liberties and taking away somebody's car keys, and saying that that person is not a safe driver. But I do think it's so much harder to do that in our society.

MK: I would also add to that that it's also dependent on your geographic situation. In a country like this where there are parts of the country where there's really no public transportation and no alternative way to get around, it becomes much more significant when someone is no longer able to drive. In smaller countries with a societal structure where a lot of people live together in the center of the town or where there is better transportation available then it can be less of an issue with respect to autonomy.

PR: Well I was struck when I was in Italy by how much more walking older people do there, and probably because they do it, it keeps them functional a lot longer. Certainly the statistics on auto crashes in the elderly are frighteningly high. We don't have any state that I'm aware of that has solved the problem of how you figure out whether someone is still competent to drive. I remember an elderly couple that I knew in Chicago; the man had been declared legally blind but was able to renew his driver's license every year. That made about as much sense as having the ATM in braille on the drive through at the bank.

Amal, maybe you could comment on what you think are some reliable indications for admission in patients like this. Or has it still got to be individualized to the point where so much depends on family structure and primary care availability, etc.?

AM: I really think it does have to be individualized. Let's take this patient with a unilobar pneumonia. If this patient looks pretty well, and the patient already has some degree of dementia, Rob brought up the concern about perhaps increasing the level of delirium related to admission. It might be very appropriate to put this patient on some good antibiotics, and send them home with a reliable family and with a nursing visit the next day. If you work in an area where you can set that up and the patient has the appropriate insurance or resources, whatever that may be, and you can set that up I think that's perfect. In my setting, I can't often arrange something like that. Therefore, this is somebody who would, in all likelihood, be either admitted to observation or just a flat out admission to the hospital. The concerns here are that, with regards to the physiologic changes, even though this person doesn't appear to be running a high fever or isn't that tachypneic or hypotensive, because of the changes that do occur in the elderly, that temperature of 99.1 would be considered febrile. The blood pressure of 105/60 mm/hg could be relative hypotension for this patient. The heart rate of 80 could be very concerning if this patient's on a beta blocker. The lack of orthostatic changes in an elderly patient doesn't even matter. This person could be essentially equivalent to a person who is significantly hypovolemic. A pulse oximetry reading of 93% clearly is a bit on the low side. If these numbers were present in a younger person, they probably wouldn't be terribly concerning. I'd still worry a bit about that 93% pulse oximetry, but everything else wouldn't be terribly concerning. Nevertheless, I would say that those are pretty remarkable numbers in an 85-year-old, and in most settings I think this justifies admitting the person unless you have the type of resources that Rob alluded to.

PR: This patient really is on the verge of decompensating, and I think she could go very rapidly downhill whether or not she's admitted.
Maura, there's been a lot of debate about whether antibiotics actually help patients once they're bacteremic. From the statistics on pneumococcal disease it would appear that antibiotics haven't changed the destiny of patients once they are bacteremic. While I think that may be true, nevertheless, I do believe that early and aggressive use of antibiotics has made an enormous difference for patients with pneumonia, and maybe our conclusions are that we've looking at the wrong end of the disease. Once they have become septic then antibiotics are not going to help much, but a patient like this who is still compensated but on the verge of being decompensated is the one who would most benefit from aggressive management. Would you comment on that please?

MK: I would agree with that. I think that, particularly in a patient who also is at risk for having more of a compromised immune system simply with respect to aging, I think that antibiotics would be a critical element in treating this infection. I also think she's at the precipice of really declining. I think it needs to be part of her care along with close evaluation of fluid management in her. I'd be very concerned about sending her home unless it was consistent with her goals of care because she already has demonstrated that she's dehydrated based on the physical examination and elevated creatinine. She has had decreased oral intake over the past week; presumably her thirst response isn't as robust as a younger person's would be. I think if she were to go home, she would be at high risk of further deterioration with or without antibiotics due to dehydration; she would probably become more hypotensive. I agree that once they're in florid septic shock, antibiotics alone are certainly not the answer. I think antibiotics early are critical in combination with other elements of treatment in this patient including close monitoring of her respiratory status. Additionally, I think her work of breathing could increase as she doesn't have as much compensatory abilities.

PR: I think that, Rob, a really important part of the management of this patient is going to be family expectations. They behave as if they expect her to live forever, and I think that their primary care hasn't done very much useful counseling in terms of her declining status. At some point they have to make a decision about how much aggressive care they want for this patient. That's something we're faced with all the time in the ED, and I don't see any particular cure for it, but certainly this is not too early to start such a discussion with this patient if you don't have the right circumstances at home. Maybe you could tell us what the final outcome of this case was since I think it's been a very interesting discussion in terms of how to manage someone like this as an outpatient.

RA: She was admitted to the hospital, and had a short stay, and was discharged home with visiting nurses and recovered from pneumonia. Beyond that, I'm not sure what happened in regards to her dementia or end of life planning.

PR: Well, the other things have to be done consistently and early or otherwise this is a patient who's going to bounce back to the ED, and then we're starting the same process all over again.

Section III: Concepts

Normal aging should have minimal effect on one's ability to enjoy the day-to-day pleasures of life, from taking a walk or reading a book to attending a play or traveling the world. But what do occur with near uniformity are ongoing slow changes that, year by year, affect our ability to respond to stress. The abundance of our youthful resources is slowly depleted, whether it is our huge stash of nephrons, pacemaker cells, neurons, or the reactive, elastic and adaptive properties of our young lungs and heart. For day-to-day needs, we continue to be well equipped and able to carry on for many decades. However, at some point, the stress of an injury or illness, which may have been a simple nuisance to us in our 20s, may be our undoing in our 80s.

Thinking about and teaching the concepts of geriatrics are confounded by several problems. First, and most importantly, is divorcing age from disease. For the most part, aging and disease go hand in hand, as most diseases have a higher prevalence with age. However, aging is not synonymous with disease. Aging is synonymous with loss of reserve to deal with disease or trauma.

Secondly, there is a strong desire to assign a number to aging. At what age are we old? The answer is not straightforward. In some studies, the trauma literature defines patients as young as 45 as elderly, whereas the medical literature suggests young (65–75), middle (75–85), and old (85+years) as categories of progressive aging. The need to assign a specific age to "geriatric" will continue as long as the important work of researching this demographic continues.

In general terms, however, it is clear from every-day practice that a sick 85 year old is different from a sick 65 year old. Understanding why or when that change happens depends on combining the knowledge of physiology, disease, pharmacology, and sociology. Table 2.1 provides a summary of the text below.

Cardiovascular system – a tired pump, hardened pipes, and frayed wires

Conduction system and the electrocardiogram

In the aging heart, there is a significant decline in the number of cells in the conduction system. Those cells that remain have reduced functionality [1]. By the age of 75, up to 90% of the sinoatrial node pacemaker cells are lost. The result is an intrinsic heart rate which decreases up to one beat per minute per decade. The duration of the PR interval is increased, with the upper limit being 220 ms in the patient older than 65 years. Atrioventricular blocks become more common and patients are more susceptible to dysrhythmogenic syncope. The ST segment flattens, and there is a decrease in the amplitude of the T wave [2]. All of these changes result in an electrocardiogram (EKG) that is less likely to be diagnostic of ischemia [3].

There is decreased sympathetic innervation as well as parasympathetic tone of the conduction system as the heart ages. With this, there is a blunted response to atropine as well as overall decreased heart rate variability [2]. This is significant, as the elderly person may not be able to mount an adequate heart rate response to a decreased stroke volume. While a sinus rhythm is the only normal rhythm in any patient, ventricular ectopy is seen more commonly in those patients older than 75 years, even without heart disease. These are usually in the form of isolated premature ventricular contractions [2]. Premature atrial contractions are also common, and their presence correlates with an increase in the size of the atria [2, 4].

By the eighth decade, the aging heart loses up to 30% of its myocytes [2]. The remaining cells hypertrophy, and the heart becomes more fibrotic. The valvular annuli and septum of the heart calcify, and cardiac amyloid deposition occurs as well as atrial dilatation. These changes increase the risk of developing dysrhythmias, the most common of which is atrial fibrillation [2, 5]. Atrial fibrillation can be seen in up to 10% of patients older than 80 years [6]. The consequences of these changes are decreased cardiac output, increased risk of stroke, and overall decreased quality of life and mental function [7].

Table 2.1 Physiologic changes with aging and clinical implications.

System	What We See …	What It Means …
Cardiovascular		
• A tired pump • Hardened pipes • Frayed wires	• Decreased heart rate • Increased incidence of blocks • Dysrhythmogenic syncope • Diastolic disease • Reliance on Starling effect to maintain stroke volume	• Think cardiac causes with syncope • Don't trust the EKG to rule out ischemia • Dehydration and atrial fibrillation have profound effects on cardiac output • Elders can be volume sensitive; fluid administration may need close monitoring
Pulmonary		
• Decreased endurance • Decreased oxygen tension	• Weak diaphragm/poor pulmonary toilet • Decreased oxygen tension • Decreased vital capacity	• Pneumonia • Failure to compensate for metabolic acidosis • Hypoxemia • Higher baseline A – a gradient • Ventilatory failure
Renal		
• A loss of mass • Drug sensitive	• Serum creatinine should stay stable • More prone to acute kidney injury • Greater effects of changes in salt and water loads • Sodium imbalance • Hyperkalemia	• Decreased renal plasma flow, but due to decreased muscle mass, a rise in creatinine is not a normal consequence of aging • Depend on sodium load to maintain volume and pressure • Easily develop hyper- or hyponatremia; watch volume status and medication interactions • Hemodynamic instability • Caution with potassium-sparing drugs or drug that affects the renin-aldosterone system • Acute kidney injury – watch out for hypovolemic states or nephrotoxic drugs • Appropriately dose renally excreted medications
Hematology/immunology		
• Waning defenses • Dull weapons	• Increased incidence of infection • More profound effects of infection • Atypical presentations of infection • Blunted WBC response to stress or infection	• Aggressively test for infection in this population • Fever in the elder may be defined as an oral temperature of 37.2 °C or rectal temperature of 37.5 °C • A decline in functional status may be the only presenting symptom of underlying infection • A normal WBC count does not rule out infection
Neurologic		
• Preserved attention • Difficulty learning new tricks	• Worsening vision • Decreased hearing • Decreased learning and problem-solving • Psychomotor slowing	• Decreased visual acuity and night vision • Eliminate background noise, speak slowly and clearly, and use hearing aids • Problem integrating new information

Table 2.1 (*continued*)

System	What We See …	What It Means …
Musculoskeletal		
• Keeping it together gets harder to do	• Decrease in muscle mass, atrophy, fatigability, and weakness • Decreased joint range of motion • Osteoporosis	• Physical disability • Increased risk of injury to bones, tendons, ligaments, and cartilage • Loss of independence
Gastrointestinal		
• Slow and uncoordinated	• Issues and complaints common from input to output	• Malnourishment • Constipation • Aspiration • Reflux • Upper gastrointestinal bleeding • GI infections • Appropriately dose medications and watch for interactions
Genitourinary		
• Incontinence is not a given	• Very common functional complaint • Increased likelihood of infections	• Incontinence • Increased incidence of UTI • Asymptomatic bacteriuria
Endocrine		
• The salt, sugar, and spice of life	• Altered mental status • Orthostatic hypotension • Generalized weakness	• Consider occult thyroid disease • Be vigilant for electrolyte and volume issues

Cardiac function

While at rest, the effects of normal aging are not detectable from the heart rate, left ventricular ejection fraction, or cardiac output. However, as the heart is stressed, the effects of aging become evident [2]. In normal aging, the left ventricular ejection fraction does not decline. However, diastolic function is significantly impaired, leading to decreased relaxation of the heart, and increased need of adequate atrial systole for filling of the left ventricle [2, 8]. The contribution of atrial systole in filling the left ventricle nearly doubles with age, from 20% to 40% in those older than 80 years [2]. Hence, when the atria are not contributing, such as is the case with atrial fibrillation, a more profound hemodynamic effect may occur than would in the younger patient presenting with atrial fibrillation. Similarly, elderly patients presenting with

a tachydysrhythmia will often present with diastolic heart failure, unlike their younger counterparts.

The aged heart is not as responsive to beta-adrenergic stimulation. Hence, the ability of the heart to respond to stress by increasing its rate and contractility is blunted [1]. The older patient must depend on stroke volume to maintain cardiac output. Unfortunately, the inotropic response is also decreased, and the elderly heart will rely more on the Starling effect to maintain stroke volume [2]. Hence, any element of dehydration or volume depletion can have profound effects on cardiac output.

Cardiac disease

Increasing age is the predominant risk factor for cardiovascular disease in the United States [9]. This fact, accompanied by the high prevalence of atherosclerotic disease and hypertension, leads to significant morbidity and mortality in the geriatric population.

Orthostatic hypotension

In the normal healthy aging individual, the ability to maintain adequate perfusion to the brain is preserved with postural changes [2]. However, in the elderly person, the underlying physiologic changes of decreased vascular compliance and decreased responsiveness to sympathetic drive lead to an increased incidence of orthostasis. Moreover, at baseline, the elderly person is commonly dehydrated, on medications that affect hemodynamics, or has comorbidities that affect their compensatory mechanisms. With that said, it should be noted that any burden on the cardiovascular system will have profound results that may lead to dizziness, falls, illness, or injury.

Vascular changes

Systolic blood pressure rises with age, and diastolic pressure plateaus, often decreasing by the sixth decade. Overall, hypertension is very common with a prevalence of greater than 50% in adults older than 60 years of age [10]. This is believed to be due to several changes that occur with age, pushing the vascular tone toward vasoconstriction. With age, comes an increased basal level of vasoconstrictive catecholamines (at the alpha receptors), as well as overall increased arterial stiffness [2]. In addition, there is the loss of the ability of the vasculature to relax or dilate due to decreased production of the smooth muscle relaxant nitric oxide and a decreased response at the vasodilatory beta-adrenergic receptors on the vessels [2, 11]. The less compliant and less responsive vasculature, coupled with the less compliant and less responsive heart, often contribute to an exaggerated drop in blood pressure in the face of dehydration or volume depletion in the elderly patient.

Pulmonary – decreased endurance and a decrease in oxygen tension

Physical changes of the aging pulmonary system include a stiffer, less compliant chest wall, and lungs that do not recoil due to increased lung tissue compliance and decreased muscle strength and endurance

[11, 12]. The diaphragm is estimated to be 25% weaker in the elderly leading to poor pulmonary toilet [12]. The elderly person is subsequently placed at risk for the development of pneumonia. In addition, successful respiratory compensation for insults such as metabolic acidosis or hypoxemia may be harder to achieve in the elderly patient.

There is a decrease in the diffusion capacity of up to 5% per decade after the age of 40 [12]. This leads to a decrease in the oxygen tension in arterial blood (PaO_2) such that the PaO_2 of a 65 year old may only reach 80 mmHg. Fortunately, the mean PaO_2 will remain relatively constant at 80 mmHg from age 65 years on [12]. The decrease in PaO_2 with aging will, if calculated, dramatically alter the difference between alveolar gas (PAO_2) and arterial blood, such that normal A–a gradient with aging will be as high as 25–30 mmHg [11, 12]. This decline in maximal oxygen uptake and decreased perception of bronchoconstriction are critical functional changes associated with aging [13]. Finally, the vital capacity, the volume of air moved between full inhalation and maximal inhalation, is lower with age; however, the total lung capacity remains relatively stable [14].

Renal – a loss of mass, altered drug sensitivity

Several changes occur within the renal system that affect the elderly person that have clinical significance. As the kidney ages, it undergoes both structural and functional changes. The renal mass decreases as a result of a decline in the number and size of the glomeruli, which are inversely proportional to age [15, 16]. After the fourth decade, the renal plasma flow decreases at a rate of 10% per decade; this means at least a 50% decline by the age of 90 [17]. It should be noted that the serum creatinine should remain constant as the loss of muscle mass is proportional to the decreased plasma flow through the glomeruli. A rise in serum creatinine is *not* a result of normal aging and should be considered a pathologic finding [18].

The ability to maintain homeostasis in terms of fluid and electrolytes is preserved, but the kidney's adaptive ability to respond to changes in salt and water load is compromised; there is impaired ability to excrete a salt or water load [18]. There is also decreased capacity of the kidney to retain sodium due to reduced levels of plasma renin and serum aldosterone [19]. There is more susceptibility to a hypernatremic dehydration due to the impaired concentrating ability of the kidney, and, conversely, the elderly person may readily develop hyponatremia if given excess fluids [15]. Fluctuations in serum sodium, which contribute to maintenance of blood volume and pressure, may predispose the elderly to hemodynamic instability. The elderly are more susceptible to developing hyperkalemia when given potassium-sparing drugs (i.e., spironolactone), potassium supplements, or drugs that affect the renin-aldosterone system [15].

The aging kidneys are susceptible to acute kidney injury, defined as a rapid reduction in kidney function resulting in a failure to maintain fluid, electrolyte, and acid–base homeostasis. This is especially true in the setting of hypovolemia or nephrotoxic agents, due to an already decreased plasma flow [20]. Renally excreted medications should be appropriately dosed and nephrotoxins avoided, if possible, in the elderly. Proteinuria is a pathologic finding, as the aging of the glomerulus is typically a sclerotic process, not a process that increases the basement membrane permeability [18].

Hematology/immunology – waning defenses, dull weapons

The process of aging does not affect the basal rate of hematopoiesis. What aging does affect is the ability of the hematopoietic system to respond to stressors or stimuli [21]. These stressors, as seen in emergency care, are often in the form of infection, trauma, neurologic catastrophe, or other illness such as acute coronary syndrome. The elderly person has a reduced reserve capacity and may not be able to mount the needed response to maintain homeostasis.

Infection is a common reason for the elderly to present to the emergency department (ED). The elderly are particularly susceptible to bacterial infection as the function of their frontline defense is compromised. The respiratory burst activity of polymorphonuclear neutrophils, which phagocytose

and kill bacteria, is decreased in those that are malnourished, which may have a higher prevalence in the elderly [21]. Cell-mediated immunity is also affected. There is a reduced T-cell repertoire in response to new antigens with a decreased ability of memory cells to proliferate. The B-cell-mediated immunity is affected by a reduced antibody response to T-cell-dependent and -independent antigens [21, 22]. There is often a suboptimal antibody response to vaccines, which is believed to be the result of a T-cell effect of the aging process [21].

Recognizing that the geriatric patient may have a muted febrile response to infection, attempts have been made to redefine fever in these patients. Elderly persons from long-term care facilities should be considered febrile with a consistent oral temp of greater than or equal to 37.2 °C or a rectal temp of greater than or equal to 37.5 °C [23]. Up to 30% of severely infected elderly patients present with an absent or blunted fever [24]. Their presentation is further complicated by nonspecific and atypical signs, such as decline in functional or mental status or anorexia with decreased oral intake [25]. Not only decreased reserve but also the presence of comorbid diseases contributes to decreased defenses and perhaps atypical presentations. The integument and mucociliary barriers are compromised and contribute to increased susceptibility to illness [25]. When an elderly person presents with a change in baseline, strongly consider infection in the differential diagnosis.

Regarding laboratory studies, the reference range for the lower limit of normal is decreased in the white blood cell (WBC) count, hematocrit, total protein, and albumin. The upper limit of normal for erythrocyte sedimentation rate increases dramatically with age to at least 20 mm/h in men and 30 mm/h in women [26].

Neurologic – preserved attention, difficulty learning new tricks

Delirium, dementia, disequilibrium, and falls will be addressed in other chapters. This section focuses on specific changes in the peripheral and central nervous systems that occur with normal aging and may affect the clinician's interaction with the elderly person or lead to increased risk of injury or illness.

Vision

By the age of 65, it is estimated that 1 in 3 elderly persons has some form of vision loss [27]. Starting at the age of 44, the lens becomes less able to accommodate for near vision (presbyopia). Cataracts form as the lens loses the ability to eliminate waste products and cellular debris. This leads to glare-related vision loss, increased light sensitivity, decreased contrast sensitivity, and decreased visual acuity [28]. The vitreous becomes more fluid, leading to the presence of "floaters" and predisposition to retinal tears and detachments. Contrast sensitivity and visual fields are diminished and there is decreased dark adaptation. Age-related macular degeneration, whose prevalence triples after the age of 70, may lead to central vision loss in the elderly [28].

Hearing

The incidence of hearing loss is estimated to double per decade, starting with 16% at 60 years, and increasing to 32% at 70 years and 64% at 80 years [28]. The loss is a bilateral high-frequency sensorineural loss [11]. The older patient also develops reduced speech discrimination that results in difficulty understanding speech when there is a high ratio of background noise, rapid speech, or poor pronunciation [28].

Changes in the brain

The brain undergoes structural changes with normal aging. There is attrition of the number of nerve cells, retraction, and, in some cases, expansion of the dendrites, loss of synapses, remodeling of synapses, and reactivity of the glial cells [29]. An amino acid peptide can form insoluble aggregates, or amyloid plaques, in the brain parenchyma and vasculature. These plaques accumulate most heavily in brain regions involved in learning and memory processes. They can cause inflammatory processes that damage the aging brain and interrupt neurotransmitter signaling pathways, leading to cognitive impairment [29]. Damage also occurs via mechanisms of oxidative stress due to the formation of free radicals.

Neurotransmitter signaling in the brain is affected by normal aging. Acetylcholine plays a key role in the memory and learning process [29]. The ability of the elderly person to reason and problem solve, "fluid

intelligence," appears to decline with age, whereas the "crystallized abilities," such as recollection of information and skills gained from past experience, remain intact [30]. This reflects the decreased ability of the elderly to adapt intellectually, not just physically, to stressors. Decreased dopamine levels play a role in deficits of motor control that occur with aging. A deficit in norepinephrine and serotonin contribute to affective disorders leading to depression [29].

Cognition

Pronounced impairment of attention is not typical of normal aging [31, 32]. Executive functions, which are defined as the ability to control and direct behavior, make meaningful inferences and appropriate judgments, plan and carry out tasks, manipulate multiple pieces of information at one time, complete complex motor sequences, and solve abstract and complex problems, should be affected minimally by normal aging [31]. Memory is also minimally affected with normal aging, with that of learning new information being the most affected [30]. Language comprehension remains intact and language production is affected mostly in the realm of spontaneous word finding [31]. If the ability of the elderly person to maintain an attention span declines, it should be taken in the context of other perceptual or sensory changes that may negatively impact them, such as loss of vision or hearing, or the presence of pain, depression, or current illness.

Psychomotor slowing is a consistent finding throughout the aging population. This may be associated with decreased dopamine activity in the brain. This will affect the elderly person's speed of cognitive processing and peripheral motor skills, that is, reaction time. This will place them at increased risk of accident and injury [31].

Musculoskeletal – keeping it together gets harder to do

The musculoskeletal system is greatly affected by aging and is one of the systems with the most noticeable changes during the normal aging process. Musculoskeletal disease is the most common cause of chronic disability in people older than 65 [33].

Muscle

The skeletal muscle mass decreases with age as does its function [11, 33]. As the muscles begin to dysfunction, the elderly try to do less with a subsequent vicious cycle of lack of use and an increase in atrophy leading to worsening dysfunction. Neuronal input to the skeletal muscle decreases due to a reduction in the number and size of spinal cord motor neurons. The axonal flow is altered, and subsequently so is the neuromuscular transmission. There is a decrease in the number of acetylcholine receptors, reduced neurotransmitter release, and a decrease in the number of nerve terminals [33]. There are alterations of the muscle itself, with injury due to contraction and alterations in signal transduction across the muscle tissue. There are oxidative stressors, vasculopathy, and mitochondrial DNA mutations that occur with aging [33]. Grossly, this all leads to decreased muscle mass, atrophy, fatigability, and weakness. It also leads to a reduced tolerance of heat and cold as well as impaired glucose homeostasis. All of these factors in turn lead to physical disability, increased risk of injury, (e.g., fractures due to a fall), and overall loss of independence.

Tendons and ligaments

The strength of tendons and ligaments is reduced with age and is related to increased cross-linking of collagen fibers, leading to stiffness as well as a decline in the water content. Changes to the tendons and ligaments impair joint range of motion by about 20–25% [33]. The tendons and ligaments are more prone to injury ranging from inflammatory damage to rupture. Due to their weakness, it takes much less force than it would in a younger counterpart to cause injury.

Cartilage

As cartilage ages, it loses its water content, the proteoglycans become smaller, and there is a change in the makeup of chondroitin sulfate. The collagen becomes stiffer with increased cross-linking (just like in the tendons and ligaments), and the chondrocytes have reduced metabolic activity, leading to reduction in, and even cessation of, proliferation [33]. These changes in cartilage lead to injury and may contribute to the formation of osteoarthritis.

Bone

Osteoporosis is one of the most common disorders affecting the elderly population. It is a result of an imbalance of bone formation and bone resorption. It affects both men and women and is a major risk factor for fractures [34]. The loss of function and independence is profound in the geriatric population once they have suffered a fracture. Almost a third are discharged to a nursing home after suffering a hip fracture [35]. Vertebral fractures are also a common finding in the elderly population, many of which may be found incidentally on radiographs. Approximately 5% of 50- to 54-year-old white women have at least one vertebral fracture found on X-ray, and that prevalence increases to greater than 35% in women aged 80–85 years [36]. Approximately two-thirds of vertebral fractures are asymptomatic with the most common locations being thoracic or lumbar [36].

Gastrointestinal – slow and uncoordinated

Aging affects all aspects of the gastrointestinal (GI) tract predisposing the elderly person to become ill and malnourished. There is impaired neuromuscular coordination of the oropharynx, which leads to dysphagia and increased risk of aspiration [37]. Dental decay and tooth loss also predispose this population to aspiration due to inability to efficiently chew food [38]. The elderly person may have an unbalanced diet related to difficulty chewing their food, leading to malnutrition. Inappropriate diet driven by finances and physical changes can lead to serious vitamin deficiencies, and scurvy is a commonly missed disease in the elderly because it is simply not considered as a cause of symptoms.

In regard to the esophagus, there is decreased upper esophageal sphincter pressure as well as peristalsis [37, 39]. This leads to dysphagia, regurgitation, and the presentation with heartburn and chest pain. The lower esophageal pressure is decreased, promoting reflux, and the stomach itself is slow to empty, further contributing to the risk of reflux [39]. There is increased susceptibility to mucosal injury from nonsteroidal anti-inflammatory agents, leading to increased incidence of gastritis, peptic ulcer disease, and upper gastrointestinal bleeding [37, 39].

23

The blood flow and perfusion of the liver decrease by about 40% with aging, which results in altered drug metabolism [37]. This places the elderly at risk of toxicity as well as drug interactions. While liver function tests are not changed with age, reserve capacity of the organ is diminished.

The incidence of cholelithiasis and choledocolithiasis increases with age and can be seen in up to 50% of patients older than the age of 70 [40]. The elderly person, whose immune response is blunted, may not show the classic signs and symptoms of biliary obstruction and infection. A clinically significant cholecystitis in the elderly may mimic the mild biliary colic seen in younger patients [40]. Unfortunately, it may produce minimal symptoms, or the patient may fail to react to the mild symptoms until the gall bladder has ruptured.

The small bowel demonstrates decreased mucosal immunity, predisposing the elderly to infections that enter the body via the gastrointestinal tract [37]. There is delayed transit of stool in the colon, predisposing to constipation [37, 41]. Diverticulosis is present in up to two-thirds of patients over 80, with approximately 10–25% of them developing diverticulitis [41]. There is overall increased mucosal proliferation in the colon, which may place the elderly person at risk of developing colon cancer [37]. There is decreased internal sphincter pressure and muscle mass of the anus, increasing the risk of fecal incontinence [41]; up to 10% of older patients are incontinent of feces or urine [37, 42].

Genitourinary – incontinence is not a given

The bladder undergoes increased involuntary contractions as it ages. This leads to increased incidence of urinary incontinence. This is especially true in the elderly man, from a combination of prostatic disease and spinal stenosis. It should be noted, however, that the majority of people remain continent into their elder years. The continence issue is not only physical but also depends on other factors such as overall mobility, dexterity, motivation, and cognition [43]. It is estimated that up to 30% of the elderly population suffer from incontinence, including up to 50% of those living in a nursing home [44].

There is increased risk of urinary tract infections (UTIs) in the elderly population as well, due to shortening of the urethra, decreased urine flow, and in men, prostate hypertrophy. Asymptomatic bacteriuria can be found in up to 50% of women and 30% of men older than 65 years [45].

Endocrine – the salt, sugar, and spice of life

The theme of loss of reserve capacity carries on to the endocrine system. While the basal plasma levels of most hormones are unchanged with normal aging, the ability of the elderly person to adapt to changes in the environment and to stressors is reduced [46].

Thyroid

There is a decreased production of T4 by the thyroid gland, which relates to lower serum T3 levels [11, 47]. The prevalence of hypothyroidism is high in those older than 60 years of age, particularly in women. It ranges from subclinical (elevated TSH (thyroid-stimulating hormone) with normal free T4) to myxedema coma and is typically due to autoimmune thyroid issues [47]. Hyperthyroidism in patients older than 65 years affects men and women equally. Up to a quarter of the cases of hyperthyroidism occur in those older than 65 [47, 48].

Clinically, one may miss the development of a thyroid disorder as the elderly person's response is often blunted or atypical. Hyperthyroidism may present without any of the hypersympathetic signs and symptoms, and the cardiac manifestation of an acute onset of atrial fibrillation or congestive heart failure may be the only sign of the disease, which has been referred to as "apathetic hyperthyroidism" [46].

Sympathoadrenal system

The sympathetic nervous system tone is increased with aging; however, the adrenergic receptor-mediated stimulation decreases [46]. Hence, the elderly do not respond as well to sympathomimetics. Nevertheless, they are more predisposed to developing essential hypertension.

Autonomic insufficiency occurs more commonly, leading to orthostatic hypotension, yet this must be investigated in the context of the medications taken by the patient, as well as their underlying comorbid conditions. A very common cause of orthostasis is due to the consumption of beta blockers even when the patient has been compliant with the recommended dosage.

The aldosterone level decreases, which predisposes the elderly person to renal sodium wasting and eventual dehydration as the thirst mechanism is blunted. The hypoaldosteronism also places the elderly person at risk of hyperkalemia, notably in those with underlying renal disease [46].

Growth hormone

Decreased growth hormone leads to changes that make the elderly person more frail and susceptible to injury and falls. There is a decrease in muscle mass as well as in bone strength [46].

Section IV: Decision-making

- Physiologic changes with aging are largely predictable and well described.
- Older adults have an impaired ability to respond to stressors that gradually worsens and is synonymous with aging.
- Acquired disease is not synonymous with aging, yet increased prevalence of acquired disease with aging accelerates loss of reserve.
- The impaired ability to respond to stressors can be evident as muted responses by almost every organ system.
- Anticipating this "atypical" response, providers may have the opportunity to detect and treat acute illness earlier.

References

1 Jamshed, N., Dubin, J., and Eldadah, Z. (2013) Emergency management of palpitations in the elderly: epidemiology, diagnostic approaches, and therapeutic options, in *Clinics in Geriatric Medicine: Geriatric Emergency Medicine*, Vol. **29** (1) (ed C.R. Carpenter), Elsevier, Philadelphia, PA, pp. 205–230.

2 Taffet, G.E. and Lakatta, E.G. (2003) Aging of the cardiovascular system, in *Principles of Geriatric Medicine and Gerontology*, 5th edn (eds W.R. Hazzard, J.P. Blass, and J.B. Jalter), McGraw-Hill, New York, pp. 403–421.

3 Glickman, S.W., Shofer, F.S., Wu, M.C. *et al.* (2012) Development and validation of prioritization rule for obtaining an immediate 12-lead electrocardiogram in the emergency department to identify ST-elevation myocardial infarction. *Am. Heart J.*, **163** (3), 372–382.

4 Aronow, W.S. (2003) Cardiac arrhythmias, in *Brocklehurst's Textbook of Geriatric Medicine and Gerontology*, 6th edn (eds R.C. Tallis and H.M. Fillit), Churchill Livingstone, pp. 425–439.

5 Lakatta, E.G. (2003) Arterial and cardiac aging: major shareholders in cardiovascular disease enterprises: part III: cellular and molecular clues to heart and arterial aging. *Circulation*, **107** (3), 490–497.

6 Kannel, W.B., Abbott, R.D., Savage, D.D., and McNamara, P.M. (1982) Epidemiologic features of chronic atrial fibrillation: the Framingham study. *N. Engl. J. Med.*, **306** (17), 1018–1022.

7 Sabatini, T., Frisoni, G.B., Barbisoni, P. *et al.* (2000) Atrial fibrillation and cognitive disorders in older people. *J. Am. Geriatr. Soc.*, **48** (4), 387–390.

8 Aronow, W.S. (2003) Effects of aging on the heart, in *Brocklehurst's Textbook of Geriatric Medicine and Gerontology*, 6th edn (eds R.C. Tallis and H.M. Fillit), Churchill Livingstone, pp. 341–348.

9 Rich, M.W. (2004) Cardiac disease, in *Current: Geriatric Diagnosis and Treatment* (eds C.S. Landefeld, R.M. Palmer, and M.A. Johnson), Lange Medical Books/McGraw-Hill, New York, pp. 156–182.

10 Meyyazhagan, S. and Messinger-Rapport, B.J. (2004) Hypertension, in *Current: Geriatric Diagnosis and Treatment* (eds C.S. Landefeld, R.M. Palmer, and M.A. Johnson), Lange Medical Books/McGraw-Hill, New York, pp. 183–190.

11 Taffett, G.E. (2003) Physiology of aging, in *Geriatric Medicine: An Evidence-Based Approach*, 4th edn (eds C.K. Cassel, R.M. Leipzig, and H.J. Cohen), Springer, New York, pp. 27–35.

12 Enright, P.L. (2003) Aging of the respiratory system, in *Principles of Geriatric Medicine and Gerontology*, 5th edn (eds W.R. Hazzard, J.P. Blass, and J.B. Jalter), McGraw-Hill, New York, pp. 511–515.

13 Connolly, M.J. (2003) Age-related changes in the respiratory system, in *Brocklehurst's Textbook of Geriatric Medicine and Gerontology*, 6th edn (eds R.C. Tallis and H.M. Fillit), Churchill Livingstone, pp. 489–493.

14 Borsboom, G.J., van Pelt, W., and van Houwelingen, H.C. (1999) Diurnal variation in lung function in subgroups from two Dutch populations: consequences for longitudinal analysis. *Am. J. Respir. Crit. Care Med.*, **159**, 1163–1171.

15 Alzahrani, A., Sinnert, R., and Gernsheimer, J. (2013) Acute kidney injury, sodium disorders, and hypercalcemia in the aging kidney: diagnostic and therapeutic management strategies in emergency medicine, in *Clinics in Geriatric Medicine: Geriatric Emergency Medicine*, Vol. **29** (1) (ed C.R. Carpenter), Elsevier, Philadelphia, PA, pp. 275–319.

16 Nyengaard, J.R. and Bendsten, T.F. (1992) Glomerular number and size in relation to age, kidney weight and body surface in normal man. *Anat. Rec.*, **232**, 194–201.

17 Wesson, L.G. (1969) Renal hemodynamics in physiological states, in *Physiology of the Human Kidney* (ed L.G. Wesson), Grune and Stratton, New York, pp. 96–116.

18 Wiggins, J. (2003) Changes in renal function, in *Principles of Geriatric Medicine and Gerontology*, 5th edn (eds W.R. Hazzard, J.P. Blass, and J.B. Jalter), McGraw-Hill, New York, pp. 543–549.

19 Bauer, J. (1993) Age-related changes in the rennin-aldosterone system. *Drugs Aging*, **3**, 238–245.

20 Beck, L.H. (2004) Renal system, fluid, and electrolytes, in *Current: Geriatric Diagnosis and Treatment* (eds C.S. Landefeld, R.M. Palmer, and M.A. Johnson), Lange Medical Books/McGraw-Hill, New York, pp. 247–256.

21 Chatta, G.S. and Lipschitz, D.A. (2003) Aging of the hematopoietic system, in *Principles of Geriatric Medicine and Gerontology*, 5th edn (eds W.R. Hazzard, J.P. Blass, and J.B. Jalter), McGraw-Hill, New York, pp. 763–770.

22 Gravenstein, S., Fillit, H.M., and Ershler, W.B. (2003) Clinical immunology of aging, in *Brocklehurst's Textbook of Geriatric Medicine and Gerontology*, 6th edn (eds R.C. Tallis and H.M. Fillit), Churchill Livingstone, pp. 113–124.

23 Norman, D.C. (2000) Fever in the elderly. *Clin. Infect. Dis.*, **31** (1), 148–151.

24 Gavazzi, G. and Kruase, K.H. (2002) Ageing and infection. *Lancet Infect. Dis.*, **2** (**11**), 659–666.

25 High, K.P. and Loeb, M. (2003) Infection in the elderly, in *Principles of Geriatric Medicine and Gerontology*, 5th edn (eds W.R. Hazzard, J.P. Blass, and J.B. Jalter), McGraw-Hill, New York, pp. 1071–1081.

26 Brigden, M.L. and Heathcote, J.C. (2000) Problems in interpreting laboratory tests. What do unexpected results mean? *Postgrad. Med.*, **107** (7), 145–146, 151-152, 155-158 passim.

27 Ganley, J.P. and Roberts, J. (1978(212)) *Eye Conditions and Related Need for Medical Care Among Persons 1–74 Years of Age, United States, 1971–72*, Vital Health Statistics, vol. **11**, pp. i–v No 228. DHHS Publication No. (PHS)83-1678.

28 Lewis, R. and Warshaw, G. (2004) Visual and hearing impairment, in *Current: Geriatric Diagnosis and Treatment* (eds C.S. Landefeld, R.M. Palmer, and M.A. Johnson), Lange Medical Books/McGraw-Hill, New York, pp. 122–137.

29 Mattson, M.P. (2003) Cellular and neurochemical aspects of the aging human brain, in *Principles of Geriatric Medicine and Gerontology*, 5th edn (eds W.R. Hazzard, J.P. Blass, and J.B. Jalter), McGraw-Hill, New York, pp. 1341–1354.

30 Horn, J. and Cattell, R. (1967) Age differences in fluid and crystallized intelligence. *J. Educ. Psychol.*, **57**, 253.

31 Craft, S., Cholerton, B., and Reger, M. (2003) Aging and cognition: what is normal?, in *Principles of Geriatric Medicine and Gerontology*, 5th edn (eds W.R. Hazzard, J.P. Blass, and J.B. Jalter), McGraw-Hill, New York, pp. 1355–1372.

32 Stuart-Hamilton, I.A. (2003) Normal cognitive aging, in *Brocklehurst's Textbook of Geriatric Medicine and Gerontology*, 6th edn (eds R.C. Tallis and H.M. Fillit), Churchill Livingstone, pp. 125–142.

33 Loeser, R.F. and Delbono, O. (2003) Aging of the muscles and joints, in *Principles of Geriatric Medicine and Gerontology*, 5th edn (eds W.R. Hazzard, J.P. Blass, and J.B. Jalter), McGraw-Hill, New York, pp. 905–918.

34 Moylan, K.C. (ed) (2004) Androgen deficiency in older men, in *The Washington Manual: Geriatrics Subspecialty Consult*, Lippincott Williams and Wilkins, Philadelphia, PA, pp. 66–70.

35 Shroff, D. and Sivaprasad, L. (2004) Osteoporosis, in *The Washington Manual: Geriatrics Subspecialty Consult* (ed K.C. Moylan), Lippincott Williams and Wilkins, Philadelphia, PA, pp. 76–80.

36 Srivastava, M. and Deal, C. (2004) Osteoporosis and hip fractures, in *Current: Geriatric Diagnosis and Treatment* (eds C.S. Landefeld, R.M. Palmer, and M.A. Johnson), Lange Medical Books/McGraw-Hill, New York, pp. 272–280.

37 Hall, K.E. (2003) Effect of aging on gastrointestinal function, in *Principles of Geriatric Medicine and Gerontology*, 5th edn (eds W.R. Hazzard, J.P. Blass, and J.B. Jalter), McGraw-Hill, New York, pp. 593–600.

38 Devlin, H. and Ferguson, M.W.J. (2003) Aging and the orofacial tissues, in *Brocklehurst's Textbook of Geriatric Medicine and Gerontology*, 6th edn (eds R.C. Tallis and H.M. Fillit), Churchill Livingstone, pp. 951–964.

39 Greenwald, D.A. and Brandt, L.J. (2003) The upper gastrointestinal tract, in *Brocklehurst's Textbook of Geriatric Medicine and Gerontology*, 6th edn (eds R.C. Tallis and H.M. Fillit), Churchill Livingstone, pp. 965–985.

40 Raimondo, M.L. and Burroughs, A. (2003) Biliary tract diseases, in *Brocklehurst's Textbook of Geriatric Medicine and Gerontology*, 6th edn (eds R.C. Tallis and H.M. Fillit), Churchill Livingstone, pp. 1019–1024.

41 Wald, A. (2003) The large bowel, in *Brocklehurst's Textbook of Geriatric Medicine and Gerontology*, 6th edn

(eds R.C. Tallis and H.M. Fillit), Churchill Livingstone, pp. 1037–1055.

42 Harari, D. (2003) Constipation and fecal incontinence in old age, in *Brocklehurst's Textbook of Geriatric Medicine and Gerontology*, 6th edn (eds R.C. Tallis and H.M. Fillit), Churchill Livingstone, pp. 1311–1322.

43 DuBeau, C.E. (2004) Urinary incontinence, in *Current: Geriatric Diagnosis and Treatment* (eds C.S. Landefeld, R.M. Palmer, and M.A. Johnson), Lange Medical Books/McGraw-Hill, New York, pp. 239–246.

44 Birge, S.J. and Lai, S.R. (2004) Approach to the geriatric patient: the comprehensive geriatric assessment, in *The Washington Manual: Geriatrics Subspecialty Consult* (eds K.C. Moylan and T.L. Lin), Lippincott Williams and Wilkins, Philadelphia, PA, pp. 1–5.

45 Anderson, R.S. and Hallen, S.A.M. (2013) Generalized weakness in the geriatric emergency department patient: an approach to initial management, in *Clinics in Geriatric Medicine: Geriatric Emergency Medicine*, Vol. 29 (1) (ed C.R. Carpenter), Elsevier, Philadelphia, PA, pp. 91–100.

46 Gruenewalk, D.A. and Matsumoto, A.M. (2003) Aging of the endocrine system and selected endocrine disorders, in *Principles of Geriatric Medicine and Gerontology*, 5th edn (eds W.R. Hazzard, J.P. Blass, and J.B. Jalter), McGraw-Hill, New York, pp. 819–835.

47 Shroff, D. and Moylan, K.C. (2004) Thyroid disease in the geriatric patient, in *The Washington Manual: Geriatrics Subspecialty Consult* (ed K.C. Moylan), Lippincott Williams and Wilkins, Philadelphia, PA, pp. 97–102.

48 Miller, M. (2003) Disorders of the thyroid, in *Brocklehurst's Textbook of Geriatric Medicine and Gerontology*, 6th edn (eds R.C. Tallis and H.M. Fillit), Churchill Livingstone, pp. 1165–1183.

3 Functional assessment of the elderly

Kirk A. Stiffler

Department of Emergency Medicine, Summa Akron City Hospital, Northeast Ohio Medical University, Akron, OH USA

Section I: Case presentation

A 78-year-old woman was brought to the emergency department (ED) by emergency medical service (EMS) with a chief complaint of a fall resulting in right wrist pain. She had gone outside to get her mail, tripped on uneven pavement, and landed on an outstretched right hand. She had no other complaint of pain and was not dizzy or lightheaded prior to the fall.

The past medical history (PMH) was significant for hypertension, hypothyroidism, and Type II diabetes mellitus. She lived alone at home since her husband's death 2 years ago. Over the past 6 months, she had a 20-lb weight loss. She felt exhausted with activity, and her activity was limited to meal preparation and shopping. She had been feeling progressively weaker over the past 6 months, and she has been using her late husband's walker for ambulation. She had no family in town, and no close friends or caregivers.

On examination, she had a "dinner fork" deformity to the right wrist. She had no other areas of tenderness, and a normal cardiopulmonary examination.

The X-ray study confirmed a mildly displaced and angulated distal radius fracture with an ulnar styloid fracture. Orthopedics recommended the application of anterior and posterior splints with follow-up in the office. As her discharge instructions were being prepared, and as she was being placed in splints, the patient asked how she would be able to use her walker, get dressed, and operate her car, which had a standard transmission. She was also concerned about how she will be able to get home, as she was brought to the ED by ambulance.

Section II: Case discussion

Dr Shamai Grossman (SG): When you hear a case like this, are you concerned about other causes of the fall? It sounds like a straightforward mechanical fall. However, given this person has gotten the mail for the last 70 years, and only fell today, does this raise any questions of whether she needs more of a workup for a fall?

Dr Amal Mattu (AM): I have to admit, I am a bit more suspicious when an elderly patient tells me about tripping and falling, and whether it were truly a mechanical fall, or whether there was some type of syncopal episode that led to the fall. Elderly patients tend to be more reluctant and stoic in reporting symptoms that they think may eventuate in having them admitted to the hospital. Before I accept that it's just a mechanical fall, I want to get as complete a history as possible. Given the comorbidities in general, I would be worried about hypoglycemia as she is diabetic, dehydration, depression, alcoholism – given her husband died not too long ago, and she doesn't have much social support. I am going to look much more in depth into her underlying medical problems than I would in a younger patient.

Dr Don Melady (DM): I would like to comment on the difficulty of getting a good history to support the conclusion of "mechanical fall." The history of the fall prodrome is almost always unreliable – simply because people are unable to accurately get those events into long-term memory before they lose consciousness. Moreover, the same applies to anytime head trauma, or following a seizure, or whenever the patient has a lot of pain. Looking to a witness or observer of the event for more detail about the prodrome is likely more helpful.

Dr Rob Anderson (RA): I would accept this as a simple mechanical fall. For me, using the term "mechanical fall" does not appropriately incorporate etiologies for the fall, nor describe the dramatic impact a fall can have on the life of an elderly patient. In this case, her fall is clearly an exclamation mark to her gradual functional decline.

SG: These are both very valid points. Let's talk about the PMH.

Dr Scott Wilber (SW): She did have a PMH significant for hypothyroidism, hypertension, and diabetes. She lived alone at home since her husband died 2 years ago. Over the past 6 months, she had a 20-lb weight loss, and she felt exhausted with any activity. Her activity had been limited to meal preparation and shopping as well as her basic activities of daily living (ADLs). She had become progressively weak. She had begun to use her husband's walker for ambulation, and she truly lacked social support, with no family in town and no close friends or caregivers.

SG: What happened when you examined this patient?

SW: She had the classic Colles fracture deformity of her wrist. She didn't have any other areas of tenderness or evidence of other injury. She had a normal cardiopulmonary examination. But also we found that she appeared to be cachectic, not a lot of muscle mass, somewhat frail and weak.

SG: Given this presentation, what would you do as far as workup?

RA: Two avenues, first, I would work up the traumatic findings with imaging. Second, I would look at this fall as a marker of something else that's going on with her. My workup would include laboratory tests, an electrocardiogram (EKG), a chest X-ray study, looking for an oncologic process with this weight loss.

AM: I would also add a metabolic workup and check her thyroid function as well. I would once again be suspicious for additional injuries besides her wrist and go over her very carefully from head to toe, looking for any additional injuries. When elderly patients fall, they have a hip fracture until proven otherwise. Certainly, you wouldn't want to miss something like that.

I would agree, you really have to look for any other probable underlying cause.

SW: I would just add that over the last couple of years I've started looking at a broader set of laboratory studies in addition to the basic metabolic panel (BMP) or chemistry 7, measuring the albumin, and total protein to look at the nutritional status. Low serum albumin is really predictive of bad adverse outcome in a lot of different scenarios, certainly in a weak and frail person.

RA: A complete metabolic panel (CMP) would be helpful in order to look at biliary diseases, which would send you down a different path. The patient may not have abdominal pain or fever but could certainly have something going on with the gallbladder.

DM: I might add calcium (occult metastatic disease), magnesium, phosphate (nutritional deficiencies), and thyroid stimulating hormone (TSH) (unexplained functional decline.)

AM: That's an interesting approach that goes against current "Choosing Wisely," to avoid overtesting, overdiagnosis, overtreatment, which is currently being recommended and enforced upon us by diverse agendas outside emergency medicine. Nevertheless, I don't believe that all the principles and assumptions of the "Choosing Wisely Movement" apply to potentially vulnerable older adults. These patients have a much higher prevalence of baseline disease, which would render broader screening tests to be very worthwhile.

SG: I would echo that in this elderly population, we have found, by broadening our workup, more disease process than we could ever imagine. If nothing else, at least checking a urinalysis on these patients would be useful as they seem to have a urinary tract infection (UTI) more often than one would think. It's interesting that the serum albumin is not part of the standard laboratory testing for any patient. I would expect this to be part of the normal spectrum of workup that a primary care physician (PCP) should be doing. This raises the question of whether this patient has any primary care coverage or whether the PCP has been involved at all in caring for this patient who has been deteriorating over the past 6 months.

DM: I would argue that expanding the search for preventable causes on this first-time faller IS choosing wisely. Our goal with older patients who have fallen needs to be not only to find the cause and treat the consequence of this fall – but also ensure safe discharge and prevent future falls. If we in the ED can do everything possible to prevent tomorrow's fall and its broken hip, everyone is well served.

RA: One more point that speaks to the history of the falls. First of all, my evaluation is different for a person who has had multiple falls. I am more aggressive with the workup for the first fall or increased frequency of falls.

AM: What's your threshold for routinely working these patients up for syncope with EKGs, mandatory monitoring, observation unit, and troponin levels?

SG: First we must ask does this patient meet criteria for syncope? If we take any of her history as being truthful, she didn't have a transient loss of consciousness. But assume that we can't trust her whatsoever because she's elderly, and we don't what her recall is. If we assume she has loss of consciousness, or near loss of consciousness, then the workup for syncope is not well evidenced by any good literature. We routinely perform EKGs because there is a 5% diagnostic yield. But that doesn't necessarily mean that we have to do them on every patient that falls. Most elderly patients in our ED get an EKG simply because they are elderly. Yet, I don't have good evidence to support doing that. Most patients will get a complete blood count (CBC), and a BMP, but there's no data to support that either. They should at least get the glucose level checked, especially in a diabetic. There isn't good data to support doing this, but there isn't good data against it either. It's such an easy, inexpensive test to do that we have not deleted it from our workup. Again, because this patient didn't clearly have syncope, I'm not sure that I would do anything more from that perspective.

SG: Let's talk about what you found with your workup.

SW: Her X-ray studies demonstrated a displaced angulated distal radius fracture and an ulnar styloid fracture. Orthopedics recommended anterior and posterior splinting and follow-up in the office. The emergency physician began to prepare discharge instructions after placing her in the splints, when she asked how she would be able to do her basic and more advanced ADLs, including how she would be using her walker, how she would be able to get dressed, and how she could drive her car that she has to use to get groceries, since the car has only a standard transmission. She was also concerned about how to get home, since she was brought to the ED by ambulance. Fairly classic concerns of older patients even though they don't always articulate them to us.

SG: This chapter is about functional assessment. What should have been done to functionally assess her?

SW: Some functional assessment was done for this patient. We did obtain the history of things that she has to do, and we did get her history of lack of social support. The functional assessment in the ED needs to be fairly focused. We have our basic activities of daily living to determine. We need to determine the things that affect her mobility and her ability to get around. For example, she may not be able to use a telephone, nor be able to use a walker to ambulate with a wrist splint. Patients need to have the ability to transfer, walk from their easy chair to the bathroom, and to the kitchen and back, to be able stay home alone. The inability to do those things requires at least 24-h care. Those to me are the minimal questions to ask. Moreover, I think we should also ask "how are you going to be able to go to the store to buy food," "do you have to do that on your own?" I also like to ask about the ability to get dressed. This is one of the things I always think about in people who are short of breath. If they are getting short of breath when they are getting dressed, that's a pretty minimal expenditure of energy, and they're probably going to have significant problems if we don't make them substantially better in the ED.

SG: In your ED, once you've done this functional assessment, how does that affect your disposition, and what options would you have for disposition?

RA: In my mind, it's all about functionality, which is almost synonymous with geriatrics. It affects everything I do. In our ED, we are fortunate to have physical therapists (PTS) who can come and see patients. I reflect on my days on inpatient medicine. I recall the medicine being done relatively quickly, and people waiting for their physical therapy or occupational therapy (PT/OT) evaluation to figure out what their safe disposition is going to be. It has always struck me as unfair that in the ED, we typically don't have that resource, yet we are asked to "road-test" someone to make sure they are safe to go home without any formal evaluation. So, we should be advocating for more presence of PT and OT in the ED to help us with this. In this case, OT evaluation would be more germane. If she would be able to go home safely, they can assist in arranging visiting nurses or outside resources to help out.

DM: I'm often struck by how a good PT/OT team can sometimes turn around someone who I initially thought would need admission – by teaching pain-relieving movement strategies, by fitting the patient with the appropriate gait aid, by establishing a list of easy modifications at home that can keep the person safe, by suggesting strategies for family and community. I agree that access to a geriatric PT/OT assessment team is essential in the ED of the future.

SG: Do you have other options, when admitting to your hospital is not really a good option, when the hospital is full, and the admitting services are adamantly resisting the admission of patients who don't have a medical problem?

CC: At Washington University, we have OT during daylight hours, but they are heavily underutilized. Our data show that only 24% of our physicians are screening for functional status to begin with and that they are not clearly recognizing patients with poor functional status. There are some things that I do know are available at other EDs around the country from our survey of 30 geriatric EDs in 2013. Some centers are using mobile angiotensin-converting-enzyme (ACE) units, and others are considering geriatric observation units for these patients or even telemedicine for some of the rural hospitals for functional assessment by a knowledgeable geriatric professional outside that ED.

RA: This would be a great opportunity for a geriatric observation unit in the ED, especially when they come in at night when resources aren't available, and to allow them a comfortable night's rest until morning when we can have people involved to help us figure out a safe disposition.

DM: We too have a protocol for holding patients through the night for further assessment in the morning when we have access to all services – PT, OT, SW, and community liaison. It has been a win–win for everyone. Patients and families like it because

it avoids the need for a hospital admission; the admitting services and the hospital like it because it decreases needless admission; and ED staff like it because we feel that we are actually doing right by the patient.

SG: I think utilizing an observation unit is a great option for these patients and that's what we routinely do in our ED. This can be done with or without a dedicated area for geriatrics. What do you do if you don't have an observation unit? Again, you have these pressures from the hospital and from the patient too, who says "I just want to go home."

AM: There are no simple answers for that. There are times when the hospital or others may not want you do the right thing purely from a financial standpoint of what is best for the hospital, but you have to put the finances behind you, and do what you think is best for the patient's health. You may get some opposition from the hospital or others. If you think the patient is not going to do well or is at some danger if they go home, then you need to keep the patient in the ED, or admit them or find some other place where the patient can go safely; whether that be a family member or some other alternative disposition where the patient is going to be taken care of. The worst-case scenario is that you cave into the pressures from the finance people, and you send the patient home, and the patient ends up sustaining some other injury, or deteriorates in some manner, and then you end up having to admit the patient in an intensive care unit with some serious injury or with sepsis. In the end, doctors need to be doctors, and do the right thing for patients, and not worry about what people who are not doctors are telling you to do because of mistaken concerns about finances.

RA: I agree passionately. We have to do the right thing for these people. An upper extremity fracture is not an inpatient diagnosis per Medicare. So patients who come in with broken arms, who can't go home safely have to be admitted to observation status, and they don't qualify for rehabilitation. It's a horrible system. But at the end of the day, we have to do the best we can and put the patient first.

SW: My suggestion is that every hospital ED look at what resources they have in town and try to make connections to resources that are available so that you're not trying to invent the wheel only at the time the patient arrives in the ED. For example, we have a homecare program owned by the hospital, where the emergency physician can actually do the face-to-face evaluation and get the home care started, and then it will transition to the PCP, which helps expedite the time to home care. We have a partially owned rehabilitation hospital. This patient would likely not meet criteria for rehabilitation. But you would be amazed at the number of patients who you think need to be placed in a skilled nursing home, but rehabilitation says they're a good candidate. We'll generally put these patients in ED observation to make sure nothing medical creeps up over the course of the next 24–48 h, and then they can go to inpatient rehabilitation. Generally, after inpatient rehabilitation in a hospital, they may qualify for skilled nursing as well.

RA: I think we can use a person's functional status to guide very important treatment decisions. A lively, active, driving 80 year old with an acute myocardial infarction (MI) should be considered for cardiac catheterization. This is in contrast to a frail, chronically ill, institutionalized 80 year old with an acute MI for whom goals of care must be sorted out with patient and family before activating the catheterization laboratory. Another example for many of the older people I care for outside the ED, I use dramatic declines in functional status as an opportunity to explore hospice.

Chris Carpenter: The new geriatric emergency medicine guidelines endorsed by ACEP, SAEM, Emergency Nurses Associations, and the American Geriatric Society clearly state that it's the policy to screen all geriatric patients for high-risk features. Those determined to be at risk should be referred to inpatient and outpatient healthcare resources to help improve overall health and functional outcome. We hope that's a crystal clear statement for the bean counters that this is not voluntary care; this is standard care for all frail older adults. We need to figure out ways to recognize them. The Canadians are working on a multinational multi-institutional instrument for patients just like this, ambulatory community dwellings for older adults after blunt trauma to try to identify those who are most likely to benefit from these interventions. That instrument is coming.

DM: As an actual Canadian here, I'd also like to amplify the comments about the importance of home-based care. We have a single-provider community-based care system with which EDs have extremely close connections (usually there is a case manager on site in the ED). Many of these "worried about discharging" situations become easy and clear if the ED can ensure prompt (like tomorrow!) follow-up care whether it be simple personal support (for bathing and toileting), or advanced nursing care (medication management, VS assessment), or PT (mobilization), or OT (cognitive assessment). I think EDs can do more to work with community partners to ensure a continuum of care from the ED.

SG: That would definitely change our practice. From everything that has been said, ours is a practice that needs to evolve, and clearly, as stated, we need to do the right thing for the patient. It helps when we have more instruments that can influence the hospital and financial administrators.

SW: One other screening tool that would be mandatory in our ED before this patient left is an informal "up and go" test. She would have to be able to get up from the bed and get around on her walker, or we would not discharge her. That's become a mandatory requirement in our department. Patients have to demonstrate their abilities. The worst thing would be to put her in an ambulance only to find out she's not able to ambulate, when she returns a few days later with other injuries or bed sores.

DM: I'm eternally surprised at how resistant physicians and trainees are to do what seems intuitive – if you are going to discharge someone home, you need to know they can walk to the door! An informal "road test" (50 m around the department) also supplies you with a wealth of information about strength, cerebellar function, executive function (can they figure out how to put on their shoes?), exertional dyspnea, heart rate, and BP variability. That's a lot of information from a 1-min test!

SG: I think that should be mandatory, and it's the correct practice. I wonder if this is being taught around the country. It needs to become routine and standard practice in every ED.

SW: In summary, this patient had a distal radius fracture plus significant concerns for functional decline. She was admitted to an observation status, where she was able to be evaluated by PT. They were able to make certain adjustments to her late husband's walker so that she was able to use it. They also were able to connect her to the geriatrics clinic and home care, and she was able to return home safely.

Functional assessment of the elderly

Functional assessment is an important aspect of geriatric emergency medical care. Limited functional capabilities can, on their own, precipitate visits to the ED, and can also be a manifestation of other serious underlying medical disease that causes patients to present to the ED. This can have an impact upon disposition decisions from the ED, and can portend future morbidity and mortality for those found to possess limited functional capacities [1]. Overall function is dependent on multiple aspects of any given patient, including medical, cognitive, affective, spiritual, and environmental issues, as well as available economic and social support mechanisms [2]. Current research demonstrates that emergency medicine providers do not properly assess nor therefore understand many an older patient's functional status [3].

Functional impairment, defined as a lack of ability to perform a particular action, is common in elderly patients and can often go unnoticed in the often hurried environment of traditional EDs. Functional impairment can lead to disability, which is the inability or limitation to perform socially defined actions [4]. EDs can cater to the special needs of such multifaceted geriatric patients by providing some of the unique aspects of geriatric patients, and this will hopefully better serve the elderly population in the future [5]. Nonetheless, there are ways in which the typical emergency physician can better identify, manage, and treat functional limitations of their geriatric patients in order to help minimize the associated morbidity and mortality. These techniques must become routine in the care of geriatric emergency patients to avoid overlooking significant subclinical limitations that may hinder appropriate recovery from acute injury or illness, while realizing that a functional limitation itself may be the reason for the presentation. Some of the more commonly used and easily implemented tools for assessing function include the ADLs scale, the instrumental ADLs scale, and various forms of physical performance testing.

Lastly, vision and hearing limitations are important issues that may limit function as well.

Activities of daily living

The basic ADLs scale can easily be used by healthcare providers to help describe baseline functioning of patients seen in the ED and can be quite helpful in understanding whether or not these patients need assistance with personal self-care and independent living. They have become routine data collection points in many national surveys of older people and are predictive healthcare resource utilization [6]. The original basic ADLs first published by Katz *et al.* and subsequently expanded Instrumental Activities of Daily Living (IADL) by Lawton and Brody encompass both basic biologic and higher functional competence activities [7, 8]. These surveys are performed in person, and the answers are typically self-reported or reported by appropriate caregivers to the healthcare personnel administering the study. Subsequent development of the Older American Resources and Services (OARS) functional measure incorporates most of these ADLs into a standardized questionnaire that can be administered either in person or via telephone interview and have been well validated for use in EDs [9, 10].

Basic ADLs include bathing, dressing, toileting, transferring, continence, and feeding [7]. These items are scored as yes or no, again by self- or caregiver report to the interviewer. As listed, these are relatively crude measures of independence and are relatively insensitive to small changes in function; nonetheless, the loss of independence on almost any one of these items should alert emergency physicians to the need to assess more fully the patient's functional status and support mechanisms before making final disposition decisions. The IADLs expand the issues to include the ability to use a telephone, shopping, food preparation, housekeeping, laundry, mode of transportation, responsibility for own medications, and the ability to handle finances [8]. The scale can be scored in various manners, with women being scored on all eight criteria, with men historically having food preparation, laundry, and housekeeping excluded. The score typically ranges from 0 to 8, with higher scores indicating more independence. Physical

ADLs include concepts such as walking, dressing, transferring, bathing, grooming, continence, and eating. Although formally administering a complete assessment of all ADLs may be beyond what most EM physicians consider easily feasible, assessing even just a few of these items, as shown by Fillenbaum, can rapidly identify elderly community residents with impaired functional capacity, which also correlates to overall physical health, mental health, and predictability of death [11]. Functional decline as measured by various ADLs is an important factor in precipitating many ED visits as well, particularly those mobility-related ADLs such as transportation, shopping, meals, housework, dressing, transferring, or walking more so than ADLs that deal with executive functions such as medicine management, money management, or telephone use [12, 13].

The Barthel Index has been in widespread use for rehabilitation purposes, but it can also be used to gain some insight into the everyday function of community-dwelling elderly people as well [14]. This assessment primarily evaluates self-care and ambulation issues, heavily weighting things such as continence and personal grooming. Other items evaluated include feeding, ambulation (including walking on level surfaces as well as stairs), and dressing oneself. Information is either self-reported by the patient or caregiver, or noted through observation during the interview. It is not very sensitive for small changes in level of functioning but continues to be used in the rehabilitation field to monitor progress on basic self-care issues [15].

Performance testing

Although the concept of ADLs and IADLs, and in particular the mobility-related ADLs of transferring and walking safely could generally be accepted to indicate a minimum requirement for discharge of someone back into the community setting, these instruments rely solely on self- (or proxy) reporting of abilities [1]. It has been increasingly recognized that more sensitive, reproducible, and feasible methods of measuring actual functional capabilities is required [16–19]. Even thorough standard neuromuscular examination techniques have been shown to be inadequate for identifying mobility problems in elderly

patients [20]. To this end, unique evaluations that can be assessed objectively, observed, or scored have been developed, and include things such as gait speed assessment, timed "up and go" testing, grip strength measurement, and balance testing. In addition, several tests that include a series of various physical tasks have been developed, each with varying feasibility and reliability for use in the ED, and include scales such as the Performance Test of Activities of Daily Living (PADL), the Timed Manual Performance Test, and the Short Physical Performance Battery (SPPB) [4, 21, 22]. Poor performance on many of the skills used in these various tests or batteries of tests have been shown to be predictors of all cause mortality in older community-dwelling adults [23].

Gait speed

In an attempt to develop and implement a simple and easily reproducible test to indicate the health and well-being of older adults, gait speed, or walking speed, has been proposed by several investigators [24–26]. Gait speed has also been shown to predict adverse outcomes in community-dwelling elderly people [27]. Studenski et al. evaluated the relationship between gait speed and overall survival on a pooled cohort of nine studies with more than 34,000 elderly patients and find that faster gait speed is associated with better 5- and 10-year survivals. This is true across the entire range of walking speeds [28]. In addition, it has been demonstrated that improvement in gait speed over a 1-year time period predicts a substantial reduction in mortality and disability [29, 30].

One of the main advantages of gait speed as an indicator of health is its ease of measurement. It can be assessed in any corridor clear of obstacles and is typically measured over a distance of 4–8 m. Patients are asked to walk at their normal speed over a predetermined distance, and the time is recorded to the nearest tenth of a second. The speed is then recorded in meters per second [30, 31]. Gait speeds above 1 m/s seem to be a minimum level for the elderly to function and participate in the community without significant support for ADLs, whereas gait speeds less than 1 m/s identify those elderly who may be at risk for adverse health-related outcomes according to current research

[25, 31]. Clinically, significant changes in gait speed seem to be 0.1 m/s, as indicated in the above study by Studenski, with incremental survival increases seen with each 0.1 m/s increase in gait speed [28]. However, admitted elderly patients may demonstrate even lower gaits speeds, with a cutoff of 0.60 m/s serving as relevant cutoff for predicting things such as hospital length of stay and ability to discharge home [32]. In the ED, it is noted that actual measurement of the gait speed is important, as self-reported slowness is a poor predictor of actual slowness [33].

Timed up and go testing

Although the Get-Up and Go Test has traditionally been used as an assessment tool for fall risk, the timed version, the Timed Up and Go (TUG) test, also correlates with functional mobility [34, 35]. In this test, patients are asked to stand up from a chair, walk 3 m, turn around, walk back to the chair, and sit back down. Those who take an average time of less than 12 s to complete the task over two attempts is considered a fast performer; less than 15 s an intermediate performer, and longer than 15 s a slow performer [36, 37]. In particular, community-dwelling older adults who are slow performers of the TUG have a greater risk of health decline, new ADLs difficulty, and falls [38]. Greater than 30 s corresponds with functional dependence [39, 40]. The test has less value in delineating the differences in risk between the intermediate and the fast performers, and overall, may not add much predictive ability to measuring gait speed alone [38]. The value of some of the more qualitative observations that can be made with the TUG test is not yet understood as well, and when used alone in the ED, it does not necessarily predict ED readmission or hospital admission [41].

Chair standing and balance testing

If gait speed cannot be readily measured for whatever reason, other brief assessments can be used, including the chair stand test or the standing balance performance test. While these tests are often used in assessing balance alone in relation to fall risk, they have been shown to be equally prognostic of adverse health events [24]. In the chair stand test, participants begin by sitting in a standard-sized chair with their arms crossed on their chest. They are then asked to stand up completely and sit back down without touching the back of the chair five times, as quickly as they can while being timed [42, 43]. Although cut points are sometimes calculated based on population percentiles for research purposes, approximately 17 s has been suggested as the best discrimination point for identifying those at increased risk [24]. Alternatively, the number of chair stand repetitions possible within a 30-s period can be assessed, with average count values ranging from 4 to 11 in 90- to 94-year-old women, to 14 to 19 in 60- to 64-year-old men [44].

In addition, standing balance tests may well be predictive of subsequent health outcomes and mortality despite a lack of standardized testing methods [45, 23]. The assessment typically involves evaluating the time that participants can perform various standing positions including side-by-side, semitandem stand (side of one heel touching great toe of other foot), tandem stand (heel of 1 ft in front of and touching the other foot), and a single-leg stand. When done in isolation (not part of a battery), it has been suggested that a time of 53 s can best discriminate elderly at risk for mobility issue and adverse outcomes [24]. This method asks the patents to hold first a semitandem stand for 30 s and then switch to a tandem stand for 30 s and finally into a single-leg stand for 30 s. The test is stopped when patients cannot hold the stand without support after two attempts.

Grip strength

Muscle strength alone may be a reasonable indicator of overall mobility and therefore function in the older population [46, 47]. Grip strength is a relatively simple, reliable, and inexpensive indicator of overall strength. Weak hand grip strength in midlife (age 45–68) has been shown to be associated with functional limitations and disabilities up to 25 years later in life, with the possible presumption that better grip strength may be protective against such disabilities and limitations [48]. Other research suggests that weak hand grip strength in middle-aged and older adults is also associated with an increased mortality, disability, and self-related mobility limitations [49, 50]. More recently, grip strength is reported to be likely a good marker of overall physical performance compared to a more extensive physical performance evaluation, though a more standardized approach and discrete cut-points are needed in order to allow more widespread use [51, 52].

Most commonly, a handheld dynamometer is used to measure the grip strength of patients in a seated position, with the elbow flexed. Patients squeeze the dynamometer for 3–5 s and then repeat the squeeze after a recovery period. Although there has been significant variability in the exact protocol to follow for recording strength, the highest value for the strongest hand was used in the largest study to date that attempted to establish discrete cut points for this test. Other protocols include recording just the dominant hand, just the strongest hand, just the right or left hand, averaging the hands, or adding the hand strengths together [49]. Sallinen *et al.* suggest a cut point of 27 kg for women and 37 kg for men in order to maximize the sensitivity and specificity in identifying mobility limitations for those older than the age of 55 years [50]. They also assessed whether body mass index (BMI) impacts these cutoffs since obesity likely alters the strength and balance requirements of those involved [53, 54]. In men, the cut points increase along with increasing BMI, up to 39 kg for overweight men and 40 kg for obese men. No such changes in the cut point for women are seen with increasing BMI. Other grip strength comparisons demonstrate various hazard ratios for each incremental 1 kg increase in recorded strength, or when comparing the lowest strength quartile to the strongest strength quartiles (HR 0.97 and 1.67, respectively) [23]. Weakness, as determined by low grip strength in the ED, is a relatively common finding in elderly patients (especially those who present with falls) and may be a reliable marker for patients at high risk for adverse outcomes [33, 55].

Formal test batteries

PADL

The PADLs was designed to objectively measure the ability of elderly patients to care for themselves [22].

It includes many activities that appear essential to living independently and correlate to either ADLs or IADLs as previously described. These include drinking from a cup, eating, grooming, dressing, making a phone call, using a key, telling time, and rising from a chair, walking and sitting back down. A total of 16 tasks are scored as 0 or 1, with lower scores representing better independence as in ADLs assessment. It is scored on the basis of the proportion of tested functions correctly performed and grouped as independent (all tasks performed without help), moderately dependent (75–99% of tasks performed without help), and dependent (less than 75% of tasks performed independently). Although this test likely has high face and content validity, as well as good reliability, it requires a significant amount of props to perform, many of which may not be readily available in the ED, as well as significant time to complete all 16 tasks. Its overall usefulness and practicality for use in the ED is therefore limited. Nonetheless, some of the insights that can be gained by asking patients to perform activities that are known requisites for survival in the community before discharge can be invaluable in helping to determine the appropriateness of such discharge or the level of additional assistance needed to make that transition successful.

TMP test

The timed manual performance test is another standardized test that may act as a proxy for functioning and correlates with future death and hospitalization (2 years) [56]. It also requires props and can be quite time-consuming (15 min for administration); therefore, shortened versions have been proposed [21]. The test consists of two types of tasks, many of which are thought to simulate several of the ADLs. The original test includes 27 items. These include opening and closing a series of wooden doors on a 2 ft × 3 ft wooden panel with various types of latches and knobs, as well as simulated eating and page turning, dexterity in handling small objects, and handwriting. The time required to perform these individual tasks seems to correlate well with overall dependency, possibly even better than traditional ADLs assessment [57]. As noted though, it is time-consuming as well as difficult to administer to seriously ill patients or those cognitively impaired given the detailed tasks that must be performed.

Short performance physical battery

The Short Performance Physical Battery (SPPB) is one of the most commonly used assessment tools. The test, safety tips, and a scoring sheet, and background information are easily accessed from the National Institute on Aging website [58]. It primarily assesses lower extremity function by measuring gait speed, balance, and chair rising [4]. It is a relatively well-validated tool having originally been studied on more than 5000 elderly patients. It is estimated to take approximately 10 min to perform the entire test. The test obviously demonstrates several aspects of physical function, but it also predicts short-term mortality, nursing home admission, and disability [4, 30, 59]. Whether or not it can be incorporated in the evaluation of elderly patients in the ED depends on many factors, including physical space limitations, staff availability and training, and the ability to appropriately identify those patients on whom the test will have the most immediate impact. In addition, although the score obtained on the SPPB does show a gradient of risk for adverse outcomes, the exact impact that any given score has on determining the need for additional care or alternative disposition has not been determined.

For the SPPB, five chair stands (without the use of arms) are timed from the start of the first rise to completion of the last rise. Ordinal scoring of 0–4 is recorded, with 0 given for inability to complete the task and 1–4 assigned based on the length of time required to complete all five chair stands. The faster the time to complete, the higher the score received, ranging from >16.7 s for a 1, to <11.1 s for a score of 4. Balance testing in the SPPB is measured by assessing semitandem standing balance, where the heel of 1 ft touches the big toe of the other foot. If participants can hold this semitandem stand for 10 s, then they are tested in the full tandem stand with a required time of 10 s. If they are unable to maintain the initial semitandem stand for a full 10 s, they are tested in the side-by-side position for 10 s. Scores of 0 (not attempted), 1 (held for <10 s), and 2 (held for 10 s) are given for each of the two stances attempted in hierarchical difficulty, for a total score of 0–4 for balance testing in the SPPB. Gait speed is measured with an 8 ft walk in an unobstructed space. Participants can use whatever normal walking aids they wish and are asked to walk at their normal pace through the end

of the 8 ft course (approximately 2.44 m) as they are timed with a stopwatch. The person administering the test may walk alongside for safety reasons if needed. Again, a score of 0–4 is given based on time required to complete the walk, with 0 indicating inability to complete the task, and a range of >5.7 s (<0.43 m/s) for a score of 1, to <3.1 s (>0.78 m/s) for a score of 4. The ordinal scores of 1–4 for gait speed (as well as chair stand time) were assigned based on the quartiles of the time required for the tasks by all of the participants. The overall score for the SPPB thus ranges from 0 to 12, with 12 representing the best performance.

The physical performance test

The physical performance test (PPT) is yet another objective measure of elderly patients' functions. As opposed to the SPPB, the PPT evaluates both upper and lower extremity functions [60]. Aspects of function assessed on the PPT include fine and coarse motor function, balance, mobility, coordination, and endurance. Several ADLs and IADLs are also simulated, or at least indirectly assessed. The scale consist of writing a sentence, simulated eating, lifting a book onto a shelf, putting on and taking off a jacket, picking a penny up off the floor, turning around 360°, a 50-ft-walk test, and stair climbing (timed one flight, and maximal number of flights climbable). Each of these items is scored on a 0–4 scale, with 4 representing the best function and 0 the inability to complete the task. A maximal score of 36 is thus achieved for the full nine-item test (a seven-item PPT exists that excludes both stair climbing assessments). The nine-item score identifies frailty, with a score of 32–36 demonstrating no frailty, 25–32 demonstrating mild frailty, 17–24 moderate frailty, and scores less than 17 suggesting the inability to function in the community without some sort of assistance [39, 61]. It has not been shown to predict future functional decline, however. As with other tests, it is difficult to administer in the ED because of length of testing (approximately 10 min), prop requirements, and lack of generalizability to significantly demented or impaired patients.

Vision and hearing assessment

Although the United States Preventive Services Task Force finds insufficient evidence to routinely screen for either vision or hearing disorders in the elderly, emergency medicine clinicians should understand the significant impact that these impairments can have on both the quality of life and overall function of many ED patients [62–64]. Impairment of both vision and hearing becomes common with advanced age [65, 66]. Combined vision and hearing losses have an even greater adverse impact than either alone despite other mental status or comorbid illness issues [67]. Visual impairment is defined as less than 20/20 corrected vision on a standard eye chart; those with less than 20/200 are considered legally blind. Increasing levels of visual impairment can lead to impairment of general function and limit independent living if not remediated [68]. In the ED, in-depth visual testing and assessment is not practical, but self-reported visual impairment with simple questions such as "How would you rate your distant and near vision?" or "In general, do you see well?", as validated within the Identification of Seniors at Risk tool, is thought to be a reliable screening tool. These types of questions in fact may capture more functional impairment issues than traditional eye chart acuity testing as it incorporates functional aspects of vision rather acuity alone [64, 69].

As with vision, hearing impairment is also thought to be predictive of impending overall functional impairment and may be worth addressing if rapid, reliable, and feasible methods are available in the ED [70]. Although several methods of screening are available and audiometry has been shown to have the highest accuracy in detecting hearing loss in the elderly, it is generally accepted that initial screening can be performed via self-reporting or a whispered voice test [71, 72]. Audiometry can then be recommended, on an outpatient basis, to those who fail either of those initial screening tests.

Frailty

In many aspects, much of what the various functional assessment tests are trying to identify relates directly to the concept of frailty, often defined as an excess vulnerability to acute and chronic stressors, with reduced ability or reserve to maintain or regain homeostasis after a destabilizing event [73–75]. Frailty is not often thought of as single clinical complaint in the ED but is often manifested or identified through deficiencies in physical function that are consequences of cumulative subclinical conditions including medical diseases, and behavioral and social risk factors [73]. Fried *et al.* define components of frailty as slowness (as tested by the 15-ft-walk test), weakness (as tested by the hand grip strength on a dynamometer), diminished physical activity (measured by assessing kilocalories expended per week), exhaustion (as self-reported), and unintentional weight loss (10 lbs or 5% of weight in 1 year). The presence of three or more of these attributes defines frailty, while one or two of these attributes identifies a subset of patients defined as pre-frail [74]. At least one study reports it to be feasible to apply this definition in the ED to identify elderly frail patients, though the evaluation takes approximately 7–8 min [33]. There are several other identification tools such as the Clinical Frailty Scale and the Frailty Index-Comprehensive Geriatric Assessment [76, 77]. All of these tools identify frailty, which consistently correlate with adverse outcomes such as functional decline, hospitalization, institutionalization, and death, including those who are recently discharged from the ED [74, 78, 79].

The geriatric emergency department

Given the complexities of evaluating geriatric patients in the ED, functional decline, among other things such as dementia and delirium, is often overlooked [80–83]. Routine emergency care of such geriatric patients typically requires more resources than similar complaints in younger ED patients [84]. The need for specific skills, instruments, and alternative models of care for this population has been recognized for some time [85, 86]. In response to this recognized need, Geriatric Emergency Department Guidelines were recently established and endorsed by several national relevant societies with vested interests in appropriate geriatric emergency care [5]. As discussed, many of the performance tests used to assess functional status of elderly patients are not feasible within the confines of a traditional ED. However, within the concept of a geriatric care in the ED, many of these tests could be performed. For example, PTs could reliably assess physical components such as gait speed, TUG testing, chair standing, balance testing, grip strength, and even the SPPB. Geriatric technicians could be used to help complete screening questionnaires regarding various ADLs, and potentially even things such as vision and hearing screening [87]. Though definitive research is still needed, this step toward a more comprehensive yet targeted multidisciplinary geriatric assessment should increase the value and quality of geriatric emergency care [5, 88, 89].

Conclusion

Fully assessing function in an elderly patient or population is no doubt a complex undertaking. The concept of function itself is multidimensional, and limitations of function will adversely affect different patients in different manners and to varying degrees. As reviewed, there are many different tools by which to assess function, each with inherent strengths, weaknesses, and underlying assumptions about the participant as well as societal norms for independence. Emergency clinicians are currently not adequately assessing functional status much of the time and must begin to incorporate additional tools into their practice in order to better understand the functional status of the elderly population they are serving [3]. In general, it is thought that performance testing is likely the best proxy for function, followed by the patients' own rating of functional limitations, followed lastly by physicians' prediction of functional status. For busy emergency physicians practicing in the often harried ED setting, selecting the right population to assess with the proper tool can be challenging. Until adequate resources become more widely available though, targeting those elderly who are being considered for discharge back into the community setting with limited support with some mobility performance testing before such discharge would be a reasonable first step.

- The functional status of geriatric patients is dependent on multiple aspects of the individual patient, including things such as medical, physical, cognitive, and environmental issues.
- Assessment of functional status in the ED is important, particularly so for those patients being considered for discharge back into the community at large because decreased function is associated with future adverse events.

- Functional impairment is common in geriatric patients and may itself be a reason for an ED visit.
- Direct observation of functional capabilities via performance testing of gait, gait speed, strength, and balance capabilities is the best method to assess such function, as both patients and physicians are poor predictors of functional limitations.
- Incorporating functional assessment into the multidisciplinary team approach such as that proposed by the new geriatric emergency department guidelines may help improve outcomes and prevent future adverse events.

References

1 Sanders, A.B. and Force SAEMGEMT (1996) *Emergency Care of the Elder Person*, Beverly Cracom Publications, St Louis, MO.

2 Halter, J., Ouslander, J., Tinetti, M. *et al.* (2009) *Hazzard's Geriatric Medicine and Gerontology*, 6th edn, McGraw-Hill Education, New York, NY.

3 Rodriguez-Molinero, A., Lopez-Dieguez, M., Tabuenca, A.I. *et al.* (2006) Functional assessment of older patients in the emergency department: comparison between standard instruments, medical records and physicians' perceptions. *BMC Geriatr.*, 6, 13.

4 Guralnik, J.M., Simonsick, E.M., Ferrucci, L. *et al.* (1994) A short physical performance battery assessing lower extremity function: association with self-reported disability and prediction of mortality and nursing home admission. *J. Gerontol.*, 49 (2), M85–M94.

5 Carpenter, C.R., Bromley, M., Caterino, J.M. *et al.* (2014) Optimal older adult emergency care: introducing multidisciplinary geriatric emergency department guidelines from the American College of Emergency Physicians, American Geriatrics Society, Emergency Nurses Association, and Society for Academic Emergency Medicine. *Ann. Emerg. Med.*, 63 (5), e1–e3.

6 Wiener, J.M., Hanley, R.J., Clark, R., and Van Nostrand, J.F. (1990) Measuring the activities of daily living: comparisons across national surveys. *J. Gerontol.*, 45 (6), S229–S237.

7 Katz, S. (1983) Assessing self-maintenance: activities of daily living, mobility, and instrumental activities of daily living. *J. Am. Geriatr. Soc.*, 31 (12), 721–727.

8 Lawton, M.P. and Brody, E.M. (1969) Assessment of older people: self-maintaining and instrumental activities of daily living. *Gerontologist*, 9 (3), 179–186.

9 George, L.K. and Fillenbaum, G.G. (1985) OARS methodology. A decade of experience in geriatric assessment. *J. Am. Geriatr. Soc.*, 33 (9), 607–615.

10 Fillenbaum, G.G. (1988) *Multidimensional Functional Assessment of Older Adults: The Duke Older Americans Resources and Services Procedures*, Erlbaum, Hillsdale, NJ.

11 Fillenbaum, G.G. (1985) Screening the elderly. A brief instrumental activities of daily living measure. *J. Am. Geriatr. Soc.*, **33** (10), 698–706.

12 Wilber, S.T., Blanda, M., and Gerson, L.W. (2006) Does functional decline prompt emergency department visits and admission in older patients? *Acad. Emerg. Med.*, **13** (6), 680–682.

13 Wilber, S.T., Stefanov, D., Gerson, L.W., and Blanda, M. (2010) Simplifying the assessment of activities of daily living in older ED patients: an exploratory factor analysis. *Acad. Emerg. Med.*, **17**, s110.

14 Mahoney, F.I. and Barthel, D.W. (1965) Functional evaluation: the Barthel index. *Md. State Med. J.*, **14**, 61–65.

15 Applegate, W.B., Blass, J.P., and Williams, T.F. (1990) Instruments for the functional assessment of older patients. *N. Engl. J. Med.*, **322** (17), 1207–1214.

16 Wilber, S.T. and Gerson, L.W. (2003) A research agenda for geriatric emergency medicine. *Acad. Emerg. Med.*, **10** (3), 251–260.

17 Studenski, S., Perera, S., Wallace, D. *et al.* (2003) Physical performance measures in the clinical setting. *J. Am. Geriatr. Soc.*, **51** (3), 314–322.

18 Elam, J.T., Graney, M.J., Beaver, T. *et al.* (1991) Comparison of subjective ratings of function with observed functional ability of frail older persons. *Am. J. Public Health*, **81** (9), 1127–1130.

19 Carpenter, C.R., Heard, K., Wilber, S. *et al.* (2011) Research priorities for high-quality geriatric emergency care: medication management, screening, and prevention and functional assessment. *Acad. Emerg. Med.*, **18** (6), 644–654.

20 Tinetti, M.E. and Ginter, S.F. (1988) Identifying mobility dysfunctions in elderly patients. Standard neuromuscular examination or direct assessment? *J. Am. Med. Assoc.*, **259** (8), 1190–1193.

21 Gerrity, M.S., Gaylord, S., and Williams, M.E. (1993) Short versions of the timed manual performance test. Development, reliability, and validity. *Med. Care*, **31** (7), 617–628.

22 Kruiansky, J. and Gurland, B. (1976) The performance test of activities of daily living. *Int. J. Aging Hum. Dev.*, **7** (4), 343–352.

23 Cooper, R., Kuh, D., Hardy, R., and Mortality Review G, Falcon, Teams HAS (2010) Objectively measured physical capability levels and mortality: systematic review and meta-analysis. *Br. Med. J. (Clin. Res. Ed.)*, **341**, c4467.

24 Cesari, M., Kritchevsky, S.B., Newman, A.B. *et al.* (2009) Added value of physical performance measures in predicting adverse health-related events: results from the health, aging and body composition study. *J. Am. Geriatr. Soc.*, **57** (2), 251–259.

25 Cesari, M., Kritchevsky, S.B., Penninx, B.W. *et al.* (2005) Prognostic value of usual gait speed in well-functioning older people--results from the health, aging and body composition study. *J. Am. Geriatr. Soc.*, **53** (10), 1675–1680.

26 Ostir, G.V., Kuo, Y.F., Berges, I.M. *et al.* (2007) Measures of lower body function and risk of mortality over 7 years of follow-up. *Am. J. Epidemiol.*, **166** (5), 599–605.

27 Abellan van Kan, G., Rolland, Y., Andrieu, S. *et al.* (2009) Gait speed at usual pace as a predictor of adverse outcomes in community-dwelling older people an International Academy on Nutrition and Aging (IANA) Task Force. *J. Nutr. Health Aging*, **13** (10), 881–889.

28 Studenski, S., Perera, S., Patel, K. *et al.* (2011) Gait speed and survival in older adults. *J. Am. Med. Assoc.*, **305** (1), 50–58.

29 Hardy, S.E., Perera, S., Roumani, Y.F. *et al.* (2007) Improvement in usual gait speed predicts better survival in older adults. *J. Am. Geriatr. Soc.*, **55** (11), 1727–1734.

30 Guralnik, J.M., Ferrucci, L., Pieper, C.F. *et al.* (2000) Lower extremity function and subsequent disability: consistency across studies, predictive models, and value of gait speed alone compared with the short physical performance battery. *J. Gerontol. A Biol. Sci. Med. Sci.*, **55** (4), M221–M231.

31 Bohannon, R.W. (1997) Comfortable and maximum walking speed of adults aged 20-79 years: reference values and determinants. *Age Ageing*, **26** (1), 15–19.

32 Ostir, G.V., Berges, I., Kuo, Y.F. *et al.* (2012) Assessing gait speed in acutely ill older patients admitted to an acute care for elders hospital unit. *Arch. Intern. Med.*, **172** (4), 353–358.

33 Stiffler, K.A., Finley, A., Midha, S., and Wilber, S.T. (2013) Frailty assessment in the emergency department. *J. Emerg. Med.*, **45** (2), 291–298.

34 Mathias, S., Nayak, U.S., and Isaacs, B. (1986) Balance in elderly patients: the "get-up and go" test. *Arch. Phys. Med. Rehabil.*, **67** (6), 387–389.

35 Podsiadlo, D. and Richardson, S. (1991) The timed "up & go": a test of basic functional mobility for frail elderly persons. *J. Am. Geriatr. Soc.*, **39** (2), 142–148.

36 Bischoff, H.A., Stahelin, H.B., Monsch, A.U. *et al.* (2003) Identifying a cut-off point for normal mobility: a comparison of the timed 'up and go' test in community-dwelling and institutionalised elderly women. *Age Ageing*, **32** (3), 315–320.

37 Nordin, E., Lindelof, N., Rosendahl, E. *et al.* (2008) Prognostic validity of the timed up-and-go test, a modified get-up-and-go test, staff's global judgement

and fall history in evaluating fall risk in residential care facilities. *Age Ageing*, **37** (4), 442–448.

38 Viccaro, L.J., Perera, S., and Studenski, S.A. (2011) Is timed up and go better than gait speed in predicting health, function, and falls in older adults? *J. Am. Geriatr. Soc.*, **59** (5), 887–892.

39 Lusardi, M.M., Pellecchia, G.L., and Schulman, M. (2003) Functional performance in community living older adults. *J. Geriatr. Phys. Ther.*, **26** (3), 14–22.

40 Bohannon, R.W. (2006) Reference values for the timed up and go test: a descriptive meta-analysis. *J. Geriatr. Phys. Ther.*, **29** (2), 64–68.

41 Walker, K.J., Bailey, M., Bradshaw, S.J. *et al.* (2006) Timed up and go test is not useful as a discharge risk screening tool. *Emerg. Med. Australas.*, **18** (1), 31–36.

42 Whitney, S.L., Wrisley, D.M., Marchetti, G.F. *et al.* (2005) Clinical measurement of sit-to-stand performance in people with balance disorders: validity of data for the five-times-sit-to-stand test. *Phys. Ther.*, **85** (10), 1034–1045.

43 Csuka, M. and McCarty, D.J. (1985) Simple method for measurement of lower extremity muscle strength. *Am. J. Med.*, **78** (1), 77–81.

44 Bennell, K., Dobson, F., and Hinman, R. (2011) Measures of physical performance assessments: Self-Paced Walk Test (SPWT), Stair Climb Test (SCT), Six-Minute Walk Test (6MWT), Chair Stand Test (CST), Timed Up & Go (TUG), Sock Test, Lift and Carry Test (LCT), and Car Task. *Arthritis Care Res.*, **63** (Suppl 11), S350–S370.

45 Cooper, R., Kuh, D., Cooper, C. *et al.* (2011) Objective measures of physical capability and subsequent health: a systematic review. *Age Ageing*, **40** (1), 14–23.

46 Rantanen, T., Guralnik, J.M., Izmirlian, G. *et al.* (1998) Association of muscle strength with maximum walking speed in disabled older women. *Am. J. Phys. Med. Rehabil./Assoc. Acad. Physiatr.*, **77** (4), 299–305.

47 Buchner, D.M., Larson, E.B., Wagner, E.H. *et al.* (1996) Evidence for a non-linear relationship between leg strength and gait speed. *Age Ageing*, **25** (5), 386–391.

48 Rantanen, T., Guralnik, J.M., Foley, D. *et al.* (1999) Midlife hand grip strength as a predictor of old age disability. *J. Am. Med. Assoc.*, **281** (6), 558–560.

49 Bohannon, R.W. (2008) Hand-grip dynamometry predicts future outcomes in aging adults. *J. Geriatr. Phys. Ther.*, **31** (1), 3–10.

50 Sallinen, J., Stenholm, S., Rantanen, T. *et al.* (2010) Hand-grip strength cut points to screen older persons at risk for mobility limitation. *J. Am. Geriatr. Soc.*, **58** (9), 1721–1726.

51 Stevens, P.J., Syddall, H.E., Patel, H.P. *et al.* (2012) Is grip strength a good marker of physical performance among community-dwelling older people? *J. Nutr. Health Aging*, **16** (9), 769–774.

52 Roberts, H.C., Denison, H.J., Martin, H.J. *et al.* (2011) A review of the measurement of grip strength in clinical and epidemiological studies: towards a standardised approach. *Age Ageing*, **40** (4), 423–429.

53 Lafortuna, C.L., Maffiuletti, N.A., Agosti, F., and Sartorio, A. (2005) Gender variations of body composition, muscle strength and power output in morbid obesity. *Int. J. Obes.*, **29** (7), 833–841.

54 Maffiuletti, N.A., Agosti, F., Proietti, M. *et al.* (2005) Postural instability of extremely obese individuals improves after a body weight reduction program entailing specific balance training. *J. Endocrinol. Invest.*, **28** (1), 2–7.

55 Crehan, F., O'Shea, D., Ryan, J.M., and Horgan, F. (2013) A profile of elderly fallers referred for physiotherapy in the emergency department of a Dublin teaching hospital. *Ir. Med. J.*, **106** (6), 173–176.

56 Williams, M.E., Gaylord, S.A., and Gerritty, M.S. (1994) The timed manual performance test as a predictor of hospitalization and death in a community-based elderly population. *J. Am. Geriatr. Soc.*, **42** (1), 21–27.

57 Williams, M.E., Hadler, N.M., and Earp, J.A. (1982) Manual ability as a marker of dependency in geriatric women. *J. Chronic Dis.*, **35** (2), 115–122.

58 Aging NIo (2013) *Assessing Physical Performance in the Older Patient*, http://www.grc.nia.nih.gov/branches/leps/sppb/ (accessed 15 November 2013).

59 Guralnik, J.M., Ferrucci, L., Simonsick, E.M. *et al.* (1995) Lower-extremity function in persons over the age of 70 years as a predictor of subsequent disability. *N. Engl. J. Med.*, **332** (9), 556–561.

60 Reuben, D.B. and Siu, A.L. (1990) An objective measure of physical function of elderly outpatients. The physical performance test. *J. Am. Geriatr. Soc.*, **38** (10), 1105–1112.

61 Brown, M., Sinacore, D.R., Ehsani, A.A. *et al.* (2000) Low-intensity exercise as a modifier of physical frailty in older adults. *Arch. Phys. Med. Rehabil.*, **81** (7), 960–965.

62 Moyer, V.A. (2012) Screening for hearing loss in older adults: U.S. Preventive Services Task Force recommendation statement. *Ann. Intern. Med.*, **157** (9), 655–61.

63 Chou, R., Dana, T., and Bougatsos, C. (2009) Screening older adults for impaired visual acuity: a review of the evidence for the U.S. Preventive Services Task Force. *Ann. Intern. Med.*, **151** (1), 44–58, w11-w20.

64 Lee, P., Smith, J.P., and Kington, R. (1999) The relationship of self-rated vision and hearing to functional status and well-being among seniors 70 years and older. *Am. J. Ophthalmol.*, **127** (4), 447–452.

65 Nelson, K.A. and Dimitrova, E. (1993) Statistical Brief #36: severe visual impairment in the United States and in each state, 1990. *J. Vis. Imp. Blind.*, **87**, 80–85.

66 Cruickshanks, K.J., Tweed, T.S., Wiley, T.L. *et al.* (2003) The 5-year incidence and progression of hearing loss: the epidemiology of hearing loss study. *Arch. Otolaryngol. Head Neck Surg.*, **129** (**10**), 1041–1046.

67 Keller, B.K., Morton, J.L., Thomas, V.S., and Potter, J.F. (1999) The effect of visual and hearing impairments on functional status. *J. Am. Geriatr. Soc.*, **47** (**11**), 1319–1325.

68 Branch, L.G., Horowitz, A., and Carr, C. (1989) The implications for everyday life of incident self-reported visual decline among people over age 65 living in the community. *Gerontologist*, **29** (3), 359–365.

69 McCusker, J., Bellavance, F., Cardin, S. *et al.* (1999) Detection of older people at increased risk of adverse health outcomes after an emergency visit: the ISAR screening tool. *J. Am. Geriatr. Soc.*, **47** (**10**), 1229–1237.

70 Reuben, D.B., Mui, S., Damesyn, M. *et al.* (1999) The prognostic value of sensory impairment in older persons. *J. Am. Geriatr. Soc.*, **47** (8), 930–935.

71 Bagai, A., Thavendiranathan, P., and Detsky, A.S. (2006) Does this patient have hearing impairment? *J. Am. Med. Assoc.*, **295** (4), 416–428.

72 Pirozzo, S., Papinczak, T., and Glasziou, P. (2003) Whispered voice test for screening for hearing impairment in adults and children: systematic review. *Br. Med. J. (Clin. Res. Ed.)*, **327** (**7421**), 967.

73 Walston, J., Hadley, E.C., Ferrucci, L. *et al.* (2006) Research agenda for frailty in older adults: toward a better understanding of physiology and etiology: summary from the American Geriatrics Society/National Institute on Aging Research Conference on Frailty in Older Adults. *J. Am. Geriatr. Soc.*, **54** (6), 991–1001.

74 Fried, L.P., Tangen, C.M., Walston, J. *et al.* (2001) Frailty in older adults: evidence for a phenotype. *J. Gerontol. A Biol. Sci. Med. Sci.*, **56** (3), M146–M156.

75 Clegg, A., Young, J., Iliffe, S. *et al.* (2013) Frailty in elderly people. *Lancet*, **381** (**9868**), 752–762.

76 Rockwood, K., Song, X., MacKnight, C. *et al.* (2005) A global clinical measure of fitness and frailty in elderly people. *Can. Med. Assoc. J.*, **173** (5), 489–495.

77 Jones, D.M., Song, X., and Rockwood, K. (2004) Operationalizing a frailty index from a standardized comprehensive geriatric assessment. *J. Am. Geriatr. Soc.*, **52** (**11**), 1929–1933.

78 Hastings, S.N., Purser, J.L., Johnson, K.S. *et al.* (2008) Frailty predicts some but not all adverse outcomes in older adults discharged from the emergency department. *J. Am. Geriatr. Soc.*, **56** (9), 1651–1657.

79 Evans, S.J., Sayers, M., Mitnitski, A., and Rockwood, K. (2014) The risk of adverse outcomes in hospitalized older patients in relation to a frailty index based on a comprehensive geriatric assessment. *Age Ageing*, **43** (1), 127–132.

80 Hustey, F.M. and Meldon, S.W. (2002) The prevalence and documentation of impaired mental status in elderly emergency department patients. *Ann. Emerg. Med.*, **39** (3), 248–253.

81 Lewis, L.M., Miller, D.K., Morley, J.E. *et al.* (1995) Unrecognized delirium in ED geriatric patients. *Am. J. Emerg. Med.*, **13** (2), 142–145.

82 Elie, M., Rousseau, F., Cole, M. *et al.* (2000) Prevalence and detection of delirium in elderly emergency department patients. *Can. Med. Assoc. J.*, **163** (8), 977–981.

83 Donaldson, M.G., Khan, K.M., Davis, J.C. *et al.* (2005) Emergency department fall-related presentations do not trigger fall risk assessment: a gap in care of high-risk outpatient fallers. *Arch. Gerontol. Geriatr.*, **41** (3), 311–317.

84 Aminzadeh, F. and Dalziel, W.B. (2002) Older adults in the emergency department: a systematic review of patterns of use, adverse outcomes, and effectiveness of interventions. *Ann. Emerg. Med.*, **39** (3), 238–247.

85 Salvi, F., Morichi, V., Grilli, A. *et al.* (2007) The elderly in the emergency department: a critical review of problems and solutions. *Intern. Emerg. Med.*, **2** (4), 292–301.

86 Hwang, U. and Morrison, R.S. (2007) The geriatric emergency department. *J. Am. Geriatr. Soc.*, **55** (**11**), 1873–1876.

87 Carpenter, C.R., Griffey, R.T., Stark, S. *et al.* (2011) Physician and nurse acceptance of technicians to screen for geriatric syndromes in the emergency department. *West. J. Emerg. Med.*, **12** (4), 489–495.

88 Platts-Mills, T.F. and Glickman, S.W. (2014) Measuring the value of a senior emergency department: making sense of health outcomes and health costs. *Ann. Emerg. Med.*, **63** (5), 525–527.

89 Conroy, S.P., Ansari, K., Williams, M. *et al.* (2014) A controlled evaluation of comprehensive geriatric assessment in the emergency department: the 'emergency frailty unit'. *Age Ageing*, **43** (1), 109–114.

4 Pharmacological issues in the elderly

Ruben Olmedo & Denise Nassisi
[1] *Department of Emergency Medicine, Division of Toxicology, Mount Sinai Medical Center, Icahn School of Medicine at Mount Sinai, New York, NY, USA*
[2] *Geriatric Emergency Department, Department of Emergency Medicine, Mount Sinai Medical Center, Icahn School of Medicine at Mount Sinai, New York, NY, USA*

Section I: Case presentation

A 79-year-old man is brought to the emergency department (ED) by family because of increasing confusion, general weakness, and lethargy. Per the patient and the family, he was in his usual state of good health, which included daily walks, until 4 or 5 days ago when he started to become more and more tired. At first he started having trouble concentrating while working on the computer and couldn't read the newspaper or complete his daily crossword puzzles. He was having difficulty walking or even getting up from a chair.

The patient's past medical history was significant for hypertension, hyperlipidemia, benign prostatic hypertrophy, and mild alcoholic cirrhosis. The patient stated and the family confirmed that he had quit drinking alcohol 7 years earlier. His medications included aspirin, lisinopril/hydrochlorothiazide (Zestoretic) 20/12.5, atorvastatin (Lipitor) 40 mg daily, and tamsulosin (Flomax) 0.8 mg daily. Of note, the patient had recently seen his primary care physician who had started him on metoprolol 50 mg twice a day for further blood pressure control.

Upon examination, he was an alert, oriented, well-developed, overweight man who was pale and mildly diaphoretic. The initial vital signs were temperature 37.2 °C (99 °F), heart rate 84 beats/min, blood pressure 84/48 mm Hg, respiratory rate 20 breaths/min, and O_2 saturation 95% on room air. The lungs were clear, the cardiovascular examination showed a regular rate and rhythm without murmurs, gallops, or rubs and the abdomen was soft and nontender. The pulses were thready on palpation.

Section II: Case discussion

Dr Jon Mark Hirshon (JMH): This was a 79-year-old man coming to the ED due to a change in function and mental status. The differential is wide open, and it's important that your initial history and physical examination elucidate what's going on. So looking for anything from a stroke to a urinary tract infection (UTI) to a GI bleed to medication change, I think the key is to approach this with a wide diagnostic lens to look at all the potential differential diagnoses. What is the acute difference that prompted this presentation?

Dr Peter Rosen (PR): You may not get a specific answer in this case because it is kind of a nondescript presentation, but I think that's helpful too. When you have the inability to put together a very specific complaint, not only do you have to think about all the concerns that Dr Hirshon just enunciated, but this may be a sign of altered mental status as well.

Dr Don Melady (DM): In regard to defining what the problem is and keeping a broad differential, a wise geriatric nurse whom I've worked with for a long time claims the single best question you can ask is "what has changed?" Moreover, you need to then decide to whom you are going to ask that question. One of this man's problems is confusion. If your only informant is

Geriatric Emergencies: A Discussion-Based Review, First Edition.
Edited by Amal Mattu, Shamai A. Grossman and Peter L. Rosen.
© 2016 John Wiley & Sons, Ltd. Published 2016 by John Wiley & Sons, Ltd.

confused, turn to other sources who are more productive of reliable information. In this case, it sounds like he was brought in by family members so that's where I would turn.

PR: Shamai, would you like to comment on the vital signs?

Dr Shamai Grossman (SG): The vital signs are rather worrisome. This is a patient who is a known hypertensive on multiple blood pressure–lowering medications, and he has a blood pressure of 84/48 mm Hg, which makes me concerned about a whole host of different problems – from sepsis to acute volume loss to medication overdose. I would put this patient into the category of patients that we need to take care of immediately given that blood pressure.

PR: One of the traps that we fall into with the elderly patient is that the vital signs are often abnormal in minor degree. This man is a little more worrisome than most given the blood pressure. Moreover, he also has a slight elevation of the temperature and respiratory rate. I think that many times we just miss these things in the elderly, because they don't appear as abnormal to us when we think in terms of young adults.

JMH: One other vital sign that we didn't mention is his heart rate of 84, which we might accept as a normal heart rate in a younger person or in a healthy older person. Nevertheless, in the presence of a significant hypotension, clearly this represents a bradycardia, which needs to be kept in mind in terms of the diagnostic process.

PR: When you see patients of this age who may be confused and have an alteration of their ability to do their daily tasks, is there an expeditious screening examination that you use to test for an acute organic brain syndrome, or are you obligated to use one of the lengthy discriminating tests that seem to take about a week to perform?

JMH: Personally, I ask the patient to follow relatively simple instructions: "Can you sit up and take a deep breath? Can you tell me where you are?" I use as my initial evaluation some basic function questions to help evaluate whether the mental status is impaired, and then for me what's important is whether this is a change from baseline. That's where I need prior records with a well-documented mental status examination or family members who can indicate to me that

there's something different. If I want something more formal, I can do a mini mental status examination.

PR: I agree with you. Waxing and waning mental capacities are a real clue – even if it's by history alone. One of the things I like to use is the patient's drawing of a clock face. I find that's a good predictor of organic brain syndrome. If they can't draw a face with a simple time, the chances are they are organic. Rob, do you have anything you like to use?

Dr Rob Anderson (RA): The clock drawing test is a test I routinely use in my geriatric work to test for executive functioning. Executive function provides clues to how a person handles tasks such as taking medications or driving. If I could emphasize why I like this case, it is because I learned from experienced geriatricians that every presentation in an old person is a medication effect until proven otherwise. I keep forgetting this lesson. You could go anywhere with this case. This patient could have anything wrong with him, but it is most probably a medication effect.

Dr Bryan Hayes (BH): This patient actually doesn't have a whole lot of medications compared to most older adults. We have a couple of blood pressure medications, and metoprolol was added recently. His tamsulosin dose is 0.8 mg daily, which is on the high end of the usual dosage range, which could cause some hypotension especially combined with that new metoprolol dose. Other things that I screen for are drug–drug interactions that could be causing altered mental status, including anticholinergic drugs. Whenever you have an older adult presenting like this person did, with a possible sepsis picture, we should also rule out salicylate intoxication as being a cause. He has a slightly elevated respiratory rate, if that's reported accurately. His temperature is a little on the high side. He's a little bit altered. Therefore, a salicylate level would well be worth sending in this guy as well.

PR: I think that's an excellent point. Chronic salicylate poisoning is common in the elderly and may be hard to identify not only from confusing salicylate levels but also from the mixed metabolic acidosis/alkalosis picture.

PR: This patient has many possible causes for an acute organic brain syndrome, one that you have identified is possible aspirin overdose and another one is beta blockade. Could you tell us a little about Flomax (tamsulosin)? Could there be some complications of that medication that could be operative here?

BH: It's a specific type of alpha blocker. So it does have, especially in this higher dosage, orthostatic, or even true hypotension from it. I was wondering if that higher dose and adding the metoprolol on top of that may have caused this picture. I like to look at possible drug interactions in the older adults who have many medications. In this case, there aren't a lot of specific interactions between any of the drugs that he's on; however, both Lipitor and Flomax are metabolized by Cyp3A4. Who knows if this person started a diet with grapefruit juice and started having higher levels of those drugs that could also be contributing to this picture?

PR: Dr Anderson, I would guess that most of this patient's workup will be unhelpful. I think that your comment earlier about remembering pharmacology is exemplified by the fact that all your tests don't show you much of anything. Perhaps this is something that we have iatrogenically induced with our pharmacologic therapies. As Dr Hayes pointed out, he's taking a rather small number of medications. Still, that doesn't rule out the medications as the source of the problem. Let's assume that we perform the entire workup, and you don't find much of anything. Where would you go next?

RA: That's a great question because we're faced with this all the time in the ED. A situation where the older patient looks better on paper than clinically, where we may not have the definitive diagnosis, and yet we feel the patient needs admission for further consideration. You know, all of outpatient medicine is based on time. Time to wait and see, time to see how our treatments work or don't work. Unfortunately, time is the one thing we don't have in the ED, and yet it is often the most valuable diagnostic tool when caring for the elderly. Assuming this patient remains hypotensive, he really needs to be admitted for further observation. Maybe as the beta-blockers wear off, his blood pressure will return to normal, maybe he will spike a fever, maybe something else will develop. Yet, it is often difficult to ask for admission for our older adults when the diagnosis and treatment plan are not clear.

JMH: The issue is not whether to admit them or not. If they come in hypotensive, even if I correct it, I'm going to watch them for a while. For me, the struggle is what level of inpatient health care will this person fit into? Part of that is going to be based on their vital signs. If they remain hypotensive, I'm going to put them into at least the step down unit. If they are correct, will I put them on the floor for 24 h? Are they admitted? Are they observation patients? These are the kind of problems we are struggling with now.

PR: Would you ever consider putting a patient like this in your observation unit? Let's say he responded to fluids whether or not you gave him calcium or glucagon, and his blood pressure came back to a less scary level. Would you be willing to watch him for 24 h in an observation unit in the ED, or do you think that he belongs to a more critical unit?

SG: I think that's a very good question. Most of that would depend on how convinced I am that this is medication related. If indeed I could somehow prove to myself that there are no other life threats than beta-blocker toxicity, then the observation unit may be wonderful place for this patient. The problem is that it's often multifactorial. Putting him in observation for 24 h often won't resolve his issue. There may be a concomitant UTI or other process that tipped the patient over so that suddenly metoprolol was no longer a safe medication for him.

PR: Dr Grossman raises a great point. As emergency physicians (EPs), we can safely escape our responsibility to be involved in discharging to outpatient care by admitting this patient. What would you do to investigate the possibility that it isn't just the prescription of beta-blocker that got him into trouble?

RA: It sounded like this patient has great baseline function, like he's doing well at home. Regardless, I have been repeatedly impressed by the confusion medications cause people when I visit them at home. Multiple prescribers, poorly written instructions, and the sheer number of pills are all factors. One of the things I hear over and over is "I don't know what these pills are, I just take what the doctor tells me to."

PR: I think this is a terrific case. Even though the cause of the drug-induced confusion may be less frequent for beta blockade, medication alterations are very very common.

DM: A lot of our discussion turns around disposition for him and around physical findings of hypotension and relative bradycardia, both of which are not suitable for discharge. I would also like to emphasize that acute confusion is *absolutely* NOT a diagnosis that you can discharge safely. When the patient is being admitted to the hospital, it's extremely important for the EP who has identified delirium to actually use that word while talking to our internal medicine colleagues.

PR: Yet, when you admit a patient to a unit who is elderly, we worry about the unit itself inducing confusion. How do you manage patients who are already confused, and not make them worse by admitting them to a part of the hospital that is well known to take normally oriented people and disorienting them?

JMH: When I approach any patient, I look at the risks and benefits of action or inaction, both in terms of intervention and nonintervention. Unless this person is doing things that are outright dangerous to himself or others, I would minimize any type of medication that has the potential to alter sensorium. When I admit them to the intensive care unit (ICU) or wherever they are going, I try to communicate my perspective to that unit. Unless this person is trying to crawl out of bed and has the risk of breaking his hip, I would be very cautious in terms of giving him any type of benzodiazepine. Especially, when he is likely to have a prolonged length of stay.

RA: There is one little pearl that I picked up recently. When we hear about medications in the elderly, we always hear "start low and go slow." I've always hated that phrase because I never knew what to do with that, until somebody added a modifier that was get somewhere. Start low and go slow but get somewhere when you're taking care of these patients.

Section III: Concepts

Background

Older adults aged ≥65 years are the most rapidly growing group in the United States, and this group constitutes the biggest consumers of medications. Emergency clinicians will see more and more older adults and will be confronted with their pharmacologic complexities. Caring for the older population can be very challenging as they have multiple morbidities that require multiple medications. In addition, there may be concerns related to frailty, functional ability, cognitive deficits, and psychosocial issues that impact their care and medical management.

Cognitive deficits, functional impairment, and caregiver issues often lead to medication errors and noncompliance. Prescribing or administering medication is the most frequent medical intervention performed by medical providers. Many older adults have several medical conditions that require the administration of multiple clinically indicated medications for their proper treatment. For example, 5% of older adults take 1 medication, whereas 40% take 5–9 medications, and 18% take more than 10 medications [1]. However, it has been estimated that 30% of drugs prescribed to the elderly are not necessary [2]. There are several factors that contribute to the manner in which older adults manage their medications. Some of these factors are intrinsic to the patient's physiologic alterations during the aging process such as the body mass, age-related drug absorption, metabolism, and disposition. Extrinsic factors that contribute to medication management are multiple and complex. They comprise the increased number of concomitant medical conditions, multiple providers, use of multiple medications including nonprescription drug and herbal products (many of which may be taken without the knowledge of the physician), impaired cognitive function, financial burden, and medication noncompliance, to name a few. All these intrinsic and extrinsic factors interact and individually or in unison have the potential to cause adverse drug effects that in the elderly may be unsafe, and, in some instances, harmful. This chapter discusses these intrinsic and extrinsic factors and the way that pharmacology impacts the medical care of older adults.

Physiologic changes in aging

The process of aging encompasses a gradual decline in the physiologic response to external stimuli. These alterations occur both in the organ and systems level as well as at the cellular level. For instance, as one ages, there are decreases in hormonal responsiveness in the endocrine system, blood vessel distensibility in the vascular system, baroreflex response, skeletal muscle mass, and renal function, to name a few [3]. This decline in maintaining homeostasis brings about disease and ultimately mortality.

Due to the physiologic changes that occur as part of the normal aging process, drug doses generally should start lower and be increased slower. This is referred to as the geriatric axiom "start low and go slow."

Pharmacokinetics

The process by which a drug gets absorbed, metabolized, and eliminated is termed pharmacokinetics. All of these steps are altered during aging, and as a result, serum levels of medications may be altered, as will be their effect on end organs.

Absorption

The first step in this process, absorption of drugs through the gastrointestinal route, changes very little for most drugs. By contrast, intramuscular drug absorption is unpredictable, and that route should be avoided in this age group.

Distribution

Once a drug is absorbed, it distributes itself throughout the body depending on its chemical nature – hydrophilic versus lipophilic. The volume the drug distributes itself in the body is called the volume of distribution (V_d). It is inversely related to its plasma concentration and directly with plasma half-life. During aging, there is a decline in total body water content, which may be further reduced by diuretics. This change in body habitus means that hydrophilic drugs will need to be adjusted, as they will distribute over a smaller volume to give the same plasma concentration. In contrast, total body fat increases during aging. This means that lipophilic drugs will need a higher dosing as they will distribute over a higher volume and will take a longer time to reach steady-state concentrations. However, as the aging process continues, the total body fat then decreases in the very old and the dosing will have to be lowered, as the same amount of medication will give a higher plasma concentration. The binding of drugs to serum albumin is not affected by aging; however, in chronically ill or poorly nourished older adults, there may be decreased levels of serum albumin. This can result in an increased amount of unbound or

free drug levels despite the total drug concentration being normal. Drugs that are highly protein bound (e.g., salicylates and warfarin) are most affected [4–6]. There are also age-related changes to the blood–brain barrier permeability that make the brain more susceptible to central nervous system (CNS) side effects with certain drugs [7, 8].

Metabolism and elimination

The next step in pharmacokinetics is drug clearance or elimination. A drug may undergo metabolic clearance via the liver or be eliminated via renal filtration. Liver function is in part dependent on its size and blood flow, both of which decrease during the aging process. In addition, the function of the enzymes that carry out phase I and phase II reactions of metabolic elimination diminish during aging. For example, CYP 450 enzymes decrease about 30% in patients older than 70 years of age [9]. The bioavailability of drugs that require extensive first-pass metabolism may be increased (e.g., propranolol and labetalol), whereas drugs that need to be activated by the liver might be slowed or reduced (e.g., enalapril) [10]. However, the overall hepatic clearance is not greatly altered with aging and does not contribute such a large effect on drug plasma concentration. Only in elders with severe frailty or liver disease, may the function of the liver be so diminished that it will require an adjustment in drug dosing [10–13].

By contrast, renal elimination plays a very significant role in drug clearance in the elderly. The decline in glomerular filtration rate (GFR) as one ages has been well established. During aging, there is a significant loss of glomeruli and renal blood flow that will retard drug elimination. Serum creatinine is not an accurate reflection of creatinine clearance because creatinine production declines in parallel with age due to age-related reduction in lean body muscle mass. The decrease in GFR as a function of age is easily observed in the Cockroft and Gault equation in which creatinine clearance varies directly with age [14]. In fact, it has been estimated that GFR may decline from 25% to up to 50% between the ages of 20 and 90 [15]. Dosing of medications that are renally eliminated need to be adjusted in the elderly population.

Drug–drug interactions

A drug–drug interaction is a pharmacologic or clinical response to a drug combination that is different from the anticipated effect of each drug if it were given solitarily. The incidence of drug–drug interactions increases with increased number of medications. Other risk factors for drug–drug interactions include visiting multiple healthcare providers and the use of multiple pharmacies. While liver metabolism does not play a major role in the availability of a single drug in the aged population, liver metabolism plays a significant role in the development of drug–drug interactions. Drug interactions involving the cytochrome P450 system are very common. When prescribing a new drug or evaluating for the possibility of a drug toxicity, an evaluation of whether the cytochrome P450 system is involved should be determined, either with induction or inhibition [12].

Pharmacodynamics

Pharmacodynamics relates the effect of a drug on the end organ or the physiologic effect of the drug. It is deemed that this is representative of a drug's action at the cellular level; how adequate is the drug receptor affinity, the number of receptors in cellular surface, how well the intracellular mechanism is carried out through its second messengers, and the homeostatic cellular regulation to the drug's effect. Age-related changes may occur at all levels of these pharmacodynamic processes.

The effectual change to drug response as part of the aging process is depicted in different organ systems. For example, in the cardiovascular system, the aged myocardium has a lower sensitivity to catecholamines. Not only is there a diminished response by the β-adrenoreceptor, but also the number of receptors is downregulated [16, 17] In the CNS, the number of dopaminergic and cholinergic neurons and dopamine D and cholinergic receptors are reduced. Similarly, the number of GABA (gamma-aminobutyric acid) receptors is diminished and its subunit composition is changed [11]. Clinically, this leads to a diminished response to the antihypertensive effects of β-adrenoreceptor antagonists in the cardiovascular system. In the CNS, it leads to an increased extrapyramidal signs and symptoms when taking dopaminergic or cholinergic/anticholinergic medications.

The significance of these changes in the elderly population is of great consequence. In this population, 5% to 33% have drug-induced orthostasis, which then leads to falls or syncope. Up to 11% of

syncope in the elderly may be drug induced. Elderly patients have diminished compensatory response in the setting of orthostatic hypotension, including diminished thirst response, and although there is increased antidiuretic hormone it is ineffective with less ability to concentrate the urine. Many medications have anticholinergic properties, and the elderly are sensitive to their side effects. A significant number of geriatric patients present with altered mental status that may be due to anticholinergic medications. The changes in pharmacokinetics and pharmacodynamics have a wide variability and depend on age, weight, gender, and pharmacogenetic makeup. Unfortunately, most premarketing clinical pharmaceutical trials do not include older adults, and approved drug doses may not be appropriate in this population.

Adverse drug-related events and potentially inappropriate medication use in older adults

Elderly patients presenting to the ED have a high incidence of using prescription medications and over-the-counter medications for the management of their chronic illnesses. Drug classes that have been identified as particularly problematic in the elderly and that should be used with caution include anticholinergics, psychotropics, anticoagulants, analgesics, hypoglycemic, and cardiovascular agents. The use and misuse of these agents often cause adverse drug-related events (ADREs) and are a principal cause of emergency patient presentation. An ADRE is any undesirable or noxious effect resulting from the use of a drug. Advanced age, frailty, and increased number of medications increase the likelihood of an ADRE. Although ADREs can occur in any age group, the elderly are more likely to develop delirium, depression, worsening dementia, orthostatic hypotension, falls, and incontinence. ADREs may account for 10.6–28% of ED visits [18]. When reviewing elderly patients' medication lists, one study finds that 31% have at least one potential adverse drug interaction. In turn, these events lead to an elevated hospital admission rate of ~30%. As many as 28% of US hospitalizations in older adults are due to drug-related problems with up to 70% of these due to an adverse reaction to the drug [19]. This is further exacerbated by the fact that EPs may not recognize a medication effect as a cause of a patient's presenting symptom. One study determined that EPs only detect 51.2%

of these ADREs. Furthermore, signs and symptoms of ADRE in the elderly are not straightforward. It is reported that 12.2% of patients presenting to the ED with nonspecific complaints are medication related.

The "prescribing cascade" is when additional medication is prescribed to treat an adverse effect of another medication. A provider fails to identify that the patient's new symptom is due to a medication, and instead of recognizing and stopping the causative medication, another medication is begun, thus further putting the patient at risk of yet additional medication side effects and adverse interactions [20–22].

Avoiding the use of the medications that may potentially cause ADRE is an approach that is used to diminish such unwanted effects. Two processes or outcome measures that assess medication-related problems are described as either explicit (criterion-based) or implicit (judgment-based).

In the explicit process or criterion-based outcome measure, a list of several medications that are to be avoided among older adults is developed by a group of expert consensus. Unfortunately, the caveat with all these studies is that they are not validated in an ED setting, but rather in ambulatory care and institutional settings. The criteria address concerns related to chronic or long-term use. In addition, there are emergency situations inherent to ED care where "inappropriate" medication may be needed on a temporary or single dose basis. The optimal drugs for such ED circumstances have not been adequately addressed or studied. Nevertheless, available guidelines do provide a foundation under which EPs can detect potential medications that are more likely to cause ADREs in the elderly. Beers and coworkers, in the United States, published and updated the most common and widely used drugs-to-avoid criteria. Fifty-three medications or medication classes were included in the latest update of the Beers criteria of 2012. These criteria include potentially inappropriate medications (PIMs) and medication classes to avoid in older adults; PIMs and classes to avoid in older adults with certain diseases and syndromes, and medications to be used with caution in older adults. A large group of the medications on this list include those that cause sedation, anticholinergic effects, orthostatic hypotension, or hypoglycemia; all of which will cause a patient to become dizzy, altered or confused, and more prone to falling. Other medications on the list include certain nonsteroidal anti-inflammatory drugs

(NSAIDs) that predispose to gastrointestinal bleeding, along with digoxin, and certain hormones that may increase cardiac problems.

Similar initiatives have been created in Canada [22, 23], Europe [24–27], and Asia [28, 29]. The STOPP (Screening Tool of Older Person's Prescriptions) and START (Screening Tool to Alert doctors to Right Treatment) criteria [24] developed in Ireland also include prescribing omission errors (e.g., failure to prescribe anticoagulant medications in older adults with chronic atrial fibrillation considered at high risk for embolic disease), which is something that the Beers criteria do not do. It is worthy to note that there are no prospectively controlled trials that specifically use the Beers criteria as an intervention to reduce ADREs in the emergency setting.

In the implicit process or judgment-based outcome measure, the appropriateness of a patient's medication regimen is assessed by single physicians. As results are not generalizable, an instrument called the Medication Appropriateness Index may be used to obtain data. It assesses each medication prescribed after considering its indication, effectiveness, duplications, correct and practical directions, drug–drug and drug–disease interactions, dosage, duration, and cost. Unnecessary polypharmacy may be detected by the topics of indication, effectiveness, and duplication. Although this method is time-consuming and does not assess underprescribing, it does have good intrarater and interrater reliability and validity [30] (Table 4.1).

While it is important to be aware of medications that are highly associated with the development of ADREs in the elderly, it should be emphasized that any medication can cause a significant ADRE. The study by Budnitz et al. that used electronic data to survey ADREs reports that most emergency hospitalizations for recognized adverse drug events in older adults result from a few commonly used medications, and relatively few are as a result of taking medications typically designated as high risk or inappropriate [31]. In another study, Budnitz et al., evaluated ED visits due to ADREs, also using electronic survey data for patients ≥65 years of age, find that drugs meeting Beers criteria for "always potentially inappropriate" account for 3.6% (95% CI 2.8–4.5%) of the estimated 178,000 visits. However, three medications not on the Beers list (warfarin, digoxin, and insulin) account for 33.3% (95% CI 27.8–38.7%) of the visits. Overall medications in the

Table 4.1 Beers criteria for potentially inappropriate medication (PIM) use in older adults (anticholinergic, antiparkinsonian, and antispasmodics).

Therapeutic Category	Drugs		
Anticholinergics	Brompheniramine	Cyproheptadine	Doxylamine
	Carbinoxamine	Dexbrompheniramine	Hydroxyzine
	Chlorpheniramine	Dexchlorpheniramine	Promethazine
	Clemastine	Diphenhydramine	Triprolidine
Antiparkinson agents	Benztropine		
	Trihexyphenidyl		
Antispasmodics	Belladonna alkaloids	Dicyclomine	Clidinium-chlordiazepoxide
	Propantheline	Hyoscyamine	
		Scopolamine	

general class of anticoagulants or antiplatelet agents, antidiabetic agents, and narrow therapeutic index agents account for nearly half of all visits for ADREs, though they were prescribed in only 9.4% of the patients seen [32].

Polypharmacy, medication reconciliation, and the brown bag checkup

Polypharmacy with its increased risk of adverse drug reactions and interactions has become an increased health threat to the older population. Aging is unfortunately accompanied by an increase in the number and severity of chronic diseases, and these diseases often require pharmacologic therapy. Polypharmacy is defined as the use of multiple medications. It is not uncommon for elder adults to be on 5–10 medications or more [33]. It is estimated that 20% of Medicare beneficiaries have five or more chronic conditions, and 50% receive five or more medications [34]. It is also important to consider the use of over-the-counter medications, herbal medications, and supplements when evaluating a patient's medication use and potential for ADREs and drug interactions.

Unfortunately, many patients experience fragmented care placing them at greater risk factor for an ADRE. Visiting multiple doctors or care settings, and using more than one pharmacy makes an ADRE more likely. Due to their multiple medical conditions, older adults commonly visit several different medical settings including EDs and specialty physicians who may not be fully aware of the other conditions and medications that the patient has.

Medication reconciliation

Medication reconciliation is a formal process for creating the most complete and accurate list possible of a patient's current medications, and comparing the list to those in the patient record or medication orders. According to the Joint Commission, medication reconciliation is the process of comparing a patient's medication orders to all of the medications that the patient has been taking. It is an important component of safe patient care. Ideally, it should be done at every transition of care in which new medications are ordered, or existing orders are rewritten to avoid medication errors such as omissions, duplications, dosing errors, or drug interactions.

The "brown bag" checkup is the less formal but effective process of going through the patient's bag of medications at the bedside with the patient and family or caregiver [35]. This process provides a key opportunity to identify potential medication errors, avoid unnecessary or redundant medications, and, therefore, prevent potential ADREs. It is an important opportunity to communicate with and educate the patient and the caregiver regarding medication use, and an excellent chance to enhance medication compliance. Confusion between generic and trade names of drugs is a common source of medication error, and the brown bag check is a good way to check for this.

Specific drugs categories

Diuretics

This class of medications is widely used in the elderly population for the management of hypertension and

Table 4.2 Beers criteria for PIM use in older adults (diuretics).

Therapeutic Categories	Drugs
	Spironolactone

congestive heart failure (CHF). However, because of the blunted compensatory cardiovascular mechanism and altered pharmacokinetics in the elderly, diuretics may cause orthostatic hypotension, general weakness, dizziness, and syncope. Also common are electrolyte abnormalities such as hyponatremia, hypokalemia, hypomagnesemia, and hyperuricemia and hyperkalemia in potassium sparing diuretics. Given the higher incidence of concomitant cardiac disease, dysrhythmias, gout, and polypharmacy, this population has a higher risk of developing these complications and the ensuing outcomes that these electrolytes abnormalities may cause (Table 4.2).

Cardiovascular agents

As a class, cardiovascular medications are the most commonly prescribed medications in the elderly, and, therefore, the most responsible cause of adverse effects. They are used to treat hypertension, myocardial ischemia and infarction, dysrhythmias, and CHF. They are also used in the treatment of headaches and anxiety.

Beta-blockers reduce mortality in patients after myocardial infarction and in patients who have CHF by a 31% margin during a 13-month follow-up. However, the pharmacokinetics of these drugs and pharmacodynamic changes that occur during aging make these drugs less effective in this population. In a study that assessed the effects of beta blockade relative to age in healthy patients, older subjects have a blunted decline in the heart rate response compared to younger participants. This effect is principally due to the action on contractility and heart rate greater than that peripheral vasodilatation. Attention must be paid to the individual type of elimination these drugs undergo as therapeutic plasma levels depend on appropriate drug clearance. For instance, some of the beta-blockers are water soluble (atenolol, nadolol, and sotalol) and thus depend on renal function for their elimination. Liver metabolism is important in metoprolol, propranolol, and pindolol. Also beware of beta-blockers that are lipophilic such as propranolol and metoprolol as they may cause CNS effects.

Calcium channel blockers do not possess the same pharmacodynamic effects as beta-blockers. Older patients don't have the blunted heart rate response found with beta-blockers nor do they have the same decrease in blood pressure and inotropy. Pharmacokinetically, all classes of calcium channel blockers undergo hepatic metabolism to nonactive metabolites, and elimination will depend on adequate hepatic blood flow. A lower dosage may be needed to attain adequate therapeutic response in the elderly.

Digoxin, a cardiac glycoside, has a long history of utilization for the treatment of CHF, and to control atrial fibrillation. Its benefits in decreasing the incidence of hospitalization compared to placebo for worsening CHF are well demonstrated [36]. However, there are certain aspects of its pharmacokinetics that make digoxin harmful in the elderly population. Digoxin has a large volume of distribution and is renally eliminated. It has a half-life of 36–48 h in patients with normal renal function. Thereby, a decrease in body habitus or renal function will elevate plasma levels and cause toxicity as it has a narrow therapeutic index. Monitoring plasma levels is not always useful since they do not reliably reflect toxicity.

Digoxin interacts with many medications that alter its effects or its plasma levels. For example, digoxin toxicity may be potentiated by electrolyte abnormalities such as hypokalemia, hypomagnesemia, or hypercalcemia, which may be caused by the concomitant use of diuretics to treat CHF. Digoxin's atrioventricular blocking effect is exacerbated by drug interactions with calcium channel blockers, amiodarone, and other antidysrhythmic medications and may produce second-degree or higher degree atrioventricular blocks. Macrolides increase digoxin levels by increasing drug absorption from the GI tract. In addition, symptoms of digoxin toxicity are nonspecific (anorexia, nausea, nonspecific abdominal pain, and altered mental status). Frequently, an elderly patient with history of CHF on digoxin and diuretics presents to the ED with confusion and a bradydysrhythmia after experiencing diarrhea and dehydration following a course of antibiotics for an upper respiratory infection (Table 4.3).

Anticoagulants

The benefit of anticoagulation therapy in patients with atrial fibrillation is well documented, as the prevalence

Table 4.3 Beers criteria for PIM use in older adults (cardiovascular).

Therapeutic Categories	Drugs		
Alpha blockers	Doxazosin		
	Prazosin		
	Terazosin		
Alpha agonists	Clonidine	Methyldopa	Reserpine
Central	Guanabenz	Guanfacine	
Antidysrhythmics	Amiodarone	Flecainide	Propafenone
	Dofetilide	Ibutilide	Quinidine
	Dronedarone	Procainamide	Sotalol
	Disopyramide		
	Digoxin		
Calcium channel blockers	Nifedipine		

of atrial fibrillation and its complications increase with age. In an analysis of 39,000–67,000 Medicare patients with atrial fibrillation aged ≥65 years over a 10-year period, warfarin reduces the hazard ratio for stroke (driven by reduction in ischemic stroke). In the BAFTA study, patients ≥75 years with atrial fibrillation, warfarin reduces the incidence of stroke, systemic embolism, or intracranial hemorrhage versus aspirin without increasing the incidence of major bleeding events [37]. However, a cohort study of patients with nonvalvular atrial fibrillation with a median age of 73 years finds that a net clinical benefit for warfarin increases with age and also shows that warfarin is underprescribed. Patients aged 65–84 years use warfarin only 60% of the time and those ≥85 years only 35% of the time [38].

The limitation to the use of warfarin is secondary to several complex factors in the elderly population. Pharmacologically, warfarin has a variable dose response, with a slow onset and offset of action. This makes starting a patient on warfarin and titrating to therapeutic levels or taking someone off back to normal levels a very slow process. Warfarin has multiple drug–drug and food–drug interactions that may alter its plasma levels. In addition, routine monitoring of a patient's coagulation profile is therefore required to assure the maintenance of a therapeutic anticoagulation level and for dose adjustments if necessary. The risk of overanticoagulation is severe bleeding, which in the elderly is already common as are falls.

New oral anticoagulants do not have many of these limitations because of their different pharmacokinetics. Their shorter half-life makes their onset and offset much shorter compared to warfarin. Dabigatran is renally eliminated, and its dose must be adjusted in patients with renal insufficiency. Although fewer drug interactions may occur with new oral anticoagulants compared with warfarin, drug interactions to be avoided with these new agents do exist. For example, dabigatran concentrations may become subtherapeutic with concomitant use of P-glycoprotein inducers such as rifampin and St John's Wort. Conversely, P-glycoprotein inhibitors (e.g., amiodarone, verapamil, quinidine, ketoconazole, and clarithromycin) will elevate dabigatran concentration and increase the risk of bleeding. Similarly, inducers of CYP3A4 (e.g., ketoconazole and itraconazole) or HIV protease inhibitors may increase plasma levels of rivaroxaban and apixaban. Although the use of new oral anticoagulants has taken away the need for routine monitoring because of their novel mechanism of action, recent studies report that the risk of bleeding from these agents is as similar to warfarin in the elderly population [39–41]. Moreover, concomitant treatment with aspirin, antiplatelet inhibitors, and NSAIDs will increase the risk of bleeding with any oral anticoagulant (Table 4.4).

Antipsychotics/antidepressants

In the past two decades, there has been a vast increase in the number of antipsychotic, antidepressant, and antiepileptic medications that treat organic as well as functional conditions of the CNS. These medications are used to treat not only symptoms related to their

Table 4.4 Beers criteria for PIM use in older adults (antithrombotics, antiplatelets, NSAIDs).

Therapeutic Categories	Drugs		
	Dipyridamole		
	Ticlopidine		
	ASA		
NSAIDs	Diclofenac	Fenoprofen	Meloxicam
	Diflunisal	Ibuprofen	Piroxicam
	Etodolac	Ketoprofen	Mefenamic acid
	Ketorolac	Naproxen	Meclofenamate
	Sulindac	Tolmentin	Nabumetone
	Oxaprozin	Indomethacin	

individual class of medications but are also to treat personality disorders, mood disorders, learning disabilities, and chronic pain.

For instance, the antipsychotics, while able to treat a variety of psychotic disorders in the elderly, are widely used to treat agitation, dementia, delirium, and combativeness. Full control is not usually possible without sedation, and adverse effects become apparent as incremental dosages are used. All antipsychotics have antimuscarinic effects that may further a patient's confusion and hallucinations. Their cardiovascular effects via alpha blocking effects cause peripheral vasodilatation and orthostatic hypotension and dizziness, making this population more prone to falls. These agents also have inwardly rectifying potassium channel (IK_r) blocking effects that cause QT_c prolongation in the electrocardiogram (ECG) and, therefore, may lead to ventricular dysrhythmias. In addition, they also cause urinary retention, which may present as abdominal discomfort or pain, and predispose the patient to UTIs after Foley catheter insertion for their treatment. Tricyclic antidepressants also possess peripheral alpha blocking and antimuscarinic side effects as do the antipsychotics. In the myocardium though, they block the sodium entrance into the cell during phase 0 of the action potential that manifests in the ECG as QRS prolongation. (SSRIs) selective serotonin reuptake inhibitors do not have this sodium channel blocking effect and have a higher safety margin (Table 4.5).

Opioids
Studies demonstrate that opioid use in the elderly with chronic pain is consistently underutilized. This practice is probably based on the fact that the elderly

are noticeably more sensitive to opioid's respiratory depressant effects given the age-related changes in respiratory function. Thus, many use this group of medications with caution in this population. However, as the sensitivity of an individual patient is determined, dosage should be titrated appropriately for full analgesic effect without the adverse effects.

When choosing an analgesic agent for the elderly population, opioids have been found to increase the risk of cardiovascular events, falls, fracture, safety events requiring hospitalization, and all-cause mortality among elderly patients when compared to NSAIDs. However, not all opioids carry the same risk. One study finds that at equianalgesic dosages, there is an elevated risk of cardiovascular events with codeine compared with hydrocodone after 180 days of exposure. There is a reduced risk of fracture for tramadol and propoxyphene after 30 and 180 days, and increased risk of all-cause mortality after 30 and 180 days for codeine and oxycodone. These results do not change by dosage category (low, medium, high, or very high) except in fractures, where in the higher dosage categories, differences between opioids became less apparent.

Diabetes agents
Diabetes mellitus is extremely common in the elderly population with more than 65% of the US population aged 65 and older having this disease [42]. Key components of diabetes management should always include lifestyle modifications and education regarding nutrition and exercise. There is limited data addressing optimal glycemic goals in the elderly population. Guidelines recommend that optimal glycemic control levels take into account the individual's

53

Table 4.5 Beers criteria for PIM use in older adults.

Central Nervous System		
Therapeutics Categories	Drugs	
Tricyclic antidepressants (TCAs)	Amitriptyline Clomipramine Doxepin Chlordiazepoxide-amitriptyline	Imipramine Trimipramine Perphenazine-amitriptyline
Antipsychotics	First and Second generation Thioridazine Mesoridazine	
Barbiturates	Amobarbital Butabarbital Butalbital Mephobarbital	Pentobarbital Phenobarbital Secobarbital
Benzodiazepines	Alprazolam Estazolam Lorazepam Oxazepam Temazepam Triazolam	Clorazepate Chlordiazepoxide Clonazepam Diazepam Flurazepam Quazepam
Non-benzodiazepine hypnotics	Eszopiclone Zolpidem Zaleplon	
Miscellaneous	Chloral hydrate	Meprobamate

overall health, functional status, and life expectancy. In a healthy elderly patient with a life expectancy over 10 years, glycemic control targets would be similar as for a younger patient. However, a higher target hemoglobin A1C level would be tolerated in a frail elderly patient whose life expectancy is less than 10 years [43].

Tight glycemic control is associated with an increase in episodes of hypoglycemia. Hypoglycemia is a dreaded complication seen with insulin, sulfonylurea agents, and meglitinides. Hypoglycemia in the elderly is associated with dizziness, weakness, falls with resulting decreased mobility and fractures, as well as with confusion, delirium, and deterioration in cognitive function [44]. The adrenergic response to hypoglycemia is blunted compared to that seen in the younger population [45]. There are also risks of hyperglycemia as well, including dehydration, visual changes, and decreased cognitive and functional status. Metformin is a frequently used agent for diabetes with the advantage of not inducing hypoglycemic

episodes. It does have the side effect of causing a rare lactic acidosis. Very important in the elderly is that metformin should not be used in patients with renal impairment, thus limiting its use. A calculated (or estimated) GFR >30 ml/min has been suggested as a safe cutoff level of renal function for the use of metformin [46].

Short-acting sulfonylureas such as glipizide are a viable alternative for those with contraindications to metformin use. The thiazolidinedione pioglitazone is of limited usefulness because of concerns of associated fluid retention, CHF, myocardial infarction, and fractures [47].

Herbal and dietary supplements
Herbal remedies and dietary supplements are also important causes of adverse reactions and herb–drug interactions. Information about the use of these substances should be sought by the medical provider. Often patients do not inform their healthcare providers about the use of these substances [48].

Common herbal supplements include ginkgo biloba, St. John's wort, echinacea, ginseng, garlic, saw palmetto, kava, valerian root, milk thistle, and glucosamine. Recognized interactions include ginkgo biloba with warfarin, St. John's wort with serotonin reuptake inhibitors and kava with sedatives.

Section IV: Decision making

Conclusion

There are multiple intrinsic and extrinsic factors that contribute to the risk of adverse drug reactions in the elderly population. Older adults have significant alterations in pharmacokinetics and pharmacodynamics that influence the way they process and respond to medications. The aging process is associated with increased chronic diseases that require treatment with multiple medications often resulting in polypharmacy. The physiologic changes and the increased number of medications increase the risk of adverse drug reactions and drug–drug interactions in this population. It is always prudent to think of drug causes of new onset changes in elderly patients' function or mental awareness.

Key points

- Evaluate whether the patient's presenting illness is caused by a medication.
- Always consider whether the benefits clearly outweigh the risks in starting a new drug. Consider alternative drugs that might be safer with less adverse effects for the elderly. Also consider whether nonpharmacologic treatment might be an option.
- Remember that the frequency of adverse drug reactions increases with the number of medications used.
- Carefully review dosage recommendations and adjust for renal impairment.
- Carefully consider potential drug–drug interactions based upon the patient's preexisting drug regimen.

References

1 Kaufman, D.W., Kelly, J.P., Rosenberg, L. *et al.* (2002) Recent patterns of medication use in the ambulatory adult population of the United States: the Slone survey. *J. Am. Med. Assoc.*, **287** (3), 337–344.

2 Lazarou, J., Pomerance, B., and Corey, P. (1998) Incidence of adverse drug reactions in hospitalized patients: a meta-analysis of prospective studies. *J. Am. Med. Assoc.*, **279** (15), 1200–1205.

3 Bowie, M.W. and Slattum, P.W. (2007) Pharmaco-dynamics in older adults: a review. *Am. J. Geriatr. Pharmacol.*, **5** (3), 263–303.

4 Avon, J., Gurwitz, J.H., and Rochon, P. (2003) Principles of pharmacology, in *Geriatric Medicine: An Evidence-Based Approach*, 4th edn (eds C.K. Cassel, R.M. Leipzig, H.J. Cohen *et al.*), Springer-Verlag, New York.

5 Dasgupta, A. (2002) Clinical utility of free drug monitoring. *Clin. Chem. Lab. Med.*, **40**, 986–993.

6 Dasgupta, A. (2007) Usefulness of monitoring free (unbound) concentrations of therapeutic drugs in patient management. *Clin. Chim. Acta*, **377**, 1–13.

7 Cusak, B.J. (2004) Pharmacokinetics in older persons. *Am. J. Geriatr. Pharmacother.*, **2**, 274–302.

8 Montamat, S.C., Cusack, B.J., and Vestal, R.E. (1989) Management of drug therapy in the elderly. *N. Engl. J. Med.*, **321** (5), 303–309.

9 Sotaniemi, E.A., Arranto, A.J., Pelkonen, O. *et al.* (1997) Age and cytochrome P450-linked drug metabolism in humans: an analysis of 226 subjects with equal histopathologic conditions. *Clin. Pharmacol. Ther.*, **3** (61), 331–339.

10 Kinirons, M.T. and O'Mahony, M.S. (2004) Drug metabolism and ageing. *Br. J. Clin. Pharmacol.*, **57**, 540–544.

11 Klotz, U. (2009) Pharmacokinetics and drug metabolism in the elderly. *Drug Metab. Rev.*, **41**, 67–76.

12 Mangoni, A.A. and Jackson, S.H. (2004) Age-related changes in pharmacokinetics and pharmacodynamics: basic principles and practical applications. *Br. J. Clin. Pharmacol.*, **57**, 6–14.

13 Schmucker, D.L. (2001) Liver function and phase I drug metabolism in the elderly: a paradox. *Drugs Aging*, **18**, 837–851.

14 Cockcroft, D.W. and Gault, M.H. (1975) Prediction of creatinine clearance from serum creatinine. *Nephron*, **16**, 31–41.

15 Turnheim, K. (2003) When drug therapy gets old: pharmacokinetics and pharmacodynamics in the elderly. *Exp. Gerontol.*, **38**, 843–853.

16 Abernethy, D.R. (1990) Altered pharmacodynamics of cardiovascular drugs and their relation to altered pharmacokinetics in elderly patients. *Clin. Geriatr. Med.*, **6**, 285–292.

17 Feldman, R.D., Limbird, L.E., Nadeau, J. *et al.* (1984) Alterations in leukocyte beta-receptor affinity with aging. A potential explanation for altered

beta-adrenergic sensitivity in the elderly. *N. Engl. J. Med.*, **310**, 815–819.

18 Hohl, C.M., Robitaille, C., Lord, V. *et al.* (2005) Emergency physician recognition adverse drug-related events in elderly patients presenting to an emergency department. *Acad. Emerg. Med.*, **12**, 197–205.

19 Col, N., Fanale, J.E., and Kronholm, P. (1990) The role of medication non-compliance and adverse drug reactions in hospitalizations in the elderly. *Arch. Intern. Med.*, **150**, 841–845.

20 Rochon, P.A. and Gurwitz, J.H. (1997) Optimizing drug treatment for elderly people: the prescribing cascade. *Br. Med. J.*, **315**, 1096.

21 Rochon, P.A. and Gurwitz, J.H. (1995) Drug therapy. *Lancet*, **346**, 32–36.

22 McLeod, P.J., Huang, A.R., Tamblyn, R.M. *et al.* (1997) Defining inappropriate practices in prescribing for elderly people: a national consensus panel. *Can. Med. Assoc. J.*, **156** (3), 385–391.

23 Naugler, C.T., Brymer, C., Stolee, P., and Arcese, Z.A. (2000) Development and validation of an improved prescribing in the elderly tool. *Can. J. Clin. Pharmacol.*, **7**, 103–107.

24 O'Mahony, D., Gallagher, P., Ryan, C. *et al.* (2010) STOPP & START criteria: a new approach to detecting potentially inappropriate prescribing in old age. *Eur. Geriatr. Med.*, 45–51.

25 Rognstad, S., Breeke, M., Fetveit, A. *et al.* (2009) The Norwegian General Practice (NORGEP) criteria for assessing potentially inappropriate prescriptions to elderly patients. *Scand. J. Prim. Health Care*, **27**, 153–159.

26 Rancourt, C., Moisan, J., Baillargeon, L. *et al.* (2004) Potentially inappropriate prescriptions for older patients in long-term care. *BMC Geriatr.*, **4**, 9.

27 Laroche, M.L., Charmes, J.P., and Merle, L. (2007) Potentially inappropriate medications in the elderly: a French consensus panel list. *Eur. J. Clin. Pharmacol.*, **63**, 725–731.

28 Chang, C.B. and Chan, D.C. (2010) Comparison of published explicit criteria for potentially inappropriate medications in older adults. *Drugs Aging*, **27** (12), 947–957.

29 Winit-Watjana, W., Sakulrat, P., and Kespichayawattana, J. (2008) Criteria for high-risk medication use in Thai patients. *Arch. Gerontol. Geriatr.*, **47**, 35–51.

30 Hajjar, E.R., Cafiero, A.C., and Hanlon, J.T. (2007) Polypharmacy in elderly patients. *Am. J. Geriatr. Pharmacother.*, **4** (5), 345–351.

31 Budnitz, D.S., Lovegrove, M.C., Shehab, N. *et al.* (2011) Emergency hospitalizations for adverse drug event in older Americans. *N. Engl. J. Med.*, **365**, 2002–2012.

32 Budnitz, D.S., Shehab, N., Kegler, S.R., and Richards, C.L. (2007) Medication use leading to emergency department visits for adverse drug events in older adults. *Ann. Intern. Med.*, **147** (11), 755.

33 Ferner, R.E. and Aronson, J.K. (2006) Communicating information about drug safety. *Br. Med. J.*, **333**, 143.

34 Tinetti, M.E., Bogardus, S.T. Jr.,, and Agostini, J.V. (2004) Potential pitfalls of disease specific guidelines for patients with multiple conditions. *N. Engl. J. Med.*, **351**, 2870.

35 Bopari, M. and Korc-Grodzick, B. (2011) Prescribing for older adults. *Mt. Sinai J. Med.*, **78** (4), 613–626.

36 The Digitalis Investigation Group (1997) The effect of digoxin on the mortality and morbidity in patients with heart failure. *N. Engl. J. Med.*, **336**, 525–533.

37 Mant, J., Hobbs, F.D., Fletcher, K. *et al.* (2007) Warfarin versus aspirin for stroke prevention in an elderly community population with atrial fibrillation (the Birmingham Atrial Fibrillation Treatment of the Aged Study, BAFTA): a randomised controlled trial. *Lancet*, **370**, 493–503.

38 Singer, D.E., Chang, Y., Fang, M.C. *et al.* (2009) The net clinical benefit of warfarin anticoagulation in atrial fibrillation. *Ann. Intern. Med.*, **151**, 297–305.

39 Patel, M.R., Mahaffey, K.W., Garg, J. *et al.* (2010) Rivaroxaban versus warfarin in nonvalvular atrial fibrillation. *N. Engl. J. Med.*, **376**, 975–983.

40 Connolly, S., Ezekowitz, M., and Yusuf, S. (2009) Dabigatran versus warfarin in patients with atrial fibrillation. *N. Engl. J. Med.*, **361**, 1139–1151.

41 Granger, C.B., Alexander, J.H., McMurray, J.J. *et al.* (2011) Apixaban versus warfarin in patients with atrial fibrillation. *N. Engl. J. Med.*, **365**, 981–992.

42 Centers for Disease Control and Prevention (2011) *National Diabetes Fact Sheet: General Information and National Estimates on Diabetes in the United States*, U.S. Department of Health and Human Services, Centers for Disease Control and Prevention, Atlanta, GA, p. 2011.

43 (a) ACCORD Study Group (2008) Effects of intensive glucose lowering in type 2 diabetes. *N. Engl. J. Med.*, **358**, 2545–2559;(b) American Diabetes Association (2012) Standards of medical care in diabetes – 2012 (Position Statement). *Diabetes Care*, **35** (**Suppl. 1**), S11–S63.

44 Kirkman, M., Briscoe, V.J., Clark, N. *et al.* (2012) Diabetes in older adults: a consensus report. *J. Am. Geriatr. Soc.*, **60**, 2342–2356.

45 Matyka, K., Evans, M., Lomas, J. *et al.* (1997) Altered hierarchy of protective responses against severe hypoglycemia in normal aging in healthy men. *Diabetes Care*, **20**, 135.

46 Johnson, J.A., Majumdar, S.R., Simpson, S.H., and Toth, E.L. (2002) Decreased mortality associated with

the use of metformin compared with sulfonylurea monotherapy in type 2 diabetes. *Diabetes Care*, **25** (**12**), 2244–2248.

47 Inzucchi, S., Bergenstal, R., Buse, J. *et al.* (2012) Management of hyperglycemia in type 2 diabetes: a patient-centered approach position statement of the American Diabetes Association (ADA) and the European Association for the Study of Diabetes (EASD). *Diabetes Care*, **35** (6), 1364–1379.

48 Eisenberg, D.M., Kessler, R.C., Foster, C. *et al.* (1993) Unconventional medicine in the United States. Prevalence, costs, and patterns of use. *N. Engl. J. Med.*, **328**, 246.

5 Altered mental status in the elderly

Josh Joseph & Maura Kennedy

Department of Emergency Medicine, Beth Israel Deaconess Medical Center, Harvard Medical School, Boston, MA, USA

Section I: Case presentation

A 93-year-old man was brought into the ED (emergency department) by his wife and daughters for confusion. He had a history of dementia with a gradual decline in his functioning over the past year. Twice in the past week, the staff at his apartment complex found him in the lobby, seemingly agitated, and brought him back to the apartment that he shared with his wife. On the day of the ED visit, he was with his wife at a restaurant when he ran into the street, flagged down a police officer, and reported that he was being imprisoned. At this stage, the family brought him to the ED for evaluation. Per his wife, he was eating well and had no vomiting or diarrhea. He had not complained to his family about abdominal pain, nausea, urinary symptoms, or chest pain. Though he had not complained of shortness of breath, his wife thought he seemed to be wheezing that morning, so she had told him to use his inhalers.

The past medical history was notable for dementia, atrial fibrillation, coronary artery disease, and COPD (chronic obstructive pulmonary disease). He was a former smoker, with a 40-pack-year history of tobacco use. He drank three glasses of wine a week. He was retired, a WWII (World War II) veteran, and lived with his family in senior housing. Medications included digoxin, warfarin, tiotropium, albuterol, fluoxetine, and lorazepam.

The vital signs were as follows: temperature 37°C, pulse 76 beats/min, blood pressure 162/81 mm Hg, respirations 24 breaths/min, and pulse oximetry 89% on room air. On examination, he was sleeping but awakened to voice and was in no acute distress. The cardiac examination was notable for an irregular rhythm but no murmurs. He was tachypneic and had diffuse wheezing in the bilateral lung fields. The abdomen was nondistended and nontender. He had no lower extremity edema or calf tenderness. On neurologic examination, cranial nerves were intact; he had full strength in his upper and lower extremities bilaterally and no clonus or rigidity. He was oriented to person, reported the year as 1909, and stated that he was in prison. He had fluent but very tangential speech, and fell asleep several times during the medical evaluation. When asked to recite the days of the week backward, he stopped at Wednesday and was not able to proceed.

A CT (computed tomography) scan of his head was obtained, and demonstrated global atrophy with periventricular and subcortical white matter hypodensities consistent with chronic small vessel disease. A chest radiograph demonstrated hyperinflation and flattening of the diaphragm but no acute infiltrate. The ECG (electrocardiogram) showed atrial fibrillation with a ventricular rate in the 70s, and a right bundle branch block that was unchanged from prior ECGs. A complete blood count (CBC), chemistries, and a urinalysis were all normal. The INR (international normalized ratio) was therapeutic at 2.4.

Conclusion

The patient was thought to have delirium, likely secondary to an acute COPD exacerbation. He was given oral steroids, nebulizer treatments, placed on supplemental oxygen, and admitted to the hospital.

Geriatric Emergencies: A Discussion-Based Review, First Edition.
Edited by Amal Mattu, Shamai A. Grossman and Peter L. Rosen.
© 2016 John Wiley & Sons, Ltd. Published 2016 by John Wiley & Sons, Ltd.

The lorazepam was discontinued. His mental status improved over several days, and he was discharged to home 4 days after his hospitalization reportedly at his baseline mental status.

Section II: Case discussion

Dr Peter Rosen (PR): When a patient like this comes in, at least in the EDs I have worked in, he's almost immediately referred to psychiatry. Is there some way you can prevent a behavioral consultation before a medical evaluation?

Dr Amal Mattu (AM): I think the information about the frequent misdiagnosis of delirium in patients like this has disseminated throughout the EM (emergency medicine) community, and emergency physicians and acute care providers have become more aware of the fact that (1) older patients who may appear to have dementia are oftentimes misdiagnosed; (2) delirium is missed; (3) even if the patient has a diagnosis of dementia, they may have delirium superimposed on top of the dementia; and (4) if you miss the delirium, they have a markedly increased morbidity and mortality.

PR: It's interesting that in San Diego this patient might have been taken directly to the psychiatric hospital by the paramedics. There, they fortunately had a very good internist at the intake end of their hospital who did very good medical workups on these patients. While we've educated the physicians, I'm not sure we've educated our triage personnel. Do you know if the patient was on home oxygen?

Dr Maura Kennedy (MK): He was not on home oxygen.

PR: Let's say this patient was brought in by family to your triage desk, and he's combative at the triage desk. How do you deal with that in your ED?

Dr Jon Mark Hirshon (JMH): It would depend on the level of how well you can coach him and guide him, and how combative he is. It's always a difficult question of how to deal with someone who's uncooperative – whether that combativeness is based on rational thought or not – as part of the initial assessment. I would try to encourage him into a room, someplace where it wouldn't be too stimulating, perhaps with

family support, and then try to assess him from there. If he is brought in with a clearly altered mental status (AMS), uncooperative and trying to run away, then I would have to provide physical or chemical restraint, but that is clearly the last measure. My preference is to work with him and his family in a collaborative manner to see if we can get him to calm down enough to the point where we can perform a more formal assessment.

PR: The problem I have with patients like this is that they frequently are even more combative in the hospital setting because it's so strange to them. They're already confused, people start touching them, which I think induces a response of violence, and they end up getting immediately sedated with a drug that just adds to their confusion. Is there any way to settle these people down without going to that negative loop?

Dr Richard Wolfe (RW): To reiterate, you may have to go to chemical sedation if you have no other choice to control the patient, but I agree with you, you want to try a quiet setting, family support, and try to gently talk the patient down a bit, but at the same time, you want to see how the patient evolves, to see if they're waxing and waning to confirm that you're dealing with an organic brain delirium as opposed to just dementia or other psychiatric problems. Nevertheless, if you're having trouble controlling the patient, I'm not sure how you can avoid chemical sedation.

PR: Are there any sedatives that are less confusion-inducing than others?

RW: I would definitely avoid benzodiazepines, and even though I think they are not ideal, neuroleptic agents are my preferred choice.

PR: In other chapters, we have discussed the broad workup that patients like this mandate when you first see them, but why don't we now discuss instead some of the obvious responses to this patient, and then perhaps some of the zebra responses that ought to be considered.

JMH: While the shotgun approach to the elderly with confusion or the general approach to the geriatric patient coming to the ED does apply here as we have discussed before, there is a broad differential that we pursue with our residents including metabolic disorders, medication-related problems, infections, and central nervous system abnormalities. We would obtain blood work, urinalysis, EKG, and likely some sort of neuroimaging whether it be a CT scan or MRI (magnetic resonance imaging), those are kind of initial things that I think should happen in any patient who presents this way. Some of the more zebra diagnoses that we should always think about in patients that present like this, especially in this age group, would be discovered in neuroimaging such as normal pressure hydrocephalus, as well as thyroid dysfunction, certain electrolyte abnormalities, or vitamin deficiencies.

PR: Given that this patient has chronic lung disease as well as his other history, how would you approach his COPD?

MK: I would establish his baseline oxygen saturation, if possible, and if he is hypoxic compared to his baseline, give him gentle supplemental oxygen. He is clearly tachypneic and has wheezes bilaterally, so going down the standard approach to treating what appears to be a COPD flare is important, meanwhile ensuring that there is not a pneumonia that set off the COPD exacerbation. If appears that he is not at his baseline given his tachypnea, he is not on home oxygen and on review of the medical records, his typical oxygen saturation is 93–94% on room air; accordingly, I would take a standard approach to treating his underlying COPD exacerbation with steroids and bronchodilators, and obtain a chest radiograph to determine if there is an acute infection contributing to it. I would then see if his mental status changes after those treatments are initiated.

PR: I think many of us wouldn't be able to resist intubating this patient, and many of us wouldn't be able to resist ordering a blood gas on this patient even though it's not going to give us any useful information because we know in advance it's going to be abnormal. I would be reluctant to start out with intubation, and I think he can probably be managed without it if we put a little bit of patience into his management.

Dr Shamai Grossman (SG): I would just add that if I see COPD on a patient's history, I will often assume that the patient has been on supplemental home oxygen, and when a patient comes in with an acute change in mental status, I might get a blood gas to make sure they are not retaining CO_2 as a missed etiology of the acute alteration in mental status.

RW: You can also look at the bicarbonate on the electrolyte panel as an indication of how chronic its elevation is, and secondly, I think you always have to assume at this stage that they are CO_2 retaining, and set your target oxygen saturations up front so you don't induce further narcosis with your oxygen.

PR: My point about not looking at an immediate blood gas is that I would assume he is a CO_2 retainer, and I would be more interested in what the response to treatment is, and then see what the blood gas is only if the patient isn't responding to treatment, as opposed to starting out with abnormal blood gases as too many people look at that initial high CO_2, and immediately reach for an endotracheal tube. I can't argue against getting a CT scan ultimately on this patient although you're going to need to get him under control behaviorally before you can send him to a scanner.

PR: We have a history here that he's a WWII veteran, and I don't know why that information was given. One of the diseases that we often miss in the elderly is tetanus. He's in an age group where tetanus immunizations were not universal, in fact, I don't think they became mandatory in our school system until after WWII. Of course, if he'd been in the service, then we know at least at one point that he had a full series of immunizations, but then again he might not have been up to date on his boosters. Tetanus can certainly be a cause of mental deterioration in these patients. Can you think of any other diseases that we forget about frequently in these elderly patients that may cause them to have a decline in their mental status?

JMH: I think that's a difficult question because the differential is so long. Because he's elderly, he's at risk for diseases that we don't see any more. Furthermore, he's at risk for cancer or infections, and just by being elderly is less able to respond to infections. Therefore, I have to systematically go through all the possibilities – infectious, oncologic, neurologic, respiratory, or cardiorespiratory – really is a long and extensive differential. I would also consider iatrogenic causes because medications are often the cause of many problems. Elderly patients almost always take a more number of medications and we need to see if they are contributing to the story.

PR: Considering some of the diseases that we don't start outthinking about in these patients, gastrointestinal (GI) bleed comes to mind. Would you do a rectal examination on this patient?

RW: Absolutely, it's even more likely to be positive in the cirrhotic patient who is presenting with AMS as here you need to think about hepatic encephalopathy triggered by a GI bleed. The rectal examination would also permit you to check the prostate for prostatitis, another potential occult infection that could be going on.

PR: He has a normal temperature, would you still go down a sepsis pathway in this patient?

SG: Absolutely, when you hear hoof beats, don't start with zebras. By far the most common trigger for an acute alteration in mental status in the elderly is infection. Moreover, the elderly often can't and don't mount a fever. I would definitely continue to pursue an infectious workup even if there is no fever. I would also check a rectal temperature as we often miss the fever because the temperature wasn't taken properly.

PR: We have obtained his head CT scan and don't find anything other than what we expected: an aged brain. I think we're at the point however where it's quite clear that our disposition on this patient is not going to be homeward bound. Do you have problems admitting patients like this? I certainly can remember when I was in Denver that the medicine service never wanted to admit such patients and thought they belonged on psychiatry, while psychiatry, of course, refused to admit any patient in whom they could find a medical excuse to admit to medicine.

AM: It might be hospital dependent. In our hospital, as well as a couple of other hospitals I've worked at, it is not a difficult thing to get these patients admitted to the medicine service or the hospitalist service for a relatively quick workup. Dr Hirshon alluded to the differential being very broad, and I think that the inpatient folks have come to understand that the full workup simply cannot be done completely in the ED. The patient needs to have a full medication reconciliation including evaluation for potential medication side effects and medication interactions. As mentioned above, elderly patients are probably on 10–20 medications on average, not to mention over-the-counter medications, which may have

antihistamine effects, cause urinary retention, or have metabolic complications. This specific patient is on a couple of medications that in themselves can cause mental status changes – fluoxetine and lorazepam. All of these things cannot be assessed within a few hours in the ED. Delirium has such a high morbidity and mortality if it is missed, that it is cost-effective and simply smart medicine to admit these patients to see if any further workup can elicit the cause of potential delirium in these patients before relegating these patients to psychiatry for psychiatric workup for the mental status issues.

PR: Would you make any effort to evaluate such patients in an observation unit as opposed to admitting them formally to an inpatient service?

SG: While we are placing more and more elderly patients in an observation unit, I can't guarantee this patient is going to be improved and dischargeable within 24 h – or 85% of the time, which is the criteria that we use for observation admission – because I don't really know what's wrong with this patient at this moment. An AMS might be a self-limiting process, particularly if it is medication related, but other causes of delirium might not resolve within 24 h, and this patient might need several days in the hospital before he is ready to go home. In addition, placing the patient in observation, instead of admitting him to the hospital, may cost the patient a significant amount of money in copays. Therefore, observation units probably have a limited role in this type of patient.

PR: Dr Wolfe you have identified that the patient is on benzodiazepines, which you indicated you would prefer not to use in an elderly patient. Do you have an idea of how long they can induce an alteration – in other words, when can you expect their effect to be worn off?

RW: The half-life is often prolonged in the elderly, so we could be looking at days before recovery if the delirium was triggered by the benzodiazepines. We have a "witches brew" of medications; not only fluoxetine, but Prozac will also induce delirium. For some reason, if we identify delirium and flag that for the colleagues upstairs, we dramatically decrease mortality. We don't know how or why that happens, but at least that's what the data seems to suggest. We don't know how to reproduce that yet in observation units. It may be that as we transform our observation process, make it longer, set it up to really deal with the things that exacerbate and worsen delirium, as well as performing the needed diagnostics, we may also see that same effect of reducing mortality, but at this point we are still uncertain, and we don't have the structure and setup to be able to do that.

PR: Is there a correlation as to where the patient is admitted to the hospital to reduce that mortality? In other words, does he need an intensive care unit (ICU) admission?

RW: I would argue quite the contrary. We think the things that worsen and trigger delirium are sleep deprivation, as well as not being able to resume normal daily activities, being in an unfamiliar setting, and the ICU seems from a delirium standpoint, one of the worst places you could be. On the other hand, you have the problems of dealing with his oxygenation, it depends on how quickly you can turn that around, and the patient needs to be able to cooperate some way with the treatment if you're going to be successful at reversing his COPD exacerbation.

SG: Did they check a digoxin level? – as this too has been implicated as one of the causes of AMS in the elderly.

MK: They did not check a digoxin level.

SG: I would add one more point, even with a normal digoxin level, or one which is therapeutic, digoxin can still be the culprit in causing delirium in the elderly. Therefore, part of the management should be holding the patient's digoxin to see if that helps clear his sensorium.

PR: Don't you think that digoxin is an odd choice of medications for this patient, he doesn't appear to have a lot of atherosclerotic disease, and it certainly doesn't do much for cor pulmonale.

SG: I suspect the patient was placed on digoxin because they were wary with his COPD of putting him on a beta-blocker, and then the choices were calcium channel blocker or digoxin. The thinking was probably that digoxin was a safe drug for rate control in a patient who may have underlying atrial fibrillation or paroxysmal atrial fibrillation, even if it's not clearly documented in his past medical history.

RW: It's interesting though because digitalis delirium was described over a 100 years ago, it's probably one of the first drugs associated with delirium. The other one obviously is the ipratropium, an anticholinergic drug that can also precipitate delirium, in his inhaler.

PR: I noticed that he was already anticoagulated, so certainly his INR and hematocrit need to be checked early because bleeding is a real inducer of mental delirium, which fortunately in this case, he did not have.

PR: We talked a couple of weeks ago about the advantage of having a pharmacist in the ED, and here is yet another wonderful example of how much help we could derive from having someone who would help you look up the interactions and help you discuss the long-term complications of medications.

MK: I think it is important to note that there was a very detailed evaluation of this individual's mental status in this case. The assessment of delirium requires an evaluation beyond just orientation to person, time, and place. In this case, recognition of his inattentiveness and his altered level of arousal (falling asleep in the middle of the medical evaluation) were critical to making the diagnosis of delirium.

PR: Do you really need a formal mental status on this patient to conclude that he's having episodes of delirium? I think his whole behavior for the past couple of days would document that.

MK: I agree – in this case you've got evidence of agitation and an acute alteration, and those are clearly elements that are suggestive of delirium, but to make the formal diagnosis the patient must be inattentive as well. A detailed evaluation of mental status is more critical in making the diagnosis in more subtle cases of delirium, such as hypoactive delirium, and is something that we don't necessarily teach well from the EM perspective.

PR: I think that's a good point, and I certainly think that helps in terms of concluding in your own mind how long you'll have to manage this patient. Still I would submit that because he's already giving you very clear signs of delirium, and that he's not going to turn around in a few hours even if you can get his COPD under control.

Section III: Concepts

Background

What is altered mental status? Definitions of AMS, delirium, and dementia

Delirium or AMS is a common presenting complaint for elderly patients in the ED, and may also present as a contributing or confounding factor of trauma or surgical disease. While approximately 7–10% of elderly ED patients have delirium, emergency physicians recognize delirium in only one out of six delirious ED patients [1–8]. Delirium is associated with high inpatient mortality, between 25% and 33%, and 1 year mortality as high as 77% by some estimates [9–11]. Unrecognized ED delirium may result in higher mortality [4]. The causes of AMS in the elderly are varied, and it is difficult, and at times impossible, to obtain a concise or coherent history without the presence of a family member or caregiver. Many causes of AMS are not discovered in the ED, but it is essential that emergency physicians know potentially life-threatening causes, as a careful clinical history and workup can rule out acute pathology and make progress toward a final diagnosis.

One of the most important components of the evaluation of AMS is defining the time course of a patient's presentation. Delirium is characterized by an acute fluctuation in consciousness or cognition lasting days to weeks, whereas dementia consists of relatively stable, progressive deficits in memory and cognition that manifest over the course of months to years [12]. This reflects the fact that delirium is caused by some insult to homeostasis, such as infection or inflammation, whereas dementia is often due to an underlying neurodegenerative process.

There are exceptions to this categorization. Some toxic and metabolic causes of delirium are very gradual, such as in chronic aspirin overdose [13, 14]. Dementias can also be acute in onset, such as in microvascular infarcts, and some forms of dementia, such as normal pressure hydrocephalus, can be reversible [15].

Clinically, patients with delirium often shift between periods of relative lucidity and extreme distractibility, which may include hallucinations, delusions, and aggressiveness, to the point of being temporarily indistinguishable from frank psychosis. Delirious patients can have profound fluctuations in wakefulness, ranging from periods of hyperactivity to drowsiness. Lethargy, stupor, and coma can be more profound manifestations of the pathologies leading to delirium, but require more rapid evaluation and aggressive management of possible threats to the airway and circulation.

Delirium can be categorized into three subtypes: primarily hyperactive or hypoactive, and mixed [16, 17]. The hyperactive subtype is characterized by agitation and increased activity (which is often purposeless), whereas the hypoactive subtype corresponds to psychomotor retardation, social withdrawal and decreased speech, and reduced situational awareness. The mixed subtype is characterized by waxing between the other two subtypes. Some authors use a Richmond Agitation-Sedation Scale (RASS) to grade the subtype of delirium, with positive scores corresponding to hyperactivity and negative scores to the hypoactive subtype [17]. While the hyperactive subtype may seem difficult to ignore, clinicians in the emergency setting frequently incorrectly assess delirium, particularly the hypoactive subtype [1, 5, 18]. Given that there are a number of brief, easily administered scoring systems to detect delirium and that delirium can be a major contributor to mortality, clinicians need to stay vigilant for the diagnosis [4, 6, 8, 19–21].

Unlike patients with delirium, patients with dementia generally maintain a baseline level of wakefulness, and their deficits tend to be fixed [12, 22]. These deficits may be dependent on context, and patients who are settled in a relatively fixed routine may be able to continue performing fairly complex tasks despite dramatic memory impairments. Removing these patients from their familiar routines and surroundings often results in significant psychological distress, and can exacerbate existing deficits. Complicating matters, patients with dementia can also be affected by "sundowning": agitation and increasing confusion spurred by the interruption of normal circadian rhythms, which often resembles delirium [23]. In addition, patients with dementia are at increased risk of developing delirium (delirium superimposed on dementia) during an acute illness [22].

From the point of view of the emergency physician, delirium should be considered the default presentation of an elderly patient with AMS. This is not only because delirium generally signals a more acute etiology, but also because it is less common for family members to bring patients due to a gradual decline. An exception is when family members who have only sporadic contact with a patient become aware of problems that have been in development over months to years, or when demented patients who have relatively fixed routines suffer an accident or trauma.

Initial altered mental status workup

Physicians evaluating a patient with AMS should take a systematic approach using a focused physical examination, including careful attention to vital sign abnormalities and screening laboratory tests and radiologic studies as appropriate. A key factor is getting a history from caregivers, as well as available nursing home and past medical record notes. It is also critical that the emergency physician perform a delirium assessment.

At the most basic level, the clinician should assess the patient's orientation as well as an attention task. Examples of attention tasks include having the patient name the days of the week or months of the year backward, or having the patient recite spans of three or more digits [24]. A more thorough measurement of cognition may include standardized tests such as the Mini-Cog (a combination of three item recall and clock drawing) [25]; however, this must be combined with a test of attention to distinguish delirium from dementia.

The Confusion Assessment Method (CAM) is the most commonly used, validated tool for diagnosing delirium, with a sensitivity (94–100%) and specificity (90–95%) and has been specifically evaluated in the ED setting [6, 26]. The CAM is applied after the provider has performed a formal cognitive evaluation. A patient is considered delirious if there are present features 1 and 2 and either 3 or 4 of the CAM (Figure 5.1). An adaptation of feature 1 of the CAM that has been used in the ED setting is acute change in mental status, or a fluctuating course, as an ED length of stay is often not long enough to observe fluctuations in a patient's mental status [5].

A number of targeted screening methods are being studied for more rapid diagnosis of delirium and may be reasonable to perform at triage in the near future. For instance, the combination of the Delirium Triage Screen [(DTS) that consists an assessment of level of consciousness and attention] with the brief CAM, an additional four questions administered to patients who have a positive DTS, shows promise in

identifying delirium within the course of an initial interview [27]. Similarly, focused, standardized methods of interviewing caregivers are being developed to help identifying patients with delirium [28].

Infection

Infection is a very common cause of delirium in patients presenting to the ED [29]. Though often reversible, the consequences of missing an infection can be severe. Elderly patients may present with the same signs and symptoms of infection as the general population, such as fever, tachycardia, rigors, and leukocytosis; however, these signs are less consistent in the elderly, and presentations with hypothermia and leukopenia can also occur [30, 31]. Elderly patients are also less likely to present with localizing complaints, such as flank pain or dysuria in pyelonephritis, and cough in pneumonia [32–35].

A number of factors may contribute to infection in the elderly. Many institutionalized elderly patients suffer from chronic bladder or bowel incontinence, which is associated with an increased likelihood of developing UTI (urinary tract infection) [36, 37]. Chronic indwelling catheters pose a significant additional risk [38, 39]. Prior strokes and dysphagia can increase the risk of aspiration pneumonia [40]. Chronic lung disease can decrease clearance of secretions, increasing the likelihood of aspiration pneumonia, as well as the morbidity of viral illnesses and postviral pneumonia [41, 42].

The physical examination findings for infection in the elderly are often difficult to gather [33]. In particular, it may be difficult to obtain a good lung examination due to a patient's unwillingness or inability to cooperate. In patients who are institutionalized or immobile, it is important to be on the lookout for decubitus ulcers and associated cellulitis, particularly in patients who are incontinent, as associated cellulitis is a risk [43, 44]. A convenient time to look for ulcers can be in conjunction with a catheterized urine specimen. A thorough abdominal examination is also essential as delirious patients may not demonstrate obvious symptoms of intra-abdominal infections.

All elderly patients presenting with fever and AMS should have a urinalysis and chest X-ray study, as well as a CBC. Routine lumbar puncture in the absence of focal findings, such as meningismus or high-grade fevers in the absence of another identified cause of infection, is not necessary. Viral nasopharyngeal

Key features of the Confusion Assessment Method

1. *Acute onset and fluctuating course*
   Is there evidence of an acute change in mental status from the patient's baseline? Did this (abnormal) behavior fluctuate during the past day, that is, tend to come and go or increase and decrease in severity?
2. *Inattention*
   Does the patient have difficulty focusing attention, for example, being easily distractible, or having difficulty keeping track of what was being said?
3. *Disorganized thinking*
   Is the patient's speech disorganized or incoherent, such as rambling or irrelevant conversation, unclear or illogical flow of ideas, or unpredictable switching from subject to subject?
4. *Altered level of consciousness*
   Overall, how would you rate this patient's level of consciousness?
   > Alert (normal)
   > Vigilant (hyperalert)
   > Lethargic (drowsy, easily aroused)
   > Stupor (difficult to arouse)
   > Coma (unarousable)

Figure 5.1 Confusion Assessment Method: the diagnosis of delirium requires a present/abnormal rating for criteria (1) and (2) and either (3) or (4). Adapted from Inouye SK, *et al.* Ann. Intern. Med. 1990; 113; 941–948. Confusion Assessment Method. Copyright 2003, Hospital Elder Life Program, LLC. Not to be reproduced without permission.

swabbing may be appropriate based on symptoms and the time of year.

Metabolic abnormality

Metabolic derangements are a frequent but sometimes subtle cause of delirium, which may be spurred by other etiologies such as infection. Metabolic abnormalities often coexist with dehydration and acute renal failure, which can exacerbate a number of chronic medical conditions that lead to delirium. Patients with diabetes may present with gradual development of hyperglycemia, which may become refractory to their established medications. Other endocrine disorders, such as hyper- or hypothyroidism, may become symptomatic as patients forget to take their medication, or experience alterations in absorption. Renal or liver disease may progress to frank encephalopathy due to dehydration or poor compliance with diet, dialysis, or medications [45, 46]. Patients with hematologic malignancies, gout, or renal disease may present with hyperuricemia, or with hyper- or hypocalcemia. Finally, healthy patients with chronically poor diets or on hydrochlorothiazide therapy may present with hyponatremia [47, 48].

Physical examination findings in metabolic disorders are often vague. Be aware of generalized signs of dehydration. Gross hyperreflexia or asterixis are easy to test for and require minimal cooperation from the patient. Be attentive to hyper- and hypoventilation.

Delirious patients should receive basic chemistry evaluations: sodium, potassium, chloride, CO_2, BUN, creatinine, and glucose as well as calcium, phosphate, and magnesium as appropriate. Patients with known gout, hematologic malignancies, or gross abnormalities on CBC should also have uric acid levels measured. Thyroid function tests should also be obtained if results will be available prior to discharge.

Neurologic disease

Direct insults to the brain leading to delirium generally fall into two categories, corresponding with their time of onset. Strokes, either ischemic or hemorrhagic, present with a rapid onset of symptoms over minutes to hours. More gradual causes may take several days or weeks, such as in subdural hematomas, or even months, such as in brain metastases or normal pressure hydrocephalus.

While the time of onset of symptoms is the most critical part of the history in these patients, it is useful to determine if patients have a history of prior stroke, vascular disease, malignancy, or anticoagulation. Patients on systemic anticoagulation, particularly vitamin K antagonists, are at a much higher risk of intracranial hemorrhage than the general population, and these bleeds may be caused by uncontrolled hypertension or even minor trauma [49–52].

The physical examination may yield focal neurologic deficits in the case of ischemic or hemorrhagic stroke. Inattentiveness may make many of the basic components of a neurologic examination difficult to test; however, close attention to speech, use of muscles of facial expression, and gait may yield important clues. Given the ease with which trauma may lead to intracranial hemorrhage, it is extremely important to search for the stigmata of trauma.

As with all potential stroke patients, elderly patients presenting with recent-onset focal neurological deficits should have emergent neuroimaging via noncontrast head CT scan, and a prompt neurologic evaluation. Similarly, providers should obtain a noncontrast head CT on patients who are anticoagulated and who present with any signs or history of trauma. A noncontrast head CT scan is a reasonable screening measure in patients with an established history of malignancy, although a contrast head CT or MRI (obtained as an inpatient) will be more sensitive.

Medication problems
Medications are frequent contributors to delirium, and delirium may result from even the appropriate use of many common medications. Also, elderly patients may abuse illicit drugs and alcohol despite living in an assisted care or nursing facility [53]. While polypharmacy is often cited as a cause of delirium, in the ED this is a diagnosis of exclusion.

Agents that have been commonly linked to delirium include antihistamines, benzodiazepines, and opiates [54–58]. Antihistamines and anticholinergic agents may be present in many ophthalmic preparations. Similarly, many medications for Parkinson's disease, such as selegiline and ropinirole, as well as many psychiatric medications, such as bupropion, have been associated with delirium. Patients with a history of severe arthritis or chronic pain may present with overdoses of acetaminophen or salicylates. Patients abusing alcohol or chronically on benzodiazepines may present in withdrawal when suffering from a concomitant illness or trauma.

While there is no single physical examination consistent with pharmacologically induced delirium, be aware of the general features of common toxidromes. In particular, anticholinergic toxicity is associated with tachycardia, dry skin and mucous membranes, urinary retention, and mydriasis. Salicylate toxicity is characterized by tinnitus, nausea, and hyperventilation, followed by tachycardia, worsening of delirium, and coma. Alcohol and benzodiazepine withdrawal are characterized by tremulousness, agitation, tachycardia, and eventually frank autonomic instability, hallucinations, and seizure.

Antihistamines, anticholinergic agents, and benzodiazepines should be held in patients with delirium unless there is a specific concern for benzodiazepine or alcohol withdrawal. All patients with a suspected pharmacologic component to their delirium should have basic chemistries, EKG, a serum toxicology screen, LFTs, arterial blood gas determination, as well as acetaminophen and aspirin levels drawn as appropriate.

Cardiovascular and pulmonary problems
Cardiovascular and pulmonary conditions may contribute significantly to delirium. While patients with obvious chest pain or respiratory distress point to cardiovascular and pulmonary problems, delirious elderly patients may present with a broad range of or vague symptoms. It is essential to talk to a caregiver about a patient's overall history of activity, any near-syncopal episodes, and to ask about whether a patient's breathing or level of arousal is consistent with their baseline.

Much of the existing literature regarding cardiac ischemia and delirium comes from the cardiology and cardiac surgery literature, where myocardial ischemia has been linked to increased prevalence of delirium, as has congestive heart failure [59–62]. Thus, it is essential to determine if the patient has a history of cardiovascular disease. COPD and obstructive sleep apnea may contribute to delirium due to both hypoxia and hypercarbia [63–65]. Pulmonary embolism (PE) may also contribute significantly by inducing hypoxia, pain, and tachycardia [66, 67]. Be particularly aware of the possibility of an embolism in patients who have had recent arthroplasty, or who are chronically immobile.

The physical examination rarely reveals whether a patient is having active ischemia or an embolism; however, tachycardia, tachypnea, and hypoxia are important clues to underlying distress. Close auscultation of the heart can help to identify important valvular pathology, such as the crescendo–decrescendo murmur at the right upper sternal border of aortic stenosis, which may contribute to congestive heart failure as well as ischemia. Similarly, both auscultation and palpation of the pulse may help alert you to the presence of dysrhythmias.

All patients with delirium should receive an EKG and chest X-ray study. Patients with a history of coronary disease, or a history at all concerning for ischemia or syncope should undergo serial cardiac enzymes measurements. Patients with chronic pulmonary disease may require a blood gas determination, and patients at risk for PE should have D-dimer testing or imaging via CTA (computed tomography angiogram).

Psychiatric disease

Psychiatric disease can contribute to delirium as well as mimic it. Unfortunately, the behavior-altering nature of psychiatric diseases may often cause caregivers who are less familiar with a patient to overlook concomitant delirium. It is essential to discuss whether a patient's symptoms are consistent with baseline, even if the baseline is depressed or otherwise abnormal.

Patients with preexisting dementia are at higher risk of developing delirium [22]. Both depression and other mood disorders are associated with a higher risk of delirium, and in the case of depression, worse outcomes [68, 69].

The physical examination of confused elderly patients with preexisting psychiatric disease should focus on the ability to concentrate and stay awake.

Patients with new AMS should receive a screen for drugs of abuse in addition to their workup. Patients with an established history of bipolar disorder on lithium should have levels checked [70].

Testing

While there are many potential causes of delirium, which will require more specific workups, several tests should be performed on all patients with delirium.

Serum chemistries

A basic chemistry panel (sodium, potassium, chloride, CO_2, BUN, creatinine, and glucose) should be obtained on all patients with delirium. Rates of hypoglycemia and acute kidney injury are high in patients with delirium and may contribute to or complicate many causes of delirium. Significant abnormalities

may point to potential metabolic, endocrine, or toxicologic causes of delirium.

Urinalysis and chest X-ray

The combination of urinalysis and chest X-ray study can diagnose up to 70% of fevers in the elderly. Patients with indwelling catheters may be chronically colonized, and their urinalysis must be interpreted in context. Urine culture is essential in these patients. Note that some pneumonias may be occult; combined with dehydration, they may not show up on an initial X-ray study, but may become visible after rehydration [71, 72].

EKG

The EKG is an essential screening tool for all patients with delirium. The EKG may help identify dysrhythmias, ischemia, PE, electrolyte abnormalities, and toxidromes.

CT scan head

In patients with acute and persistent changes, neurologic deficits, a history of stroke, or on anticoagulation with any report of trauma, a CT scan of the head is important. It is less useful in the general population of delirious patients.

Delirium treatment and management

Critical to the management of delirium is identification and treatment of the precipitating cause(s) [73]. Adjunctive nonpharmacologic treatments may also be initiated, including frequent reorientation, enabling family to remain with the patient, and normalizing the sleep–wake cycle [74]. Verbal de-escalation techniques should be first line for the management of delirious patients with mild-to-moderate agitation. When verbal de-escalation techniques are unsuccessful, or patients are severely agitated and at risk of injuring themselves or others or interfering with critical medical treatment, low-dose antipsychotics may be administered, such as haloperidol, risperidone, olanzapine, quetiapine, or ziprasidone. Benzodiazepines may precipitate or worsen delirium in geriatric patients and should be limited to patients with delirium secondary to alcohol or benzodiazepine withdrawal, or if a delirious patient requires sedation for diagnostic procedures such as CT imaging or lumbar puncture [75].

Disposition

Most patients with delirium should be admitted. Delirium carries a high risk of mortality, and its continued presence suggests the presence of underlying disease. Delirious patients should not be discharged, due to the significantly elevated risk of mortality in untreated delirium, and because delirium may interfere with a patient's ability to understand the discharge planning and compliance with treatment [76]. If a patient lives in a supervised environment, such as a nursing facility, and has a generally reassuring workup and for whom there is not concern for infection, ischemia, or congestive heart failure, discharge may be considered but only after consultation with the patient's outpatient providers.

Section IV: Decision Making

Decision-making

- Delirium is often a sign of serious underlying disease and is linked to significantly increased mortality.
- Careful consideration must be given to the following diagnoses:
  - Infection
  - Hyper- or hypoglycemia
  - Dehydration and acute renal failure
  - Ischemic stroke
  - Intracranial hemorrhage
  - Medication overdose or withdrawal.
- The cornerstone of the evaluation of delirium is obtaining a history from a caregiver, as well as past medical records, and performing a detailed physical examination including a structured assessment for delirium that includes a formal test of attention.
- All patients presenting with delirium should have a basic chemistry, EKG, chest X-ray study, and urinalysis.
- A head CT scan is indicated in any patient with focal neurologic deficits, a history of stroke, or anticoagulation use with any concern for trauma, even minor.
- Patients with delirium should be admitted due to the high risk of mortality.

References

1 Élie, M., Rousseau, F., Cole, M. *et al.* (2000) Prevalence and detection of delirium in elderly emergency department patients. *Can. Med. Assoc. J.*, **163** (8), 977–981.

2 Han, J.H., Morandi, A., Ely, E. *et al.* (2009) Delirium in the nursing home patients seen in the emergency department. *J. Am. Geriatr. Soc.*, **57** (5), 889–894.

3 Hustey, F.M. and Meldon, S.W. (2002) The prevalence and documentation of impaired mental status in elderly emergency department patients. *Ann. Emerg. Med.*, **39** (3), 248–253.

4 Kakuma, R., Fort, D., Galbaud, G. *et al.* (2003) Delirium in older emergency department patients discharged home: effect on survival. *J. Am. Geriatr. Soc.*, **51** (4), 443–450.

5 Lewis, L.M., Miller, D.K., Morley, J.E. *et al.* (1995) Unrecognized delirium in ED geriatric patients. *Am. J. Emerg. Med.*, **13** (2), 142–145.

6 Monette, J., Galbaud du Fort, G., Fung, S.H. *et al.* (2001) Evaluation of the Confusion Assessment Method (CAM) as a screening tool for delirium in the emergency room. *Gen. Hosp. Psychiatry*, **23** (1), 20–25.

7 Naughton, B.J., Moran, M.B., Kadah, H., and Longano, J. (1995) Delirium and other cognitive impairment in older adults in an emergency department. *Ann. Emerg. Med.*, **25** (6), 751–755.

8 Hustey, F.M., Meldon, S.W., Smith, M.D., and Lex, C.K. (2003) The effect of mental status screening on the care of elderly emergency department patients. *Ann. Emerg. Med.*, **41** (5), 678–684.

9 Leslie, D.L., Zhang, Y., Holford, T.R. *et al.* (2005) Premature death associated with delirium at 1-year follow-up. *Arch. Intern. Med.*, **165** (14), 1657.

10 Inouye, S.K., Schlesinger, M.J., and Lydon, T.J. (1999) Delirium: a symptom of how hospital care is failing older persons and a window to improve quality of hospital care. *Am. J. Med.*, **106** (5), 565–573.

11 Siddiqi, N., House, A.O., and Holmes, J.D. (2006) Occurrence and outcome of delirium in medical in-patients: a systematic literature review. *Age Ageing*, **35** (4), 350–364.

12 Association, A.P. (2013) *Diagnostic and Statistical Manual of Mental Disorders*, 5th edn, American Psychiatric Publishing, Arlington, VA.

13 O'Malley, G.F. (2007) Emergency department management of the salicylate-poisoned patient. *Emerg. Med. Clin. North Am.*, **25** (2), 333–346.

14 Bailey, R.B. and Jones, S.R. (1989) Chronic salicylate intoxication: a common cause of morbidity in the elderly. *J. Am. Geriatr. Soc.*, **37** (6), 556–561.

15 Graff-Radford, N.R. (2007) Normal pressure hydrocephalus. *Neurol. Clin.*, **25** (3), 809–832.

16 Meagher, D.J., O'Hanlon, D., O'Mahony, E. *et al.* (2000) Relationship between symptoms and motoric subtype of delirium. *J. Neuropsychiatry Clin. Neurosci.*, **12** (1), 51–56.

17 Peterson, J.F., Pun, B.T., Dittus, R.S. *et al.* (2006) Delirium and its motoric subtypes: a study of 614 critically ill patients. *J. Am. Geriatr. Soc.*, 54 (3), 479–484.

18 Han, J.H., Zimmerman, E.E., Cutler, N. *et al.* (2009) Delirium in older emergency department patients: recognition, risk factors, and psychomotor subtypes. *Acad. Emerg. Med.*, 16 (3), 193–200.

19 Ely, E.W., Shintani, A., Truman, B. *et al.* (2004) Delirium as a predictor of mortality in mechanically ventilated patients in the intensive care unit. *J. Am. Med. Assoc.*, 291 (14), 1753–1762.

20 Witlox, J., Eurelings, L.S., de Jonghe, J.F. *et al.* (2010) Delirium in elderly patients and the risk of postdischarge mortality, institutionalization, and dementia. *J. Am. Med. Assoc.*, 304 (4), 443–451.

21 Carpenter, C.R., DesPain, B., Keeling, T.N. *et al.* (2011) The Six-Item Screener and AD8 for the detection of cognitive impairment in geriatric emergency department patients. *Ann. Emerg. Med.*, 57 (6), 653–661.

22 Fick, D.M., Agostini, J.V., and Inouye, S.K. (2002) Delirium superimposed on dementia: a systematic review. *J. Am. Geriatr. Soc.*, 50 (10), 1723–1732.

23 Kim, P., Louis, C., Muralee, S., and Tampi, R.R. (2005) Sundowning syndrome in the older patient. *Clin. Geriatr.*, 13 (4), 32–36.

24 Inouye, S.K., Westendorp, R.G., and Saczynski, J.S. (2014) Delirium in elderly people. *Lancet*, 383 (9920), 911–922.

25 Borson, S., Scanlan, J., Brush, M. *et al.* (2000) The Mini-Cog: a cognitive' 'vital signs' measure for dementia screening in multi-lingual elderly. *Int. J. Geriatr. Psychiatry*, 15 (11), 1021–1027.

26 Wei, L.A., Fearing, M.A., Sternberg, E.J., and Inouye, S.K. (2008) The Confusion Assessment Method: a systematic review of current usage. *J. Am. Geriatr. Soc.*, 56 (5), 823–830.

27 Han, J.H., Wilson, A., Vasilevskis, E.E. *et al.* (2013) Diagnosing delirium in older emergency department patients: validity and reliability of the delirium triage screen and the brief confusion assessment method. *Ann. Emerg. Med.*, 62 (5), 457–465.

28 Steis, M.R., Evans, L., Hirschman, K.B. *et al.* (2012) Screening for delirium using family caregivers: convergent validity of the Family Confusion Assessment Method and interviewer-rated Confusion Assessment Method. *J. Am. Geriatr. Soc.*, 60 (11), 2121–2126.

29 Wilber, S.T. (2006) Altered mental status in older emergency department patients. *Emerg. Med. Clin. North Am.*, 24 (2), 299–316.

30 Chassagne, P., Perol, M.B., Doucet, J. *et al.* (1996) Is presentation of bacteremia in the elderly the same as in younger patients? *Am. J. Med.*, 100 (1), 65–70.

31 Tiruvoipati, R., Ong, K., Gangopadhyay, H. *et al.* (2010) Hypothermia predicts mortality in critically ill elderly patients with sepsis. *BMC Geriatr.*, 10 (1), 70.

32 Baldassarre, J. and Kaye, D. (1991) Special problems of urinary tract infection in the elderly. *Med. Clin. North Am.*, 75 (2), 375–390.

33 Crossley, K.B. and Peterson, P.K. (1996) Infections in the elderly. *Clin. Infect. Dis.*, 22 (2), 209–214.

34 Lieberman, D. and Lieberman, D. (2000) Community-acquired pneumonia in the elderly. *Drugs Aging*, 17 (2), 93–105.

35 Metlay, J.P., Schulz, R., Li, Y.-H. *et al.* (1997) Influence of age on symptoms at presentation in patients with community-acquired pneumonia. *Arch. Intern. Med.*, 157 (13), 1453.

36 Beck-Sague, C., Banerjee, S., and Jarvis, W.R. (1993) Infectious diseases and mortality among US nursing home residents. *Am. J. Public Health*, 83 (12), 1739–1742.

37 Shortliffe, L.M.D. and McCue, J.D. (2002) Urinary tract infection at the age extremes: pediatrics and geriatrics. *Am. J. Med.*, 113 (1), 55–66.

38 Tal, S., Guller, V., Levi, S. *et al.* (2005) Profile and prognosis of febrile elderly patients with bacteremic urinary tract infection. *J. Infect.*, 50 (4), 296–305.

39 Hazelett, S.E., Tsai, M., Gareri, M., and Allen, K. (2006) The association between indwelling urinary catheter use in the elderly and urinary tract infection in acute care. *BMC Geriatr.*, 6 (1), 15.

40 Martino, R., Foley, N., Bhogal, S. *et al.* (2005) Dysphagia after stroke incidence, diagnosis, and pulmonary complications. *Stroke*, 36 (12), 2756–2763.

41 Langmore, S.E., Skarupski, K.A., Park, P.S., and Fries, B.E. (2002) Predictors of aspiration pneumonia in nursing home residents. *Dysphagia*, 17 (4), 298–307.

42 Soriano, J.B., Visick, G.T., Muellerova, H. *et al.* (2005) Patterns of comorbidities in newly diagnosed COPD and asthma in primary care. *Chest J.*, 128 (4), 2099–2107.

43 Farage, M.A., Miller, K.W., Berardesca, E., and Maibach, H.I. (2007) Incontinence in the aged: contact dermatitis and other cutaneous consequences. *Contact Dermatitis*, 57 (4), 211–217.

44 Strausbaugh, L.J., Sukumar, S.R., Joseph, C.L., and High, K.P. (2003) Infectious disease outbreaks in nursing homes: an unappreciated hazard for frail elderly persons. *Clin. Infect. Dis.*, 36 (7), 870–876.

45 Frederick, R.T. (2011) Current concepts in the pathophysiology and management of hepatic encephalopathy. *Gastroenterol. Hepatol.*, 7 (4), 222.

46 Seifter, J.L. and Samuels, M.A. (eds) (2011) Uremic encephalopathy and other brain disorders associated with renal failure. *Semin. Neurol.*, 31 (2), 139–143.

47 Tareen, N., Martins, D., Nagami, G. *et al.* (2005) Sodium disorders in the elderly. *J. Natl. Med. Assoc.*, 97 (2), 217.

69

48 Chow, K., Szeto, C., Wong, T.-H. *et al.* (2003) Risk factors for thiazide-induced hyponatraemia. *Q. J. Med.*, **96** (**12**), 911–917.

49 Spektor, S., Agus, S., Merkin, V., and Constantini, S. (2003) Low-dose aspirin prophylaxis and risk of intracranial hemorrhage in patients older than 60 years of age with mild or moderate head injury: a prospective study. *J. Neurosurg.*, **99** (**4**), 661–665.

50 Fang, M.C., Chang, Y., Hylek, E.M. *et al.* (2004) Advanced age, anticoagulation intensity, and risk for intracranial hemorrhage among patients taking warfarin for atrial fibrillation. *Ann. Intern. Med.*, **141** (**10**), 745–752.

51 Callaway, D.W. and Wolfe, R. (2007) Geriatric trauma. *Emerg. Med. Clin. North Am.*, **25** (**3**), 837–860.

52 Hart, R.G., Tonarelli, S.B., and Pearce, L.A. (2005) Avoiding central nervous system bleeding during antithrombotic therapy recent data and ideas. *Stroke*, **36** (**7**), 1588–1593.

53 Benshoff, J.J., Harrawood, L.K., and Koch, D.S. (2003) Substance abuse and the elderly: unique issues and concerns. *J. Rehabil.*, **69** (**2**), 43–48.

54 Pisani, M.A., Murphy, T.E., Araujo, K.L. *et al.* (2009) Benzodiazepine and opioid use and the duration of ICU delirium in an older population. *Crit. Care Med.*, **37** (**1**), 177.

55 Alagiakrishnan, K. and Wiens, C. (2004) An approach to drug induced delirium in the elderly. *Postgrad. Med. J.*, **80** (**945**), 388–393.

56 Iseli, R., Brand, C., Telford, M., and LoGiudice, D. (2007) Delirium in elderly general medical inpatients: a prospective study. *Intern. Med. J.*, **37** (**12**), 806–811.

57 Rothberg, M.B., Herzig, S.J., Pekow, P.S. *et al.* (2013) Association between sedating medications and delirium in older inpatients. *J. Am. Geriatr. Soc.*, **61** (**6**), 923–930.

58 Greenberg, D.B. (2003) Preventing delirium at the end of life: lessons from recent research. *Prim. Care Companion J. Clin. Psychiatry*, **5** (**2**), 62.

59 Uguz, F., Kayrak, M., Cíçek, E. *et al.* (2010) Delirium following acute myocardial infarction: incidence, clinical profiles, and predictors. *Perspect. Psychiatr. Care*, **46** (**2**), 135–142.

60 Rudolph, J.L., Jones, R.N., Levkoff, S.E. *et al.* (2009) Derivation and validation of a preoperative prediction rule for delirium after cardiac surgery. *Circulation*, **119** (**2**), 229–236.

61 Bucerius, J., Gummert, J.F., Borger, M.A. *et al.* (2004) Predictors of delirium after cardiac surgery delirium: effect of beating-heart (off-pump) surgery. *J. Thorac. Cardiovasc. Surg.*, **127** (**1**), 57–64.

62 Heckman, G.A., Patterson, C.J., Demers, C. *et al.* (2007) Heart failure and cognitive impairment: challenges and opportunities. *Clin. Interv. Aging*, **2** (**2**), 209.

63 Zheng, G.-Q., Wang, Y., and Wang, X.-T. (2008) Chronic hypoxia-hypercapnia influences cognitive function: a possible new model of cognitive dysfunction in chronic obstructive pulmonary disease. *Med. Hypotheses*, **71** (**1**), 111–113.

64 MacLullich, A.M., Ferguson, K.J., Miller, T. *et al.* (2008) Unravelling the pathophysiology of delirium: a focus on the role of aberrant stress responses. *J. Psychosom. Res.*, **65** (**3**), 229–238.

65 Lombardi, C., Rocchi, R., Montagna, P. *et al.* (2009) Obstructive sleep apnea syndrome: a cause of acute delirium. *J. Clin. Sleep Med.*, **5** (**6**), 569.

66 Balas, M.C., Happ, M.B., Yang, W. *et al.* (2009) Outcomes associated with delirium in older patients in surgical ICUs. *Chest J.*, **135** (**1**), 18–25.

67 Laurila, J.V., Laakkonen, M.-L., Laurila, J.V. *et al.* (2008) Predisposing and precipitating factors for delirium in a frail geriatric population. *J. Psychosom. Res.*, **65** (**3**), 249–254.

68 Givens, J.L., Jones, R.N., and Inouye, S.K. (2009) The overlap syndrome of depression and delirium in older hospitalized patients. *J. Am. Geriatr. Soc.*, **57** (**8**), 1347–1353.

69 McAvay, G.J., Van Ness, P.H., Bogardus, S.T. Jr., *et al.* (2007) Depressive symptoms and the risk of incident delirium in older hospitalized adults. *J. Am. Geriatr. Soc.*, **55** (**5**), 684–691.

70 Shulman, K.I., Sykora, K., Gill, S. *et al.* (2005) Incidence of delirium in older adults newly prescribed lithium or valproate: a population-based cohort study. *J. Clin. Psychiatry*, **66** (**4**), 424–427.

71 Bartlett, J.G. and Mundy, L.M. (1995) Community-acquired pneumonia. *N. Engl. J. Med.*, **333**, 1618–1624.

72 Hash, R.B., Stephens, J.L., Laurens, M.B., and Vogel, R.L. (2000) The relationship between volume status, hydration, and radiographic findings in the diagnosis of community-acquired pneumonia. *J. Fam. Pract.*, **49** (**9**), 833–837.

73 Arora, V.M., McGory, M.L., and Fung, C.H. (2007) Quality indicators for hospitalization and surgery in vulnerable elders. *J. Am. Geriatr. Soc.*, **55** (**Suppl. 2**), S347–S358.

74 Inouye, S.K., Westendorp, R.G., and Saczynski, J.S. (2014) Delirium in elderly people. *Lancet*, **383** (**9920**), 911–922.

75 American Psychiatric Association (1999) Practice guideline for the treatment of patients with delirium. *Am. J. Psychiatry*, **156** (**Suppl. 5**), 1–20.

76 Han, J.H., Bryce, S.N., Ely, E.W. *et al.* (2011) The effect of cognitive impairment on the accuracy of the presenting complaint and discharge instruction comprehension in older emergency department patients. *Ann. Emerg. Med.*, **57**, 662–671.

6

Geriatric psychiatric emergencies

Josh Joseph & Maura Kennedy

Department of Emergency Medicine, Beth Israel Deaconess Medical Center, Harvard Medical School, Boston, MA, USA

Section I: Case presentation

An 82-year-old woman was brought into the emergency department (ED) by her family for concerns of weakness and weight loss. She had had months of decreased appetite, insomnia, and anhedonia. She lived with her husband in senior housing, and stated that she rarely left the house, as she was afraid to leave him alone. She rarely participated in the activities held in their apartment complex. She had stopped cooking and lost about 40 lb. Their children prepared meals for them. She also had difficulty sleeping. Over the past few days, the family reported that she had acutely deteriorated, with increasing anxiety and weeping. They called her primary care physician (PCP) who referred them to the ED for evaluation. The patient reported that her husband had been unwell and that she has been very anxious because of his health, and worried that she was not able to adequately care for him. She denied fevers, chest pain, shortness of breath, abdominal pain, nausea, or vomiting.

The past medical history was notable for depression and anxiety. She took a daily vitamin and stool softener. Her husband had terminal cancer, and had a home health aide come in several hours every day, and VNA (Visiting Nurse Assistance) services weekly. She did not use tobacco, alcohol, or illicit drugs.

The vital signs were as follows: temperature 36.5°C, pulse 86 beats/min, blood pressure 121/82 mm Hg, respirations 16 breaths/min, and pulse oximetry 96% on room air. The cardiac, pulmonary, and abdominal examinations were normal. The neurologic examination including cranial nerves, motor, muscle tone, and reflexes was normal. She was oriented to person, place, and time, recalled 3/3 objects at 5 min, and could recite months of the year backward, though slowly. Overall she had a flat affect, and became tearful when discussing care of her husband. She denied suicidal and homicidal thoughts.

A complete blood count, chemistries, thyroid stimulating hormone (TSH), and urinalysis were obtained and were normal. She demonstrated no signs of delirium. Psychiatry was consulted, and she was diagnosed with major depressive disorder, anxiety, and significant caregiver burden. Psychiatry recommended starting mirtazapine for depression and poor appetite, melatonin for sleep regulation, and referred her to outpatient geri-psychiatry. The patient did not meet the criteria for inpatient psychiatric care, and neither the patient nor her family wanted her to be hospitalized in a psychiatric facility. The case manager also arranged additional home social services for the patient and her husband.

Section II: Case discussion

Dr Peter Rosen (PR): Why did the PCP need an emergency evaluation?

Dr Maura Kennedy (MK): One of the concerns was whether this was delirium superimposed on depression, and whether her anxiety might actually be more of a delirium state. It was also a Friday afternoon, and the office was closing. Given the concern for acute delirium and drastic change over the course of 2 days, she was referred to the ED.

Geriatric Emergencies: A Discussion-Based Review, First Edition.
Edited by Amal Mattu, Shamai A. Grossman and Peter L. Rosen.
© 2016 John Wiley & Sons, Ltd. Published 2016 by John Wiley & Sons, Ltd.

PR: I noted you had ordered a TSH and also noticed the temperature was lower than normal. There are a number of differential diagnoses that can cause this, including sepsis and hypothyroidism in a patient this age. You mentioned the reflexes were normal, which argues against hypothyroidism producing significant behavioral changes. Are there other acute medical causes that could explain these behavioral changes?

Dr Jon Mark Hirshon: With any change in behavior, I always worry about intercurrent infections, such as a urinary tract infection (UTI). With elderly patients, because they often don't present in a typical manner for a disease, behavioral changes could be caused by almost anything. Prior to deciding this is a nonorganic brain disease, that is, primarily a psychiatric problem, I would want to make sure there aren't other types of infections, but additionally, make sure there aren't any cardiac symptoms or abdominal symptoms. The hidden infection that I always think of first in the elderly is a UTI.

JMH: We often don't think about psychiatric disease in the elderly. What are some clues that would make you consider that this is perhaps an exacerbation of a potential lifelong problem for this patient?

Dr Ula Hwang (UH): It's reported that she had a past history of depression and anxiety. Many of the clues are to be found in the recent history. I would say it's not an exacerbation if it's occurring acutely within the last 2 days, but in this case it seems to be a worsening or progression over some time. This was really good history delving into what's going on in her life, noting what was going on with her husband and his terminal illness, the stress this caused in taking care of him. This history coupled with a past psychiatric history gives us an idea that she is having a worsening of her underlying condition.

PR: I worry about things that we don't ordinarily look into when we see depression, such as medical causes. When I hear of a history of 40 lb weight loss, I think of occult malignancy. How diligently would you search for a hidden cancer in this patient?

Dr Scott Wilber: Forty pounds is a considerable amount of weight loss to be associated with about 2 months of decreased appetite making malignancy a reasonable thought. I'm not sure how extensively we can evaluate for an occult cancer in the ED. Certainly,

if she was a former smoker, a chest X-ray study would be reasonable as well as fecal occult blood testing. The 40 lb weight loss is generally concerning from any perspective and is going to affect her muscle strength and her ability to get around.

PR: Maybe her children are just terrible cooks. I think at least a stool guaiac is in order. If she is thin, a careful physical examination can reveal a tumor mass that would not be palpable in a more obese patient. What kind of cardiac diseases would give you this type of presentation?

Dr Shamai Grossman: The ED is sometimes the patient's only gateway to health care. Sometimes, we are stuck doing a workup that should really be done in the outpatient setting, for example, searching for an occult malignancy or other long-term disease processes. A cardiac workup may be appropriate based on the past medical history and the symptoms of the present illness. That her present failure to thrive reflects occult angina or ischemic symptoms is conceivable, but one would think the patient would have some sort of complaint that would suggest this; for example, they can't walk or they have weakness. Certainly vital sign and physical examination findings, such as tachypnea, hypoxia, bradycardia, or tachycardia, may lead us to obtain more of a cardiac workup. In patients unable to give us a history due to dementia, we may need to perform a shotgun approach in which we obtain many tests, and look for many diseases. For this patient, I would start with basic laboratory tests and an electrocardiogram (EKG). The results might then lead you to a further cardiac workup.

PR: Psychiatry is one of the places in which we usually obtain a consultation more for help with disposition rather than help with diagnosis. We have often already decided that the patient needs admission before we ask the psychiatrist to see the patient, and the issue is how and where to get the patient admitted? What do you use as your own personal criteria for recommending admission in an elderly patient who is clearly depressed?

MK: From the history provided, it is clear she has a major depressive disorder, with anhedonia, weight loss, decreased appetite, and at the time of her evaluation had no outpatient psychiatric providers and was not on any psychiatric medications. She wasn't expressing any suicidality or any thoughts of suicide, and her role as the primary caregiver for her husband is probably a protective factor against suicide. Typically, I consult psychiatry when I feel a patient requires inpatient psychiatric hospitalization. Inpatient hospitalization likely would have been the worst option for her – being away from her husband may have exacerbated her anxiety about her husband's well-being, and this acute change in environment would pose a risk of delirium development. Had we been able to ensure close follow-up with an outpatient psychiatric provider, then we likely would have discharged her without an emergency psychiatric consultation. This patient, however, did not have established care with a psychiatrist and we were concerned that she might be lost to follow-up. The psychiatry consultation was to make sure we had established care for after we had discharged her. We also involved our social worker and case manager in her care. One of the potential options included getting a social worker to come into the home to address her and her husband's needs concomitantly.

JMH: From my perspective, one of the critical factors you mentioned above is family engagement. It is very important that if she does go back home, she has family who are going to help with the follow-up. The social circumstances are clearly a strong component in this case both in terms of her husband's condition and the family support. That would give me a strong assurance that if I were to discharge her home, there would be appropriate incentive and motivation for follow-up.

PR: One of the most important parts of the evaluation of a depressed patient is whether the patient is suicidal or homicidal. I think we skirt asking this question directly, sometimes in fear that it will induce suicidal thoughts in an otherwise nonsuicidal patient. But I think that's an error and that these questions need to be asked directly. What would you do if this woman said in fact that she is fed up with being old, with taking care of her husband, and watching her husband die, and she is strongly considering killing herself?

SW: I think you would have to take that very seriously. She would require involuntary hospitalization. Even though the group that successfully completes suicide most often is elderly men, I think we would have to take this threat very seriously, even in a woman.

The caregiver burden can sometimes cause people to act in an otherwise noncharacteristic manner. A quick example is a case in town where an elderly man entered an Intensive Care Unit (ICU) and shot his wife because he didn't want to see her suffer any longer. We must take thoughts of suicide and thoughts of self-harm or harming others very seriously in this patient population, especially in men.

PR: It seems that today we don't like to hospitalize people for anything, including serious depression, and think we can control them with pharmacology. Do you have any experience with psychiatric drugs in the elderly? Do they have as many side effects as many of the other drugs we give to elderly patients? Moreover, there is always the concern of "when are they going to kick in," and "are things going to get worse before they get better."

UH: In general, whether it's older or even younger adults, we are not in the best position to start anyone on any type of chronic medication, especially psychiatric medications for depression. These are not medications that tend to work right away. They do require a longer period to be effective. In all likelihood, all of these medications will have greater side effects and greater risk of impact. In this case, in particular, the patient was very fortunate that a geriatric psychiatry outpatient referral was able to be arranged. In general, geriatric psychiatrists are fewer in number, and as the population ages, the opportunity to have a geriatric psychiatrist to consult, and manage medications is going to be increasingly rare.

SG: I would add that mirtazapine is probably a good choice, and from what I recall, the onset at 1 week is shorter than that of other agents. It also has less antidysrhythmic effects than most of the older agents on the market and, therefore, is less likely to interact with the other concurrent medications the elderly patients are already taking.

PR: We know that older spouses are quite dependent on each other and that death in one is frequently followed by death in the other. There seems to be a part of aging that is to feel that "life is complete" and that we don't want to go on with it anymore. It's not necessarily depression, as much as "it's time to die." Our society, in particular the young population, doesn't understand that. But I think a lot of older people feel this way. How do you distinguish between major depression, and when someone feels like "I have come to the end of my life?"

JMH: Before making a decision about a psychiatric illness, I need to exclude medical causes. Once you've worked through psychiatric and medical causes, and looking at the life circumstances, one can understand the individual's perspective on life. I think our society has issues with death as a general rule. Everyone is going to die at some point. Allowing someone the decision as to how they are going to get there may not be a bad thing. In this instance, there are so many circumstantial concerns, in particular with her husband as well as her past history, that I think need to be addressed and discussed in an open manner before making a decision on "how they want to go." Nevertheless, there has to be a respect for this individual.

PR: I do think there comes a time for the elderly when they have the right to say they don't want to keep living for all kinds of reasons that are at least valid for them personally, and we need to respect that as well.

SG: The converse is also true. We do have to keep in mind that just because they are old, doesn't mean they need or wish to die. They are elderly patients, but still patients. They have treatable diseases that require intervention. Our perspective should be that we should treat the disease while keeping the patient's wishes in mind.

PR: These are particularly difficult cases, because even with motivated family, being around someone who is very depressed is in itself very depressing. This quickly changes the relatives' enthusiasm for voluntarism. This can be a big management problem in someone like this. It's nice she is already in some sort of assisted living, and it's wonderful we had the capacity to get her social service support that is not available in many parts of our country. So I think this is an almost ideal management of this case, which would be almost impossible to duplicate throughout most of our cities.

JMH: At my facility, which is an academic center, we have those kinds of resources. If you are out in the community, getting a psychiatric consult is sometimes a huge burden. You're the one that ends up doing the initial evaluation and deciding on disposition. I think we need to acknowledge there are many situations in which getting even a psychiatric and

much less likely a geriatric psychiatric evaluation can be problematic.

PR: There are many community health centers that don't have psychiatrists even on call. The consultation will be performed by a psychiatric worker of some level and educational background but without the ability to prescribe psychiatric medications for you. Sometimes, you have to compromise the optimal management of the patient that was exemplified here by admitting the patient until a psychiatrist can be obtained, or at least admitting the patient under observation until you can obtain some help in starting the psychiatric medication. How did the patient end up doing over time?

MK: According to her primary care notes, she did well mainly because of the social supports. The social workers were able to get day-care options for her husband, which then gave the patient the opportunity to participate in more social activities. Even though she continued to express a lot of anxiety regarding her husband's illness and well-being, there was definite improvement in her depression particularly with increased social activity.

Section III: Concepts

Background

Psychiatric disorders are a prevalent but often subtle cause of morbidity and mortality in the elderly. The interplay of psychiatric disorders and medical and neurologic disease is complex, and there can be considerable overlap between conditions. Elderly patients suffering from underlying psychiatric conditions such as depression often present with more general somatic complaints such as fatigue, weakness, poor appetite, or poor sleep [1]. While definitive management of these conditions is rarely provided in the ED, early identification is important because a number of these conditions – such as depression, substance abuse, and suicidality – are serious but preventable contributors to mortality.

Initial psychiatric workup

Physicians evaluating elderly patients should strongly consider psychiatric comorbidity for any elderly patient presenting to the ED. This does not mean that all elderly patients need a comprehensive neuropsychiatric evaluation; rather that emergency physicians should perform a focused screening of patients based on history and examination findings. For instance, it is important to ascertain whether patients who have suffered falls or other trauma are confused, as well as to ask them (and their caregivers) about substance use.

Dementia

Dementia affects a large portion of the elderly population and is a significant cause of disability as well as accidents and trauma [2–4]. Dementia is an independent risk factor for falls, and many demented patients who live independently or quasi-independently will present to the ED for traumatic injuries when there is some change in their routine or environment to which they cannot easily adapt (such as icy roads or sidewalks) [5–8]. Since most dementias progress gradually, family members who have had infrequent contact with the patient may bring in a patient with previously undiagnosed dementia for seemingly "new" mental status changes. Critically, dementia differs from delirium based on its stable, rather than fluctuating course, although this can be very difficult to discern without the aid of a caregiver who is very familiar with the patient [9–11].

The most common dementias, Alzheimer's disease and vascular dementia, are likely multifactorial in nature, whereas many other dementias, such as Lewy body disease, are largely genetic in etiology. However, there are several potentially reversible causes of dementia of which physicians should be aware, among them normal pressure hydrocephalus (NPH), Wernicke–Korsakoff syndrome, and B12 deficiency [4, 12]. Most cases of NPH are idiopathic in nature (the only known risk factor is increasing age). This condition can also occur as a sequelae of prior head trauma, neurosurgery, or intracranial hemorrhage, though the time course between the instigating event and the development of symptoms can be variable [13, 14]. Wernicke's encephalopathy and Korsakoff's syndrome are two related clinical entities that are caused by a chronic deficiency of thiamine. Due to the very limited reserves of thiamine in the body, clinically significant levels of thiamine deficiency can develop within a few weeks. Within the general population,

the deficiency is most commonly linked to alcohol consumption. However, particularly relevant to the geriatric population is that thiamine deficiency can also be brought on by chronic malnutrition, illnesses with prolonged diarrhea or vomiting, malignancies, and dialysis [15]. Chronic deficiency of vitamin B12 is common in the elderly population and is directly linked to the development of neuropsychiatric symptoms [16]. A number of potential risk factors exist for B12 deficiency, including chronic malnutrition (such as the "tea and toast" diet or a strict vegetarian diet), bowel surgeries such as ileal resection, chronic alcohol consumption, chronic H. Pylori infection, and a number of genetic mutations that predispose patients to poor B12 absorption. Another risk factor for B12 deficiency affecting a large segment of the elderly population is long-term antacid use (both H2 blockers and PPIs (proton pump inhibitors)) [17].

Features common to all dementias are anterograde amnesia, followed by the eventual development of poor concentration and attention, and the gradual loss of executive function and inhibition. While this order fits many types of dementia, some forms of dementia, such as Lewy body dementia, exhibit changes in cognition and personality much earlier in the disease course [18].

NPH is clinically manifested by impaired cognition (particularly poor memory and concentration), a shuffling gait, and urinary or fecal incontinence. The gait found in NPH is characterized by a broad base with turned-out toes, small steps, and en bloc turning (turning around in three or more steps) [12].

Wernicke's encephalopathy is characterized by a triad of ophthalmoplegia, ataxia, and confusion; however, a minority of patients with Wernicke's encephalopathy actually present with the full triad. The most common presentation is some form of confusion or mental status changes [19]. The nature of the mental status changes is quite broad and can encompass diminished levels of attention, hallucinosis suggestive of psychosis, to stupor and even coma [15, 20]. In addition, there are many different kinds of ophthalmoplegia that may manifest with this syndrome, ranging from nystagmus to focal palsies of extraocular motions [21]. The combination of symptoms can often be difficult to distinguish from alcohol intoxication or delirium. In fact, it is estimated that the great majority of cases of Wernicke's encephalopathy are missed by clinicians [22].

Korsakoff's syndrome (or psychosis) is the irreversible end-state of thiamine deficiency. It is characterized by anterograde amnesia and a loss of working memory that is significantly out of proportion to deficits in concentration and attention, while established long-term memories tend to be preserved. Also notable are an apathetic or flat affect and a tendency toward confabulation, although the degree of confusion can be lesser than that of acute Wernicke's encephalopathy [15, 23].

Vitamin B12 deficiency presents with a constellation of symptoms, most commonly extremity paresthesias and weakness. More acute myelopathies, such as subacute combined degeneration of the dorsal column of the spinal cord, can result in a much more profound loss of sensation and proprioception as the disease progresses [24]. A variety of neuropsychiatric symptoms, including depression, memory loss, poor concentration, and even frank psychosis, may develop as a result of B12 deficiency and independently of other symptoms [25].

Although the diagnosis of dementia is primarily drawn from the history and clinical examination, there are a variety of useful screening tools. The Mini-Mental State Examination is a well-validated test for cognitive impairment with good sensitivity and specificity [26], but at 5–10 min to perform, can be quite time-consuming in the emergency setting [27]. Notably, as the test is standardized, it can be administered by a midlevel practitioner or other provider with adequate training. A shorter test with immediate application to the emergency setting is the Blessed Orientation Memory Concentration test, which consists of only six items and does not require drawing or other written input from the patient [28, 29].

NPH is primarily diagnosed via neuroimaging, such as a noncontrast head computed tomography (CT) scan imaging study. Lumbar puncture has been used historically as a means of diagnosing NPH, with evaluations of gait before and directly after removal of high volumes of cerebrospinal fluid (CSF). Improvement after lumbar puncture has a high positive-predictive value for patients who will improve with further surgical management; however, this procedure has a very high false-negative rate and should not be used as the definitive test for NPH [30].

Megaloblastic anemia suggests the possibility of thiamine or B12 deficiency, but significant neurologic and psychiatric effects may be present without anemia, particularly in B12 deficiency [31]. While there is no universally agreed on regimen for thiamine supplementation in patients suffering from Wernicke's encephalopathy, admission for multiple doses of parenteral thiamine is recommended [32–34].

Depression

Depression is the most widespread psychiatric condition affecting the elderly and is found in a significant number of elderly patients presenting to the ED. Although its exact prevalence remains debated, it has been proved to be a significant contributor to all-cause mortality and the increased use of health-care resources, even when controlling for comorbidities and in subjects who did not meet full diagnostic criteria for major depression [35–40].

Depression can be hard to recognize in the acute setting and is frequently missed by nonpsychiatrists, including emergency physicians [38, 41]. Depressed patients will often present with generalized medical complaints such as weakness, poor sleep, or lack of appetite rather than explicitly mentioning depression [42]. Furthermore, pre-existing dementia or cognitive impairment may significantly hinder patients' abilities to communicate their symptoms [43, 44].

Poor health and disability are general risk factors for depression. In particular, cancer and Parkinson's disease are linked to significantly higher rates of depression than the general population, as well as coronary artery disease, stroke, and myocardial infarction (MI) (particularly within 1 year of the event) [45, 46]. Significant psychosocial stressors include bereavement (particularly after the loss of a spouse), physical disability, trauma or interpersonal violence, and a general lack of social contact and support [47].

The formal diagnosis of a major depressive episode encompasses five or more of the following symptoms for 2 weeks: depressed mood, anhedonia (loss of interest in or enjoyment of desirable activities), change in appetite, change in sleep habits, change in motor activity, decreased feelings of self-worth, poor concentration, and thoughts of death or suicide [9]. While these are the formal criteria, a patient with any of these signs should be assessed seriously, as minor episodes of depression can contribute to poor health and even suicide. A notable change from previous guidelines is that recent bereavement is no longer considered to be an exclusion from the diagnosis of depression [48].

Just as patients with depression need not meet all of the formal criteria, screening for depressed elderly patients does not need to encompass an exhaustive psychiatric evaluation by the physician. A number of tools have been developed for the rapid recognition of depression in the ED, such as the Emergency Department Depression Screening Instrument (ED-DSI). The ED-DSI is composed of three yes-or-no questions – Do you often feel sad or depressed? Do you often feel helpless? Do you often feel downhearted and blue? – a yes to any question constitutes a positive screen. A positive screen should trigger a more in-depth evaluation of a patient's symptoms, supports, substance use, and risks for suicidality [49, 50].

Substance abuse

Substance abuse remains prevalent throughout the elderly population; however, its diagnosis and detection can be extremely difficult. It has been widely held that substance abuse problems tend to "age out" of the population over time, and while some studies estimate rates of alcoholism in the elderly as lower than the general population, these estimates vary substantially, and alcohol is a significant factor in many hospitalizations for this population.

Substance abuse often manifests as falls and other accidents. Unfortunately, these are common presenting complaints in a population with increasing sarcopenia and declining motor control, thus physicians should not be in the habit of assuming that all falls are the result of mere decrepitude. Similarly, more serious complications of substance abuse, such as alcoholic hallucinosis, can be mistaken for manifestations of more chronic issues, like "sundowning" in dementia.

Alcohol abuse in the elderly reflects two major populations of drinkers, early-onset and late-onset. Early-onset drinkers often have significant comorbid psychiatric disease, and frequently experience major chronic complications of their alcohol consumption. These drinkers may have adapted to hiding their addictions well over time or may simply have advantageous genetics. Late-onset drinkers are much more likely to begin their abuse around the time of significant stressors, such as bereavement, retirement, or disability [51].

Elderly patients are at particular risk of harm from prescription medication abuse or misuse. Both opiates and benzodiazepines are frequently prescribed for the elderly, despite the fact that the elderly are less able to metabolize these drugs and more likely to suffer significant psychiatric and neurologic side effects [52].

Although rates of alcoholism and illicit drug use among the elderly are much lower than that of the general population, a number of authors theorize that this is fundamentally a cultural phenomenon and that these rates may shift significantly over time with the aging of the baby boom generation, which has a much more permissive attitude toward substance use [51, 53].

The fundamental means by which physicians can identify substance abuse problems in elderly patients is to look for them. All geriatric trauma patients should be asked directly about substance use. While there are many validated methods of assessing alcohol abuse, the established four-question CAGE screening test (Have you ever tried to cut down on your drinking? Do you become annoyed when others ask you about your drinking? Do you ever feel guilty about your drinking? Have you ever used alcohol in the morning as an "eye-opener?") remains a brief but useful tool for screening, and longer, more specific questionnaires such as the Short Michigan Alcohol Screening Test–Geriatric Version (SMAST-GV) may be used when suspicion is high [52]. Unfortunately, a similarly validated screening tool for screening for the use of cocaine or other illicit substances in the elderly does not exist, thus a careful history remains essential [54].

Caregivers and family members should be asked straightforward questions about patients' substance use in a nonthreatening manner. Caregivers may serve as unwitting enablers of substance abuse and may either fail to recognize problematic behavior or perceive it as a natural response to the ills of growing old [51]. For demented patients, caregivers should be asked about substance use as it can lead to an even higher likelihood of falling in this population [55].

Comatose patients may be suffering from opiate or benzodiazepine overdose. Do not hesitate to undertake a trial of narcan in these patients. Similarly, consider alcohol or benzodiazepine withdrawal in all patients with delirium, particularly when there is an evidence of significant autonomic instability.

While elderly patients who present with significant falls should undergo neuroimaging (generally a noncontrast head CT), this is doubly important when alcohol use is suspected due to the high correlation of alcoholism and the development of subdural hematomas. Do not hesitate to send blood and urine screens for drugs of abuse. Scrutinize basic chemistries for evidence of hyponatremia, hypokalemia, and hypomagnesemia, as well as complete blood counts for evidence of megaloblastic anemia, all of which may result from alcohol abuse.

Psychosis

Although psychosis is a more common manifestation of psychiatric disease in the elderly population than the general population, as it is prevalent in many serious medical illnesses, new psychosis in elderly patients merits a comprehensive medical workup [56].

Psychosis is characterized by a persistent disruption of logical thought and bizarre behavior. This often manifests as delusions (fixed, false beliefs), hallucinations (unusual sensory input), illogical thought processes and speech, and agitation. Psychosis may be a primary symptom of schizophrenia, the result of medical disease as a manifestation of delirium, or they may accompany psychiatric conditions such as major depression or bipolar disorder. A correct diagnosis of new schizophrenia after age 65 is quite rare. Psychosis is much more common in patients with dementia, and hallucinations, delusions, and paranoid behavior may also occur throughout the progression of dementia [1, 57].

While the greatest risk factor for geriatric psychosis is dementia, a number of risk factors are potentially reversible. Social isolation has been closely linked to geriatric psychosis. Similarly, persistent auditory and visual impairment has been implicated in the risk for psychosis [58]. Together, these suggest that both social and sensory deprivation are critical risks for the development of geriatric psychosis [59]. Polypharmacy and substance abuse are also strongly linked to psychosis risk [58].

In the acute setting, psychosis and agitation are best managed via a combination of environmental and pharmacologic interventions. Patients with psychotic symptoms should have as few invasive lines and leads (tethers) as possible. These patients should similarly be evaluated in quieter and less stimulating areas of the ED, if feasible. Family members and caregivers should remain with the patient, and every effort should be made to ensure that these patients are able to use assistive devices such as glasses and hearing aids when needed [60].

Although psychosis is more common in the geriatric population, new onset psychosis is the result of a medical or toxicologic cause until proven otherwise. Patients with new onset psychosis should undergo a broad infectious workup (e.g., urinalysis and chest X-ray study), as well as serum chemistries, EKG, and neuroimaging.

Suicide

Suicidal ideation should be considered an imminent threat to elderly patients, on par with chest pain. Up to 70% of elderly patients who subsequently commit suicide will visit a physician in the month leading up to the event [61]. Despite this, older patients are much less likely to disclose their plans than younger patients who are having thoughts of suicide [62]. This is compounded by the fact that elderly patients who attempt to commit suicide do so with a much greater degree of planning than do younger patients and choose significantly more lethal means [63].

Depression and substance abuse are significant risk factors for suicide [61, 64]. Many chronic medical conditions are also risk factors and foremost among them is cancer. CHF (congestive heart failure), COPD (chronic obstructive pulmonary disease), and other illnesses leading to physical impairment are also associated with suicide [65, 66]. Suicide is generally more common among elders who are white, male, and unmarried or widowed [62].

Suicidal elders will often withhold suicidal ideation or plans and may not even admit depression [63]. Providers must ask patients who appear to be depressed or who demonstrate evidence of substance abuse directly about suicide. While there remain common misconceptions that asking about suicide may "plant" the idea in patients' heads, there is no evidence to support this idea [67]. Patients who acknowledge any ideation must be asked specifically whether they have a plan to commit suicide. Patients should also be asked about access to firearms, even if they do not mention thoughts of using them, due to the remarkable lethality of firearms and the frequency with which they are used in completed suicides [68].

A number of assessment methods have been developed for assessing suicide risk, including the modified SAD PERSONS score and the Manchester Self-Harm Rule. While both scales have been shown to help identify low-risk patients with suicidal ideation, they are limited by a lack of validation in multiple populations [69–71], and by the fact that geriatric patients are inherently at higher risk than the general population. More in-depth scales have been shown to have a greater accuracy, but they are limited by the need for truthful self-reporting. Furthermore, the most accurate assessments are likely those performed by an experienced psychologist or psychiatrist [69, 72].

Testing

In any patient with significant depression, psychosis, or suicidality, a full infectious and metabolic workup (encompassing basic chemistries, complete blood count, and urinalysis) is indicated in addition to a psychiatric evaluation. Patients with recent falls, new difficulty with gait, or significant changes in cognition or speech should undergo a noncontrast head CT scan, even if the onset of changes is gradual in nature.

Serum vitamin B12 and folate levels may be significantly reduced in their respective deficiencies; however, levels should not be used to guide initial therapy in the ED. Patients may have symptomatic B12 deficiency with normal serum B12 levels, and folate levels are unlikely to return in time to prevent the potentially irreversible progression of Wernicke's encephalopathy. Clinicians concerned for either deficiency should initiate treatment prior to the availability of test results [24, 73].

Disposition

Patients with newly diagnosed dementia or cognitive impairment may often benefit from the intervention of a caseworker or social worker in order to assess the need for assistive services and the relative safety of their home environment; however, in the absence of infection or significant trauma, they do not require admission for immediate evaluation of their dementia. Although it might seem commonsense, patients who are found to have dementia or any other significant cognitive impairment should not be driving, and this should be emphasized with their family or caregivers [74].

Patients with depression and evidence of an inability to care for themselves – such as significant malnutrition – should either be admitted to an inpatient facility or arrangements made for thorough and immediate medical and psychiatric care. Patients with depression but without suicidal ideation may be discharged, but primary care and psychiatric follow-up is essential [75].

Patients with frank suicidal ideation should either be directly admitted to a psychiatric facility or at least fully evaluated by a psychiatrist or psychologist. While the practice of having a patient sign a "safety contract" to determine if safe for discharge is widespread, there is minimal evidence to support the efficacy of this practice in preventing suicide, or in providing legal protection to physicians [76].

Section IV: Decision-making

- Patients with evidence of new mental status changes should have a comprehensive infectious and metabolic workup (basic chemistries, complete blood count, and urinalysis) and consideration of neuroimaging.
- NPH is diagnosed via CT scan and via clinical examination – lumbar puncture results should not be the primary means of diagnosis.
- B12 and thiamine deficiency should be treated without awaiting serum levels. Thiamine deficiency is time-sensitive, and clinicians should not hesitate to begin parenteral thiamine supplementation.
- Screen for substance use when interviewing all elderly patients and their caregivers. Consider substance abuse as a potential contributor to all geriatric traumas. Send a toxicology screen when you are concerned for substance abuse, and do not assume that a patient is "too old" to use drugs or alcohol.
- Suicidal ideation or planning in elderly patients is a critical element of the history and patients expressing either should be seen by a mental provider.
- Patients with newly diagnosed dementia or cognitive impairment should not drive.

References

1 Piechniczek-Buczek, J. (2006) Psychiatric emergencies in the elderly population. *Emerg. Med. Clin. North Am.*, 24 (2), 467–490.
2 Harlein, J., Dassen, T., Halfens, R.J., and Heinze, C. (2009) Fall risk factors in older people with dementia or cognitive impairment: a systematic review. *J. Adv. Nurs.*, 65 (5), 922–933.

3 Keene, J., Hope, T., Fairburn, C.G., and Jacoby, R. (2001) Death and dementia. *Int. J. Geriatr. Psychiatry*, **16** (**10**), 969–974.

4 Thies, W. and Bleiler, L. (2013) 2013 Alzheimer's disease facts and figures Alzheimer's Association. *Alzheimers Dement.*, **9** (**2**), 208–245.

5 Van Doorn, C., Gruber-Baldini, A.L., Zimmerman, S. *et al.* (2003) Dementia as a risk factor for falls and fall injuries among nursing home residents. *J. Am. Geriatr. Soc.*, **51** (**9**), 1213–1218.

6 Gillespie, L. and Handoll, H. (2009) Prevention of falls and fall-related injuries in older people. *Inj. Prev.*, **15** (**5**), 354–355.

7 Talbot, L.A., Musiol, R.J., Witham, E.K., and Metter, E.J. (2005) Falls in young, middle-aged and older community dwelling adults: perceived cause, environmental factors and injury. *BMC Public Health*, **5** (**1**), 86.

8 Ytterstad, B. (1999) The Harstad injury prevention study: the characteristics and distribution of fractures amongst elders--an eight year study. *Int. J. Circumpolar Health*, **58** (**2**), 84.

9 American Psychiatric Association (2000) *Diagnostic and Statistical Manual of Mental Disorders: DSM-IV-TR*, American Psychiatric Publishing.

10 Fick, D.M., Agostini, J.V., and Inouye, S.K. (2002) Delirium superimposed on dementia: a systematic review. *J. Am. Geriatr. Soc.*, **50** (**10**), 1723–1732.

11 Inouye, S.K. (2006) Delirium in older persons. *N. Engl. J. Med.*, **354** (**11**), 1157–1165.

12 Graff-Radford, N.R. (2007) Normal pressure hydrocephalus. *Neurol. Clin.*, **25** (**3**), 809–832.

13 Mazzini, L., Campini, R., Angelino, E. *et al.* (2003) Post-traumatic hydrocephalus: a clinical, neuroradiologic, and neuropsychologic assessment of long-term outcome. *Arch. Phys. Med. Rehabil.*, **84** (**11**), 1637–1641.

14 Tribl, G. and Oder, W. (2000) Outcome after shunt implantation in severe head injury with post-traumatic hydrocephalus. *Brain Inj.*, **14** (**4**), 345–354.

15 Sechi, G. and Serra, A. (2007) Wernicke's encephalopathy: new clinical settings and recent advances in diagnosis and management. *Lancet Neurol.*, **6** (**5**), 442–455.

16 Pennypacker, L.C., Allen, R.H., Kelly, J.P. *et al.* (1992) High prevalence of cobalamin deficiency in elderly outpatients. *J. Am. Geriatr. Soc.*, **40**, 1197–1204.

17 Andres, E., Loukili, N.H., Noel, E. *et al.* (2004) Vitamin B12 (cobalamin) deficiency in elderly patients. *Can. Med. Assoc. J.*, **171** (**3**), 251–259.

18 McKeith, I., Mintzer, J., Aarsland, D. *et al.* (2004) Dementia with Lewy bodies. *Lancet Neurol.*, **3** (**1**), 19–28.

19 Cook, C. (2000) Prevention and treatment of Wernicke–Korsakoff syndrome. *Alcohol Alcohol.*, **35** (**Suppl. 1**), 19–20.

20 Jiang, W., Gagliardi, J.P., Raj, Y.P. *et al.* (2006) Acute psychotic disorder after gastric bypass surgery: differential diagnosis and treatment. *Am. J. Psychiatry*, **163** (**1**), 15–19.

21 Kulkarni, S., Lee, A.G., Holstein, S.A., and Warner, J.E. (2005) You are what you eat. *Surv. Ophthalmol.*, **50** (**4**), 389–393.

22 Isenberg-Grzeda, E., Kutner, H.E., and Nicolson, S.E. (2012) Wernicke–Korsakoff-syndrome: under-recognized and under-treated. *Psychosomatics*, **53** (**6**), 507–516.

23 Kopelman, M.D. (1985) Rates of forgetting in Alzheimer-type dementia and Korsakoff's syndrome. *Neuropsychologia*, **23** (**5**), 623–638.

24 Oh, R. and Brown, D.L. (2003) Vitamin B12 deficiency. *Am. Fam. Physician*, **67** (**5**), 979–986.

25 Chatterjee, A., Yapundich, R., Palmer, C.A. *et al.* (1996) Leukoencephalopathy associated with cobalamin deficiency. *Neurology*, **46** (**3**), 832–834.

26 Folstein, M.F., Folstein, S.E., and McHugh, P.R. (1975) "Mini-mental state": a practical method for grading the cognitive state of patients for the clinician. *J. Psychiatry Res.*, **12** (**3**), 189–198.

27 Adelman, A.M. and Daly, M.P. (2005) Initial evaluation of the patient with suspected dementia. *Am. Fam. Physician*, **71** (**9**), 1745–1750.

28 Goring, H., Baldwin, R., Marriott, A. *et al.* (2004) Validation of short screening tests for depression and cognitive impairment in older medically ill inpatients. *Int. J. Geriatr. Psychiatry*, **19** (**5**), 465–471.

29 Hustey, F.M. and Meldon, S.W. (2002) The prevalence and documentation of impaired mental status in elderly emergency department patients. *Ann. Emerg. Med.*, **39** (**3**), 248–253.

30 Walchenbach, R., Geiger, E., Thomeer, R., and Vanneste, J. (2002) The value of temporary external lumbar CSF drainage in predicting the outcome of shunting on normal pressure hydrocephalus. *J. Neurol. Neurosurg. Psychiatry*, **72** (**4**), 503–506.

31 Lindenbaum, J., Healton, E.B., Savage, D.G. *et al.* (1988) Neuropsychiatric disorders caused by cobalamin deficiency in the absence of anemia or macrocytosis. *N. Engl. J. Med.*, **318** (**26**), 1720–1728.

32 Day, E., Bentham, P.W., Callaghan, R. *et al.* (2013) Thiamine for prevention and treatment of Wernicke-Korsakoff Syndrome in people who abuse alcohol. *Cochrane Database Syst. Rev.*, **7** (Art No.: CD004033). doi: 10.1002/14651858.CD004033.pub3

33 Galvin, R., Bråthen, G., Ivashynka, A. *et al.* (2010) EFNS guidelines for diagnosis, therapy and prevention of Wernicke encephalopathy. *Eur. J. Neurol.*, **17** (**12**), 1408–1418.

34 Thomson, A., Cook, C.C., Touquet, R. *et al.* (2002) The Royal College of Physicians report on alcohol: guidelines

for managing Wernicke's encephalopathy in the accident and emergency department. *Alcohol Alcohol.*, 37 (6), 513–521.

35 Borson, S., Barnes, R.A., Kukull, W.A., and Okimoto, J.T. (1986) Symptomatic depression in elderly medical outpatients: I. Prevalence, demography, and health service utilization. *J. Am. Geriatr. Soc.*, 34, 341–347.

36 Katon, W.J. (2003) Clinical and health services relationships between major depression, depressive symptoms, and general medical illness. *Biol. Psychiatry*, 54 (3), 216–226.

37 Luber, M.P., Meyers, B.S., Williams-Russo, P.G. *et al.* (2001) Depression and service utilization in elderly primary care patients. *Am. J. Geriatr. Psychiatry*, 9 (2), 169–176.

38 Meldon, S.W., Emerman, C.L., Schubert, D.S. *et al.* (1997) Depression in geriatric ED patients: prevalence and recognition. *Ann. Emerg. Med.*, 30 (2), 141–145.

39 Penninx, B.W., Geerlings, S.W., Deeg, D.J. *et al.* (1999) Minor and major depression and the risk of death in older persons. *Arch. Gen. Psychiatry*, 56 (10), 889.

40 Press, Y., Tandeter, H., Romem, P. *et al.* (2012) Depressive symptomatology as a risk factor for increased health service utilization among elderly patients in primary care. *Arch. Gerontol. Geriatr.*, 54 (1), 127–130.

41 Cole, M.G. (2008) Recognition of depression by non-psychiatric physicians, a systematic literature review and meta-analysis. *J. Gen. Intern. Med.*, 23 (1), 25–36.

42 Gallo, J.J., Rabins, P., and Anthony, J. (1999) Sadness in older persons: 13-year follow-up of a community sample in Baltimore, Maryland. *Psychol. Med.*, 29 (2), 341–350.

43 Jones, R.N., Marcantonio, E.R., and Rabinowitz, T. (2003) Prevalence and correlates of recognized depression in US nursing homes. *J. Am. Geriatr. Soc.*, 51 (10), 1404–1409.

44 Starkstein, S.E., Jorge, R., Mizrahi, R., and Robinson, R.G. (2005) The construct of minor and major depression in Alzheimer's disease. *Am. J. Psychiatry*, 162 (11), 2086–2093.

45 Carney, R.M. and Freedland, K.E. (2008) Depression in patients with coronary heart disease. *Am. J. Med.*, 121 (11), S20–S27.

46 Spiegel, D. and Giese-Davis, J. (2003) Depression and cancer: mechanisms and disease progression. *Biol. Psychiatry*, 54 (3), 269–282.

47 Bruce, M.L. (2002) Psychosocial risk factors for depressive disorders in late life. *Biol. Psychiatry*, 52 (3), 175–184.

48 Pies, R.W. (2009) Depression and the pitfalls of causality: implications for DSM-V. *J. Affect. Disord.*, 116 (1), 1–3.

49 Fabacher, D.A., Raccio-Robak, N., McErlean, M.A. *et al.* (2002) Validation of a brief screening tool to detect depression in elderly ED patients. *Am. J. Emerg. Med.*, 20 (2), 99–102.

50 Lee, V., Wong, T., and Lau, C. (2006) Validation of a 3-item screening tool for geriatric depression in the observation unit of an emergency department. *Hong Kong J. Emerg. Med.*, 13 (1), 17–23.

51 Benshoff, J.J., Harrawood, L.K., and Koch, D.S. (2003) Substance abuse and the elderly: unique issues and concerns. *J. Rehabil.*, 69 (2), 43–48.

52 Culberson, J.W. (2006) Alcohol use in the elderly: beyond the CAGE. Part 2: screening instruments and treatment strategies. *Geriatrics*, 61 (11), 20.

53 Gfroerer, J., Penne, M., Pemberton, M., and Folsom, R. (2003) Substance abuse treatment need among older adults in 2020: the impact of the aging baby-boom cohort. *Drug Alcohol Depend.*, 69 (2), 127–135.

54 Burgos-Chapman, I. and Piechniczek-Buczek, J. (2013) Cocaine use in elder adults: a focus on recognition and risk factors. *Am. J. Geriatr. Psychiatry*, 21, S125.

55 Ataollahi Eshkoor, S., Hamid, T.A., Hassan Nudin, S.S., and Yoke Mun, C. (2014) Does substance abuse contribute to further risk of falls in dementia. *Aging Neuropsychol. Cogn.*, 21 (3), 317–324.

56 Solai, L.K.K. (2013) Late-life psychosis, in *Geriatric Psychiatry* (eds M.D. Miller and K.S. Laith Kumar), Oxford University Press, New York, pp. 237–247.

57 Holroyd, S. and Laurie, S. (1999) Correlates of psychotic symptoms among elderly outpatients. *Int. J. Geriatr. Psychiatry*, 14 (5), 379–384.

58 Zayas, E.M. and Grossberg, G.T. (1998) The treatment of psychosis in late life. *J. Clin. Psychiatry*, 59, 5–10.

59 Madhusoodanan, S., Ibrahim, F.A., and Malik, A. (2010) Primary prevention in geriatric psychiatry. *Ann. Clin. Psychiatry*, 22 (4), 249–261.

60 Karim, S. and Byrne, E.J. (2005) Treatment of psychosis in elderly people. *Adv. Psychiatr. Treat.*, 11 (4), 286–296.

61 Conwell, Y. (2001) Suicide in later life: a review and recommendations for prevention. *Suicide Life Threat. Behav.*, 31 (s1), 32–47.

62 Conwell, Y., Duberstein, P.R., and Caine, E.D. (2002) Risk factors for suicide in later life. *Biol. Psychiatry*, 52 (3), 193–204.

63 Pearson, J.L. and Brown, G.K. (2000) Suicide prevention in late life: directions for science and practice. *Clin. Psychol. Rev.*, 20 (6), 685–705.

64 Blow, F.C., Brockmann, L.M., and Barry, K.L. (2004) Role of alcohol in late-life suicide. *Alcohol. Clin. Exp. Res.*, 28 (s1), 48S–56S.

65 Juurlink, D.N., Herrmann, N., Szalai, J.P. *et al.* (2004) Medical illness and the risk of suicide in the elderly. *Arch. Intern. Med.*, 164 (11), 1179.

66 Miller, M., Mogun, H., Azrael, D. *et al.* (2008) Cancer and the risk of suicide in older Americans. *J. Clin. Oncol.*, **26** (**29**), 4720–4724.

67 Buzan, R.D. and Weissberg, M.P. (1992) Suicide: risk factors and therapeutic considerations in the emergency department. *J. Emerg. Med.*, **10** (**3**), 335–343.

68 Conwell, Y., Duberstein, P.R., Connor, K. *et al.* (2002) Access to firearms and risk for suicide in middle-aged and older adults. *Am. J. Geriatr. Psychiatry*, **10** (**4**), 407–416.

69 Cochrane-Brink, K.A., Lofchy, J.S., and Sakinofsky, I. (2000) Clinical rating scales in suicide risk assessment. *Gen. Hosp. Psychiatry*, **22** (**6**), 445–451.

70 Hockberger, R.S. and Rothstein, R.J. (1988) Assessment of suicide potential by nonpsychiatrists using the SAD PERSONS score. *J. Emerg. Med.*, **6** (**2**), 99–107.

71 Ronquillo, L., Minassian, A., Vilke, G.M., and Wilson, M.P. (2012) Literature-based recommendations for suicide assessment in the emergency department: a review. *J. Emerg. Med.*, **43**, 836–842.

72 Pokorny, A.D. (1983) Prediction of suicide in psychiatric patients: report of a prospective study. *Arch. Gen. Psychiatry*, **40** (**3**), 249.

73 Donnino, M.W., Vega, J., Miller, J., and Walsh, M. (2007) Myths and misconceptions of Wernicke's encephalopathy: what every emergency physician should know. *Ann. Emerg. Med.*, **50** (**6**), 715–721.

74 Rapoport, M.J., Herrmann, N., Molnar, F. *et al.* (2008) Psychotropic medications and motor vehicle collisions in patients with dementia. *J. Am. Geriatr. Soc.*, **56** (**10**), 1968–1970.

75 Bruce, M.L., Ten Have, T.R., Reynolds, C.F. III, *et al.* (2004) Reducing suicidal ideation and depressive symptoms in depressed older primary care patients. *J. Am. Med. Assoc.*, **291** (**9**), 1081–1091.

76 Garvey, K.A., Penn, J.V., Campbell, A.L. *et al.* (2009) Contracting for safety with patients: clinical practice and forensic implications. *J. Am. Acad. Psychiatry Law Online*, **37** (**3**), 363–370.

Acute abdominal pain in the elderly: Surgical causes

Katren Tyler & Maura Kennedy

[1] *Emergency Medicine Department, University of California, UC Davis Medical Center, Sacramento, CA, USA*
[2] *Department of Emergency Medicine, Beth Israel Deaconess Medical Center, Harvard Medical School, Boston, MA, USA*

Section I: Case Presentation

A 72-year-old man presented to the emergency department (ED) at 6:15 a.m. complaining of abdominal pain. The pain started overnight after eating Indian food. It was located in the midabdomen and did not radiate. On a 10-point scale, he rated his pain a "2," or mild. He denied nausea, vomiting, diarrhea, black or bloody stools. He was passing flatus. He denied chest pain, shortness of breath, and fever. As he felt "gassy," he tried taking simethicone, but it did not relieve his symptoms. He was accompanied by his wife, who had dinner at the same restaurant the prior night and felt well.

His past medical history was notable for hypertension, hypercholesterolemia, and COPD (chronic obstructive pulmonary disease). He had no prior abdominal surgeries. He was a former smoker, reported drinking one glass of wine daily, and denied any illicit drug use.

The vital signs were as follows: temperature 37.5°C, pulse 62 beats/min, blood pressure 155/78 mm Hg, respirations 16 breaths/min, and pulse oximetry 98%. The cardiac examination was notable for an irregular heart rhythm without obvious murmur. The pulmonary examination was normal. The abdomen was soft, nontender, and nondistended. There was mild edema of the lower extremities bilaterally. The rest of the physical examination was normal. An electrocardiogram (EKG) was obtained that demonstrated

sinus rhythm with frequent premature ventricular contractions (PVCs) but no acute ischemia. A CBC (complete blood count), complete metabolic panel with liver function tests, lipase, and UA (urinalysis) were normal. Chest and abdominal radiographs were normal.

Conclusion

The patient presented with mild abdominal pain, which he thought was related to the Indian food he had eaten the night prior. Laboratory and initial radiographs were normal. These tests were reported approximately 3 h after his arrival. On reevaluation, he reported the abdominal pain had increased in severity, and was now radiating to his back. On repeat physical examination, he now had moderate tenderness to palpation in his midabdomen. A CT (computed tomography) scan of the abdomen and pelvis was subsequently obtained, which demonstrated a 5.5 cm leaking abdominal aortic aneurysm (AAA). He was started on an esmolol drip and transferred to a tertiary referral center, where he successfully underwent endovascular aneurysms repair (EVAR) of the AAA.

Section II: Case discussion

Peter Rosen: I think the first obligation in trying to deal with abdominal pain in the elderly is to try and get some impression of how well they look. It doesn't sound like this guy looked very sick at all.

Maura Kennedy No, he looked quite well. He said that he had experienced symptoms like this before when he'd eaten Indian food. He figured it was the Indian food, but he decided he would just get checked out. He did not appear at all uncomfortable and was sitting in bed quite comfortably with his wife at his bedside.

PR: You said he had no vomiting or diarrhea?

MK: Correct.

PR: Well, we all like to ascribe GI (gastrointestinal) upset to ethnic foods, particularly if we're not fond of that particular ethnic food, and our spouse is. But, in fact, it's pretty rare for food to cause prolonged symptoms unless it's accompanied by vomiting and diarrhea, and is a true case of food poisoning, which it does not sound like this case is. Amal, do you want to comment on how you distinguish between a specific entity in a geriatric patient, or whether you have a general approach to these patients that is more global?

Amal Mattu: The elderly patient's initial evaluation can be very misleading, and the patients that come in looking really sick are oftentimes the easier patients. This is a more challenging patient because the patient doesn't look sick, and the real challenge is trying to figure out whether there is some disastrous condition underlying his apparent well appearance. In younger people, I think clinical appearance is probably more reliable. A quick history and physical examination can oftentimes give you a fairly reliable risk-stratification of a person whom you could probably send home safely. But elderly patients are very deceiving in terms of what may appear to be a benign physical examination. Therefore, I have a much lower threshold to shotgun my workup in elderly patients who are coming in with abdominal pain, even if they may look relatively benign in appearance. I noticed that an EKG was done, and also an X-ray study was done early. We wouldn't do those in younger people with no complaints of chest pain. Nevertheless, in elderly patients, I would definitely get an EKG almost as part of the physical examination and also an early X-ray study looking for signs of a perforation even though the abdominal examination may not be all that bad.

PR: It's certainly a good policy to remember that acute MI (myocardial infarction) in the elderly often doesn't present with chest pain. As a matter of fact, when President Eisenhower had his first heart attack, he was treated for indigestion for 3 days, before cardiac problem finally declared itself. It is common for the elderly patient to complain of fatigue or abdominal pain or something totally unrelated to the cardiac system. Maura, one other physical examination question, was a rectal examination performed?

MK: A rectal examination was performed, it was guaiac negative.

PR: Rob, would you discuss whether we need to do rectal examinations on every patient with abdominal pain?

Rob Anderson: A chief complaint of abdominal pain in the elderly is really a big deal and is associated with a significant mortality just coming through the door. This person is probably going to need laboratory tests, and at least two physical examinations at a minimum. What about a rectal examination in every patient with abdominal pain? It seems reasonable, especially in the elderly.

PR: Anyone else have an opinion about that?

Jon Mark Hirshon: I think that in a patient like this in whom you don't know which way he is going to go, you need to quickly collect as much data as possible. There's no reason not to do a rectal examination on this person based on what we have right now. You don't know if the patient is having a GI bleed, for example, and a certain number of rectal tumors are within reach of the examining finger.

PR: I think I overemphasize the importance of a rectal examination in younger patients, especially when the concern is appendicitis. I don't believe that anyone ever made the diagnosis of appendicitis from a rectal examination, unless the patient already had many other findings and a history to suggest that the patient was clearly perforated, and had an abscess long before the rectal was done. In the elderly patient, however, I would submit that it is mandatory. GI bleeding can be very subtle. I've seen many patients who have presented with what seemed like purely respiratory problems were actually having GI bleeds. We also have to understand that many older patients don't perceive pain quite as reliably as younger patients. That may be one of the reasons that appendicitis is so often perforated in the elderly patient before it's diagnosed.

Andrew Chang In elderly patients, their pain perception changes, and probably decreases, and tends to be more visceral and poorly localized, compared to younger patients. It is much less dramatic, which makes it more difficult for us as clinicians to localize and diagnose the pain. This is another reason to keep a broad differential diagnosis.

PR: I think the only useful historical finding for appendicitis that I've been able to determine is pain that starts somewhere and moves somewhere else. Elderly patients often present without much pain at all, but may suddenly complain of constipation and sometimes obstipation. That is, they want to have a bowel movement but can't. Vaishal, would you like to comment on how you would next sort out this case. Is there going to be anything that puts us on the right track in a hurry?

Vaishal Tolia: If the patient is well known to our system, I like to see what they've had done recently, especially when it comes to imaging. A lot of these patients will have had multiple CT scans or other evaluations – endoscopies, and so on. In general, I agree with the shotgun approach, but I think getting some of that prior data can be particularly helpful. Especially to assess the anatomy and to see if there's been any abnormality noted in the past. Getting that EKG right away is important.

PR: Maura, often elderly patients have been advised not to have surgery because they are deemed to be "too old to have elective surgery." I never understood why it was thought to be safer to have to do emergent rather than elective procedures. Did this patient ever have any such condition that he was told that he possessed but advised not to have surgery? I'm thinking in particular of the gallbladder or other vascular problems.

MK: No, he actually had never sought care for any significant abdominal issues. He denied any history of known gallstones. Per his report, he had never been diagnosed with diverticulitis or other intra-abdominal medical condition and had no prior abdominal surgeries, nor had he ever been referred to a surgeon for elective abdominal surgery.

PR: Amal, what do you feel about doing a screening ultrasound (US) examination on elderly patients with abdominal pain?

AM: I think that's a fantastic idea. Ultrasound has become second nature for so many emergency physicians so as to become a part of the initial evaluation. I would say it's something that I would highly recommend in any elderly patient presenting with abdominal pain. The most life-threatening thing that you're looking for is any evidence of AAA. Even if it doesn't tell you whether the patient's got a leaking AAA, simply knowing that somebody has an AAA and is symptomatic may provide enough justification for the surgeons to move aggressively with that patient. You can also take a look at the gallbladder and a few other abdominal structures. You can also take a look in the thorax for fluid and at the heart for pericardial effusions.

Shamai Grossman: Ultrasound findings might actually be enough to prompt the surgeon to take someone directly to the operating room. The other thing that I want to add to your prior comment is that elderly patients, I find, are particularly stoic, and they often have a sense of denial as to the severity of their symptoms. Often they delay presentation because of this. Often they will deny what prior physicians may have told them requires surgical intervention. For those reasons, I sometimes find that the history that the patient gives me needs to be taken "with a grain of salt." It is necessary to assume the worst as we generally do in emergency medicine, and even more so in the elderly, and conclude that an early aggressive approach must be made to diagnosis and management.

PR: We've been told that over 50% of patients that present to the ED with abdominal pain will never have a diagnosis made. I think that tends to be truer of younger patients. I think that what is true of older patients is that there's a much higher percentage of surgically prominent causes of abdominal pain and that many of these patients are, in fact, much sicker than they appear. Rob, would you like to comment on how you diagnose aneurysm in addition to the ultrasound?

RA: In elderly folks presenting with abdominal pain, a third of them will need surgery. The most important step in diagnosing aortic aneurysm is to think of it and look for it. I had an 85-year-old woman who came in after a fall complaining of flank pain. It was tempting to have written her off as musculoskeletal pain, but we put the ultrasound probe on her belly, and her aorta was rupturing under our probe. She immediately went to the OR (open repair) and survived. Just thinking about the possibility is the most important first step. Ultrasound is great, but you often need to go to CT scan to make the definitive diagnosis, often with contrast. I would not use an magnetic resonance imaging (MRI) in the ED to make the diagnosis.

PR: The physical examination is not as helpful as one would wish. Purportedly 25% of aneurysms are palpable, but I believe that the true incidence of palpable aneurysms is much lower than that. The reason is that the aneurysm is quite soft. It's filled with kind of a toothpaste-like material, and even though there can be a large mass, it can be difficult to palpate. They also often don't present with a diminution of peripheral pulses as you do with some other vascular problems, although the distal pulses are certainly worth feeling to see if they are equal. When you look at the plain film of the abdomen, you can sometimes see the wall of the aorta in an aneurysm because it's calcified, although it may not show up on a posterior-anterior (PA) view, and we often forget to do a lateral on our plain abdominal films. It is sometimes hard to see the aneurysm on the ultrasound because of the patient's obesity. In answer to Shamai's point about it's very hard to get the surgeons to go directly to the operating room, I think that's an essential truth, but since we're not the ones that have to take responsibility for doing the surgery, my approach has been to not try to get too upset about this, but certainly to communicate the seriousness of what we're looking at, and leave it up to the surgeon whether they want other imaging studies prior to taking the patient to the operating room.

MK: The newest treatment of AAA involves an increasing use of endovascular repair. From the perspective of many of our vascular surgeons, a CT scan provides them with really important information for preoperative planning. While an ultrasound might be a quick way to make the diagnosis, the CT imaging is needed in order to decide the size of the graft to use, and other information that will help them in their planning.

VT: One of the questions you should ask the patient early on in taking your history is whether he's ever had an ultrasound study. He is 72, and he has a smoking history. The United States Preventive Services Task Force says that anyone over the age of 65 should have a screening ultrasound, especially if they have a smoking history.

AC: Sometimes calcification of an AAA can be picked up on a lateral abdominal X-ray study, but we are more often going to rely on ultrasound images or CT scan to make the diagnosis.

PR: Rob, I would like you to comment on the other vascular problem that is much more devastating in many ways than an aneurysm, and that is mesenteric thrombosis or mesenteric embolization. These patients are often difficult to diagnose. Do you have any particular clues on when you would select angiography to look for them?

RA: There are multiple different causes of ischemia that can occur in the GI tract. They all often present with diarrhea as their primary presentation. The four different types of ischemia would be chronic mesenteric ischemia with pain after eating, acute mesenteric ischemia that you're referring to, venous thrombosis, and finally ischemic colitis. What is common to all of them is that they can present with diarrhea.

AM: This is another place where the EKG is helpful to assess for atrial fibrillation in a patient like this, with an irregular heart rate, which would put him at a much higher risk of mesenteric ischemia from an embolism if he is not anticoagulated.

PR: Thank you, that's an excellent point. The only clue that I've been able to determine is that many of these patients with mesenteric vascular disease look sicker than their abdominal examination would support. Often it's just a matter of thinking of the disease. Maura, you had said earlier, the possibility of diverticulitis. I find that this is a diagnosis that seems to be much more commonly made, perhaps now that we have CT scans that find the disease earlier, but this would not be a bad presentation for someone with diverticulitis. Would you just speak briefly on what you would do next to support that diagnosis?

MK: In retrospect, there are a lot of diagnoses including diverticulitis that this patient could be having. With visceral pain being more common than somatic pain in geriatric patients, it may not localize to the left lower quadrant like you might expect. I think this is just another indication of why early use of CT scans is probably warranted in many older patients with abdominal pain. Ultimately, a CT scan can markedly change the disposition, both in terms of whether someone needs to be admitted, needs an operation, or can be discharged home. The downside is that the geriatric patient is at a higher risk of renal complications from intravenous contrast. Looking back on this case, an earlier CT scan would have been helpful in diagnosing the etiology of his abdominal pain, including diverticulitis.

RA: I just want to say a quick thing about early closure with a UA on older folks too. With diverticulitis, you can have irritation of the bladder or ureter causing pyuria, and hematuria, and if you get that UA and think you're dealing with a urinary tract issue rather than something more serious, it can cause you to miss the more serious entity.

SG: Moreover, there are many patients in whom the UA shows what appears to be a simple urinary tract infection, and yet the patient turns out to have a far more serious and ominous diagnosis.

JMH: I think one of the important things that this case highlights is the assistance of the tincture of time and serial examinations. Therefore, we will do a lot of imaging on someone like this who has a relatively non-specific but concerning type of story, but we also have a little time to watch them and see how they progress. On the initial presentation, they will be neither black nor white, so in my gray box I'm going to be aggressive in working them up. Moreover, this is one of the patients who I'm going to go back to multiple times to see how he is doing, and to be sure that his clinical status hasn't changed for the worse.

PR: Amal, would you comment on routine placement of intravenous lines in the elderly, and also, are there any other useful laboratory tests that you need early on in order to get a direct impression on which way to turn in a patient's care?

AM: Again, I'd again reemphasize my shotgun approach to elderly patients with abdominal pain. I have a very low threshold for testing broadly because the initial history and physical examination can oftentimes be very misleading. Moreover, I'd advocate IV placement early on, especially since you might end up needing to emergently resuscitate the patient if something disastrous happens. In terms of additional laboratory testing beyond the norm, in any patient with moderate-to-severe abdominal pain, I'd get a lactate level. I think in general that even though we are now overordering lactate levels, and

I've jokingly referred to lactate as the "white count of this decade," lactate levels in elderly patients are useful. They give you an indication of hypoperfusion even before the vital signs start going bad. Moreover, it turns out to be an early and sensitive marker for mesenteric ischemia as well. Certainly, I would agree with obtaining a CBC, chemistry, liver function tests, and a lipase.

PR: The only one that I would add, Amal, is a type and cross match. It will save time in the patient who has unrecognized active bleeding. Also, I would like to suggest that just as we have a broad approach to imaging and laboratory testing in these patients, we should just as routinely get the blood going in case the patient has an aneurysm that will require surgery.

AM: That's a great point.

PR: Maura, would you comment on how the course of this patient went, and what you would suggest on next for therapy other than definitive care?

MK: It fortunately took a number of hours for all of his X-ray studies and laboratory tests to be reported. Approximately 3 h after his arrival, all of his results were back and were normal. On reevaluation, he said that the pain had actually increased markedly, and he was now reporting pain radiating to his back and had moderate abdominal tenderness in the midabdomen. At that time, a CT scan of the abdomen and pelvis was obtained with IV contrast that showed a 5.5 cm leaking AAA. He was still mildly hypertensive and was started on an esmolol drip per the recommendations of the vascular surgeons. He was transferred to a tertiary referral center where he successfully underwent an endovascular repair of the aneurysm.

PR: Well, I think that's a rather small aneurysm to have suddenly bled, but that just shows that you can't totally rely on the size of the aneurysm for these patient's safety. Here is one of the places in which we're better off doing these patients electively as opposed to waiting for them to become emergencies. Does anyone else want to make some comments on final management for the patient? I think it was a very interesting case.

SG: Someone had asked whether to do a troponin on this patient prior to our discovering the etiology. I think it's a good question. We rule out patients often for truly trivial reasons particularly given older patients have frequent atypical presentations for myocardial ischemia. If I find that the EKG is unrevealing, and there is a compelling alternative diagnosis, then I wouldn't do serial troponins. On the other hand, if I don't have another more compelling diagnosis, then I'd be more inclined to ensure that this is not an acute myocardial event by doing serial troponin testing.

PR: Well, I think that the summary I would choose is that old people don't always look sick, they are much frailer than we think they are, they more often have serious disease as explanation for acute abdominal pain than younger patients, and they more often have surgical disease as an explanation for that. Therefore, we need to be quicker to be concerned about them, and we need to be more thorough in their imaging studies early on if we are going to hope to salvage them. Any last thoughts from anyone else?

RA: I think this is a fantastic case for that very reason; one could have easily been led down the incorrect "indigestion" pathway especially if a repeat physical examination by same provider had been skipped. An older person with abdominal pain will likely need at least two things: (1) they're probably going to need some sort of workup whether it's laboratory tests or imaging studies and (2) they're definitely going to need a reevaluation.

Section III: Concepts

Background

Abdominal pain is common in older patients, representing 5–10% of all ED visits in this age group [1, 2] and is in the top three presenting complaints for older adults [3]. As patients over 65 represent 15–20% of all ED visits [3], nontraumatic abdominal pain in the older patient population accounts for about 1% of all ED visits. The assessment of the cause of abdominal pain is complicated in older patients by many factors such as confounding comorbidities and medication use, challenges in history taking, age-related changes in pain sensation, and a broad differential diagnosis that includes both surgical and nonsurgical conditions [4–6]. This chapter focuses on surgical causes of abdominal pain.

Comorbidities are very common in the older population and have been reported in up to 94% of older patients presenting to the ED [7]. Some comorbidities come with warning bells: for instance, atrial fibrillation and abdominal pain raise the possibility of mesenteric ischemia. Other risks are less obvious: patients with chronic kidney disease have long-standing platelet dysfunction, which increases the risk of GI bleeding [8]. Obesity in older adults can obscure physical examination findings, increase the risk of chronic pain syndromes [9], and contribute to other comorbidities such as Type 2 diabetes mellitus, gastroesophageal reflux disease, and potentially cancer [10]. Delirium, dementia, and psychiatric illnesses such as depression may have an impact upon the evaluation of an elderly patient with acute abdominal pain.

Medication use may mask, precipitate, or complicate an acute abdominal pain presentation [2]. Oral anticoagulant and antiplatelet agents and nonsteroidal anti-inflammatory drugs (NSAIDs) may precipitate GI bleeding, and chronic opioid use may cause significant GI motility problems. In patients who are dehydrated, the use of biguanides such as metformin may cause life-threatening lactic acidosis, and NSAIDs and angiotensin-converting-enzyme (ACE) inhibitors can cause impairment of renal function [11].

As clinicians, we expect abdominal pain to be a cardinal feature in acute abdominal pathology; however, older patients with critical acute abdominal pathology may not complain of significant abdominal pain. Several life-threatening conditions such as peptic ulcer disease and acute MI are more likely to present "silently" in the older population compared with younger patients [12]. Visceral and somatic pains are subsets of nociceptive pain, which arises from actual or threatened damage to nonneural tissue and activation of pain receptors [13]. Visceral pain is usually caused by stretching, distention, inflammation, or ischemia, tends to be poorly localized, and is often associated with other systemic symptoms such as nausea and diaphoresis. Elderly patients are vulnerable to complex changes in the nervous system that mean visceral distension or inflammation may be less likely to be perceived as painful [12]. Somatic pain tends to be well localized and is caused by actual or threatened damage to tissues such as skin, muscle, tendon, joint capsules, fasciae, and bone. Older patients presenting with abdominal pain are more likely to have vague pain characteristic of visceral pain than with somatic pain. Somatic pain in the context of abdominal pain usually reflects local inflammation of the parietal peritoneum, and this will often cause localized peritoneal signs. The "surgical abdomen" is classically used to refer to a patient who presents with a rigid abdomen from peritonitis. As abdominal musculature is diminished with age, the older patient may not develop typical peritoneal signs of rebound and guarding. Nevertheless, most patients with acute surgical conditions will continue to have abdominal tenderness even in the absence of abdominal pain, reinforcing the value of the clinical examination. The presentation is often more subtle for a retroperitoneal process, such as AAA, posterior duodenal ulceration, acute pancreatitis, and renal pathology.

The oft-cited report of surgical intervention rates of 40% in the older population with abdominal pain predates the modern CT era and is unlikely to be seen with current imaging strategies [14]. More recent studies [15] support a 40% admission rate, a 20% rate of surgical intervention and a 2 week mortality of about 5%. A recent European study [16] reported 3% mortality in patients over 65 years of age with acute abdominal pain (4.7% for those over 80 years of age).

Initial workup

In the initial evaluation of abdominal pain in an older person, the emergency provider should consider time-dependent problems such as vascular catastrophes and acute myocardial ischemia, in addition to less-time critical intra- and extra-abdominal causes of acute abdominal pain. Laboratory studies and radiologic imaging will be determined by the history of present illness, physical exam findings, and differential diagnosis.

Appendicitis

Patients over 65 years of age account for 5–10% of patients with appendicitis. Older patients are more likely to present with symptoms for longer than 2 days and with complications of appendicitis such as perforation and abscess formation [17–20]. Less than one third of elderly patients with appendicitis will present with classic symptoms of anorexia, fever, right lower quadrant pain, and leukocytosis [19, 21, 22].

Most will have abdominal pain and the majority of older patients with appendicitis will have localized tenderness in the right lower quadrant [20, 22]; however, localized tenderness is surprisingly easy to overlook if appendicitis is not on the differential diagnosis.

Although usually obtained, a WBC or other inflammatory markers are nonspecific even if elevated. A CT scan of the abdomen and pelvis is the preferred diagnostic modality in the elderly patient with right lower quadrant tenderness in whom appendicitis is suspected. Liberal CT scan use has likely resulted in a decrease in perforation rates at the time of presentation [22], which is important because perforation is associated with a more complicated course and a prolonged length of stay for older patients [19, 23]. Octogenarians are more likely to present with complicated appendicitis, such as perforation, local abscess formation, or widespread peritonitis. For patients over 80, the complicated presentation rate is nearly 65% and the length of stay is nearly 8 days [22].

Laparoscopic appendectomy (LA) is increasingly the preferred surgical approach. In a large database study published in 2012 [24], LA has better outcomes in older patients with and without perforation at the time of presentation. In elderly patients presenting with perforated appendicitis, LA is associated with lower overall complication rate, in-hospital mortality, mean hospital charges, and shorter mean length of stay. Percutaneous drainage, on the other hand, is typically the preferred initial intervention for patients with a concomitant large abscess.

Biliary disease

By the age of 70, about 15% of men and 25% of women have gallstones [25]. Older age, female gender, and obesity are the primary risk factors for the development of gallstones. Clinical conditions that increase the risk of a patient with cholelithiasis developing acute cholecystitis include cardiovascular disease, diabetes mellitus, and a history of a stroke [26]. Advancing age is also a risk factor for the development of malignancy of the biliary tract including carcinoma of the head of the pancreas and cholangiocarcinoma. Included under the umbrella of biliary disease is symptomatic cholelithiasis (biliary colic), acute and chronic cholecystitis, acute cholangitis, acute gallstone pancreatitis, biliary malignancies including gallbladder carcinoma and cholangiocarcinoma, and obstructed common bile duct disease from a calculus or malignancy at the head of the pancreas.

Patients with abdominal pain from biliary causes present with symptoms and signs that cause the presenting condition to range from benign to critically ill. Biliary disease may present with abdominal pain localized in the right upper quadrant (RUQ). Patients with cholelithiasis typically present with RUQ pain and tenderness, commonly after a high-fat meal. The duration of symptoms partially depends on how long the cystic duct is occluded. Patients with acute cholecystitis will have persistent abdominal tenderness and elevation of inflammatory markers, or evidence of hepatic obstruction with transaminitis. Acute cholangitis presents with fever, jaundice, and abdominal pain (Charcot's triad) and is due to partial or complete obstruction of the common bile duct with bacterial infection [27]. Painless jaundice and a palpable gallbladder suggest obstruction of the common bile duct, often due to a malignancy, particularly of the pancreatic head [25–27].

Laboratory markers should include CBC, hepatic panel, lipase, basic metabolic panel, international normalized ratio (INR), and lactic acid for patients with suspected sepsis. For biliary colic, an abdominal ultrasound study is the diagnostic imaging study of choice. Criteria used to diagnose acute cholecystitis include the presence of gallstones with a sonographic Murphy sign, significant gallbladder wall thickening over 3 mm, pericholecystic fluid, impacted stone, or a combination of these [28]. A retrospective study finds that US is better at detecting biliary sludge and gallbladder inflammation, whereas a CT scan is better at detecting pericholecystic fluid [29]. For complicated biliary disease, including acute cholecystitis, acute cholangitis, acute gallstone pancreatitis, and obstructive disease, the patient should usually get an abdominal CT scan in addition to the US [29]. The CT scan offers better evaluation of the complications of acute cholecystitis such as gangrenous cholecystitis and perforation of the inflamed gallbladder, and may identify alternative causes of the patient's abdominal pain [28–30]. Cholescintigraphy evaluates only the gallbladder and ducts; its use is limited to patients suspected of having acute cholecystitis with an equivocal ultrasound study [28].

Patients with uncomplicated biliary colic may be managed as outpatients after immediate successful treatment of pain and exclusion of complicated disease, or they may have immediate surgery depending on time course, surgeon preference, and comorbidities. Complicated biliary disease including acute cholecystitis, acute cholangitis, acute gallstone pancreatitis, and other forms of biliary obstruction are typically admitted to the hospital with local institutional practice directing the admission service. Patients with obstruction of the common bile duct by calculus, malignancy, or stricture are usually admitted for endoscopic retrograde cholangiopancreatography (ERCP) [27, 31]. About a quarter of Medicare recipients do not undergo cholecystectomy during an admission with acute cholecystitis. Lack of definitive therapy is associated with a 38% gallstone-related readmission rate over the subsequent 2 years, compared with only 4% in patients who undergo cholecystectomy [25], suggesting that cholecystectomy should not be delayed following a diagnosis of acute cholecystitis [32, 33] in patients of all ages. Moreover, the mortality after emergency surgery is much higher than after elective surgery.

Small bowel obstruction

The classic features of small bowel obstruction (SBO) are visceral pain with nausea and diaphoresis, abdominal distension, and decreased passage of stool and flatus, which eventually results in obstipation where neither stool nor flatus is passing through the rectum. The primary risk factors for an SBO are prior abdominal surgery and external abdominal wall hernias (inguinal, femoral, and umbilical); however, SBO can develop de novo.

SBO is one of the few conditions wherein a plain abdominal series may be useful in establishing a diagnosis. Multiple air-fluid levels are usually seen. A plain abdominal series will not, however, reveal a transition point within the small bowel. Identification of a transition point is the leading indication for performing an abdominal CT scan with oral contrast for patients with SBO, as this may be an early indicator that the patient will not improve with bowel rest and may require operative repair [34, 35]. Consensus radiology guidelines suggest that abdominal CT scan with oral contrast should be avoided if a high-grade obstruction is present or suspected as it adds additional patient discomfort, wastes time, adds expense, and can lead to complications such as vomiting or aspiration. Perhaps most saliently, an abdominal CT scan with oral contrast is unlikely to improve diagnostic accuracy in patients with high-grade obstructions as the contrast will not reach the site of the obstruction [35]. Consideration should be given to an abdominal CT scan without oral contrast if high-grade or proximal obstruction is a concern [35].

Patients with SBO are usually managed nonoperatively, but there are a few conditions that require surgical correction such as an incarcerated inguinal or femoral hernia that cannot be reduced, or a focal transition point. In addition, increasing abdominal tenderness, laboratory signs of inflammation, and fever may push for surgical relief of the obstruction. Patients with an SBO should be admitted to the hospital and have a nasogastric tube placed and suction drainage commenced.

Large bowel obstruction and volvulus

The majority of patients with a large bowel obstruction (LBO) will present with abdominal distension and pain. The classic symptom is obstipation, where flatus does not pass. Vomiting is a late sign. Causes of colonic obstruction are broadly divided into benign and malignant causes. Most causes of colonic obstruction are malignant, including colorectal cancer and external compression from other malignancies within the abdominal cavity including peritoneal carcinomatosis [36]. About 50% of all LBOs are due to colorectal cancers, and about 10% of colorectal cancers present with an LBO. Benign causes of colonic obstruction include diverticulitis, diverticular stricture, fecal impaction, inflammatory bowel disease, volvulus, and functional obstructions from ileus and pseudo-obstruction [36–38]. Colonic volvulus, which occurs when a mobile part of the colon twists around a fixed base leading to a closed-loop obstruction, accounts for between 10% and 17% of LBOs [37, 38]. Patients with volvulus are at particular risk of a delayed presentation as they are often institutionalized and are dependent on caregivers noticing an acute change in bowel habit, which may be difficult in the chronically constipated [36–38]. Chronic constipation, prior surgery, prior volvulus, institutionalization, and neuropsychiatric conditions are the major risk factors for the development of sigmoid or cecal volvulus in older patients [37].

Laboratory tests may reveal anemia, leukocytosis, renal impairment, and metabolic acidosis [36]. A plain abdominal series may be helpful in determining the degree of distention and presence of volvulus or free air. A sigmoid or cecal volvulus is apparent on 60–75% of plain abdominal series [37] – a sigmoid volvulus is often described as having a "coffee bean" shape, whereas a cecal volvulus has a "bird beak"[38]. The addition of a contrast enema in patients with volvulus can increase the diagnostic accuracy of plain films significantly and is occasionally therapeutic [37]. Most patients with an LBO, however, have an obstructing malignancy, and in the absence of indications for an emergency laparotomy, will require advanced imaging, most commonly in the form of an abdominal CT scan. It is extremely important to distinguish between functional obstruction seen in pseudo-obstruction (usually managed with bowel rest and replacement of electrolytes) from anatomic obstruction, but even with advanced imaging studies, this can be difficult [38].

Colonic obstruction used to be almost exclusively managed surgically, but now many patients are treated acutely with interventional radiology and gastroenterology assistance, and may not require immediate operation [36]. Sigmoid volvulus is managed with endoscopic de-torsion typically by colonoscopy, followed by placement of a rectal tube, though semielective sigmoid resection is usually indicated as volvulus can recur in up to 90% of patients [37]. Endoscopic techniques are rarely successful for cecal volvulus, and operative repair is standard [37]. Severe cecal distension from any cause places the patient at increased risk of perforation. The often quoted 12 cm cecal diameter should be regarded as a guideline [36]. The risk of perforation is likely related to the rate of the distension, and patients with an acute cecal volvulus are at particularly high risk for perforation [37, 38]. Patients with peritonitis, strangulation, necrosis, or perforated viscus may be taken directly to the operating room. For LBO due to obstructing colorectal malignancy, the clinical decision-making can be complex. Patients with perforation or peritonitis will almost always require operative management with the exact surgery determined by the location of the cancer [36, 39]. For patients who have not perforated and do not have peritonitis, decisions can include the staging of the tumor and overall tumor burden. In the last decade, colonic stents have been used as a bridge to surgery and as a means to facilitate palliative chemotherapy and radiotherapy [38]. Patients with functional LBO require bowel rest, management of electrolytes, and treatment of the underlying condition [36, 38].

Hernias

Hernias are usually classified by anatomic location and whether they are internal or external. External hernias are through the abdominal wall and internal hernias are within the abdominal cavity. External hernias include inguinal, femoral, umbilical and paraumbilical, incisional, and lateral abdominal wall hernias. Internal hernias include diaphragmatic hernias such as hiatal hernias and the paraesophageal hernias, and mesenteric hernias that include many postsurgical hernias. Inguinal hernias account for about 75% of all hernias and are most common in men. Incarcerated hernias, in which the hernia bulge cannot be reduced, are surgical emergencies as they are at risk of strangulation, which can result in ischemia, infarction, and gangrene [40, 41].

If an abdominal wall hernia is not incarcerated, then the patient usually complains of an intermittent bulge in the groin or beside the surgical incision. This is often painful and frequently described as a dragging sensation. If the hernia is incarcerated, the patient frequently notices that the hernia can no longer be reduced and has become more painful. If the hernia is strangulated, the patient is likely to present with an increasingly painful irreducible hernia mass, and with progressive symptoms of bowel ischemia or infarction. The patient may have noticed a change in color of the hernia bulge, especially for umbilical hernias. As strangulated bowel within incarcerated hernias progresses from ischemia to infarction, an increase in systemic symptoms such as anorexia, nausea, and hemodynamic instability develops. In older patients, an incarcerated inguinal or femoral hernia may not be appreciated by the patient or caregiver, and the patient may present with symptoms of a bowel obstruction, including abdominal distension, nausea, and vomiting.

The majority of external hernias present a straightforward diagnosis, with a bulge at an anatomically consistent site. If possible, the patient should stand and cough during examination as this is an effective method to temporarily increase the intra-abdominal pressure in the groin and improve recognition of a hernia. The defect in the abdominal wall musculature is easily appreciated in most cases. Internal and obturator [42] hernias present more of a diagnostic challenge and are usually identified on abdominal CT scan or other abdominal imaging. A plain film of the chest can often reveal the presence of a hiatal hernia. With the exception of a known hiatal hernia, many obstructed or strangulated internal hernias may only be definitively identified on CT scan or at operation [40, 41].

If an external hernia such as an inguinal or femoral hernia is easily reducible in the ED, then the patient is usually referred for outpatient repair. If the external hernia is not easily reducible in the ED, then an attempt is usually made at reduction with the assistance of procedural sedation and positioning, usually with the contralateral side dependent to relieve pressure on the hernia. If this is not successful, or there is evidence of strangulation and bowel ischemia, then the patient is referred for immediate surgical repair [40, 41]. It is prudent to have surgical consultation for all incarcerated hernias to avoid a mass reduction that reduces the bulge, but not the obstruction of the hernia sac. This is more common with direct (through the abdominal wall), than with indirect (persistent peritoneal sac), hernias. Direct hernias are the most common in elderly patients.

Abdominal aortic aneurysm (AAA)

The diagnosis of an AAA occurs almost exclusively in older patients. Patients may present to the ED with abdominal pain due to a leaking, ruptured, or rapidly expanding AAA; or an AAA may be an incidental finding during ED imaging. The risk factors for the development of an AAA are male sex, tobacco use, hypercholesterolemia, hypertension, and family history [43]. The risk factors for expansion of an AAA are advanced age, severe cardiac disease, prior stroke, tobacco use, and cardiac or renal transplantation [43]. The risk factors for a ruptured AAA are female gender, larger aneurysm, current tobacco use, duration of tobacco use, and prior cardiac or renal transplant [43].

The classic presentation of a ruptured AAA is abdominal pain, hypotension, and a pulsatile abdominal mass. Alternatively, AAA may mimic ureterolithiasis, presenting with ipsilateral flank pain and hematuria [44]. Physical examination only reveals an AAA in 30–40% of cases, increasing as the aneurysm enlarges, and limited by obesity [43]. Hypotension in the presence of a known or suspected AAA necessitates an emergent quest to establish if the AAA is leaking into the retroperitoneum, or into the peritoneal cavity. Since the signs and symptoms of AAA are subtle and often obscure, one must think of the diagnosis and aggressively look for the presence of an aneurysm. The majority of patients with a ruptured AAA are not aware they have an AAA. The prehospital mortality of patients with ruptured AAA is estimated to be 30–80% [43, 45].

The rapid diagnosis of the presence of an AAA in the ED patient has been greatly facilitated by the widespread use of bedside US. ED bedside US can quickly reveal the AAA and the presence of free fluid in the abdomen. It is less useful at detecting retroperitoneal hemorrhage. The preferred imaging modality for a ruptured AAA is a CT (scan) angiogram that can both confirm the rupture and assist the vascular surgery team in planning the operative repair. The use of intravenous contrast becomes crucial to the surgical planning for endovascular repair. A ruptured AAA is an unfortunate diagnosis to make since patients may progress quickly to profound hypotension, shock, and death. Rupture into the peritoneal cavity is associated with high prehospital mortality [45]. Retroperitoneal rupture is more likely to partially tamponade, facilitating the possibility of surgical repair. The overall mortality for ruptured AAA, including the patients who do not survive to hospital, exceeds 80% [45].

Surgical repair of an AAA, either electively or emergently, occurs through the traditional operating room (OR) repair or endovascular aneurysm repair (EVAR). The mortality rate associated with a ruptured AAA undergoing open surgical repair is between 40% and 50% [46]. For patients over 80 years of age who present with a ruptured AAA, clinical evidence of shock and a low hemoglobin level, the mortality rate for OR is 95% [47]. Several studies show significantly improved outcome with EVAR when compared with OR [48]. The increasing use of EVAR has implications for the emergency physician in the management of ruptured AAA. If the local vascular surgery practice routinely uses EVAR, then a patient with a ruptured AAA requires an emergent CT scan with intravenous contrast to facilitate surgical planning.

The incidental finding of an aneurysmal abdominal aorta is an important diagnosis to make, and critical to communicate to the patient, as well as to ensure that the patient receives adequate follow-up. In male patients, the rate of rupture per year is small, until the aneurysm reaches 5.5 cm. In women, aneurysm diameter indexed to body size is the most important determinant of rupture, whereas aneurysm diameter alone is most predictive of rupture for men. Women with the largest diameter aneurysms and the smallest body sizes are at the greatest risk of rupture [49]. Above 7 cm, the risk of rupture is between 20% and 50% per year. Elective repair of AAA in patients over 80 carries a significant mortality risk of about 6% for OR and just under 2% for EVAR, and there is a correspondingly high morbidity risk (between 15% and 30%) [50]. The risk of emergent repair mortality as described above approaches 90%.

Mesenteric ischemia

The four major types of mesenteric ischemia are acute superior mesenteric artery (SMA) thromboembolic occlusion, mesenteric arterial thrombosis, mesenteric venous thrombosis, and nonocclusive mesenteric ischemia, including ischemic colitis [51]. When emergency physicians refer to mesenteric ischemia, they are usually referring to acute mesenteric ischemia with bowel infarction.

Acute mesenteric ischemia is most commonly due to acute embolism to the SMA, which accounts for 40–50% of all episodes, with thrombosis of the SMA accounting for 20–30% of cases [52]. Nonocclusive mesenteric ischemia accounts for about 25% of cases and thrombosis of the portal or mesenteric veins about 5–10% [52]. Chronic arterial thrombosis is almost always associated with extensive atherosclerotic disease [52, 53]. Mesenteric venous thrombosis is typically seen with hypercoagulable states. Nonocclusive mesenteric ischemia is the type typically seen in critically ill patients with profound hypoperfusion and carries an extremely high mortality [51, 52].

The classic presentation is an older patient with abdominal pain with severe pain and few or minimal focal abdominal findings. This patient is often described as having "pain out of proportion to the examination." Intra-arterial thrombosis can also present with stuttering symptoms, with meals being a precipitant for insufficient mesenteric arterial flow, often referred to as abdominal angina [51, 52]. The SMA is particularly vulnerable to embolic and arterial thrombotic events because of its acute angle as it courses over the left renal vein. Complete occlusion of the SMA is devastating because it supplies the entire small bowel and half of the colon (to the splenic flexure). Conditions that are particularly associated with the development of mesenteric ischemia are those with increased likelihood of embolic disease, local factors that predispose to local thrombosis, systemic low flow states, and hypercoagulable states. Conditions predisposing to embolic ischemia or infarction of the mesentery include atrial fibrillation, left ventricular aneurysms following acute MI, endocarditis, and patent foramen ovale that enable venous emboli to enter the systemic circulation.

In the older patient with severe abdominal pain, who has a nonfocal abdominal examination with the classic "pain out of proportion to examination," most probably has an acute SMA thromboembolic occlusion. This diagnosis carries a mortality greater than 50%. Abdominal tenderness, peritoneal signs, and the findings of blood in the stool only develop once transmural necrosis has developed, a finding that portends a grave prognosis [51]. Delays in diagnosis are common and are associated with higher morbidity and mortality. Abdominal CT scanning with IV contrast, ideally timed as an angiographic study, is the imaging study of choice [52, 53]. The classic finding is a filling defect within the SMA.

Intervention prior to development of extensive bowel necrosis is the goal. An ECG may be helpful in identifying atrial fibrillation or ventricular aneurysm. Early in the course of the disease, the lactate will be normal and could falsely reassure a physician. An elevated lactate signifies the development of mesenteric infarction. Once frank bowel necrosis has developed, the patient will require bowel resection to survive, yet the prognosis is grave with mortality rates exceeding 50% [51–53]. Prior to the development of full thickness bowel necrosis, interventional radiology may be able to provide targeted thrombolysis or local arterial stenting, with or without damage control surgery [53]. However, there is insufficient evidence to clearly recommend surgical embolectomy, angiography and transcatheter thrombolytics, or angiography and suction embolectomy, and therapy should be based on the availability of local expertise

[52]. The treatment of mesenteric venous thrombosis is systemic anticoagulation. The treatment of the low flow states associated with nonocclusive mesenteric ischemia is directed at the underlying cause.

Testing

Laboratory evaluation

It is uncommon that a laboratory test will provide the definitive diagnosis for a patient with a surgical cause of abdomen pain. Leukocytosis is common and nonspecific, and older patients are less likely to develop a leukocytosis than younger patients even in the presence of peritoneal irritation.

Imaging

For evaluation of acute abdominal pain in older patients the options are CT scan, ultrasound imaging, and plain radiograph studies. The choice of imaging is dependent on the clinician's differential diagnosis and the patient's hemodynamic stability.

CT scanning utilization has increased significantly since the early 1990s. About 50–60% of ED patients over 65 years of age with abdominal pain have an abdominal CT scan as part of their evaluation. Abdominal CT scan appears to alter the diagnosis in about 50% of elderly patients with abdominal pain [54, 55]. It is likely that this has contributed to earlier diagnosis of surgical conditions, a reduction in exploratory laparotomies, and to an overall reduction in mortality. In 2004, Esses *et al.* [56] published a study demonstrating that CT scan significantly changed the disposition of older ED patients with abdominal pain. Following the CT scan, surgical intervention was found to be necessary in 10 out of 104 patients, 8 of whom were not suspected of having a surgical condition prior to CT scan. This included two patients with a perforated viscus.

Abdominal CT scans usually involve the administration of contrast to improve the images of the structures being examined. Intravenous contrast provides important information about vascular structures and inflammatory processes within the abdominal cavity. Intravenous contrast is usually withheld for renal dysfunction, with the absolute level and protocols determined by individual institutions. If there is concern for an acute vascular catastrophe, then the IV contrast should be given regardless of renal function. For patients on renal replacement therapy, the recommendation is dialysis within 24 h to limit the risk of converting a patient with oliguric renal failure to one with anuric renal failure, and to reduce the impact of the osmotic load [57]. Oral contrast is being used less frequently in the evaluation of acute abdominal pain than in previous years. If the patient has had a surgical procedure within the last 30 days, then consideration should be given to an intra-abdominal abscess, and the patient should have enteral contrast (oral or rectal) [34]. Barium is usually reserved for stable clinical situations without the possibility of perforation. Iodinated water-soluble contrast media is primarily limited to select situations. These include patients in whom there is suspected bowel perforation or leak (including bowel fistula, sinus tract, or abscess). Less commonly, water-soluble oral contrast media may be preferred to barium contrast media in patients with likely SBO in whom timely surgery is anticipated [57]. Radiation exposure from CT scans is less concerning in older patients than in younger patients, although older patients remain vulnerable to contrast-induced nephropathy.

Ultrasound imaging remains extremely useful in the evaluation of older patients with abdominal pain. Point of care or bedside ultrasound has revolutionized the emergency physician's ability to direct care, and this is particularly true when evaluating the acute abdomen. Point-of-care US facilitates the identification of AAA in the unstable patient, and whether there is free fluid to suggest a leaking AAA and hemoperitoneum [58]. Ultrasound imaging also remains the study of choice for the identification of gallstones and is extremely useful for identifying the complications of gallstones such as acute cholecystitis. The CT scan is not as sensitive at identifying gallstones, many of which are radiolucent, but it is extremely sensitive at identifying the complications of biliary disease, including many of the features that are traditionally thought of as belonging to the ultrasound modality such as pericholecystic fluid and gall bladder wall thickening [30]. A CT scan is particularly useful for identifying pancreatic pathology that is variably seen on ultrasound.

Plain film studies are of limited utility in the evaluation of acute abdominal pain in any age group. A study involving 1000 patients does not recommend routine abdominal films in the evaluation of acute abdominal pain in all patients [59]. Depending on institutional practice, plain abdominal film studies may function as an early diagnostic test for SBO, and be diagnostic for an LBO and suspected radiopaque foreign bodies. Plain film studies lack sensitivity for detecting free air regardless of age [34, 60]. CT scans are more likely to detect free air and to detect transition points in SBO [34, 60].

Disposition

Almost all patients with a surgical abdominal condition will be managed as inpatients, and most, by definition, will proceed to the OR. For vascular emergencies, this is a very time-dependent process, and the patients should be quickly evaluated in the ED in conjunction with the vascular surgery team. Patients with reducible external hernias are referred for outpatient surgery with detailed return precautions. Between these two extremes lie much of the inflammatory conditions that cause abdominal pain in the elderly population.

Emergency laparotomy is associated with an overall mortality risk of 14% in all patients, and this risk increases with age and frailty [61, 62]. Patients older than 90 years of age, with an American Society of Anesthesiologists class V, septic shock, dependent functional status, and abnormal white blood cell count have a less than 10% probability of survival from emergency laparotomy [61]. Emergency laparotomy, especially laparotomy requiring bowel resection is associated with very high mortality rates in octogenarians. Bowel resection was required in 51 out of 100 patients in a recent retrospective case series with an overall mortality of 45% [39].

Section IV: Decision-making

- The differential diagnosis of abdominal pain in older adults is broad and includes numerous life-threatening surgical conditions.
- The assessment of abdominal pain in the older adult may be obfuscated by changes in pain perception, cognitive impairment, and confounding comorbidities and medications.
- Careful serial abdominal *examinations* are essential as most patients with acute surgical abdominal

pathology will have focal tenderness even in the absence of abdominal pain.

- Ultrasound is the imaging study of choice for biliary disease. Bedside ultrasound is used in the evaluation of hemodynamically unstable patients, looking for evidence of ruptured AAA.
- CT scans are the usual study of choice for undifferentiated abdominal pain, or for surgical conditions with inflammatory, obstructive, or ischemic etiologies.
- Though IV CT contrast may contribute to nephropathy, IV contrast is necessary for the diagnosis of acute mesenteric arterial occlusion, or to facilitate an endovascular repair of an AAA, regardless of the renal function.
- Emergency laparotomy is associated with a high mortality in all age groups and is extremely high in older patients with serious comorbidities.

References

1 Lowenstein, S.R., Crescenzi, C.A., Kern, D.C., and Steel, K. (1986) Care of the elderly in the emergency department. *Ann. Emerg. Med.*, **15** (5), 528–535 (Epub 1986/05/01).

2 Yeh, E.L. and McNamara, R.M. (2007) Abdominal pain. *Clin. Geriatr. Med.*, **23** (2), 255–270, v (Epub 2007/04/28).

3 Pines, J.M., Mullins, P.M., Cooper, J.K. *et al.* (2013) National trends in emergency department use, care patterns, and quality of care of older adults in the United States. *J. Am. Geriatr. Soc.*, **61** (1), 12–17.

4 Platts-Mills, T.F., Esserman, D.A., Brown, D.L. *et al.* (2012) Older US emergency department patients are less likely to receive pain medication than younger patients: results from a national survey. *Ann. Emerg. Med.*, **60** (2), 199–206 (Epub 2011/10/29).

5 Hwang, U. and Platts-Mills, T.F. (2013) Acute pain management in older adults in the emergency department. *Clin. Geriatr. Med.*, **29** (1), 151–164 (Epub 2012/11/28).

6 Samaras, N., Chevalley, T., Samaras, D., and Gold, G. (2010) Older patients in the emergency department: a review. *Ann. Emerg. Med.*, **56** (3), 261–269 (Epub 2010/07/14).

7 Singal, B.M., Hedges, J.R., Rousseau, E.W. *et al.* (1992) Geriatric patient emergency visits. Part I: comparison of visits by geriatric and younger patients. *Ann. Emerg. Med.*, **21** (7), 802–807 (Epub 1992/07/01).

8 Galbusera, M., Remuzzi, G., and Boccardo, P. (2009) Treatment of bleeding in dialysis patients. *Semin. Dial.*, **22** (3), 279–286.

9 Ray, L., Lipton, R.B., Zimmerman, M.E. *et al.* (2011) Mechanisms of association between obesity and chronic pain in the elderly. *Pain*, **152** (1), 53–59 (Epub 2010/10/12).

10 Wang, Y.C., McPherson, K., Marsh, T. *et al.* (2011) Health and economic burden of the projected obesity trends in the USA and the UK. *Lancet*, **378** (9793), 815–825 (Epub 2011/08/30).

11 American Geriatrics Society 2012 Beers Criteria Update Expert Panel (2012) American Geriatrics Society updated Beers Criteria for potentially inappropriate medication use in older adults. *J. Am. Geriatr. Soc.*, **60** (4), 616–631 (Epub 2012/03/02).

12 Moore, A.R. and Clinch, D. (2004) Underlying mechanisms of impaired visceral pain perception in older people. *J. Am. Geriatr. Soc.*, **52** (1), 132–136 (Epub 2003/12/23).

13 Woolf, C.J. (2010) What is this thing called pain? *J. Clin. Invest.*, **120** (11), 3742–3744 (Epub 2010/11/03).

14 Bugliosi, T.F., Meloy, T.D., and Vukov, L.F. (1990) Acute abdominal pain in the elderly. *Ann. Emerg. Med.*, **19** (12), 1383–1386.

15 Lewis, L.M., Banet, G.A., Blanda, M. *et al.* (2005) Etiology and clinical course of abdominal pain in senior patients: a prospective, multicenter study. *J. Gerontol. A Biol. Sci. Med. Sci.*, **60** (8), 1071–1076.

16 Laurell, H., Hansson, L.E., and Gunnarsson, U. (2006) Acute abdominal pain among elderly patients. *Gerontology*, **52** (6), 339–344.

17 Hui, T.T., Major, K.M., Avital, I. *et al.* (2002) Outcome of elderly patients with appendicitis: effect of computed tomography and laparoscopy. *Arch. Surg.*, **137** (9), 995–998; discussion 999–1000.

18 Southgate, E., Vousden, N., Karthikesalingam, A. *et al.* (2012) Laparoscopic vs open appendectomy in older patients. *Arch. Surg.*, **147** (6), 557–562.

19 Harbrecht, B.G., Franklin, G.A., Miller, F.B. *et al.* (2011) Acute appendicitis – not just for the young. *Am. J. Surg.*, **202** (3), 286–290.

20 Augustin, T., Cagir, B., and Vandermeer, T.J. (2011) Characteristics of perforated appendicitis: effect of delay is confounded by age and gender. *J. Gastrointest. Surg.*, **15** (7), 1223–1231 (Epub 2011/05/11).

21 Horattas, M.C., Guyton, D.P., and Wu, D. (1990) A reappraisal of appendicitis in the elderly. *Am. J. Surg.*, **160** (3), 291–293.

22 Storm-Dickerson, T.L. and Horattas, M.C. (2003) What have we learned over the past 20 years about appendicitis in the elderly? *Am. J. Surg.*, **185** (3), 198–201.

23 Gurleyik, G. and Gurleyik, E. (2003) Age-related clinical features in older patients with acute appendicitis. *Eur. J. Emerg. Med.*, **10** (3), 200–203 (Epub 2003/09/16).

24 Masoomi, H., Mills, S., Dolich, M. *et al.* (2012) Does laparoscopic appendectomy impart an advantage over open appendectomy in elderly patients? *World J. Surg.*, **36** (7), 1534–1539.

25 Riall, T.S., Zhang, D., Townsend, C.M. Jr., *et al.* (2010) Failure to perform cholecystectomy for acute cholecystitis in elderly patients is associated with increased morbidity, mortality, and cost. *J. Am. Coll. Surg.*, **210** (5), 668–677.

26 Cho, J.Y., Han, H.S., Yoon, Y.S., and Ahn, K.S. (2010) Risk factors for acute cholecystitis and a complicated clinical course in patients with symptomatic cholelithiasis. *Arch. Surg.*, **145** (4), 329–333; discussion 333 (Epub 2010/04/21).

27 Ferreira, L.E. and Baron, T.H. (2013) Acute biliary conditions. *Best Pract. Res. Clin. Gastroenterol.*, **27** (5), 745–756 (Epub 2013/10/29).

28 Blaivas, M. and Adhikari, S. (2007) Diagnostic utility of cholescintigraphy in emergency department patients with suspected acute cholecystitis: comparison with bedside RUQ ultrasonography. *J. Emerg. Med.*, **33** (1), 47–52 (Epub 2007/07/17).

29 McGillicuddy, E.A., Schuster, K.M., Brown, E. *et al.* (2011) Acute cholecystitis in the elderly: use of computed tomography and correlation with ultrasonography. *Am. J. Surg.*, **202** (5), 524–527.

30 Yarmish, G.M., Smith, M.P., Rosen, M.P. *et al.* (2014) ACR appropriateness criteria right upper quadrant pain. *J. Am. Coll. Radiol.*, **11** (3), 316–322 (Epub 2014/02/04).

31 Fogel, E.L. and Sherman, S. (2014) ERCP for gallstone pancreatitis. *N. Engl. J. Med.*, **370** (2), 150–157 (Epub 2014/01/10).

32 Gutt, C.N., Encke, J., Koninger, J. *et al.* (2013) Acute cholecystitis: early versus delayed cholecystectomy, a multicenter randomized trial (ACDC study, NCT00447304). *Ann. Surg.*, **258** (3), 385–393 (Epub 2013/09/12).

33 de Mestral, C., Rotstein, O.D., Laupacis, A. *et al.* (2014) Comparative operative outcomes of early and delayed cholecystectomy for acute cholecystitis: a population-based propensity score analysis. *Ann. Surg.*, **259** (1), 10–15 (Epub 2013/08/28).

34 Yaghmai, V., Rosen, M.P., and Lalani, T. (2012) American College of Radiology Appropriateness Criteria Acute (nonlocalized) Abdominal Pain and Fever or Suspected Abdominal Abscess. (Epub 12/11/2013).

35 Ros, P.R. and Huprich, J.E. (2006) ACR Appropriateness Criteria on suspected small-bowel obstruction. *J. Am. Coll. Radiol.*, **3** (11), 838–841 (Epub 2007/04/07).

36 Sawai, R.S. (2012) Management of colonic obstruction: a review. *Clin. Colon Rectal Surg.*, **25** (4), 200–203 (Epub 2013/12/03).

37 Gingold, D. and Murrell, Z. (2012) Management of colonic volvulus. *Clin. Colon Rectal Surg.*, **25** (4), 236–244 (Epub 2013/12/03).

38 Yeo, H.L. and Lee, S.W. (2013) Colorectal emergencies: review and controversies in the management of large bowel obstruction. *J. Gastrointest. Surg.*, **17** (11), 2007–2012 (Epub 2013/09/21).

39 Green, G., Shaikh, I., Fernandes, R., and Wegstapel, H. (2013) Emergency laparotomy in octogenarians: a 5-year study of morbidity and mortality. *World J. Gastrointest. Surg.*, **5** (7), 216–221 (Epub 2013/07/31).

40 Kingsnorth, A. and LeBlanc, K. (2003) Hernias: inguinal and incisional. *Lancet*, **362** (9395), 1561–1571 (Epub 2003/11/15).

41 Matthews, R.D. and Neumayer, L. (2008) Inguinal hernia in the 21st century: an evidence-based review. *Curr. Probl. Surg.*, **45** (4), 261–312 (Epub 2008/03/25).

42 Tateno, Y. and Adachi, K. (2014) Sudden knee pain in an underweight, older woman: obturator hernia. *Lancet*, **384** (9938), 206.

43 Chaikof, E.L., Brewster, D.C., Dalman, R.L. *et al.* (2009) The care of patients with an abdominal aortic aneurysm: the Society for Vascular Surgery practice guidelines. *J. Vasc. Surg.*, **50** (4, Suppl), S2–S49 (Epub 2009/10/14).

44 Coursey, C.A., Casalino, D.D., Remer, E.M. *et al.* (2012) ACR Appropriateness Criteria(R) acute onset flank pain–suspicion of stone disease. *Ultrasound Q.*, **28** (3), 227–233.

45 Reimerink, J.J., van der Laan, M.J., Koelemay, M.J. *et al.* (2013) Systematic review and meta-analysis of population-based mortality from ruptured abdominal aortic aneurysm. *Br. J. Surg.*, **100** (11), 1405–1413 (Epub 2013/09/17).

46 Bown, M.J., Sutton, A.J., Bell, P.R., and Sayers, R.D. (2002) A meta-analysis of 50 years of ruptured abdominal aortic aneurysm repair. *Br. J. Surg.*, **89** (6), 714–730 (Epub 2002/05/25).

47 Biancari, F. and Venermo, M. (2011) Open repair of ruptured abdominal aortic aneurysm in patients aged 80 years and older. *Br. J. Surg.*, **98** (12), 1713–1718 (Epub 2011/10/29).

48 Reimerink, J.J., Hoornweg, L.L., Vahl, A.C. *et al.* (2013) Endovascular repair versus open repair of ruptured abdominal aortic aneurysms: a multicenter randomized controlled trial. *Ann. Surg.*, **258** (2), 248–256 (Epub 2013/04/04).

49 Lo, R.C., Lu, B., Fokkema, M.T. *et al.* (2013) Relative importance of aneurysm diameter and body size for predicting abdominal aortic aneurysm rupture in men and women. *J. Vasc. Surg.* (Epub 2014/01/07).

50 Raval, M.V. and Eskandari, M.K. (2012) Outcomes of elective abdominal aortic aneurysm repair among the elderly: endovascular versus open repair. *Surgery*, **151** (2), 245–260 (Epub 2011/01/20).

51 Sise, M.J. (2014) Acute mesenteric ischemia. *Surg. Clin. North Am.*, **94** (1), 165–181 (Epub 2013/11/26).

52 Oliva, I.B., Davarpanah, A.H., Rybicki, F.J. *et al.* (2013) ACR Appropriateness Criteria (R) imaging of mesenteric ischemia. *Abdom. Imaging*, **38** (4), 714–719 (Epub 2013/01/09).

53 Acosta, S. and Bjorck, M. (2014) Modern treatment of acute mesenteric ischaemia. *Br. J. Surg.*, **101** (1), e100–e108 (Epub 2013/11/21).

54 Gardner, R.L., Almeida, R., Maselli, J.H., and Auerbach, A. (2010) Does gender influence emergency department management and outcomes in geriatric abdominal pain? *J. Emerg. Med.*, **39** (3), 275–281 (Epub 2008/11/11).

55 Lewis, L.M., Klippel, A.P., Bavolek, R.A. *et al.* (2007) Quantifying the usefulness of CT in evaluating seniors with abdominal pain. *Eur. J. Radiol.*, **61** (2), 290–296.

56 Esses, D., Birnbaum, A., Bijur, P. *et al.* (2004) Ability of CT to alter decision making in elderly patients with acute abdominal pain. *Am. J. Emerg. Med.*, **22** (4), 270–272.

57 ACR Committee on Drugs and Contrast Media (2013) *ACR Manual on Contrast Media v9*, American College of Radiology.

58 Mazzei, M.A., Guerrini, S., Cioffi Squitieri, N. *et al.* (2013) The role of US examination in the management of acute abdomen. *Crit. Ultrasound J.*, **5** (**Suppl. 1**), S6 (Epub 2013/08/02).

59 van Randen, A., Laméris, W., Luitse, J.S. *et al.* (2011) The role of plain radiographs in patients with acute abdominal pain at the ED. *Am. J. Emerg. Med.*, **29** (6), 582–589.e2.

60 Yeung, K.W., Chang, M.S., Hsiao, C.P., and Huang, J.F. (2004) CT evaluation of gastrointestinal tract perforation. *Clin. Imaging*, **28** (5), 329–333 (Epub 2004/10/09).

61 Al-Temimi, M.H., Griffee, M., Enniss, T.M. *et al.* (2012) When is death inevitable after emergency laparotomy? Analysis of the American college of surgeons national surgical quality improvement program database. *J. Am. Coll. Surg.*, **215** (4), 503–511.

62 Vester-Andersen, M., Lundstrøm, L.H., Møller, M.H. *et al.* (2014) Mortality and postoperative care pathways after emergency gastrointestinal surgery in 2904 patients: a population-based cohort study. *Br. J. Anaesth.*, **112** (5), 860–870.

8

Nonsurgical abdominal pain in the elderly

Katren Tyler & Maura Kennedy

[1] *Department of Emergency Medicine, UC Davis Medical Center, University of California, Sacramento, CA, USA*
[2] *Department of Emergency Medicine, Beth Israel Deaconess Medical Center, Harvard Medical School, Boston, MA, USA*

Section I: Case presentation

A 71-year-old woman presented to the emergency department (ED) with abdominal pain. The pain started the evening prior and had gradually worsened over the course of the past day and was now severe. The pain was maximal in the right upper quadrant and epigastric regions without radiation. She denied any clear precipitating factors. She had tried both acetaminophen and antacids on the day prior but had no relief with these medications. She also reported nausea starting the day before and started vomiting several hours prior to coming to the ED. On review of systems, she reported shortness of breath. She denied fever, cough, chest pain, urinary symptoms, black or bloody stools, or diarrhea.

The past medical history included a history of hypertension, asthma, and a remote history of lung cancer. The past surgical history was notable for a partial lobectomy years ago; she had no abdominal surgery. She did not use tobacco, alcohol, or illicit drugs.

The vital signs were as follows: temperature 36°C, pulse 89 beats/min, blood pressure 116/48 mmHg, respirations 32 breaths/min, and pulse oximetry of 92% on room air. On examination, she appeared uncomfortable, was tachypneic, and was actively vomiting. The cardiac examination was normal, but on pulmonary auscultation, she had decreased breath sounds on the right and scattered wheezes bilaterally. The abdomen was nondistended, with mild epigastric tenderness and a negative Murphy's sign. The rest of the physical examination was normal.

Section II: Case discussion

Dr Shamai Grossman (SG): Elderly patients are more inclined to delay coming into the ED – do you have any explanation?

Dr Scott Wilber (SW): There are probably a few reasons. Physiologically, many diseases present atypically in older individuals and with vague symptoms. For example, rather than getting crushing substernal chest pain with myocardial infarction (MI), they are more likely to present with shortness of breath. Thus, atypical presentations are one cause. Also, the older we are, the more life experience we have, and we tend to relate our symptoms to other things that we've had that may have been fairly benign. So an older person may say the chest pain is the acid reflux that they typically got when they were 25 years old, or the same symptoms experienced before the cholecystectomy performed years ago. Thus, minimizing and attributing symptoms to a prior, less serious problem is another cause.

Dr Rob Anderson (RA): Many elderly patients will do anything to stay out of the hospital, either because of prior admissions that they didn't enjoy, or because

Geriatric Emergencies: A Discussion-Based Review, First Edition.
Edited by Amal Mattu, Shamai A. Grossman and Peter L. Rosen.
© 2016 John Wiley & Sons, Ltd. Published 2016 by John Wiley & Sons, Ltd.

of fear of a serious diagnosis, such as cancer, so they often try to stay home as long as they can, rather than present to the ED.

Dr Jon Mark Hirshon (JMH): There's a certain amount of effort required to go to the hospital; many elderly simply can't mount the energy to organize the trip. Moreover, often with older men, there's a real tendency to minimize and deny symptoms to try to make come true the hope there is nothing seriously wrong.

SG: What was your differential diagnosis?

Dr Maura Kennedy (MK): Initially, it was quite broad. The fact that she was tachypneic, short of breath, and hypoxic put pulmonary etiologies high on our differential, including pneumonia and pulmonary embolism. We were also concerned about an atypical presentation of an acute MI, and entertained intra-abdominal etiologies including pancreatitis with an associated pleural effusion, hepatitis, biliary colic, and bowel obstruction.

SG: We often see patients who come in with abdominal pain who say "I'm just constipated." This produces a knee-jerk reflex on the part of house staff and nursing to attribute it to constipation. How do you approach this patient?

JMH: I'll often say that my job is to make sure it's not something acutely life-threatening or limb-threatening, and even though it may feel like constipation, it's my job to make sure it's not something else. Particularly, in the elderly patient in whom symptoms can be misleading, I want to have a relatively broad differential to start with, and not immediately dismiss the problem as a recurrence of something benign from the past. I also express my concern to the patient and family.

SG: What hints on this patient's history would help sway you one way or the other when creating a pathway of where to go in working the patient up?

RA: First of all, this is a relatively acute presentation, and you need to marshal your resources and have situational awareness as to what you think might be going on. In my department, I would probably want to move this patient to a more acute area if they ended up in the fast track by an optimistic triage. The respiratory rate is a real tip off that this patient is quite sick, and in the elderly patient, this may be one of your first markers that something bad is going on. Thus, the first question must be "is this patient sick, or do I have some time to work on them?" There's nothing to do except start getting data as fast as you can because the differential is so huge.

SG: Beyond the tachypnea, are there elements of the physical examination that you should be looking for or things that really stood out?

SW: Commonly, your history and examination can provide you clues, but oftentimes they won't be specific. In this patient, we had a number of findings that didn't lead to any one diagnosis, but merely confirmed the patient was acutely ill. Thus, the differential was still quite broad. There were vital sign abnormalities and borderline hypoxia with tachypnea. There were diminished breath sounds, so that makes us think of some pulmonary pathology as a potential contributor. Finally, there was abdominal tenderness. Sometimes, patients even with a perforated hollow viscus have fairly benign abdominal examinations and appear to be resting comfortably. Elderly patients don't seem to mount the severe peritoneal response that we see in younger patients. If a patient does have severe tenderness, you want to take that seriously, but the absence of peritoneal signs should not make you think that there is no significant disease inside the abdomen.

Dr Peter Rosen (PR): Even in younger patients, there may be a lag period between the actual time of perforation and the onset of peritoneal findings. It is especially easy to underestimate the degree of illness in elderly patients as they may minimize symptoms, don't perceive pain so severely as younger patients, or may be used to being uncomfortable and don't react to pain as much. We have all been taught that the patients with mesenteric vascular occlusions may appear sick without having much in the way of abdominal findings on physical examination.

JMH: I would emphasize that the vital signs are quite important. The fact that she has a history of hypertension and her blood pressure 116/48 is significant. She's also on beta-blocker therapy for hypertension – so while her heart rate of 89 is technically in the normal range, it may actually be a lack of an appropriate response as opposed to being normal.

RA: This is a case that has a very broad differential, nevertheless I sometimes see residents anchoring prematurely on a diagnosis, such as immediately concluding this must be pancreatitis or pneumonia. This is the kind of patient where you have to be flexible, and as data comes in, you may change and focus your differential. I think it is not only intellectually interesting but also challenging.

PR: I think sometimes the anchoring prematurely is a means of fixing on a diagnosis that will permit early discharge.

SG: Where do you go with this patient? The history is diffuse and nonspecific, the examination has a number of different findings that are suggestive of pulmonary and abdominal processes and perhaps more. What tests would you order?

RA: Obviously, you can get things going quickly by ordering an immediate ECG, portable chest X-ray study, and placing an ultrasound probe on the abdomen. Just think of all the things that you can do quickly to start evaluating this patient, simultaneously sending off all the laboratory tests that you think will be helpful. This patient requires a shotgun kind of approach.

SG: Please discuss what happened with this patient.

MK: The patient was brought back to one of our resuscitation bays. We ordered a full set of laboratory tests including liver function tests and a lipase. We also ordered an abdominal CT scan, a portable chest X-ray study, and we were preparing for both an ECG and ultrasound at the bedside.

SG: Is there anyone who wouldn't have ordered a CT scan for this patient?

RA: I think you're still in the initial resuscitation phase with this patient. If they make it long enough, then a CT scan would be great, but they're obviously pretty sick to begin with.

SW: You also need to consider whether you use IV or oral contrast for your CT scan as all of those things take a different amount of time. The location of your CT scanner is also important. It's easier and safer to get the patient to a CT scanner that is in the ED than to transport them outside the ED for imaging. There is also varied decision-making about the chest X-ray study. I would make sure that the chest X-ray

study was done as an upright chest X-ray. You will never see free air under the hemidiaphragm on a supine view.

SG: There is a classic adage that bad things happen in the CT scanner. Even if we send them on telemetry with someone accompanying them, they are still out of our immediate grasp, and beyond our ability to easily resuscitate. What happened next?

MK: The portable chest X-ray study was the first test completed and demonstrated complete opacification of the right lung. She was being hooked up to obtain an ECG when she vomited.

SG: When you saw opacification of the right lung, what did you think then?

MK: We weren't entirely sure. She had this history of a lobectomy, so we thought about metastatic or recurrent disease causing a pleural effusion. Pleural effusion secondary to pancreatitis was also on our differential. While we didn't hear a murmur on cardiac examination, we considered valvular dysfunction causing asymmetric pulmonary edema, as well as pneumonia. It didn't actually help us to narrow our differential; rather it expanded our pulmonary differential.

SG: What happened next?

MK: While we had the leads on for the ECG, she vomited and probably aspirated. Her mental status declined, and she became hypoxic, bradycardic and lost pulses in less than 5 min after arrival in the ED. She was intubated immediately, and chest compressions were started. After one round of epinephrine, she had return of spontaneous circulation. The postarrest ECG showed 3 mm of ST elevations in II, III, and aVF with reciprocal ST depression in I and aVL and V1–V3.

SG: Did she have an ECG prior to the cardiac arrest?

MK: Unfortunately, no. Ultimately, we thought the ST-elevation MI was the cause of vague abdominal pain and cardiac arrest, although we did consider whether it could be secondary to demand ischemia with an existing lesion.

SG: Do you have other thoughts about where you might take this patient at this point?

SW: As she was acutely ill upon arrival, the goal is to collect data as quickly as possible, while starting the resuscitation process. Post-cardiac arrest, you've got ST elevations, a clear pathway to pursue with activation of the cardiac catheterization laboratory or other interventions depending on the resources at your facility.

RA: This is an opportunity for readers of this text to think about system changes they can make within their own system. Considering that about one third of women over 65 present with abdominal pain as their presentation of an acute MI, instituting ECG for all older women with abdominal pain in triage might be a good idea. In our hospital, we do get an ECG on every elderly patient who presents with epigastric abdominal pain.

MK: The patient was subsequently emergently taken to the cardiac catheterization laboratory. She had 100% occlusion of the mid-RCA (right coronary artery), but while undergoing cardiac catheterization and angioplasty she developed ventricular fibrillation and deteriorated into a systole. Despite CPR (cardiopulmonary resuscitation) and defibrillation, she expired.

SG: I am not sure whether this was an unusual presentation of an acute MI or whether this was demand ischemia. Inferior wall AMIs (acute myocardial infarctions) generally have the best prognosis of any myocardial lesion. In a patient who appeared to be relatively well to start with, it is an unusual outcome. Unfortunately, this could be the nature of disease in the elderly where symptoms are hard to pick up because they're not typical. Is there something that could have been done to turn the tide in this case?

MK: I think the critical issue would have been doing the ECG earlier. While it was obtained in the first 5 min of her ED course, she deteriorated quite rapidly. Had we obtained the ECG prior to her aspiration, we may have been able to differentiate between a primary cardiac event and demand ischemia after the aspiration.

SW: One system change that we have in our large tertiary catchment area is to do prehospital ECGs. The paramedics are very good at doing them even on older patients with abdominal pain, shortness of breath, or even just older people who fall down. Perhaps had we had the benefit of a prehospital ECG 15 min earlier, she might have spent just a few minutes in the

ED and gone straight to the cardiac catheterization laboratory.

SG: I think that's an excellent point. Part of the problem with this patient is that she just walked in on her own rather than calling an ambulance. That brings us back to the original question we had: "Why is it that patients, when they get old, don't seem to want to come to the ED for evaluation?"

PR: In addition to all the reasons we discussed above, there may be a subconscious desire to be done with a difficult life, without being suicidal or depressed, that contributes to a person's reluctance to go to the ED.

JMH: When this happens it's hard for everybody. It's hard not only for the patients and the families but also for the physicians. When you have someone come in talking and then dies in front of you or pretty close to it, it can be quite a turbulent and emotionally challenging type of event. I think it's important to have a postarrest debriefing or conference to attempt to see what could have been done, to help look at system changes, but also to help the junior clinicians process how they're feeling, and to decompress the impact of something like this.

RA: In younger people, you usually have two findings that lead to a diagnosis: you usually have pain, either on history or physical examination, plus abnormal objective data that leads you to the diagnosis. In the elderly, you may only have one of those two findings. You either have pain with objective data that looks fine or you have no pain with objective data that looks abnormal. I think that the challenge is to try to figure out who you're going to work up further. If you have somebody with pain but normal laboratory studies, you might do some more workup in terms of imaging. But if you have somebody with no pain but abnormal laboratory tests we're stuck trying to figure out what we're going to do next. With the elderly, you need to be more aggressive and pursue other imaging based on what you think is going on.

SG: One of the programs we've developed in Boston uses vital signs as a trigger for acute care. This patient, with a respiratory rate of 32 breaths/min, would have been triggered. In our department, this means that the attending physician, one or two resident physicians, one or two nurses, and a technician are at the bedside within 1–2 min to evaluate this patient and create a plan of care together. As mentioned before, when you have an organized approach that includes the evaluation early on, you often can get things done in a much more efficient manner and sometimes save a life.

Section III: Concepts

Introduction

Abdominal pain is a very common chief complaint in the ED in all age groups. The immediate evaluation of an older patient with abdominal pain is aimed at excluding time-dependent conditions that will require an intervention. The differential for abdominal pain in the elderly is broad as it may be the presenting symptom for illnesses involving intraperitoneal, extraperitoneal, and nonabdominal structures. Extraperitoneal structures such as the genital-urinary tract and pelvic organs may present with abdominal, flank, or pelvic pain, although acute primary infections of the genital tract and pelvic organs are less common in the older population than in younger patients [1, 2]. Older patients are more likely to have a malignant process from a pelvic organ than younger patients. Nonabdominal conditions that may present as abdominal pain in older patients include life-threatening intrathoracic conditions such as acute myocardial infarction, pneumonia, and aortic dissection.

About 20% of older patients presenting with abdominal pain will require an emergent surgical procedure, and about 40% are admitted to the hospital [3]. Therefore, the majority of older patients presenting to the ED with abdominal pain will not require immediate surgery in the traditional sense of going to the operating room (OR) directly from the ED. The line between what constitutes an acute surgical condition and what does not has become blurred in recent years with the rise of interventional radiology procedures, including the emergent stenting of occluded vessels, placement of nephrostomy tubes, and percutaneous drainage of intra-abdominal abscesses. In some instances, fragile older patients may be able to tolerate a limited interventional radiology procedure when they would not be able to tolerate a procedure in the OR. This chapter focuses on nonsurgical causes of acute abdominal pain in the elderly. Chapter 7 discusses surgical causes of acute abdominal pain and explores in more depth how confounding comorbidities, challenges in history taking, and age-related changes in pain sensation impact the assessment of the older adult with abdominal pain.

Initial evaluation

The history and physical examination remain the cornerstone of the clinical evaluation, but can be challenging in the older patient with comorbidities. In addition, cognitive impairment, including dementia, makes the history taking problematic, and a baseline cognitive impairment may be complicated by the development of delirium. The physical examination is also less reliable in older patients with abdominal pain since they are more likely to have vague visceral pain and less likely to have peritoneal signs of rebound and guarding due to changes in the nervous system [4].

Peptic ulcer disease

Peptic ulcer disease is broadly divided into gastric and duodenal ulceration and also includes other acid-related diagnosis such as gastritis. Peptic ulcer disease can be uncomplicated, presenting with local pain and minor symptoms, or complicated by perforation or upper gastrointestinal bleeding (UGIB). Since the recognition of the role and treatment of *Helicobacter pylori* (*H. pylori*) in acid-related disease and the widespread availability of medication that manage gastric acid levels such as histamine-2 (H2) blockers and proton pump inhibitors (PPIs), the incidence of perforation associated with peptic ulceration has fallen; however, perforation continues to have a high mortality in older patients [5, 6]. Complicating the diagnosis, nearly 90% of patients with a perforated peptic ulcer do not have a preexisting history of peptic ulceration [6]. Advancing age, medication use (nonsteroidal anti-inflammatory drugs (NSAIDs), steroids, and aspirin), tobacco smoking, *H. pylori* infection, and salt use all affect secretion of gastric acid and increase the risk of peptic ulcer disease. Advancing age is an independent predictor of poor outcomes following perforation of a peptic ulcer or bleeding from a peptic ulcer [6]. In addition, older patients may be on medications that increase the risk of bleeding (such as warfarin or clopidogrel) or impair the normal cardiovascular responses to hemorrhage (beta-blockers and calcium channel blockers). Moreover, since the elderly patients are often delayed in their presentation to seek help, they increase the morbidity and mortality of perforation, which is critically time dependent.

The majority of patients will present with a burning epigastric discomfort, reflecting both the inflammatory nature of the pain and the foregut origin of the celiac plexus. A perforated peptic ulcer will usually present with the sudden onset of epigastric pain and symptoms of peritoneal irritation; however, as abdominal musculature is diminished with age, the older patient may not manifest the typical signs of abdominal rigidity, rebound, or guarding [4].

A complete blood count (CBC) may reveal a leukocytosis in peptic ulcer perforation or anemia in a significant UGIB. Serial hemoglobin and hematocrits may be used as a marker for the bleeding rates although there are multiple confounders such as dilution from resuscitation fluids. The blood urea nitrogen (BUN) to creatinine ratio may help differentiate between an upper and lower source for gastrointestinal bleeding with a BUN/creatinine ratio of >30 having a positive likelihood ratio of 7.5 for UGIB [7]. An INR (International Normalized Ratio) should be tested if the patient is known to be on an oral anticoagulant, or if they present with UGIB, especially in the context of known or suspected liver disease. While plain abdominal radiographs have been recommended for detection of free air from a perforated viscus, they lack the specificity and sensitivity to be relied upon in the high-risk elderly population. An abdominal CT scan is extremely sensitive for free air, indicates the perforation site, and is the study of choice if a perforated peptic ulcer is the suspected diagnosis [8].

Uncomplicated peptic ulcer disease can usually be managed with an oral H2 blocker or PPI and outpatient follow-up with gastroenterology; *H. pylori* testing may be performed at the discretion of the ED provider, but in most institutions will not result during the ED stay. Complicated peptic ulcer disease typically necessitates admission to the hospital and will often require invasive procedures, monitoring, and ICU level of care. Perforated peptic ulceration is managed surgically. PPIs are frequently administered while waiting for endoscopy but do not affect rebleeding, surgery, or mortality rates [9].

Pancreatitis

Gallstone- or bile-duct-stone-associated pancreatitis accounts for over 50% of all cases of acute pancreatitis and is the most common etiology in the older population. The gallstones that precipitate gallstone pancreatitis are generally small (<5 mm), and the exact etiology by which gallstones produce pancreatitis remains elusive [10]. Increasing age is a predictor for increased severity of pancreatitis. Alcohol abuse is also a risk factor for acute pancreatitis, but only about 5% of alcoholics develop pancreatitis, and alcoholic pancreatitis tends to develop prior to age 65. Older patients who have survived recurrent episodes of alcohol-induced acute pancreatitis may have chronic pancreatitis manifesting as pain, malabsorption, and diabetes. Many medications have been implicated in precipitating acute pancreatitis, and among the more frequent offenders are types of antiretroviral therapy.

For mild acute pancreatitis, the most common feature is abdominal pain, usually perceived in the epigastrium, with pain radiating into the midthoracic region, consistent with the formation of the pancreas and the biliary ducts from the embryonic foregut, and the location of the pancreas as a retroperitoneal organ. Other conditions that present similarly include other retroperitoneal pathologies such as abdominal aortic aneurysm (AAA), posterior duodenal ulceration, and occasionally renal pathology. Severe acute pancreatitis, particularly necrotizing pancreatitis, is associated with systemic complications including multisystem organ failure and electrolyte and chemical abnormalities, of which the most well described is hypocalcemia. Hypoglycemia, hyperglycemia, and ketoacidosis are also seen, and hyperlipidemia can be both the cause and the effect of acute pancreatitis [10–12].

Laboratory testing for a patient with suspected acute pancreatitis typically includes a CBC, chemistry including a calcium level, hepatic panel, and lipase.

For most patients presenting with an initial episode of pancreatitis, an upper abdominal ultrasound study (US) will help evaluate the biliary tract. An abdominal CT scan with IV contrast will provide diagnostic confirmation and exclude other serious and acute pathologies, and as well, confirm complications of pancreatitis such as pseudocyst formation [8].

The majority of patients with bile-duct stone pancreatitis improve with conservative management. A minority will progress to life-threatening severe pancreatitis. Differentiating between patients with acute pancreatitis who will progress to severe disease is not straightforward. The Ranson criteria and the Acute Physiology and Chronic Health Examination II score predict only about 50% of patients who go on to develop severe pancreatitis [12]. Other scoring systems may be easier to use, but may also not be any more helpful in predicting severe disease [11]. The timing of endoscopic interventions including endoscopic retrograde cholangiopancreatography (ERCP) with or without endoscopic sphincterotomy continues to be debated in the gastroenterology literature [12]. Most agree that the indications for ERCP for bile-duct stone associated acute pancreatitis include presence of cholangitis (fever, jaundice, and sepsis), obstructing stone seen on imaging, persistent biliary obstruction, or clinical deterioration. Contraindications to ERCP in acute pancreatitis include severe clinical or hemodynamic instability and severe coagulopathy [10, 12].

Diverticulitis

The majority of patients with acute diverticulitis present with left lower-quadrant pain, usually associated with systemic signs and symptoms such as nausea, fever, and chills. Advanced age, chronic constipation, and low dietary fiber are all risk factors for the development of diverticulitis [13].

Although abdominal-pelvic CT scan with oral or rectal contrast to facilitate bowel lumen visualization has traditionally been the preferred study for the identification of diverticulitis today many institutions will rely on IV contrast alone [1]. Patients with uncomplicated diverticulitis are usually managed with oral antibiotics as outpatients. Patients with complicated diverticulitis, such as phlegmon, abscess, peritonitis, or with systemic symptoms such as vomiting require hospitalization. Patients with diverticulitis with phlegmon only, or with a small abscess (less than 4 cm) (Stage IA or IB), are managed with intravenous antibiotics and bowel rest. Patients with an abscess greater than 4 cm diameter (Stage IIB) should be considered for percutaneous drainage. Patients with diverticulitis with purulent peritonitis (Stage III) or feculent peritonitis (Stage IV) are managed operatively; these conditions are associated with high morbidity and mortality [13].

Urinary tract infections

Urinary tract infections (UTIs) are common in the older patient population, but diagnosis can be difficult

in the ED. Independent community-dwelling older patients will typically manifest the classic symptoms of a UTI including dysuria, frequency, urgency, suprapubic pain, or flank pain. Patients with cognitive issues may not be able to recognize early UTI symptoms and may present with more global dysfunction including malaise, fatigue, and delirium [14]. Thus, it is always prudent to search for a UTI in the presence of an acute organic brain syndrome. Older patients are at risk for UTI for many reasons. They are more likely to have incomplete bladder emptying, or a neurogenic bladder associated with comorbidities such as diabetes, dementia, or Parkinson's disease, and they are more likely to have a long-standing urinary catheterization, which is associated with urinary colonization [15]. In men, prostatic enlargement contributes to obstructed flow of urine and increases the risk of urinary infection [14].

Older patients are at risk for developing asymptomatic bacteriuria (ASB), which, in turn, increases the risk of developing a UTI. For community-dwelling older patients, about 10% of men and 30% of women over 65 have ASB. The incidence is greater in patients residing in long-term care facilities and reaches 55% in some series [14–16]. There is good evidence that treating ASB is not helpful and can be harmful, exposing patients to the risks of antibiotic therapy and resistance [14, 15] ASB is defined in women as two consecutive clean-catch midstream urine samples growing $>10^5$ CFU/ml of the same uropathogen (no more than two species), in a patient without symptoms of a UTI and no indwelling urinary catheter within 7 days of the first urine culture. In men, a single midstream specimen is required [14]. The diagnosis of ASB depends on the passage of time and the reporting of a culture result, something that is unavailable to the treating emergency physician.

A midstream clean-catch urine sample should be obtained for urinalysis with microscopy to make the diagnosis of a UTI in the ED. An in-and-out catheter is preferred if the patient cannot provide a midstream sample. For patients with long-standing catheters, the catheter should be changed prior to sending a culture. Though the main CDC (Centers for Disease Control and Prevention) definition of UTI requires a culture result, its alternative definition includes two of the following: temperature $>38\,°C$ (fever is not seen in uncomplicated cystitis), dysuria, frequency, urgency, or suprapubic pain, and at least one of the following: positive Gram stain, pyuria (>10 white blood cells (WBCs)/ml³), positive leukocyte esterase, or nitrite by dipstick method, or two positive urine cultures with the same uropathogen (>10²) in a nonvoided sample [14]. These guidelines rely heavily on new urinary symptoms. Given the frequency of ASB in the older patient, the firm diagnosis of a UTI depends upon the patient being able to provide a history consistent with an infectious inflammatory process of the urinary tract, something that is often impossible in older patients, especially in the ED. Surrogates for a history of urinary symptoms include recent decline in functional status, acute delirium, and systemic signs of infection. When considering catheter-associated UTIs (CA-UTIs), it becomes even more confusing, as these are extremely difficult to distinguish from catheter-associated ASB on the basis of urinalysis [17]. The symptoms of the patient become the most important factor in considering whether to initiate antibiotic therapy. A special case involves patients with spinal cord injury, in whom increased spasticity, autonomic dysreflexia, and a sense of unease are markers of CA-UTI [17].

UTIs are classified as uncomplicated or complicated, or as lower UTI or upper UTI. Uncomplicated UTIs occur in nonpregnant women without urinary catheterization or urinary tract abnormalities. All UTIs in men, in patients with a catheter, or in patients with systemic symptoms are complicated. Lower UTIs have symptoms limited to the bladder or urethra. Any other UTI is a complicated (or an upper) UTI and includes all those UTIs with systemic symptoms [15]. Up to one third of older patients will not mount a fever in response to an infection, and up to 10% of older patients with severe infections will be hypothermic [18]. In patients who are unable to provide a history of acute urinary symptoms, the diagnosis of a complicated UTI should be considered where there is fever (or hypothermia), altered mental state, malaise, and focal signs consistent with UTI including costovertebral angle tenderness.

Guidelines suggest empiric antibiotic therapy for the acutely ill and treatment based upon culture results for those who are not acutely ill; however, this distinction is often less than clear in the ED particularly in patients with cognitive impairment [15]. Patients with uncomplicated UTIs can be treated with 3 days of antimicrobial therapy directed at *Escherichia coli*, and managed as an outpatient with return precautions. Very few older women will meet this definition, and no older men, as by definition any UTI in a man is complicated. For all complicated UTIs, the standard duration of treatment is 7 days [14–16]. For patients with a long-term catheter, the decision to treat an infection should be based upon symptoms and not the appearance or odor of the urine, macroscopically or on urinalysis. In selected patients with a long-term catheter and without any acute symptoms of infection, it may be appropriate to defer antimicrobial treatment until urine culture results are available. Current recommendations include avoiding prophylactic antibiotics for patients with long-term catheters or at the time of catheter changes. Urinary catheters should only be placed for strict indications, and removed as soon as possible [17], as a urinary catheter acts as a tether, and is often associated with the development of delirium [14, 19]. Systemic illness in older patients with a complicated or upper UTI will typically trigger admission. The 28-day mortality associated with bacteremia of urinary origin is about 5% in older patients [15].

Nonabdominal causes of abdominal pain

Clinicians must also search for serious nonabdominal causes of abdominal pain in older adults. Any intrathoracic pathology can present with upper abdominal pain, including pneumonia, pulmonary embolism, pleural effusion, congestive heart failure (CHF) with hepatic congestion, and particularly inferior AMIs. Increasing age and female gender are associated with atypical presentations of AMI [20], and abdominal pain may be the presenting complaint for up to one third of older women with an AMI [21]. Herpes zoster (HZ) and diabetic ketoacidosis can also present with abdominal pain as the chief complaint. One in three people will develop HZ in their lifetime, and more than half occur in individuals over 60 years of age. Older age is also associated with increased morbidity and mortality from HZ. Once the diagnostic dermatomal vesicular rash has developed, the diagnosis is usually straightforward. However, a prodrome that includes pain, pruritus, and dysesthesia may precede the development of the pathognomonic rash by several days, complicating the diagnosis [22].

Testing

Laboratory tests

In older patients, obtaining a CBC, routine chemistry, lipase, and hepatic panels are generally considered to be the most useful, although they will rarely be diagnostic in isolation. Serial lactate levels are helpful to monitor responses to resuscitation, or in the evaluation of a patient who is suspected of having mesenteric infarction or sepsis [23]. Cardiac markers are useful if the patient is suspected of acute myocardial ischemia, evidence of demand ischemia, or if the patient has significant sustained tachycardia or episodes of hypotension. Serial CBCs may need to be performed if patients are suspected of having gastrointestinal bleeding. Urinalysis (UA) should almost always be done in older patients, but directing care at a positive result can be more complicated than in younger patients since older patients are less likely to have the classic symptoms of a UTI and may have colonization of the urinary bladder [14–16].

Electrocardiography

An electrocardiogram should be obtained in any older adult presenting with upper abdominal pain or vague, nonlocalizing abdominal pain.

Diagnostic imaging

Diagnostic imaging studies are driven by the clinician's clinical assessment and differential diagnosis; however, the history and physical examination of the older patient with abdominal pain is often less specific than in younger patients. Accordingly, diagnostic imaging is often critical to the diagnosis of the underlying cause of the patient's abdominal pain. The most important decision is whether to obtain an abdominal CT scan. About 60% of older patients who present to EDs with abdominal pain have an abdominal CT scan as part of their evaluation [24]. Abdominal CT scan appears to alter the diagnosis in about 50% of elderly patients with abdominal pain and alters admission decision in one-quarter of patients [24–26]. The specific CT scan protocol chosen will be dependent on the clinicians' differential diagnosis. For example, proper timing of intravenous contrast is critical in the evaluation of the abdominal vasculature when mesenteric ischemia is high on the differential diagnosis, whereas rectal contrast may aid in the evaluation of distal colonic abscesses.

While the radiation exposure and risk of subsequent malignancy is less concerning in older patients, many older patients have comorbidities and long-term medications that increase their risk of developing contrast nephropathy in association with intravenous contrast administration. While intravenous contrast for CT scans should generally be avoided in patients with acute or chronic renal impairment, although patients receiving regular hemodialysis can usually receive intravenous contrast as long as they have dialysis within 24 h.

Disposition

Once it has been established that a patient does not require an emergent procedure (either through interventional radiology, gastroenterology, or in the operating room), attention turns to whether the patient is safe for discharge, or if the patient requires admission. Many patients with "nonsurgical" abdominal pain will still require admission to the hospital, and some will still require admission to the surgical service. Some patients may need admission for intravenous antibiotics, fluids, or ongoing monitoring of associated conditions such as acute renal failure. Other patients can be discharged home with clear return precautions and follow-up plans. Critical decision points include the patient's ability to tolerate oral intake, including prescribed medications, the normalization of vital signs, and an ability to perform activities of daily living at a level that is consistent with baseline function. A patient with limited mobility, who usually lives independently, may require admission to the hospital when presenting with diarrhea and mild cramping abdominal pain because of an inability to get to the bathroom in a timely fashion. ED observation units may be utilized for patients who do not clearly require an admission, but who may be at risk for deterioration after a premature discharge from the ED.

Section IV: Decision-Making

- The differential diagnosis for abdominal pain in the elderly is broad and includes intraperitoneal, extraperitoneal, and nonabdominal pathologies.
- Abdominal CT scans remain an extremely useful diagnostic test and are potentially therapeutic when utilized with CT-guided drainage.

- ASB is common in older adults and is easily confused with UTI in the ED. For patients who are systemically unwell (including delirium), empiric therapy is recommended. For patients with no urinary symptoms, waiting for culture results is advised.
- Up to one third of older women with an acute MI will present atypically with abdominal pain as the presenting symptom.

References

1 Hammond, N.A., Nikolaidis, P., and Miller, F.H. (2010) Left lower-quadrant pain: guidelines from the American College of Radiology appropriateness criteria. *Am. Fam. Physician*, 82 (7), 766–770 (Epub 2010/10/01).

2 Jackson, S.L. and Soper, D.E. (1999) Pelvic inflammatory disease in the postmenopausal woman. *Infect. Dis. Obstet. Gynecol.*, 7 (5), 248–252 (Epub 1999/10/19).

3 Lewis, L.M., Banet, G.A., Blanda, M. *et al.* (2005) Etiology and clinical course of abdominal pain in senior patients: a prospective, multicenter study. *J. Gerontol. A Biol. Sci. Med. Sci.*, 60 (8), 1071–1076.

4 Moore, A.R. and Clinch, D. (2004) Underlying mechanisms of impaired visceral pain perception in older people. *J. Am. Geriatr. Soc.*, 52 (1), 132–136 (Epub 2003/12/23).

5 Thorsen, K., Soreide, J.A., Kvaloy, J.T. *et al.* (2013) Epidemiology of perforated peptic ulcer: age- and gender-adjusted analysis of incidence and mortality. *World J. Gastroenterol.*, 19 (3), 347–354 (Epub 2013/02/02).

6 Christensen, S., Riis, A., Norgaard, M. *et al.* (2007) Short-term mortality after perforated or bleeding peptic ulcer among elderly patients: a population-based cohort study. *BMC Geriatr.*, 7, 8 (Epub 2007/04/19).

7 Srygley, F.D., Gerardo, C.J., Tran, T., and Fisher, D.A. (2012) Does this patient have a severe upper gastrointestinal bleed? *J. Am. Med. Assoc.*, 307 (10), 1072–1079 (Epub 2012/03/15).

8 Yaghmai, V., Rosen, M.P., Lalani, T. *et al.* (2012) *American College of Radiology Appropriateness Criteria Acute (Nonlocalized) Abdominal Pain and Fever or Suspected Abdominal Abscess*, American College of Radiology (ACR), Reston, VA. 12/11/2013.

9 Lu, Y., Loffroy, R., Lau, J.Y., and Barkun, A. (2014) Multidisciplinary management strategies for acute non-variceal upper gastrointestinal bleeding. *Br. J. Surg.*, 101 (1), e34–e50 (Epub 2013/11/28).

10 Ferreira, L.E. and Baron, T.H. (2013) Acute biliary conditions. *Best Pract. Res. Clin. Gastroenterol.*, 27 (5), 745–756 (Epub 2013/10/29).

11 Mounzer, R., Langmead, C.J., Wu, B.U. *et al.* (2012) Comparison of existing clinical scoring systems to predict persistent organ failure in patients with acute pancreatitis. *Gastroenterology*, 142 (7), 1476–1482; quiz e15-6.

12 Fogel, E.L. and Sherman, S. (2014) ERCP for gallstone pancreatitis. *N. Engl. J. Med.*, 370 (2), 150–157 (Epub 2014/01/10).

13 Moore, F.A., Catena, F., Moore, E.E. *et al.* (2013) Position paper: management of perforated sigmoid diverticulitis. *World J. Emerg. Surg.*, 8 (1), 55 (Epub 2013/12/29).

14 Matthews, S.J. and Lancaster, J.W. (2011) Urinary tract infections in the elderly population. *Am. J. Geriatr. Pharmacother.*, 9 (5), 286–309.

15 Beveridge, L.A., Davey, P.G., Phillips, G., and McMurdo, M.E. (2011) Optimal management of urinary tract infections in older people. *Clin. Interv. Aging*, 6, 173–180 (Epub 2011/07/15).

16 Arinzon, Z., Shabat, S., Peisakh, A., and Berner, Y. (2012) Clinical presentation of urinary tract infection (UTI) differs with aging in women. *Arch. Gerontol. Geriatr.*, 55 (1), 145–147 (Epub 2011/10/04).

17 Hooton, T.M., Bradley, S.F., Cardenas, D.D. *et al.* (2010) Diagnosis, prevention, and treatment of catheter-associated urinary tract infection in adults: 2009 International Clinical Practice Guidelines from the Infectious Diseases Society of America. *Clin. Infect. Dis.*, 50 (5), 625–663.

18 Mallet, M.L. (2002) Pathophysiology of accidental hypothermia. *Q. J. Med.*, 95 (12), 775–785.

19 Inouye, S.K., Westendorp, R.G., and Saczynski, J.S. (2014) Delirium in elderly people. *Lancet*, 383 (9920), 911–922 (Epub 2013/09/03).

20 Gupta, M., Tabas, J.A., and Kohn, M.A. (2002) Presenting complaint among patients with myocardial infarction who present to an urban, public hospital emergency department. *Ann. Emerg. Med.*, 40 (2), 180–186 (Epub 2002/07/26).

21 Lusiani, L., Perrone, A., Pesavento, R., and Conte, G. (1994) Prevalence, clinical features, and acute course of atypical myocardial infarction. *Angiology*, 45 (1), 49–55 (Epub 1994/01/01).

22 Sampathkumar, P., Drage, L.A., and Martin, D.P. (2009) Herpes zoster (shingles) and postherpetic neuralgia. *Mayo Clin. Proc.*, 84 (3), 274–280 (Epub 2009/03/03).

23 Andersen, L.W., Mackenhauer, J., Roberts, J.C. *et al.* (2013) Etiology and therapeutic approach to elevated lactate levels. *Mayo Clin. Proc.*, **88** (10), 1127–1140 (Epub 2013/10/02).

24 Lewis, L.M., Klippel, A.P., Bavolek, R.A. *et al.* (2007) Quantifying the usefulness of CT in evaluating seniors with abdominal pain. *Eur. J. Radiol.*, **61** (2), 290–296.

25 Esses, D., Birnbaum, A., Bijur, P. *et al.* (2004) Ability of CT to alter decision making in elderly patients with acute abdominal pain. *Am. J. Emerg. Med.*, **22** (4), 270–272.

26 Gardner, R.L., Almeida, R., Maselli, J.H., and Auerbach, A. (2010) Does gender influence emergency department management and outcomes in geriatric abdominal pain? *J. Emerg. Med.*, **39** (3), 275–281 (Epub 2008/11/11).

Back pain

Nicholas Santavicca[1] & Michael E. Winters[2]

[1] Department of Emergency Medicine, University of Maryland Medical Center, Baltimore, MD, USA
[2] Departments of Emergency Medicine and Medicine, University of Maryland School of Medicine, Baltimore, MD, USA

Section I: Case presentation

A 63-year-old man presented to the emergency department (ED) with a chief complaint of "low back pain." He stated that the pain began insidiously and was progressive over the preceding 3 weeks. He denied any precipitating event or trauma. The patient localized his discomfort to the paraspinal upper lumbar and lower thoracic regions. He denied bowel or bladder dysfunction. He denied lower extremity numbness, tingling, or weakness. There was no fever, polyuria, dysuria, hematuria, constipation, diarrhea, or abdominal pain. He denied saddle anesthesia. The patient reported a history of hypertension, hyperlipidemia, diabetes mellitus, and a remote history of prostate cancer that had been treated with radiation therapy. His medications included hydrochlorothiazide, lisinopril, metformin, and simvastatin. He denied medication allergies, tobacco use, or intravenous drug use. He occasionally drank alcohol during social events.

The patient's vital signs were significant for a blood pressure of 155/81 mmHg, a heart rate of 88 beats/min, a respiratory rate of 19 breaths/min, and a temperature of 37.1 °C. Physical examination of the back was normal in appearance with mild tenderness to palpation in the T10 to L2 segments. Neurologic examination, including gait, revealed normal strength, sensation, and reflexes. The prostate was nodular but nontender to palpation. Rectal tone was normal. There was no CVA (costovertebral angle) tenderness to percussion. The patient underwent an

X-ray study of the lumbar spine that was interpreted as degenerative joint disease. He was given analgesics and discharged with a diagnosis of "musculoskeletal low back strain."

The patient returned to the ED 3 days after his initial visit. At the time of the second presentation, the patient was unable to ambulate secondary to bilateral lower extremity weakness, and he was incontinent of urine. He subsequently underwent an emergent diagnostic study that revealed the diagnosis.

Section II: Case discussion

Dr Peter Rosen (PR): This sounds like a rather common ED visit that we all see at least once or twice per shift. Dr Bond I'm sure you've never done it, but I know I have – and that's when I see the complaint of back pain I think "oh God, another drug seeker." I'm sure that part of that is relieved when I see the age of the patient. Because, while I have actually seen a drug seeker who was in her 80s, I think it's pretty rare, and most often drug seekers are younger. But I do think it colors our vision of how we approach patients – whether we want it to or not. What is your basic workup for a patient with back pain – assuming you can get past the immediate distaste for having to deal with possibly another drug seeker?

Dr Michael Bond (MB): Well, my worst patient is a back pain patient who also has dental pain. If they just have back pain, I think the workup should

Geriatric Emergencies: A Discussion-Based Review, First Edition.
Edited by Amal Mattu, Shamai A. Grossman and Peter L. Rosen.
© 2016 John Wiley & Sons, Ltd. Published 2016 by John Wiley & Sons, Ltd.

consist of a comprehensive history and physical examination, which was done in this case. The big mistake that people make is that they don't undress the patient – including taking off their shoes – so they can perform a complete examination. Physicians often forget to examine the end of the human body – which is our perineum. In this case, they did a rectal examination, which probably is over and above what is necessary, as they could have just ensured that perineal sensation was intact. Once you have a complete examination and history, then additional testing is not needed unless a red flag is noted. This gentleman, though, has a history of prostate cancer that was reported as being remote and had been treated with radiation therapy. If it was really remote, like a decade ago, you could make an argument that no further testing is needed. However, because of his age I would get plain films of his spine, and if these were normal I would treat his pain, since most of back pain will be musculoskeletal – degenerative joint disease, herniated disc, or pulled muscle – and most of these causes are going to get better regardless of what we do. I think this workup was appropriate. The most important element, again, is a good physical examination.

Dr Ula Hwang (UH): I think disrobing the patient is a very important point. Seeing their functional status, what was being impacted motor- and sensory-wise. Looking at the skin with older adults, look for zoster rashes. That could cause pain. This patient's pain was much more diffuse, and no zoster rash was noted.

PR: I don't do a rectal examination on every patient with back pain. However, there is a reason here, which is not present in most patients. I think the history of prostatic cancer, no matter how remote, justifies a rectal examination or testing for perineal sensation by feeling the perineum. If they can feel my hand squeezing their perineum that's almost as good as a rectal examination, as it gives you sensation but doesn't give you motor function, which rectal sphincter tone can do. I also do not do lumbar films as a routine. Can you summarize for us your indications for plain lumbar spine films on patients with back pain?

Dr Maura Kennedy (MK): Plain lumbar spine films are challenging. In our older patients, we need to consider compression fractures that can happen without much trauma, and if there is focal tenderness,

they can be informative on occasion. The challenge is in a trauma situation with back pain, as plain films can be misleadingly reassuring. In a traumatic event, what appears to be a compression fracture on plain radiographs may actually be an unstable burst fracture. One of the concerning aspects of this history is that his pain has been progressing over several weeks and not improving. For this reason, imaging is very reasonable in him; however, he had diffuse tenderness at numerous levels, but imaging was only done of the lumbar spine. I think there are elements of the history and examination missing here but could better distinguish between perhaps a simple musculoskeletal cause of back pain versus more concerning cause. These include whether he had any abdominal tenderness and whether his pain is worse when he's ambulating and improves when he's resting.

MB: I think that's a really good point as far as the abdominal examination; when I first read the case, I was thinking an abdominal aortic aneurysm (AAA) could easily be a cause in this patient. A thorough abdominal examination is definitely warranted. I'd also like to know whether he has more pain while sleeping as opposed to while he's up and about, as this would suggest a nonmechanical cause of his back pain. In this age group, I would also worry about spinal stenosis. I would ask "is this pain relieved by bending over and walking with a carriage in the shopping mall as opposed to regular walking?"

PR: Related to spinal stenosis I would ask, "does the patient have pain while he walks, and what's the pain like?" this suggests pseudoclaudication – It's still a very hard diagnosis to prove in the ED, however, even though you think you're seeing it. I would also presume that a man of this age would have osteoarthritis, and that is also a clue to spinal stenosis.

PR: All of us would be a little more concerned about this patient because of his age. That to me puts him in a category that needs imaging. I think that any history of trauma, and as you've suggested, whether or not this pain is worsening with position warrants imaging. Did that interpretation of that X-ray study come from the emergency physician or from the radiologist? Many times, we don't see our own films simply because we are given a report, and if it's a film we're not especially interested in, we don't go to the extra

111

labor of pulling up the digital image. As clinicians, we often do a slightly better job of looking for the pathology we're interested in because we have the clinical history rather than the radiologist who's just reading the films.

UH: The emergency physician interpreted the film at that time.

PR: It's probably accurate then. We have a fair bit of information about his past history. Do we have a PSA (prostate-specific antigen) level?

UH: We don't have the PSA level.

Dr Shamai Grossman (SG): Do we at least know whether he followed up regularly with his oncologist?

UH: That information wasn't available to me at the time, but I would assume that he did not.

PR: Let me ask a couple of laboratory questions. Years ago, we used to do an acid phosphatase level to both look for possible prostatic cancer and to look for metastatic disease. It was pretty accurate for both. It was, of course, replaced by the PSA, which is probably more accurate for prostate cancer, but not more accurate for metastases. Do you know if we can still readily obtain an acid phosphate in the ED?

SG: Alkaline phosphatase we certainly can, it's part of our routine liver function tests, but I've never ordered an acid phosphatase and believe it's unlikely that it's available – and certainly not on an emergent basis.

PR: Alkaline phosphatase is actually a fairly easy test to obtain, but my guess is that you're quite correct, most EDs don't have it available as a test. Maybe it's something we ought to be looking into because I think this is exactly the kind of patient in whom it would be useful. Remember to send your study before you do your prostate examination because the prostate contains alkaline phosphatase, and you artificially elevate the level if you do your rectal examination before you get your study. I do think we can obtain PSA pretty readily. I might be inclined to order a PSA if I can't obtain that information from his primary care or from his medical record. I always worry about in a patient this age is prostatic metastases.

PR: I liked your thought about aortic aneurysm as certainly that is a common cause of back pain before it's ruptured, or even as it's rupturing. Plain films can demonstrate one because of the calcification in the wall of the aneurysm. It can also miss it. Palpation of an aneurysm is not as commonly possible as we would like to believe it is. I would do a bedside ultrasound as well as obtain lumbar films because I think that's a very strong possible diagnosis in this patient.

SG: One of the questions I routinely ask, when patients come in with back pain that's not clearly from trauma, is what they were doing when it started. If they tell me it began while they were sleeping, it at least gives me some thought that it's from some nondescript trauma that occurred while they were in bed. If the pain occurred while they were simply sitting and doing absolutely nothing, it would make me a bit more worried.

PR: The only trauma I can think of in bed besides sex is seizure. I think that's a good historical point, regardless we're all concerned about this patient more than we're concerned about most of our back pain patients. I think he had a terrific workup that leaves you with absolutely no place to go, because there really isn't any reason to go any further based on what you've already found in this case unless you can find some other special information. I do think that given that his pain was a little more diffuse than localized, and sounded a little more musculoskeletal than discogenic, would you have considered, in retrospect, adding a thoracic spine to your lumbar spine X-ray? Sometimes, we can see metastases on the thoracic spine that we can't see in the lumbar spine.

UH: I think in this case just because his examination did reveal more tenderness diffusely and up into the thoracic region, in retrospect adding thoracic images could have been of some utility. But again, if it is our ED reading of the films and potentially not having old ones for comparison, you may not discover what we later find out is metastatic disease in his vertebral bodies. The history, in addition to these comorbidities – hypertension, hyperlipidemia – will make you think along the lines of not just metastatic cancer pain but also AAA, or dissection. The duration of his pain implies – this is a disease process that's been progressive for the last 3 weeks. It didn't happen acutely, yesterday. Nevertheless, we must ask, despite no history of trauma, did something happen? With a shorter duration of onset, you also should start to consider an infectious etiology. As patients get older, they're going to be at a greater risk for things that can cause back pain (more) than younger patients. I don't know if I would necessarily do laboratory testing for all patients, but if you have a suspicion for some type of cancerous lesion, you could also check to see if the calcium levels are elevated.

PR: Good point, particularly in patients with breast cancer because they can present with serious complications of hypercalcemia, and we tend to forget that it's treatable even if they have metastatic disease. I suspect that the diagnosis in this case could only have been made with an MRI (magnetic resonance imaging), and I don't see any indication for one on this presentation. My indication to obtain an MRI in the ED is a cord obstruction syndrome, and that was not present when you first saw this patient.

MB: I definitely don't see any indication for MRI in the ED at this point. Referral for an outpatient MRI to evaluate for a herniated disc or other causes of his pain is reasonable if he is not getting better with conservative therapy. With no neurological symptoms at all, it's really hard to justify an MRI acutely.

SG: The key to this case is the follow-up. As long as you're very clear that this patient is going to follow up with either his primary care physician or his oncologist within the next couple of days he should be safe for discharge. While I do think this patient needs an MRI, I don't think this patient needs an MRI in the ED. That needs to be communicated to both the patient and the person who is following the patient. It also needs to be well documented. In your notes, you can't say this is clearly musculoskeletal in a patient who has a history of prostate cancer.

MB: I would disagree with that somewhat. I would say as long as he has good follow-up – follow-up with his primary care provider, as long as he's getting good follow-up for his prostate cancer, like yearly PSA levels, then I don't know if he needs an MRI. I definitely don't want to set the standard that everybody with any history of cancer over the age of 60 with back pain needs an MRI, because the majority of these cases are still going to be musculoskeletal back pain. The older you get, the more likely you are to throw out your back.

SG: I agree. I think he's entitled to a short course of therapy to see how the patient does. But, very

clearly, we shouldn't brush the pain off and say it's musculoskeletal.

MB: I would just say with caution that he does not absolutely need an MRI. He needs a great follow-up; he needs to have in his discharge instructions that say "we're treating you for musculoskeletal back pain, but this could be something more serious, and you need to follow up with your doctor. You need to make sure your cancer is being appropriately followed."

PR: At this point, I also don't think an MRI is indicated. On the other hand, this is a patient who concerns me because we don't really have a diagnosis that I'm totally comfortable with. Would you be inclined to bring this patient back to the ED? The reality of our medical delivery system is that for him to follow up with his primary care provider or his oncologist is probably not going to happen within this week. I'd be surprised if you could get an appointment for him in 48 h. I'd be surprised if you could get an appointment for him in the next month. But the reality is you can always bring him back to the ED. Would you be inclined to do that, or would you be inclined to put him in observation for a little while to see if you can get rid of his pain, and, if you can't get rid of his pain, then maybe you have to use that as an indication for doing further workup?

MK: I think it depends really on how he looks and how severe his pain is. Before I would consider discharging him, I would want to make sure he can ambulate and can function at home. In terms of whether I would keep him overnight would depend upon if his pain is well controlled with oral medications. I would probably just start with acetaminophen. I think the key here is discussing with him what his outpatient care is. Does he have a primary care physician? Is it someone that he regularly follows up with? If he hasn't seen one of his outpatient providers in a long time, I'd say he needs to be reevaluated within 2 days, and if he cannot get an outpatient clinic appointment in this time frame, he should return to the ED. My general instruction for people is that if their symptoms are getting worse or markedly severe, or if they develop new symptoms, then they should absolutely return to the ED.

PR: We've talked in the past about pain medicine for the elderly. Even though as you've pointed out, 63 is hardly elderly, how would you approach managing his discomfort in the ED? While Tylenol purportedly is as good as anything else for pain relief, I believe that's only true of the people who get pain relief from it, and that's probably only 40% of the people who take it. Many other patients get zero pain relief with Tylenol. Where would you go for this patient if he did not respond to acetaminophen, or would you use something else initially?

UH: Whenever approaching a patient with regard to pain management, I ask "what have you already used at home?" Has this patient already tried acetaminophen, and what dosing is he using? If not, I would, as Maura suggested, try that initially. If that isn't effective, then I might consider moving onto NSAIDs (nonsteroidal anti-inflammatory drugs). This patient doesn't really have any significant concomitant diseases. Although he does have hypertension, he doesn't have a history of renal disorder, nor a history of GERD (gastroesophageal reflux disease) or GI (gastrointestinal) disorders that may be a contraindication. Given our initial impression that this is musculoskeletal back strain, I might consider short-term NSAIDs on this man. Thereafter, I move up to opiate medications. It all depends on how severe the pain is. If he calls the pain a 10/10 and is completely not physically functional because of this pain, that will also dictate how aggressively I go. I might start with an IV opiate rather than initially try an oral opiate. But again, the goal would be, and this would be discussed with the patient, "what do you expect with pain relief? Do you expect 0 pain or do you expect functional relief? Is your pain so bad that you can no longer ambulate? If we can get you to ambulate and get your pain from a 9 to a 6, would that be appropriate for you?" Discussing the patient's expectations, how we plan to try to manage his pain treatment, and how to get to those goals is critical in these patients. With older adults, the ultimate ED goal is to manage with oral analgesics. In this case, if we send them out on an opiate analgesic, we should also offer a bowel regimen.

PR: To go back toward our MRI discussion just a little bit further, if you found that this patient was not responding to a pain regimen and you even had to add opiates but despite adding opiates the patient still wasn't comfortable in the ED, would you consider that as an indication for an MRI?

MB: This might be my very jaded Baltimore opinion, but I think that most of the time the people that I see who can't get good pain relief for are mostly the drug seekers. Even people with epidural abscesses and AAA's most of the time respond to even a small dose of narcotics. I don't know that pain relief is the best indication for an MRI. A lot of the time, just like with patients with fever in whom I don't expect the fever to go completely away in the ED, with pain I'm just trying to make them comfortable. My rule is that they have to be able to eat and they have to be able to walk; then they can go home with follow-up.

PR: What I meant was not the patient whose pain was not totally relieved, but one whose pain is getting worse despite opiates. I have found a couple of spinal cord obstructive syndromes in those particular patients before they develop neurologic findings, one of whom actually developed rectal sphincter tone loss as he went for his MRI. Sometimes, if your first examination is negative, you don't repeat it, particularly if it's a rectal examination. But I would in a patient who is not getting pain relief and who is getting worse.

MB: If he's getting worse I would definitely do the MRI. But, a lot of times, I am very jaded with our Baltimore population who are "allergic" to Tylenol, but can take Percocet. Some of them don't get pain relief because of their secondary gain issues. But if I think it's a stoic, 63-year-old Vietnam veteran who never complains about anything – then absolutely.

PR: I start out having to overcome a bias against back pain. But, having overcome it, these are patients that do worry me because it's so hard to prove their diagnosis.

PR: Can you tell us what happened to this poor patient?

UH: This patient returned 3 days later after his initial visit. Now he wasn't able to ambulate secondary to bilateral lower extremity weakness and was also incontinent of urine. He then underwent an emergent MRI and was found to have metastatic involvement, most notably at the L2 level with evidence of cord compression. He was immediately given a dose of IV dexamethasone to try to relieve the swelling, and was admitted and underwent emergent radiation therapy to the L-spine and surgical decompression, but unfortunately, his neurologic symptoms did not improve. This patient's diagnosis was malignant spinal cord compression, likely from his prostate cancer, and he died approximately 5 months later from complications of his advanced cancer.

PR: In retrospect, were his metastases observable on that lumbar spine film, or did they only show up on the MRI?

UH: They were observable. In retrospect, it's much easier to go back and look for subtle disease after you know the diagnosis.

PR: Well, again I wouldn't fault anyone for missing it. It's not that obvious – it's not like multiple myeloma washout of metastatic areas, and they can be easy to miss. I don't know what else you could have done on that first visit short of the special laboratory testing that might have given you a clue. I'm not sure that it would have made any difference anyway because it doesn't sound like he responded to either radiation or steroids. He just had a very bad disease. Perhaps for the future, would you be at all inclined to do a PSA as part of your general workup of the older patient with back pain?

SG: The problem with tests, such as PSA or other infrequently ordered emergent labs, is that they will not get run in an expeditious manner and are often batched and run only a couple of times per week. With results unavailable for 1–2 days post visit, their utility in emergency medicine is severely limited. In addition, any test that does not result during the patient's ED visit becomes a liability when faced with the difficulties in ensuring the results are appropriately followed up.

PR: Do you have any final thoughts?

UH: I think that this is a very good example of a case where, in older patients, the diagnoses will not be written across their foreheads, they're going to be subtle. I don't think there was anything in the management of this patient during the first ED visit that was incorrect. I think this patient was very well managed, and a very thorough examination was documented, and the appropriate studies were done. The point is that with older adults, they present with atypical presentations, complex histories, and one has to be aware of subtle diagnoses.

PR: I would just remind people again that getting follow-up for these patients is much harder in most institutions than we ever think it is. Perhaps I'm more tuned in because of some personal experiences in trying to get follow-up, and I think that this is a place where we can use the ED profitably. In the 3 days before he returned, we don't know what his efforts were to follow up, whether or not he was compliant with instructions. With the older patient in whom we don't have a clear diagnosis, we can do that patient a great service by simply demanding that he come back to the ED for that first post follow-up visit.

MB: The biggest challenge is that we have to change the mentality of a lot of EDs. Many of my staff seem to approach these patients with hostility when we've seen them just a couple of days before. I never get push-back if I go to Starbucks more than once a week, but we do that to our patients way too often. We need to change the whole culture of emergency medicine so that we are the place for frequent follow-ups for some of these patients that have conditions that are undiagnosed, and that could be potentially deadly. If they are coming back then, we, the medical establishment, have perhaps not yet met their needs, and we have to take another look at how to best treat them.

PR: I get tired of hearing my colleagues saying "this is an inappropriate visit." There is no such thing, even if it's a drug seeker. Every patient who comes in is somebody that guarantees that I have a job. The reality is, if I've asked a patient to come back in 2 days, then why should another physician scorn the patient because it's a "too frequent visit, and inappropriate." I do think we have to change our attitudes, and the only way to do that is to communicate this to your residents not to tolerate complaints about inappropriate visits, and try to convince them that they are just shortening their own careers and their own enjoyment of their careers if they start judging patients so harshly. It's a hard thing to change, however.

Section III: Concepts

Background

Acute back pain is experienced by more than 90% of adults during their lifetime and is the second most common reason to visit a physician [1]. For the majority of patients, the cause of back pain is not life threatening, and symptoms typically resolve in 4–6 weeks. Unfortunately, up to 10% of patients with acute back pain have a critical condition that requires immediate diagnosis and emergent therapy [2]. These "back pain emergencies" can be grouped into vascular, infectious, and malignant conditions. Accurate diagnosis of these emergencies can be challenging in the elderly, as numerous factors affect the signs and symptoms of these critical diagnoses. The following chapter will focus on the clinical presentation, diagnosis, and treatment of select life-threatening emergencies in elderly patients with acute back pain.

Vascular catastrophes

Aortic dissection

Acute aortic dissection (AD) is estimated to affect 5–30 patients per million per year and accounts for 0.003% of patients who come to an ED with acute back, chest, or abdominal pain [3, 4]. AD is a true vascular emergency that carries a high mortality rate. In fact, the rate increases 1–2% *for every hour* of delay in diagnosis and treatment [5]. Unfortunately, delays in diagnosis are common and adversely affect patient outcome [4, 6, 7].

Not surprisingly, AD affects elderly patients more commonly than younger age groups. In fact, its peak incidence is between the ages of 60 and 80 years [8]. Risk factors for AD among the elderly include hypertension, hyperlipidemia, smoking, male gender, preexisting aortic abnormalities, previous cardiac surgery, and connective tissue disorders such as Marfan's and Ehlers–Danlos syndromes [8–10].

The clinical presentation of AD in elderly patients is highly variable. The classic textbook description of tearing or ripping back or chest pain is present infrequently [11]. More often, patients describe the abrupt onset of severe pain that reaches maximal intensity soon after onset [11, 12]. Moreover, up to 53% of patients with AD present with back pain, especially patients with dissection of the descending aorta [6]. The pain might also be described as migratory, such as back pain that moves to the chest or abdomen. Importantly, neurologic symptoms are present in up to 30% of patients with AD [6]. They include lower extremity weakness, sensory abnormalities, and paraplegia. It is easy to see how the diagnosis of AD can be delayed in elderly patients presenting with

back pain and neurologic symptoms in the legs. In contrast to the textbook presentation that includes markedly elevated blood pressure, elderly patients with AD more commonly present with normal, or even low, blood pressure [1, 8]. In addition, pulse and blood pressure differentials between the extremities are present in only 20–40% of patients [9, 10]. One cannot exclude the diagnosis of AD based on normal blood pressure readings or the absence of pulse differentials between the extremities.

Definitive diagnosis of AD requires imaging. Often, a chest radiograph (CXR) is ordered as an initial screening study. The most common radiographic abnormality in patients with AD is a widened mediastinum (>8 cm.) However, this abnormality is present in only 63% of ascending dissections and just 56% of descending dissections [12]. Additional radiographic abnormalities include left pleural effusion, elevation of the right main bronchus, and tracheal deviation [13]. Overall, the sensitivity of a CXR for AD can be as low as 80% [4, 12].

Computed tomography (CT) with intravenous contrast has become the diagnostic study of choice to confirm AD. The sensitivity and specificity of CT for AD approach 94% [14]. For elderly patients who are too unstable to be sent for CT, a transesophageal echocardiogram (TEE) can be performed at the bedside. Depending on the operator's experience and ability to visualize the entire aorta, the sensitivity of TEE for AD can reach 98% [14].

The ED management of elderly patients with AD centers on control of the heart rate and blood pressure. The primary goal is to decrease shear forces on the torn aortic wall to prevent further propagation of the dissection or aortic rupture. To achieve this goal, rapidly decrease the heart rate to approximately 60 beats/min with beta-blocker medication [15, 16]. Recommended beta-blocker medications for AD include esmolol and labetalol [15–17]. Once the heart rate is controlled, rapidly reduce the systolic blood pressure (SBP) to approximately 100–120 mmHg. A number of antihypertensive medications can be used to achieve SBP reduction: labetalol, combination of nicardipine and esmolol, and combination of sodium nitroprusside and esmolol [15–18]. Following stabilization of the heart rate and SBP, shift the treatment to interventional management with endovascular devices or open surgical repair.

Abdominal aortic aneurysm

Similar to AD, AAA is more common in elderly patients. It is estimated that 5% of people over the age of 65 years have an AAA, and this estimate is projected to rise [19]. The incidence of AAA increases by 2–4% each decade beyond 65 years [4]. Risk factors for AAA are similar to those for AD: smoking, hypertension, male gender, connective tissue disorders, and a family history of AAA [19–22]. Of these risk factors, smoking is the strongest risk factor and is present in approximately 70% of elderly men with AAA [19, 20]. For the emergency physician, the most important complication of an AAA is rupture, the risk of which increases if the aneurysm is increasing in size, and the blood pressure is elevated [22, 23]. Aneurysms less than 5 cm in diameter have a risk of rupture of 1% per year, whereas those greater than 6 cm have a rupture rate of 25% per year [21, 22, 24]. Aneurysms larger than 8 cm have a rupture rate of 25% within 6 months [24].

Older patients with ruptured AAA can present with a myriad of symptoms. The classic triad of abdominal pain, hypotension, and a pulsatile abdominal mass is present in fewer than 50% of patients with a ruptured AAA [25]. More often, patients present with the acute onset of pain that can be localized to the back or flank. Additional complaints can include nausea, vomiting, urinary retention, and lower extremity sensory or motor abnormalities. Hypotension is absent in up to 40% of patients with ruptured AAA [10]. Furthermore, the sensitivity of a physical examination in detecting an AAA greater than 5 cm is just 75% [26]. As a result of these varied presentations, ruptured AAA is often misdiagnosed as nephrolithiasis, diverticulitis, or acute musculoskeletal back pain.

Emergent abdominal ultrasound performed is invaluable in evaluating the elderly with suspected AAA. The sensitivity and specificity of ultrasound performed by an emergency physician for the detection of AAA are 97% and 94%, respectively [27]. Unfortunately, ultrasound is not sensitive for AAA rupture, as most ruptures bleed into the retroperitoneum. Nevertheless, older patients with acute back or flank pain with an AAA on bedside ultrasound should be considered to have a rupture until proven otherwise. For stable patients with an inconclusive ultrasound examination, CT scan of the abdomen remains the imaging modality of choice for confirming AAA and evaluating for rupture. The sensitivity of CT scan for diagnosing AAA approaches 100%, whereas its sensitivity for detecting retroperitoneal hemorrhage is approximately 75% [28].

Unstable older patients with an AAA should be taken to the operating room emergently [10]. For patients who are hemodynamically stable and undergoing diagnostic imaging to confirm a ruptured AAA, establish large-bore intravenous access and request a type and cross for packed red blood cells, platelets, and fresh frozen plasma. As in the management of AD, the blood pressure should be controlled to limit shear stress on the aneurysm wall and contain a hematoma if rupture is present [10]. Once the diagnosis is confirmed, operative repair remains the treatment of choice for AAA rupture although more and more institutions are performing aortic stenting rather than open surgery.

Infectious catastrophes

Spinal epidural abscess

The incidence of spinal epidural abscess (SEA) is increasing [1]. Reasons for this increase are multifactorial and include the increasing prevalence of human immunodeficiency disease, diabetes mellitus, malignancy, spinal procedures, and intravenous drug abuse [29]. Older adults are at particular risk for SEA because of the higher prevalence of diabetes, malignancy, and other comorbid conditions that result in immunosuppression [29].

SEA occurs through three primary mechanisms: hematogenous spread, direct extension from an adjacent source, and direct inoculation from a spinal procedure [30]. The most common sources of infection for hematogenous spread in people who are not intravenous drug users are the urinary tract, respiratory tract, skin, and soft tissue [29, 31]. Though SEA may occur in any location of the spine, the majority of them occur in the thoracolumbar spine. Approximately 60% of cases are caused by *Staphylococcus aureus* [32]. Gram-negative bacteria (e.g., *Pseudomonas aeruginosa*) account for an increasing number of cases, especially among intravenous drug abusers and patients with end-stage renal disease who are receiving hemodialysis [33]. Unfortunately, the diagnosis of SEA is often missed, resulting in a mortality rate approaching 15% [34].

The classic triad of fever, back pain, and neurologic symptoms is present in fewer than 20% of patients at initial presentation [35]. Back pain, the most common complaint, occurs in up to 85% of cases [32, 34]. The majority of patients with SEA are afebrile at their initial presentation. Many older persons cannot mount an adequate immune response to infection, and many others take medications that have antipyretic properties; therefore, the diagnosis of SEA cannot be excluded based on the absence of a fever. Neurologic symptoms at the time of presentation are an ominous finding and occur in up to 35% of patients [32, 34]. Neurologic symptoms imply spinal cord compression and occur along a spectrum from paresthesia to motor dysfunction, and finally bowel and bladder incontinence. Bladder incontinence is characterized as an overflow incontinence due to acute retention.

Laboratory studies have low diagnostic yield for patients with suspected SEA. More than a third of patients with SEA do not have leukocytosis. Although the erythrocyte sedimentation rate (ESR) and C-reactive protein (CRP) have higher sensitivities than the white blood cell count, normal values for them cannot be used to exclude the diagnosis. Though often obtained, blood cultures fail to identify a pathogen in approximately 40% of patients with SEA [32].

MRI with gadolinium remains the study of choice for the diagnosis of SEA. The sensitivity of MRI for SEA exceeds 90% [36]. An MRI is useful to evaluate the extent of disease and the degree of spinal cord compression. Because SEA can span several spinal segments and up to one third of patients have multiple abscesses, the entire spine should be included in the image [31]. When MRI is contraindicated or not available, CT myelography can be performed; however, it is invasive and carries the risk of spreading infection if the needle pierces the abscess.

Patients with SEA who are unstable or who have neurologic symptoms should receive broad-spectrum antibiotics as soon as possible, and a neurosurgeon should be consulted regarding emergent decompression of the abscess. Steroids are not indicated for cord compression caused by SEA [37]. For hemodynamically stable patients with a SEA and a normal neurologic examination, antibiotics may be administered after appropriate tissue samples have been obtained in the operating room, or, more commonly, by CT-guided biopsy.

Vertebral osteomyelitis

Vertebral osteomyelitis (VOM) occurs in approximately 5.3 per million patients per year [38]. Similar to SEA, the incidence is increasing in response to the increasing prevalence of intravenous drug use, spinal instrumentation, and immunosuppressive conditions. The risk factors, mechanism of infection, and most common location for VOM are identical to those for SEA. Endocarditis accounts for up to 12% of cases of VOM [39]. Bacterial pathogens for VOM are also similar to those for SEA and include both gram-positive (e.g., *S. aureus*) and gram-negative (e.g., *E. coli, Pseudomonas)* bacteria [40].

Back pain, seen in approximately 90% of patients with VOM, is its most common presenting symptom [40]. The pain can be described as localized or radicular and is often worse at night or with recumbency. In fact, when an older patient describes back pain that is worse at night or the supine position, SEA, VOM, and malignancy should come to mind. Fever is seen in less than half of patients with VOM at initial presentation. Neurologic symptoms of paresthesia, weakness, or bowel or bladder dysfunction are uncommon in patients with VOM, unless an abscess has formed, and is causing cord compression [39, 40].

Laboratory evaluation of the older adult patient with suspected VOM often includes a complete blood count, ESR, CRP, and blood cultures. As with SEA, an elevated white blood cell count is seen in only 50% of patients [40]. Though the sensitivity of ESR and CRP is higher than the white blood cell count, up to 20% of patients can have normal values in the setting of VOM [41]. Similarly, blood cultures identify a pathogen in only 60% of patients. Quite simply, in patients at high risk for VOM, do not exclude the diagnosis based on a normal white blood cell count, ESR, or CRP.

MRI remains the diagnostic test of choice for VOM, with a sensitivity of approximately 95% [1, 42]. In addition to identifying abnormalities of the intervertebral disc and disc space, MRI can identify fluid collections and spinal cord compression. A CT scan of the spine can evaluate the vertebrae, but is unable to identify cord abnormalities or SEA accurately. Therefore, a CT scan of the spine is less sensitive than MRI for VOM. Plain films of the spine might demonstrate bone abnormalities such as erosions; however, these changes take weeks to develop, making plain films useless in the early diagnosis of VOM.

The ED treatment of patients with VOM centers on antibiotic therapy and consultation with either neurosurgery or orthopedic surgery. For the patient with hemodynamic instability and neurologic symptoms, broad-spectrum antibiotics that treat both gram-positive and gram-negative bacteria should be initiated immediately. With the rising incidence of methicillin-resistant *S. aureus*, antibiotics should be sensitive to this pathogen. For the hemodynamically stable older patient with VOM and a normal neurologic examination, tissue cultures should be obtained prior to antibiotic administration, if possible. Tissue cultures can be obtained via CT-guided biopsy or from samples taken in the operating room. The duration of antibiotic therapy depends on the individual patient, the organism causing infection, and the response to initial antibiotic therapy. Though ESR and CRP should not be used to confirm or exclude the diagnosis of VOM, these tests can be used to evaluate the response to treatment [43].

Malignant spinal cord compression

In 2000, the World Health Organization estimated a 50% growth in the incidence of cancer over the next 20 years [44]. Currently, cancer is the second most common cause of death in the United States [45].

Spinal cord compression from metastatic malignancies is a back pain emergency that must be diagnosed promptly to prevent further disability and death. It has been reported that up to 50% of patients with advanced cancer have spinal metastases [46]. Up to 5% of patients with terminal cancer have metastatic spinal cord compression (MSCC) [47]. In fact, MSCC is the initial presentation of cancer in up to 20% of patients [48]. Lung, breast, and prostate cancers have the highest incidence of spinal metastasis and account for up to 70% of cases of MSCC [49]. Non-Hodgkin's lymphoma, renal cell carcinoma, and multiple myeloma account for most of the remaining cases [49, 50]. The thoracic spine is the most common location of metastatic disease, accounting for approximately 60% of cases, followed by the lumbosacral and cervical spine [51, 52].

Back pain is the most common presenting symptom in patients with MSCC, occurring in up to 95% of cases [49]. Typically, the back pain of metastatic disease begins gradually and slowly worsens. Patients ultimately diagnosed with MSCC complain of back pain an average of 2 months before the diagnosis is confirmed [53]. The majority of patients report that the back pain is worse at night and when they lie down [49]. As the disease progresses, the pain can be described as mechanical, worsening with movement. Neurologic symptoms are late findings and indicate a grave prognosis. Motor weakness is typically the first neurologic symptom of MSCC, present in 60–85% of patients at the time of diagnosis [54]. Weakness can be subtle, described by patients as "clumsiness" or "heaviness." Sensory abnormalities usually occur following the onset of motor weakness and are present in up to 50% of patients at the time of diagnosis [52]. Late findings of MSCC include bowel or bladder incontinence and autonomic dysfunction.

As in the assessment of other back pain emergencies, laboratory studies are generally not helpful in the diagnosis of MSCC. A complete blood count might demonstrate shifts in select cell lines, indicative of hematologic malignancies. Hypercalcemia seen on an electrolyte panel suggests malignancies such as multiple myeloma and lung or breast cancer, but this finding is not specific for these diseases. The ESR or CRP could also be elevated; however, these findings are also nonspecific for malignant disease.

MRI is the imaging modality of choice for the diagnosis of MSCC, with a sensitivity and specificity of 93% and 97%, respectively [55]. Since up to one third of patients have multiple sites of metastatic spinal involvement, MRI of the entire spine should be obtained. Radiographs of the spine might demonstrate vertebral body abnormalities, but the false-negative rate of plain films is as high as 17% [1, 51]. The diagnosis of MSCC based on a normal radiograph of the spine should not be excluded. CT scans are more useful than plain films and can be obtained when MRI is contraindicated or unavailable. As discussed in relation to infectious causes of acute back pain, CT of the spine cannot determine thecal sac compression or spinal cord signal changes.

The ED treatment of patients with MSCC centers on corticosteroid therapy and is based on the presenting neurologic examination. Administer corticosteroids as soon as possible for patients with suspected MSCC and neurologic abnormalities. Corticosteroids decrease vasogenic edema and have been shown to shorten hospital length of stay and delay the onset of paralysis [53, 56]. Dexamethasone is the recommended corticosteroid of choice [57]. In addition to its ability to reduce vasogenic edema, this drug provides analgesia and has tumoricidal effects on select malignancies, namely, leukemias, lymphomas, and breast cancer [58]. Though controversy remains as to the optimal dose, 10 mg can be administered intravenously as soon as the diagnosis is considered. Depending on the malignancy, some patients with MSCC can be treated emergently with radiation therapy. Following the administration of dexamethasone, consult radiation oncology and neurosurgery so that radiation therapy or surgical decompression can be arranged, as warranted.

Section IV: Decision-making

- Back pain is a common complaint among older patients.
- Although most causes are benign, up to 10% of patients harbor a back pain emergency.
- Careful consideration must be made of critical back pain differential diagnoses including the following:
  - Vascular (aortic dissection and aortic aneurysm)
  - Infectious (spinal epidural abscess and vertebral osteomyelitis)
  - Malignancy-related spinal cord compression.
- Evaluation for these disastrous conditions begins with a risk-factor assessment and history of present illness, followed by the appropriate diagnostic imaging modality (MRI).
- For the majority of cases, laboratory studies are not helpful.
- Specific actions can be taken in the ED to facilitate the diagnosis, intervene in the disease process, and stabilize the patient in preparation for the next phase of care.
- Management of patients with back pain emergencies usually requires specialty consultation.

Acknowledgment

The manuscript was copyedited by Linda J. Kesselring, MS, ELS, the technical editor/writer in the Department of Emergency Medicine at the University of Maryland Medical Center.

References

1 Winters, M.E., Kluetz, P., and Zilberstein, J. (2006) Back pain emergencies. *Med. Clin. North Am.*, **90**, 505–523.

2 Corwell, B. (2010) The emergency department evaluation, management, and treatment of back pain. *Emerg. Med. Clin. North Am.*, **28**, 811–839.

3 von Kodolitsch, Y., Schwartz, A.G., and Nienaber, C.A. (2000) Clinical prediction of acute aortic dissection. *Arch. Intern. Med.*, **160**, 2977–2982.

4 Souza, D. and Ledbetter, S. (2012) Diagnostic errors in the evaluation of nontraumatic aortic emergencies. *Semin. Ultrasound CT MR*, **33**, 318–336.

5 Hirst, A.E. Jr., Johns, V.J. Jr., and Kime, S.W. Jr. (1958) Dissecting aneurysm of the aorta: a review of 505 cases. *Medicine (Baltimore)*, **37**, 217–279.

6 Ranasinghe, A.M., Strong, D., Boland, B., and Bonser, R.S. (2011) Acute aortic dissection. *Br. Med. J.*, **343**, d4487.

7 Spittell, P.C., Spittell, J.A. Jr., Joyce, J.W. *et al.* (1993) Clinical features and differential diagnosis of aortic dissection: experience with 236 cases (1980 through 1990). *Mayo Clin. Proc.*, **68**, 642–651.

8 Mehta, R.H., O'Gara, P.T., Bossone, E. *et al.* (2002) Acute type A aortic dissection in the elderly: clinical characteristics, management, and outcomes in the current era. *J. Am. Coll. Cardiol.*, **40**, 685–692.

9 Sandridge, L. and Kern, J.A. (2005) Acute descending aortic dissections: management of visceral, spinal cord, and extremity malperfusion. *Semin. Thorac. Cardiovasc. Surg.*, **17**, 256–261.

10 Gupta, R. and Kaufman, S. (2006) Cardiovascular emergencies in the elderly. *Emerg. Med. Clin. North Am.*, **24**, 339–370.

11 Tsai, T.T., Trimarchi, S., and Nienaber, C.A. (2009) Acute aortic dissection: perspectives from the International Registry of Acute Aortic Dissection (IRAD). *Eur. J. Vasc. Endovasc. Surg.*, **37**, 149–159.

12 Hagan, P.G., Nienaber, C.A., Isselbacher, E.M. *et al.* (2000) The International Registry of Acute Aortic Dissection (IRAD): new insights into an old disease. *J. Am. Med. Assoc.*, **283**, 897–903.

13 Mehta, R.H., Bossone, E., Evangelista, A. *et al.* (2004) Acute type B aortic dissection in elderly patients: clinical features, outcomes, and simple risk stratification rule. *Ann. Thorac. Surg.*, **77**, 1622–1629.

14 Nienaber, C.A., von Kodolitsch, Y., Nicolas, V. *et al.* (1993) The diagnosis of thoracic aortic dissection by noninvasive imaging procedures. *N. Engl. J. Med.*, **328**, 1–9.

15 Rodriguez, M.A., Kumar, S.K., and De Caro, M. (2010) Hypertensive crisis. *Cardiol. Rev.*, **18**, 102–107.

16 Salgado, D.R., Silva, E., and Vincent, J.L. (2013) Control of hypertension in the critically ill: a pathophysiological approach. *Ann. Intensive Care*, **3**, 17.

17 Marik, P.E. and Rivera, R. (2011) Hypertensive emergencies: an update. *Curr. Opin. Crit. Care*, **17**, 569–580.

18 Johnson, W., Nguyen, M.L., and Patel, R. (2012) Hypertension crisis in the emergency department. *Cardiol. Clin.*, **30**, 533–543.

19 Lederle, F.A. (2011) The rise and fall of abdominal aortic aneurysm. *Circulation*, **124**, 1097–1099.

20 Lederle, F.A., Johnson, G.R., Wilson, S.E. *et al.* (2000) The aneurysm detection and management study screening program: validation cohort and final results. Aneurysm Detection and Management Veterans Affairs Cooperative Study Investigators. *Arch. Intern. Med.*, **160**, 1425–1430.

21 Lederle, F.A., Johnson, G.R., Wilson, S.E. *et al.* (1997) Prevalence and associations of abdominal aortic aneurysm detected through screening. Aneurysm Detection and Management (ADAM) Veterans Affairs Cooperative Study Group. *Ann. Intern. Med.*, **126**, 441–449.

22 Brown, L.C. and Powell, J.T. (1999) Risk factors for aneurysm rupture in patients kept under ultrasound surveillance. UK Small Aneurysm Trial Participants. *Ann. Surg.*, **230**, 289–297.

23 Bengtsson, H. and Bergqvist, D. (1993) Ruptured abdominal aortic aneurysm: a population-based study. *J. Vasc. Surg.*, **18**, 74–80.

24 Reed, W.W., Hallett, J.W. Jr., Damiano, M.A., and Ballard, D.J. (1997) Learning from the last ultrasound: a population-based study of patients with abdominal aortic aneurysm. *Arch. Intern. Med.*, **157**, 2064–2068.

25 Steele, M.A. and Dalsing, M.C. (1987) Emergency evaluation of abdominal aortic aneurysms. *Indiana Med.*, **80**, 862–864.

26 Lederle, F.A. and Simel, D.L. (1999) The rational clinical examination: does this patient have abdominal aortic aneurysm? *J. Am. Med. Assoc.*, **281**, 77–82.

27 Rubano, E., Mehta, N., Caputo, W. *et al.* (2013) Systematic review: emergency department bedside ultrasonography for diagnosing suspected abdominal aortic aneurysm. *Acad. Emerg. Med.*, **20**, 128–138.

28 Weinbaum, F.I., Dubner, S., Turner, J.W., and Pardes, J.G. (1987) The accuracy of computed tomography in the diagnosis of retroperitoneal blood in the presence of abdominal aortic aneurysm. *J. Vasc. Surg.*, **6**, 11–16.

29 Broder, J. and Snarski, J.T. (2007) Back pain in the elderly. *Clin. Geriatr. Med.*, **23**, 271–289.

30 Darouiche, R.O. (2006) Spinal epidural abscess. *N. Engl. J. Med.*, **355**, 2012–2020.

31 Solomou, E., Maragkos, M., Kotsarini, C. *et al.* (2004) Multiple spinal epidural abscesses extending to the whole spinal canal. *Magn. Reson. Imaging*, **22**, 747–750.

32 Pradilla, G., Ardila, G.P., Hsu, W., and Rigamonti, D. (2009) Epidural abscesses of the CNS. *Lancet Neurol.*, **8**, 292–300.

33 Huang, C.R., Lu, C.H., Chuang, Y.C. *et al.* (2011) Clinical characteristics and therapeutic outcome of Gram-negative bacterial spinal epidural abscess in adults. *J. Clin. Neurosci.*, **18**, 213–217.

34 Reihsaus, E., Waldbaur, H., and Seeling, W. (2000) Spinal epidural abscess: a meta-analysis of 915 patients. *Neurosurg. Rev.*, **23**, 175–205.

35 Davis, D.P., Wold, R.M., Patel, R.J. *et al.* (2004) The clinical presentation and impact of diagnostic delays on emergency department patients with spinal epidural abscess. *J. Emerg. Med.*, **26**, 285–291.

36 El Sayed, M. and Witting, M.D. (2011) Low yield of ED magnetic resonance imaging for suspected epidural abscess. *Am. J. Emerg. Med.*, **29**, 978–982.

37 Witham, T.F., Khavkin, Y.A., Gallia, G.L. *et al.* (2006) Surgery insight: current management of epidural spinal cord compression from metastatic spine disease. *Nat. Clin. Pract. Neurol.*, **2**, 87–94; quiz 116.

38 Modic, M.T., Feiglin, D.H., Piraino, D.W. *et al.* (1985) Vertebral osteomyelitis: assessment using MR. *Radiology*, **157**, 157–166.

39 Gasbarrini, A.L., Bertoldi, E., Mazzetti, M. *et al.* (2005) Clinical features, diagnostic and therapeutic approaches to haematogenous vertebral osteomyelitis. *Eur. Rev. Med. Pharmacol. Sci.*, **9**, 53–66.

40 Mete, B., Kurt, C., Yilmaz, M.H. *et al.* (2012) Vertebral osteomyelitis: eight years' experience of 100 cases. *Rheumatol. Int.*, **32**, 3591–3597.

41 Beronius, M., Bergman, B., and Andersson, R. (2001) Vertebral osteomyelitis in Goteborg, Sweden: a retrospective study of patients during 1990–1995. *Scand. J. Infect. Dis.*, **33**, 527–532.

42 Mylona, E., Samarkos, M., Kakalou, E. *et al.* (2009) Pyogenic vertebral osteomyelitis: a systematic review of clinical characteristics. *Semin. Arthritis Rheum.*, **39**, 10–17.

43 Roblot, F., Besnier, J.M., Juhel, L. *et al.* (2007) Optimal duration of antibiotic therapy in vertebral osteomyelitis. *Semin. Arthritis Rheum.*, **36**, 269–277.

44 Hayat, M.J., Howlader, N., Reichman, M.E., and Edwards, B.K. (2007) Cancer statistics, trends, and multiple primary cancer analyses from the Surveillance, Epidemiology, and End Results (SEER) Program. *Oncologist*, **12**, 20–37.

45 Minino, A.M., Murphy, S.L., Xu, J., and Kochanek, K.D. (2011) Deaths: final data for 2008. *Natl. Vital Stat. Rep.*, **59**, 1–126.

46 Ortiz Gómez, J.A. (1995) The incidence of vertebral body metastases. *Int. Orthop.*, **19**, 309–311.

47 Barron, K.D., Hirano, A., Araki, S., and Terry, R.D. (1959) Experiences with metastatic neoplasms involving the spinal cord. *Neurology*, **9**, 91–106.

48 Schiff, D., O'Neill, B.P., and Suman, V.J. (1997) Spinal epidural metastasis as the initial manifestation of malignancy: clinical features and diagnostic approach. *Neurology*, **49**, 452–456.

49 Cole, J.S. and Patchell, R.A. (2008) Metastatic epidural spinal cord compression. *Lancet Neurol.*, **7**, 459–466.

50 Oberndorfer, S. and Grisold, W. (2012) Spinal cord involvement. *Handb. Clin. Neurol.*, **105**, 767–780.

51 Bach, F., Larsen, B.H., Rohde, K. *et al.* (1990) Metastatic spinal cord compression: occurrence, symptoms, clinical presentations and prognosis in 398 patients with spinal cord compression. *Acta Neurochir. (Wien)*, **107**, 37–43.

52 Helweg-Larsen, S. (1996) Clinical outcome in metastatic spinal cord compression: a prospective study of 153 patients. *Acta Neurol. Scand.*, **94**, 269–275.

53 Prasad, D. and Schiff, D. (2005) Malignant spinal-cord compression. *Lancet Oncol.*, **6**, 15–24.

54 Helweg-Larsen, S., Sorensen, P.S., and Kreiner, S. (2000) Prognostic factors in metastatic spinal cord compression: a prospective study using multivariate analysis of variables influencing survival and gait function in 153 patients. *Int. J. Radiat. Oncol. Biol. Phys.*, **46**, 1163–1169.

55 Li, K.C. and Poon, P.Y. (1988) Sensitivity and specificity of MRI in detecting malignant spinal cord compression and in distinguishing malignant from benign compression fractures of vertebrae. *Magn. Reson. Imaging*, **6**, 547–556.

56 Lee, K., Tsou, I., Wong, S. *et al.* (2007) Metastatic spinal cord compression as an oncology emergency: getting our act together. *Int. J. Qual. Health Care*, **19**, 377–381.

57 Loblaw, D.A., Mitera, G., Ford, M., and Laperriere, N.J. (2012) A 2011 updated systematic review and clinical practice guideline for the management of malignant extradural spinal cord compression. *Int. J. Radiat. Oncol. Biol. Phys.*, **84**, 312–317.

58 Loblaw, D.A., Perry, J., Chambers, A., and Laperriere, N.J. (2005) Systematic review of the diagnosis and management of malignant extradural spinal cord compression: the Cancer Care Ontario Practice Guidelines Initiative's Neuro-Oncology Disease Site Group. *J. Clin. Oncol.*, **23**, 2028–2037.

10 Headache

Benjamin W. Friedman & Rebecca Nerenberg

Department of Emergency Medicine, Montefiore Medical Center, Albert Einstein College of Medicine, Bronx, NY, USA

Section I: Case presentation

A 70-year-old woman presented with 5 days of a headache that she reported as diffuse, pressure-like, and 10 out of 10 in intensity. She denied head trauma, fever, and vomiting but did have mild neck pain. She stated that she rarely suffered from headaches. She had no associated photophobia or phonophobia. She tried over-the-counter acetaminophen and ibuprofen, but it didn't help her. She noted the headache was better when she was reclining and worse when she sat up.

The past medical history is significant for coronary artery disease and hypertension; the daily medications were a baby aspirin daily as well as lisinopril.

On examination, she was visibly uncomfortable and preferred to lie flat on the gurney. She was afebrile with a heart rate of 78 beats/min, a blood pressure of 155/85 mmHg, and a respiratory rate of 10 breaths/min. The physical examination was unremarkable, including the neurological examination. There was no facial rash. Routine blood work was normal, which included an ESR (erythrocyte sedimentation rate) of 20 mm/h. The head CT scan was normal. She received metoclopramide and diphenhydramine without effect. A lumbar puncture (LP) was performed, which showed an opening pressure of 5 mm H_2O, zero WBCs (white blood cells), and zero RBCs (red blood cells). Despite intravenous morphine, she was still in significant pain.

Neurology was consulted, and she was admitted for further inpatient management as part of her inpatient workup.

Section II: Case discussion

Dr Peter Rosen (PR): Was there any reporting of funduscopic examination?

Dr Andrew Chang (AC): I didn't look at her fundi, but I do not believe the neurologist documented papilledema.

PR: Is there any particular diagnosis in a geriatric patient with acute onset of headache that would be more likely compared to a young adult woman, say, who came in with the first bad headache of her life?

AC: I guess one diagnosis to consider in the elderly, which I don't usually put in the differential for a younger patient, would be temporal arteritis, but this patient had a sedimentation rate that was normal. I would also be concerned about any recent trauma, and hopefully the history would help you determine that. Particularly, if there are cognitive issues in an older patient, then I would search for possible occult head trauma-related causes of headache.

PR: The patient was worked up apparently for a subtle subarachnoid hemorrhage (SAH). Is there anything in this age group that you are particularly concerned with that, again, you might not be concerned with in a younger patient?

Dr Maura Kennedy (MR): Headaches in the elderly are in general less common than in younger patients. This includes chronic headaches and migraine. Certainly, new onset migraine would be atypical, and I share Dr Chang's thoughts about temporal arteritis

Geriatric Emergencies: A Discussion-Based Review, First Edition.
Edited by Amal Mattu, Shamai A. Grossman and Peter L. Rosen.
© 2016 John Wiley & Sons, Ltd. Published 2016 by John Wiley & Sons, Ltd.

and SAH. I would also think that malignancy is a "do not want to miss" cause of headache. Other things about this case: the history does not seem consistent with trigeminal neuralgia, which is more common in geriatric patients. I would expect if this were a herpes zoster–related headache it would be more unilateral, and would probably have the typical rash by now. Some medications that are commonly used in geriatric patients can cause headache. Tension headaches can be precipitated by degenerative changes in the cervical spine as well.

AC: As Dr Kennedy mentioned, the prevalence of headaches declines with age, and it's pretty atypical to develop a primary headache disorder after age 50 (although this is hardly elderly, it is considered the cutoff). Despite this decreasing prevalence of primary headaches with age, secondary causes of headache have an increasing incidence with age. So as you get older, you are much less likely to have a primary headache disorder such as migraine or tension, and much more likely to have something like temporal arteritis, cerebral venous sinus thrombosis, or carotid dissection.

PR: What I was also driving at is that I think as you get older, you have to think more about brain tumor. In particular, a patient who has not had headaches before would be concerning to me for a structural abnormality. This patient was taking aspirin every day. Would that count in your mind as an anticoagulant that would indicate a need for a CT scan independent of everything else?

Dr Scott Wilbur (SW): I think that we often don't think of aspirin as an anticoagulant, but as you mention, it really is. It does increase your bleeding risk slightly. I do know that patients taking other antiplatelet agents such as Plavix have a substantially increased risk. Perhaps not as high as warfarin, but certainly more than someone who is not on those medications. So yes, I would consider aspirin in placing patients at an increased risk of hemorrhage.

AC: I am quick to obtain a CT scan in the elderly, in part because even if they aren't on an anticoagulant, even a seemingly trivial injury that they might not even recall can cause subdural hematomas.

PR: I think that it's very important to try to elicit a history of trauma, but I have personally seen at least

a half dozen patients who have had subdurals, who had no memory of the trauma or the fall. In a couple of cases, someone else had observed it, but the patient himself or herself had no memory of the event. You have to assume that something like that is always in the equation. Dr Chang, you indicated the patient had received an LP after the CT scan was negative. How common do you find an SAH in an elderly patient whose CT is negative, or was your reason for the LP to look for subtle infection?

AC: The general rule of thumb for considering an LP is for any "first, worst, or changed" headache. This patient was just so uncomfortable, and despite not having a "thunderclap" onset, we were still concerned about a possible SAH. We weren't all that concerned at the time for infection because she was afebrile and didn't have a stiff neck. So the main motivation for this case was SAH. In terms of how likely an LP will identify an SAH in the face of a negative CT scan, one study suggests it is as high as 10%, though I don't think that study included elderly patients [1].

PR: I'm not sure I still believe that, even in young patients given our more sensitive CT scanners. I think an elderly patient with an acute SAH has an increased incidence not from aneurysms so much as from other vascular causes. I also think it is probably worthwhile seeing if there is xanthochromia. I know our British colleagues don't do the LP until at least 12 h after the onset of the headache, but we don't wait that long in our ED. I wonder if that would be a worthwhile addition to our diagnostic procedures. In this patient's case, it's been 5 days, but what if this was an acute onset, and had just started that morning?

Dr Shamai Grossman (SG): There are a couple of issues I would consider before I answer this question. First, the older you get, the less distinct the history is, and also the less reliable, and we often can't rely, or we shouldn't rely on history. When we do have a history that actually gives us some very specific direction, we should probably head in that direction. That said, if the patient comes in with an immediate onset of a headache, it's probably very low value if any at all in doing an LP unless you're really worried about an acute infectious process. I think more often than not, our patients come in somewhat later in the time frame from the onset of their symptoms, and, therefore, we do the LP because we think we're going to get xanthochromia. Going back to this case though, the headache is better lying down and worse sitting up. This should make you start thinking about some sort of cerebrospinal fluid (CSF) leak, or something like what we see very commonly in post-LP headaches, but she had a headache before she had the LP. Then you have to worry, is she being vague about her symptoms, was there unrecognized or unremembered trauma that could have induced a CSF leak? That's a very unusual comment to have from a patient prior to actually having an LP. That's probably where I would want to head in this case given that the nature of the remaining history seems rather vague, and the workup thus far seems negative and fairly extensive.

AC: Dr Grossman brings up an excellent historical point, which is that the history is consistent with a CSF leak, though as he pointed out, this started prior to the LP. In this patient's case, since the LP came back negative, we tried to discharge her but she couldn't sit up because she was in so much pain. This postural worsening brings up another point I'd like to mention, which is the importance of taking an opening pressure during the LP, which is something I do routinely now as I get older. In this case, her opening pressure was pretty low, and this provides a clue to her diagnosis. In emergency medicine, we tend to do LPs to rule out SAH and meningitis. In this case, we did it to rule out SAH. One reason why the opening pressure is important is because if you do a head CT and it's negative, and then you follow that with an LP that shows zero red cells, then you've essentially ruled out an SAH. But if the patient is miserable and can't be discharged, then the opening pressure might be able to guide you to an alternative diagnosis. If it's really high, you might think of pseudotumor cerebri or cerebral venous sinus thrombosis. If it's really low, as it was in this case (it was 5 mmH$_2$O), then it can suggest a spontaneous CSF leak, which fits with the postural history that Dr Grossman alluded to earlier.

PR: I have to say that those are fascinating points. I don't believe I've ever seen any spinal fluid leak that wasn't visible in the nose or the ear other than in patients who have already had some kind of neurosurgical procedure, but I think it is an interesting piece of history in this patient. Dr Chang, you make another very important point that I think we ought to stress, not just for geriatric patients but in emergency

medicine. We tend to worry about one or two critical diagnoses, and when we've ruled those out we think our job is finished, and we're ready to discharge the patient. But, in point of fact, all we've done is eliminate a couple of possibilities, and without an explanation of what is causing the patient's problem, our job definitely isn't done and we need to keep looking. Are there other disease processes that we should consider here?

Dr Amal Mattu (AM): I think we've gone through a pretty good differential thus far. I'm not sure I would add any more to our differential at this point.

PR: Would anybody feel an early MRI (magnetic resonance imaging) was indicated for this patient? We've become somewhat blasé about not obtaining MRIs except for spinal cord obstruction syndromes. Are there any neurologic presentations that could be identified with an MRI that it would be useful to find earlier rather than later?

AM: There is another possible consideration for a unilateral type of headache and that is carotid artery or vertebral artery dissections. It's not necessarily just a disease of elderly patients, but they almost invariably tend to be unilateral headaches. This might be worth adding to the differential, and also a reason an MRA (magnetic resonance angiography) or CTA (computed tomography angiography) might be indicated as well.

PR: I think that temporal arteritis is another interesting possibility that doesn't necessarily need to present with localized tenderness over the temporal artery since it is really more of a diffuse phenomenon. However, all the patients I've ever seen with temporal arteritis have presented with some visual impairment. I don't recall that she had any such visual impairment, and although I don't think that rules it out completely, think it certainly puts it lower down on our list.

AC: She did not have any visual complaints. With temporal arteritis, the ESR is usually elevated, often over 100, although it can be normal in about 1% of the population.

PR: You know, we're going to see patients who refuse to give us any of the criteria of a disease, and in that case, I don't think we can be faulted for not making the diagnosis. I'd like to proceed with this patient's diagnosis and management.

SW: I think this was a perplexing case because it seems as though the workup we typically do to identify a cause of the headache has mostly been done. I'll throw in one other very unusual cause of headache in this age group, and that would be acute angle glaucoma, so I might consider checking intraocular pressures. Other than that, I'm at a loss for further diagnostic studies, and I don't know that an MRI would be terribly helpful in this patient with no neurologic findings to suggest stroke or vascular disease with the exception of what Dr Mattu mentioned. In terms of management, medications should be used with caution in the elderly. The patient was treated with metoclopramide and diphenhydramine. Both of these medications are on the Beers criteria list for potentially inappropriate medications in the elderly. Metoclopramide can cause extrapyramidal effects that are increased in older patients, especially older women, and diphenhydramine is highly anticholinergic and can cause delirium, urinary retention, and other medical conditions.

AC: Do you have a suggestion on what alternative medication to administer to this patient? We wanted to avoid ketorolac because of the potential antiplatelet effect in someone who could have a subarachnoid or subdural, and she did eventually get morphine because she was still in so much pain. Would a single dose of metoclopramide 10 mg still be relatively contraindicated in a patient like this?

SW: It's a tough position to be in, and I think opioids are really one of the only reasonable choices in a patient such as this. I agree with your concern with ketorolac; the risk of bleeding and the risks for other GI (gastrointestinal) side effects are going to be higher in this age group. If NSAIDs (nonsteroidal anti-inflammatory drugs) are going to be used, you need to be using GI protection as well. I also agree with you on the single dose issue, although I would still say they should be used with caution, recognizing that there is the potential for adverse effects. Certainly, even if she had relief from the metoclopramide, sending her home with a prescription for it might not be the best approach.

PR: I think that you articulated some very important drug issues although I can't think of any drug we can give her for pain relief that doesn't run the risk of producing some confusion in an elderly patient.

Dr Ula Huang (UH): I think Beers criteria of inappropriate medications in the elderly are something that is probably new to the emergency medicine world. It is a list of expert consensus recommended drugs that shouldn't be used, or are potentially inappropriate, for older adults. Ketorolac is also on the Beers criteria list. That being said, in the ED, and with a one-time use, we have to weigh the risks and benefits. In this case, the patient was admitted. Metoclopramide and diphenhydramine, or Reglan and Benadryl, are typical migraine concoctions. I think opiates are our only last line of defense. Acetaminophen is the first line of pain medication that is relatively safe in older adults, and after that, even ibuprofen is considered inappropriate. I tend to reach for morphine when patients are uncomfortable.

UH: I think that Dr Kennedy had mentioned earlier that pain medications may potentially cause confusion, and I think that is true, but at the same time, the pain itself may actually cause the patient to be confused. Blood pressure medications might be another cause of medication-related headache.

PR: You mentioned earlier that there are medications that can cause headaches. Can you mention a couple, since I am having trouble thinking of any off the top of my head?

MK: Vasodilators are common causes of medication-induced headache in the geriatric population. Tamoxifen may do this as well, although I don't think you'll see a 65-year-old or older person taking tamoxifen. I'd like to emphasize again that while the potential side effects of pain medications include delirium, not treating pain can result in delirium as well, so I do think it is important that we aggressively treat pain.

PR: I didn't mean to imply that because analgesics can cause confusion, we shouldn't relieve pain. I think there are many instances in emergency medicine where we have to basically choose the lesser of two evils. In my mind, not treating pain is a greater evil than treating pain, and having subsequently having some confusion. I think we are more likely to induce confusion in the elderly by our hospital practices, such as waking people every few hours for vital signs, having them in a strange environment, and not letting them have the usual familiar cues that help them from getting confused at home. Why don't you tell us what evolved with this patient upon admission. Were they able to relieve her pain with opiates?

AC: Opiates did not relieve her pain in the ED, and so she had to be admitted. She eventually had an inpatient MRI with gadolinium that showed diffuse dural enhancement, which locked in the diagnosis of spontaneous intracranial hypotension, which is caused by a spontaneous CSF leak. It is an interesting diagnosis, and one of the clues is that it's postural, as Dr Grossman picked up on. It just happens to be spontaneous and not as a complication of an LP. Again, this is where the opening pressure can give us a clue. We usually measure this to see if it's a high pressure, but, as this case demonstrates, a low pressure can be helpful as well. In our hospital and I believe in many others, MRIs are being ordered more and more frequently in both the ED and inpatient setting, and as a result, I think this diagnosis will be made more frequently. To review: spontaneous intracranial hypotension is a spontaneous CSF leak that typically occurs at the low cervical or cervicothoracic junction. When you lose about 10% of your CSF volume, the brain actually displaces downward, which stretches the pain-sensitive vascular structures, and that's what leads to the headache. There is a formula where the intracranial volume is equal to your brain volume plus the CSF volume plus the intracranial blood volume. Since your intracranial volume and your brain volume have to remain constant, if you lose CSF volume from a leak then you have to compensate it by increasing the intracranial blood volume, and that is done by the venous system. So when gadolinium contrast is administered during the MRI, more of the gadolinium collects in the venous system resulting in diffuse dural enhancement. This shows up as a hyperdense signal that surrounds the outside border of the entire brain. Treating spontaneous intracranial hypotension is generally similar to a post-LP headache. IV caffeine can be tried followed by a blood patch, which is typically placed in the lumbar area, even though the leak is up higher in the cervical region as it would be dangerous to place the patch in the cervical region. The anesthesiologists use a large volume blood patch, and they tilt the patient in Trendelenburg to attempt to get the blood up to where the leak is in the neck. I didn't know about this diagnosis at the time that I

admitted her, but I have since had one other case, and I think it's going to become a more common diagnosis as MRIs are ordered with greater frequency.

PR: One of the other diagnoses I was thinking about was whether this could have been a superior sagittal thrombosis? The patients I have seen with this were younger, but they didn't have any neurologic findings. They just had a severe and unremitting headache that was increasing, and without a CTA you would never make this diagnosis.

SW: I've actually seen cerebral venous sinus thrombosis quite frequently now, and even had a case just a few days ago.

UH: I wondered if both of Dr Chang's cases were older adults?

AC: This case as you know was 70 years of age. The other case was younger. I don't remember her exact age, but I think she was in her 50s.

AC: Cerebral venous sinus thrombosis is an excellent thought, and another situation where the opening pressure might be helpful, though in that case it would be very high.

PR: I wonder what would make you develop a spontaneous leak. But again, everyone responds to LPs with a headache, and perhaps it has to do with your body's ability to reconstitute spinal volume as opposed to an actual leak.

Section III: Concepts

Background

Headache is the fifth leading cause of ED visits, accounting for 5 million visits to US EDs annually [2]. It is also common among older adults, reported by 14% of older women and 7% of older men [3]. Headache etiology encompasses a broad range of diagnoses including many that threaten life or limb.

The goal of emergency care is twofold: first to determine whether the headache is a secondary headache (symptomatic of an underlying infectious, inflammatory, ischemic, or space-occupying lesion) or a primary headache (a headache attributable to a recurrent underlying headache disorder, such as migraine). The second goal is to treat the patient's pain, though secondary headaches also require prompt diagnosis and treatment directed at the underlying condition. Among older adults who present with new onset headache, most are diagnosed ultimately with a benign headache etiology but should be referred onward for continuing care. However, the risk of a malignant process in older adults is markedly increased. In one series, 15% of new headache types in older adults are due to a malignant process [4]. In the next section, we describe features of the primary and secondary headaches that are most common in older adults.

Primary headaches

Migraine, tension-type, and cluster headaches are the most prevalent of the primary headache disorders, while classical trigeminal neuralgia, a common cause of facial pain, is also common in geriatric patients. Hypnic headache is an uncommon cause of primary headache, but is, for the most part, a disease of older adults and so will be described here as well.

The unifying features among these various disorders include (1) episodic recurrence, which can range from a few distinct isolated episodes to frequent and chronic episodes and (2) ultimately, a benign course. Prevalence of primary headaches peaks in middle-aged adults and declines in the geriatric population, driven mostly by marked reductions in the frequency of tension-type headache and migraine. This decline in prevalence is caused by a decreased incidence as patients get older and by an aging sun-setting of symptoms, in which patients with established migraine or tension-type headache no longer develop acute attacks. Though the primary headache usually begins in late adolescence or early adulthood, one population-based study demonstrates that 17% of older adults with a primary headache disorder report their first onset of the primary headaches at age 65 years or older [5].

Tension-type headache

Tension headache, the most prevalent type of the headache disorders, is characterized by the absence of most remarkable headache features [6]. Rather than the unilateral, pulsating pain of migraine, or the severe periorbital boring pain of cluster headache, tension headache patients describe their pain as a bilateral squeezing or pressure-like pain. It is defined by the absence of nausea and vomiting. Either photophobia or phonophobia may be present, but the combination of these two features excludes the diagnosis. Similarly, autonomic symptoms such as ptosis, conjunctival injection, or lacrimation do not occur with tension-type headache. Commonly, patients with tension headache report pericranial muscle tenderness and tightness, involving the muscles of the head and neck, leading some to call this headache a muscle contraction headache. Because of its generally bland nature, tension headache is often described as a regular or plain headache. Tension headaches may be brief, lasting no more than several hours, or they may linger for more than 1 week. Diagnostic guidelines define tension headache as a chronic episodic disorder, characterized by acute exacerbations of the typical headache [6]. Subtypes include chronic tension headache, which requires the presence of headache on more than 15 days per month, and episodic versions, in which the exacerbations are less frequent [6]. Though prevalence rates in Americans between the ages of 60 and 65 are nearly 25%, this disease is actually less prevalent in those older than 60 years of age than in any other adult age bracket [7]. Among the population of patients older than 65, the prevalence of tension headache continues to decline with every passing decade. Despite its substantial population prevalence, the pain intensity of tension headache is generally no worse than mild or moderate, and, therefore, tension headache is an infrequent cause of ED visit among older adults. Patients with tension headache are often less interested in the treatment of the headache and more interested in diagnosis and reassurance that their headache does not represent a malignant process.

Migraine headache

Though much less prevalent than tension headache, migraine in the elderly is a more common cause of ED visits, and has a greater impact from a population perspective because of associated functional disability [8]. Patients with an acute migraine attack are less likely to participate fully in work, recreational, and social activities, and much more likely to remain at home.

Acute migraine attacks are characteristically described as a unilateral throbbing or pulsating headache, associated with phonophobia, photophobia, osmophobia, and nausea or vomiting. Migraine typically lasts between 4 and 72 hours [6]. Longer lasting unremitting migraine attacks are called "status migrainosus."

Fifteen percent of patients with migraine have an aura, which are abnormal neurological features, particularly visual or sensory disturbances that precede the acute headache by up to 1 hour. Aura may be perceived as positive features, such as complex geometric images, or negative features, such as scotoma. Similarly for sensory symptoms, patients may describe positive features such as tingling sensations or negative features such as numbness. In the elderly, a migraine aura may occur without a headache, thus making differentiation from transient ischemic attacks difficult. Characteristics of migraine aura without headache that may help differentiate it from ischemic events include the predominance of visual symptoms such as a scintillating scotoma, a gradual build-up or expansion of symptoms, a slow progression of visual symptoms through visual fields, a march of sensory symptoms through the body, and an evolution of symptoms from one modality to the next, such as visual followed by sensory and then speech symptoms [9]. A migraine prodrome may precede the headache by several days. The prodrome consists of changes in mood, appetite, attention, and sleep patterns. Similar symptoms may follow the migraine as well. Migraine is much less common in patients 60 years and older, with prevalence rates in men of 2% and in women of 6%, compared to rates of 8% and 26% in middle-aged adults [10].

Historically, migraine has been considered a vascular headache, primarily because of its throbbing nature. More current thinking attributes migraine to abnormal sensory processing and dysfunctional activation of various regions of the brain stem. The trigeminal nerve is key to migraine pathogenesis, as it activates in response to intracranial stimuli and transmits nociceptive stimuli through brain stem nuclei, and onward to thalamic relays [11]. Vascular involvement, when it occurs, is likely a secondary process. Cortical spreading depression, the gradual gap-junction-based depolarization of brain cortex, likely underlies migraine aura, though its role in the migraine headache itself is controversial [11].

Cluster headache

Much less prevalent than either migraine or tension headache, cluster headache is a devastatingly painful headache series characterized by recurrent, relatively brief bouts of a severe unilateral headache that occur daily, or multiple times every day, clustered within a discrete time period lasting from weeks to months. It is associated with abnormal activation of the ipsilateral posterior hypothalamus.

Cluster headache is typically accompanied by autonomic symptoms ipsilateral to the pain, such as ptosis, facial edema, lacrimation, or conjunctival injection. Unlike migraine, patients with cluster do not prefer to lie down, but instead will characteristically pace the floor restlessly. The severity of the pain and associated restlessness have caused it to be regarded as a suicide headache, though reports of suicide during an acute cluster attack are rare [12].

Cluster attacks often begin during sleep, and, similar to migraine, may also be triggered by alcohol consumption or intense odors. By definition, cluster attacks last no longer than 3 h [6]. Thus, the headache may have resolved or be resolving by the time the patient presents for medical attention. Though tempting to diagnose these headaches as "headache, resolved," the emergency physician should strive to identify the cluster pattern, and to provide treatment to prevent the next headache in the cluster. Unlike migraine, which has a strong predilection for women, cluster headache is three times more common in men [13].

Trigeminal neuralgia

Trigeminal neuralgia, also known as tic douloureux, is characterized by severe paroxysms of lancinating unilateral pain in the distribution of the trigeminal nerve, usually involving the second or third branches [14]. It is often precipitated by a seemingly innocuous stimulus to the face, such as a gust of wind or chewing gum [6]. Unlike the primary headaches discussed earlier, trigeminal neuralgia is more common in older age groups as prevalence is correlated directly with age [15]. The duration of attacks and remissions between attacks vary and may increase with more established disease.

Trigeminal neuralgia is typically divided into symptomatic and classical, the former referring to those patients with an identifiable lesion causing the symptoms, such as malignancy or multiple sclerosis, whereas the latter referring to those patients without an apparent anatomical cause. Increasingly, vascular contact with the trigeminal nerve is thought to be a cause in select cases of classical trigeminal neuralgia. For these patients, microvascular decompression (a neurosurgical procedure to distance the nerve from the vasculature) may eliminate symptoms. However, the neurosurgical mortality associated with this procedure is significant in the elderly, so patients need to consider carefully whether medical management can suffice [16]. A variety of generally low-morbidity surgical procedures are available, including peripheral techniques, which target the postganglionic trigeminal nerve, and percutaneous procedures that target the ganglion itself. Some patients may benefit from radiotherapy. Many patients enjoy headache relief with these procedures, though up to 50% will experience recurrent pain at 1 year [14].

Hypnic headache

Hypnic headache is an uncommon disorder that primarily affects patients over the age of 50. It is characterized by frequently recurring headaches (>10 days per month) that occur only during sleep and awaken the patient. The duration of the headache is more than 15 min, and in some cases, may last up to 4 h. The character of the headache is usually tension like, though migraine-like hypnic headaches have also been described. As with all headaches that occur for the first time in patients older than 50, these patients require a diagnostic workup to exclude secondary causes of headache [17].

Secondary headaches

Unlike younger patients, who usually present with an exacerbation of a primary headache disorder or a benign secondary cause of headache, geriatric patients presenting with a new headache are much more likely to present with a secondary headache, many of which are potentially life or limb threatening.

Giant cell arteritis

Among older adults presenting to medical attention with a headache, giant cell arteritis is as common as migraine [3]. It is a systemic large vessel vasculitis, with a predilection for branches of the aortic arch, such as the carotid and vertebral arteries. Though it can affect patients as young as the sixth decade of life, it is predominantly a disease of the geriatric population. Women are affected two to three times more frequently than men [18].

Headache is the most common symptom; vision loss and ischemic stroke are the most feared sequelae. Other common symptoms include fatigue, weight loss, and fever, as well as scalp tenderness and jaw claudication. Formal diagnostic criteria require three of the following five features: (1) age at onset ≥ 50 years, (2) new onset or new type of headache, (3) temporal artery tenderness or decreased pulsation, (4) ESR ≥ 50 mm/h, or (5) abnormal temporal artery biopsy [19]. Since only three criteria are required, biopsy negative patients may still meet diagnostic criteria. False-negative biopsies occur because affected arteries are often involved intermittently rather than continuously. While neither an ESR nor a C-reactive protein is sufficiently sensitive to exclude the disease from consideration, the combination of these two tests is quite sensitive and can be used to exclude the need for biopsy in all but the highest risk patients [20].

Corticosteroids are the treatment of choice for giant cell arteritis, and particularly in the setting of visual symptoms, should be initiated immediately, rather than waiting for confirmatory biopsy [21]. Thoracic aortic aneurysm is a late manifestation of this illness. Polymyalgia rheumatica, a disease of older adults characterized by bilateral morning aching and stiffness of the neck, shoulder, or pelvic girdle, is associated with giant cell arteritis, and is also corticosteroid responsive.

Brain tumor headache

The majority of patients with intracranial tumors report headaches at the time of diagnosis, though as many as 40% of patients with intracranial tumors will not [22]. Primary brain tumors occur at an incidence of 10–12/100,000. Brain metastases of non-CNS (central nervous system) malignancies are more common than primary CNS tumors, but only rarely are the symptoms of the brain metastasis the presenting manifestation of a non-CNS cancer [22]. Underlying headache disorders should not automatically be attributed to the brain tumor, especially if the headaches predate the tumor time frame. As per classification guidelines, headaches experienced in association with a brain tumor are attributable to a brain tumor if they resolve after surgical removal or volume reduction of the mass [6]. The clinical manifestation of brain tumor–related headaches can be divided into two types of symptoms: focal headaches, traditionally thought to be related to tumor location, and generalized headaches, thought to be related to increased intracranial pressure, which can develop if the tumor bulk occludes the flow of CSF [23].

Headaches associated with brain tumors are often described as severe in intensity, worse upon awakening, and are associated with nausea and vomiting. However, headaches associated with brain tumors are quite variable in character. Most commonly, they are intermittent, develop and resolve within hours, are of moderate intensity, and are not specific in location [24–26]. Headaches associated with brain tumors commonly fulfill diagnostic criteria for tension headache, and some meet criteria for migraine [27]. Headache as the sole presenting symptom of an intracranial tumor is relatively uncommon. Most patients will present with other neurological symptoms or signs such as seizures or focal deficits [22]. A personal susceptibility to headache or family history of headaches may increase the risk of headaches associated with brain tumors. Tumor type appears to contribute to the likelihood of headache. Increasing size of tumor leads to increasing headache frequency in younger patients. In older adults, brain atrophy allows tumors more space to grow prior to headache onset [22]. American College of Emergency Physicians (ACEP) guidelines recommend brain imaging in all patients older than 50 with a new headache type [28].

Cervical artery dissection

Cervical artery dissection encompasses both internal carotid artery and vertebral artery dissections. Both are more common in middle-aged patients than in older adults [29]. Overall, the incidence of carotid dissection is 2.5–3/100,000 patients. Vertebral dissection has traditionally been thought of as less common, although more recent work describes more comparable incidence rates [30, 31]. Tears occur in the inner intimal layer, resulting in an intramural hematoma, which can lead to blood flow obstruction, stenosis, or aneurysmal dilatation. Brain ischemia occurs due to thrombotic or embolic blood flow obstructions. Cervical artery dissection is classified as spontaneous or traumatic. Spontaneous dissection has been associated with connective tissue disease, migraines, and acute infection, although atherosclerosis is an important contributing factor [32]. Preceding hyperextension or rotation of the neck are proximate causes of traumatic dissection. Mechanisms of traumatic dissection include direct injury to the neck, such as seat belt injuries in motor vehicle collisions, strangulation, and chiropractic manipulation. A forceful Valsalva maneuver that

occurs with coughing, vomiting, and heavy lifting may also contribute to dissection.

The classical presentation of cervical artery dissection involves headache, neck pain, and signs of brain ischemia. Headache is often the first presenting symptom and often precedes neurologic findings by hours to days. Carotid dissection most often presents with a gradual onset of ipsilateral frontal or frontotemporal throbbing headache or with facial or ocular pain. Patients may experience cranial nerve palsies, transient monocular blindness, tinnitus, or distortion of taste. A partial Horner's syndrome, consisting of ptosis and miosis, in the setting of neck or facial pain, is highly concerning for carotid dissection. In contrast, patients with vertebral dissection often have occipital headache that may be either unilateral or bilateral. Patients may also have neck pain, vertigo, nausea, vomiting, unilateral facial numbness, and unsteady gait [33].

Historically, diagnosis of cervical dissection required conventional angiography with visualization of a double lumen and intimal flap. More recently, MRA and CTA have become the dominant imaging modalities. Diagnostic neuroimaging patterns include stenosis, occlusion, and dissection. Color duplex ultrasound can also be used in some situations that do not involve major trauma. Findings indicating dissection can include an echogenic intimal flap, a thrombus floating in the intraluminal space, and an abrupt tapering of the arterial lumen.

Treatment of cervical artery dissection most often involves anticoagulation for 3–6 months, or antiplatelet agents alone. Limited evidence suggests that anticoagulants are associated with low risk of death or disability when used as treatment for cervical artery dissection [34]. Surgical treatment or endovascular therapy are considered when medical management is insufficient or symptoms continue to progress.

Subarachnoid hemorrhage

Blood in the subarachnoid space is an important secondary cause of headache. The majority of SAH is traumatic, and this is discussed in the following traumatic headache section. Of patients with nontraumatic SAH, approximately 85% have a ruptured intracranial aneurysm. The remainders have arteriovenous malformation, other vascular malformations, or intracranial lesions with a propensity for bleeding. Intracranial aneurysms most commonly occur at areas of high wall sheer stress, along the arteries that make up the Circle of Willis. There are 30,000 cases of nontraumatic, aneurysmal SAH annually in the United States [35]. The classic headache of SAH is described as "thunderclap" or sudden onset, often during exertion, with maximal intensity at onset, and is often described as the "worst headache of one's life." Associated symptoms may include nausea, vomiting, loss of consciousness, meningismus, and focal or generalized neurologic findings. However, in 40% of cases, headache alone may be the only symptom [36].

SAH can be fatal or cause substantial morbidity. Earlier diagnosis leads to better outcomes [4, 5]. The workup to establish the diagnosis is a noncontrast CT of the head followed by spinal fluid analysis if the CT scan is noncontributory. While highly specific, the sensitivity of noncontrast head CT for subarachnoid blood declines rapidly with time. The sensitivity approaches 100% if performed within 6 hours, remains 90–95% within 24 h, and may be no better than 50% after several days have elapsed [37]. CT angiography is highly sensitive for larger and more concerning aneurysms, and, in the acute setting, may follow a noncontrast head CT. Noncontrast head CT followed by CTA of the brain is a diagnostic protocol that first excludes subarachnoid blood and then excludes aneurysm. There is some controversy, however, regarding the use of CTA to exclude SAH since CTA can only diagnose an aneurysm, but the aneurysm may not necessarily be the cause of the headache. MRI is most useful for excluding blood in the subarachnoid space once the sensitivity of CT scan is no longer sufficient [38].

In SAH, a spinal fluid analysis will reveal elevated opening pressures, erythrocytes, or xanthochromia. Blood is present within the spinal fluid within minutes after SAH. While there is no specific threshold for the number of RBCs seen, most patients with true SAH will have thousands of RBCs/mm^3. Xanthochromia may take up to 12 h to develop, and as such may be absent in a patient with SAH who has a spinal fluid analysis performed soon after headache onset.

Supportive treatment of the patient with SAH includes management of the airway, modest blood pressure control, and homeostatic support. Preventing vasospasm with oral nimodipine improves outcomes [39]. Seizure prophylaxis may be useful. Hypotension should be avoided. Hypertension can be managed with labetalol, nicardipine, or esmolol in the setting of markedly elevated blood pressure. Neurosurgical consultation should be sought to evaluate for surgical clipping versus endovascular coiling of the aneurysm if that is the cause. Early intervention reduces the rate of rebleeding, which may occur within 24 hours of the initial bleed. Outcomes are optimized when aneurysm repair is completed early [40].

Traumatic headache
Blunt head trauma can result in a variety of injuries, many of which cause headache. Bleeding in the subarachnoid, subdural, or epidural spaces or within the brain parenchyma itself may be life threatening. In older adults, intracranial hemorrhage can be quite subtle and present without focal neurological signs making it difficult to exclude neurosurgical emergencies based on physical examination alone [41].

Similarly, the traumatic mechanism of the intracranial hemorrhage in older adults may be so minor such that the patient may not readily relay relevant history regarding a potential traumatic event. Even with the absence of radiographically visible injury, patients may experience headache in the setting of recent or distant head trauma. It is clear that minor head trauma can cause isolated headache or headache in conjunction with a postconcussive syndrome [42]. These headaches may initiate at the time of the trauma or may be delayed in onset for days or weeks. Some are short-lived, whereas others persist for years. These so-called posttraumatic or postconcussive headaches may take on the form of migraine or tension-type headache and are commonly treated as such. There are no proven interventions to prevent or treat acute posttraumatic headache [43]. Reasonable recommendations include "brain rest," in which patients avoid bright or noisy stimuli and electronic devices.

Meningitis
The classic combination of symptoms for meningitis includes headache, fever, meningismus, and altered mental status. However, up to 50% of elderly patients with bacterial meningitis may present without all four of these signs and symptoms. Therefore, the absence of one of them cannot be used to exclude meningitis from the differential diagnosis. In one case series, 93% of patients had fever, 77% had altered mental status, and 62% had meningismus [44, 45]. Even though meningitis is rare in the elderly, the

diagnosis must be pursued unless there is another readily identifiable source of infection [46, 47].

It may be difficult to distinguish bacterial from nonbacterial CNS infection, especially in older adults. Treatable causes of aseptic meningitis, such as Lyme disease or Cryptococcus, must be considered in at-risk patients, such as those that are immuno-compromised. Lyme neuroborreliosis should be considered in endemic regions during warm weather. Patients usually present with headache, meningismus, nondermatomal paresthesias, and facial nerve palsies. The classic erythema migrans rash almost always appears in patients with CNS Lyme disease, though it usually precedes the headache by several weeks [48]. Cryptococcal meningitis is classically a disease of the immunocompromised. It often presents as an indolent subacute meningitis that one is tempted to call a tension headache. Look for this disease when the CD4 counts are lower than 100 cells/mm^3. As the disease progresses, elevated intracranial pressure may cause alterations in consciousness, papilledema, cranial nerve palsies, and seizures [49]. Common viral causes of meningitis include enterovirus, varicella-zoster virus, and herpes simplex virus; varicella virus and herpes simplex virus are more likely to cause encephalitis [50].

Cerebral venous sinus thrombosis

Relatively uncommon, cerebral venous sinus disease is difficult to diagnose because it is often not apparent on conventional ED testing (i.e., brain CT) and usually requires MRI. Cerebral venous sinus thrombosis may present as a "thunderclap" headache, though more commonly, it will present as a worsening nonspecific headache. Conventional thromboembolic risk factors, such as use of exogenous estrogen or genetic thrombophilia, increase a patient's risk of this disease. Similarly, recent cranial or facial surgery place patients at risk, as do proximate facial or sinus infections. In older adults, however, nearly one third of patients who develop this disease do not have an identifiable risk factor [51].

Thrombosed sinuses include the transverse, superior sagittal, the left and right lateral, and the straight sinuses. Patients may present with isolated headache, signs of intracranial hypertension, focal neurological signs including seizure, and encephalopathy causing alterations in mental status [51]. As with other thromboembolic diseases processes, a d-dimer has been used to exclude patients at low risk of sinus thrombosis, though the test has inadequate sensitivity to exclude patients in whom sinus venous thrombosis is strongly suspected [52]. A noncontrast CT scan is generally insensitive to this disease process though occasionally one will see a dense triangular sign, indicating hyperacute thrombosed blood in the superior sagittal sinus. MRI with a focus on the venous circulation is often necessary to exclude cerebral venous sinus thrombosis. Anticoagulation with heparin improves outcomes [53].

Though quite rare, cavernous sinus thrombosis is often a devastating illness, usually less subtle than thrombosis of sinuses located more posteriorly, and more likely to result from bacterial infection rather than aseptic thrombosis. In cavernous sinus thrombosis, chemosis, proptosis, and restricted ocular mobility become more apparent as the disease progresses, with lateral gaze at most risk due to the susceptible position of cranial nerve VI.

Headache attributable to a substance or its withdrawal

Since a wide-ranging variety of medications are known to cause headache (Box 10.1), it is important to scrutinize an older adult's medication regimen as a potential cause of the headache. Diagnosis can be suggested by a temporal relation to medication initiation, though it may require substitution of the suspected medication before the diagnosis can be confirmed. Some medications, such as nitroglycerin, are well known to cause headache, and do so in such close proximity to medication administration that the clinician is left with little doubt about headache etiology [54]. When the causal pathway is not clear-cut, it is often appropriate to first rule out malignant etiologies. The insidious diagnosis of medication overuse headache is attributable to a gradual increase in analgesic medication, most often analgesic medication that has been used specifically to treat a headache. These patients usually report an episodic headache disorder at baseline that has gradually become chronic over time. Common culprits are opioids and barbiturate-containing migraine preparations. Other classes of medication that have been implicated in medication overuse headache include triptans, NSAIDs, and even acetaminophen. Management of these patients requires substitution of the causative analgesic with a new headache medication regimen, consisting of acute and preventive medications [55]. This can be particularly tricky if the analgesic is also being used for a different condition, such as arthritis or low back pain.

Overuse of ethanol can cause headache acutely, as can withdrawal from chronic ethanol use. Caffeine is sometimes used as a treatment of headache, but withdrawal from this substance can cause headache as well [6].

Box 10.1 Medications that are known causes of headache

Nitrates
Phosphodiesterase inhibitors
Digitalis
Hydralazine
Nifedipine
Dipyridamole
Amiodarone
Lithium
Thyroid hormone replacement
Estrogen
Antihistamines
Selective serotonin reuptake inhibitors
Opioids
Barbiturates

Hypertensive headache

High blood pressure is often present in patients who present to an ED with headache. This is particularly true in older adults given their higher prevalence of hypertension. It remains unclear if the headache is associated with elevated blood pressure or merely present coincidently. International guidelines attribute headaches to elevated blood pressure if the systolic blood pressure rises rapidly to ≥ 180 mmHg or if the diastolic rises to ≥ 120 mmHg, and if the headache resolves with normalization of blood pressure [6]. Treatment of moderately elevated blood pressure is unlikely to result in headache improvement. It is not yet known whether severely elevated blood pressure ought to be lowered rapidly in patients with an acute headache. Also, it is not clear which hypertensive patients are at risk for hypertensive encephalopathy or whether these patients with headache and elevated blood pressure are at risk of acute stroke. The Posterior Reversible Encephalopathy Syndrome (PRES) is defined by the presence of abnormal imaging findings in conjunction with elevated blood pressure, headache, and focal neurological findings, seizure, or encephalopathy. Patients on immunomodulatory therapy appear to be at particular risk. For patients with neurological deficits or imaging findings consistent with hypertensive insult, moderate blood pressure reduction is an appropriate goal [56].

Cervicogenic headache

The upper cervical sensory neurons innervate the scalp and often terminate within the trigeminal nucleus caudalis, the putative relay nucleus for migraine nociception that lies at the junction of the lower brain stem and upper cervical spine. Spinal pathology, including arthropathies and degenerative disease, can therefore cause pain that will be perceived as a headache or even as migraine. Confirming these diagnoses, however, may be tricky, particularly in older adults, as arthropathies and degenerative disease are near ubiquitous on imaging studies. Diagnosis may be suggested by the reproduction of pain with upper neck palpation or repositioning of the head. Cervicogenic headache can be differentiated from a tension headache by its characteristic side-locked, unilateral location. Definitive diagnosis requires confirmation by relieving the pain with cervical nerve blockade. ED treatment with NSAIDs, muscle relaxants, and opioids is appropriate [57].

Ophthalmological causes of headache

A variety of ailments originating from the eye may cause periorbital pain in older adults, mandating an ocular examination in elderly patients when they present with headache. Most notable among these disease processes is angle closure glaucoma, which, when it develops acutely, may present with severe periorbital pain, nausea and vomiting, and thus be confused with migraine. Recent use of anticholinergic or sympathomimetics may suggest the diagnosis, as will the classic history of pain onset upon exiting a darkened room. An ocular examination will reveal conjunctival injection and a dilatated and fixed or sluggish pupil. Diagnosis can be confirmed with an assessment of intraocular pressure. Subacute or intermittent angle closure may not be apparent on physical examination. Keratitis, uveitis, and iritis may also present as headache and may require a fluorescein or slit lamp exam for diagnosis [58].

Testing for patients with headache

Imaging

Regardless of the patient's age, the appropriate use of imaging remains an integral part of ED management of headache. However, as the age of the patient increases, the malignant risk of ionizing radiation becomes less pronounced, and the potential benefit increases. Guidelines recommend a noncontrast head CT in patients older than 50 years of age presenting with a novel headache [28]. While MRI offers increased sensitivity for a variety of pathological processes including ischemic stroke, its routine use in the ED for older adults with headache is not indicated. The combination of a noncontrast head CT with neurovascular imaging can be used to exclude many of the pathological processes discussed earlier. CT vascular imaging requires contrast, and therefore may not be appropriate for patients with impaired renal function, whereas MRI vascular imaging does not.

Laboratory testing

Laboratory tests only rarely help differentiate primary from secondary headaches. Features of the history and physical examination are usually much more useful with regard to providing valuable information for the emergency physician.

One notable exception is giant cell arteritis. For this disease, an elevated ESR is part of the diagnostic criteria, and a normal sedimentation rate and C-reactive protein help exclude the disease. Serum testing for cryptococcal antigen and Lyme disease can help exclude these disease processes too, though positive serum tests will require confirmatory spinal fluid analysis. Spinal fluid analysis is useful for identifying infectious headache etiologies, noninfectious causes of meningitis such as malignancy, and for identifying subtle subarachnoid bleeds. Spinal fluid analysis should be considered in older adults when a headache etiology remains unclear.

Treatment

Treatment of secondary headaches depends on the underlying disease process. For primary headaches, a variety of treatment options are available though patients will often have a history of successful treatment with a particular agent. Triptans and dihydroergotamine, which are two frequently used evidence-based classes of parenteral primary headache disorder medications, are associated with increased risk of cardiovascular events in patients with cardiovascular risk factors, including advanced age. Therefore, they should be used cautiously if at all in older adults, preferably reserved for those with a history of good response and no prior adverse events after receiving the medication [59].

Migraine

Management of the acute migraine is directed toward relief of the headache, functional disability, and other symptoms associated with the acute attack. Two thirds of patients with migraines suffer recurrent or persistent pain within 24 hours of ED discharge. Nonspecific parenteral analgesics such as NSAIDs and opioids are effective for relief of acute migraine attacks [60]. Though commonly used, opioids are felt merely to mask the pain of the acute headache rather than treating the underlying pathophysiologic process, and, therefore, place patients at a higher risk of headache recurrence after ED discharge. Opioids may also be associated with ED recidivism and worsening of the underlying episodic migraine disorder [61]. Migraine-specific parenteral treatments that include dopamine receptor antagonists, such as prochlorperazine, metoclopramide, or droperidol, are highly effective for acute migraines and generally well tolerated. Second-line parenteral medication treatment options include the antiepileptic valproate and magnesium. Corticosteroids, though unlikely to provide quick relief, are useful for decreasing recurrence of headache after ED discharge [60]. For some patients, regional anesthesia utilizing a greater occipital nerve blockade with local anesthetics may provide benefit with little risk of systemic medication effects [62].

Tension headache

Scant evidence exists to guide parenteral management of tension headache. For those who have not responded to oral analgesics such as acetaminophen, NSAIDs, or opioid combinations, parenteral dopamine antagonists or parenteral NSAIDs are likely to help [63].

Cluster headache

High flow oxygen is an evidence-based therapy for acute cluster headache. Parenteral NSAIDs or dopamine antagonists may be useful as well. Patients with acute cluster headache refractory to these therapies should be given parenteral opioids. Because patients with acute cluster headaches are very likely to continue to suffer similar acute headaches over the days and weeks after the acute attack, the emergency physician should initiate therapy with corticosteroids and calcium channel blockers at the time of ED discharge [13].

Trigeminal neuralgia

Antiepileptic drugs such as carbamazepine or oxcarbazepine successfully diminish the frequency and intensity of pain paroxysms, though they are unlikely to help acutely. Regional nerve blocks with long-acting local anesthetics often provide temporary relief, particularly in the infraorbital region of the trigeminal nerve. NSAIDs and opioids may also be used to afford short-term relief [14].

Hypnic headache

Caffeine appears to be the most effective treatment of hypnic headache. Caffeine, lithium, melatonin, and NSAIDs have all been tried as prophylactic treatments with varying efficacy [17].

Section IV: Decision-making

- New onset of a primary headache disorder is less common in the elderly. A diagnostic workup is often indicated in elderly headache patients without an established history of similar headaches.
- Diagnostic workup of headache should be tailored to the disease in question. Laboratory tests, LP, and noncontrast head CT each have limitations that must be recognized.
- Giant cell arteritis is as common as migraine in the elderly. ESR and C-reactive protein can be used to exclude this disease.
- Many medications can cause headache. Temporal relationships should be sought between headache onset and initiation and discontinuation of elderly headache patient's medications.

- Treating primary headaches in the elderly can be challenging because of age-related contraindications. Antidopaminergics such as metoclopramide or prochlorperazine are useful first-line therapies.
- When treating primary headaches, opioids are best avoided if possible.

References

1 Perry, J.J., Spacek, A., Forbes, M. *et al.* (2008) Is the combination of negative computed tomography result and negative lumbar puncture result sufficient to rule out subarachnoid hemorrhage? *Ann. Emerg. Med.*, **51** (6), 707–713.

2 McCaig, L.F. and Nawar, E.W. (2006) National Hospital Ambulatory Medical Care Survey: 2004 emergency department summary. *Adv. Data*, **372**, 1–29.

3 Solomon, G.D., Kunkel, R.S. Jr., and Frame, J. (1990) Demographics of headache in elderly patients. *Headache*, **30** (5), 273–276.

4 Pascual, J. and Berciano, J. (1994) Experience in the diagnosis of headaches that start in elderly people. *J. Neurol. Neurosurg. Psychiatry*, **57** (10), 1255–1257.

5 Prencipe, M., Casini, A.R., Ferretti, C. *et al.* (2001) Prevalence of headache in an elderly population: attack frequency, disability, and use of medication. *J. Neurol. Neurosurg. Psychiatry*, **70** (3), 377–381.

6 Headache Classification Subcommittee of the International Headache Society (2004) The International Classification of Headache Disorders: 2nd edition. *Cephalalgia*, **24** (**Suppl. 1**), 1–151.

7 Schwartz, B.S., Stewart, W.F., Simon, D., and Lipton, R.B. (1998) Epidemiology of tension-type headache. *J. Am. Med. Assoc.*, **279** (5), 381–383.

8 Friedman, B.W., Serrano, D., Reed, M. *et al.* (2009) Use of the emergency department for severe headache. A population-based study. *Headache*, **49** (1), 21–30.

9 Fisher, C.M. (1986) Late-life migraine accompaniments-further experience. *Stroke*, **17** (5), 1033–1042.

10 Lipton, R.B., Bigal, M.E., Diamond, M. *et al.* (2007) Migraine prevalence, disease burden, and the need for preventive therapy. *Neurology*, **68** (5), 343–349.

11 Goadsby, P.J., Charbit, A.R., Andreou, A.P., and Akerman, S. (2009) Neurobiology of migraine. *Neuroscience*, **161** (2), 327–341.

12 Torelli, P. and Manzoni, G.C. (2005) Behavior during cluster headache. *Curr. Pain Headache Rep.*, **9** (2), 113–119.

13 Nesbitt, A.D. and Goadsby, P.J. (2012) Cluster headache. *BMJ*, **344**, e2407.

14 Cruccu, G., Gronseth, G., Alksne, J. *et al.* (2008) AAN-EFNS guidelines on trigeminal neuralgia management. *Eur. J. Neurol.*, **15** (10), 1013–1028.

15 Koopman, J.S., Dieleman, J.P., Huygen, F.J. *et al.* (2009) Incidence of facial pain in the general population. *Pain*, **147** (1-3), 122–127.

16 Rughani, A.I., Dumont, T.M., Lin, C.T. *et al.* (2011) Safety of microvascular decompression for trigeminal neuralgia in the elderly. Clinical article. *J. Neurosurg.*, **115** (2), 202–209.

17 Holle, D., Naegel, S., Krebs, S. *et al.* (2010) Clinical characteristics and therapeutic options in hypnic headache. *Cephalalgia*, **30** (12), 1435–1442.

18 Lawrence, R.C., Felson, D.T., Helmick, C.G. *et al.* (2008) Estimates of the prevalence of arthritis and other rheumatic conditions in the United States. Part II. *Arthritis Rheum.*, **58** (1), 26–35.

19 Bloch, D.A., Michel, B.A., Stevens, M.B. *et al.* (1990) The American College of Rheumatology 1990 criteria for the classification of giant cell arteritis. *Arthritis Rheum.*, **33** (8), 1122–1128.

20 Kermani, T.A., Schmidt, J., Crowson, C.S. *et al.* (2012) Utility of erythrocyte sedimentation rate and C-reactive protein for the diagnosis of giant cell arteritis. *Semin. Arthritis Rheum.*, **41** (6), 866–871.

21 Salvarani, C., Cantini, F., Boiardi, L., and Hunder, G.G. (2002) Polymyalgia rheumatica and giant-cell arteritis. *N. Engl. J. Med.*, **347** (4), 261–271.

22 Kirby, S. (2010) Headache and brain tumours. *Cephalalgia*, **30** (4), 387–388.

23 Boiardi, A., Salmaggi, A., Eoli, M. *et al.* (2004) Headache in brain tumours: a symptom to reappraise critically. *Neurol. Sci.*, **25** (**Suppl. 3**), S143–S147.

24 Vazquez-Barquero, A., Ibáñez, F.J., Herrera, S. *et al.* (1994) Isolated headache as the presenting clinical manifestation of intracranial tumors: a prospective study. *Cephalalgia*, **14** (4), 270–272.

25 Valentinis, L., Tuniz, F., Valent, F. *et al.* (2010) Headache attributed to intracranial tumours: a prospective cohort study. *Cephalalgia*, **30** (4), 389–398.

26 Schankin, C.J., Ferrari, U., Reinisch, V.M. *et al.* (2007) Characteristics of brain tumour-associated headache. *Cephalalgia*, **27** (8), 904–911.

27 Forsyth, P.A. and Posner, J.B. (1993) Headaches in patients with brain tumors: a study of 111 patients. *Neurology*, **43** (9), 1678–1683.

28 Edlow, J.A., Panagos, P.D., Godwin, S.A. *et al.* (2008) Clinical policy: critical issues in the evaluation and management of adult patients presenting to the emergency department with acute headache. *Ann. Emerg. Med.*, **52** (4), 407–436.

29 Kim, Y.K. and Schulman, S. (2009) Cervical artery dissection: pathology, epidemiology and management. *Thromb. Res.*, **123** (6), 810–821.

30 Schwartz, N.E., Vertinsky, A.T., Hirsch, K.G., and Albers, G.W. (2009) Clinical and radiographic natural history of cervical artery dissections. *J. Stroke Cerebrovasc. Dis.*, **18** (6), 416–423.

31 Lee, V.H., Brown, R.D. Jr., Mandrekar, J.N., and Mokri, B. (2006) Incidence and outcome of cervical artery dissection: a population-based study. *Neurology*, **67** (10), 1809–1812.

32 Rubinstein, S.M., Peerdeman, S.M., van Tulder, M.W. *et al.* (2005) A systematic review of the risk factors for cervical artery dissection. *Stroke*, **36** (7), 1575–1580.

33 Schievink, W.I. (2001) Spontaneous dissection of the carotid and vertebral arteries. *N. Engl. J. Med.*, **344** (12), 898–906.

34 Lyrer, P. and Engelter, S. (2010) Antithrombotic drugs for carotid artery dissection. *Cochrane Database Syst. Rev.*, **10**, CD000255.

35 Zacharia, B.E., Hickman, Z.L., Grobelny, B.T. *et al.* (2010) Epidemiology of aneurysmal subarachnoid hemorrhage. *Neurosurg. Clin. N. Am.*, **21** (2), 221–233.

36 Edlow, J.A. and Caplan, L.R. (2000) Avoiding pitfalls in the diagnosis of subarachnoid hemorrhage. *N. Engl. J. Med.*, **342** (1), 29–36.

37 Perry, J.J., Stiell, I.G., Sivilotti, M.L. *et al.* (2011) Sensitivity of computed tomography performed within six hours of onset of headache for diagnosis of subarachnoid haemorrhage: prospective cohort study. *Br. Med. J.*, **343**, d4277.

38 Ward, M.J., Bonomo, J.B., Adeoye, O. *et al.* (2012) Cost-effectiveness of diagnostic strategies for evaluation of suspected subarachnoid hemorrhage in the emergency department. *Acad. Emerg. Med.*, **19** (10), 1134–1144.

39 Dorhout Mees, S.M., Rinkel, G.J., Feigin, V.L. *et al.* (2007) Calcium antagonists for aneurysmal subarachnoid haemorrhage. *Cochrane Database Syst. Rev.*, **3**, CD000277.

40 Larsen, C.C. and Astrup, J. (2013) Rebleeding after aneurysmal subarachnoid hemorrhage: a literature review. *World Neurosurg.*, **79** (2), 307–312.

41 Stiell, I.G., Wells, G.A., Vandemheen, K. *et al.* (2001) The Canadian CT Head Rule for patients with minor head injury. *Lancet*, **357** (9266), 1391–1396.

42 Blyth, B.J. and Bazarian, J.J. (2010) Traumatic alterations in consciousness: traumatic brain injury. *Emerg. Med. Clin. North Am.*, **28** (3), 571–594.

43 Comper, P., Bisschop, S.M., Carnide, N., and Tricco, A. (2005) A systematic review of treatments for mild traumatic brain injury. *Brain Inj.*, **19** (11), 863–880.

44 Domingo, P., Pomar, V., de Benito, N., and Coll, P. (2013) The spectrum of acute bacterial meningitis in elderly patients. *BMC Infect. Dis.*, **13**, 108.

45 Cabellos, C., Verdaguer, R., Olmo, M. *et al.* (2009) Community-acquired bacterial meningitis in elderly patients: experience over 30 years. *Medicine*, **88** (2), 115–119.

46 Marco, C.A., Schoenfeld, C.N., Hansen, K.N. *et al.* (1995) Fever in geriatric emergency patients: clinical features associated with serious illness. *Ann. Emerg. Med.*, 26 (1), 18–24.

47 Choi, C. (2001) Bacterial meningitis in aging adults. *Clin. Infect. Dis.*, 33 (8), 1380–1385.

48 Pachner, A.R. and Steiner, I. (2007) Lyme neuroborreliosis: infection, immunity, and inflammation. *Lancet Neurol.*, 6 (6), 544–552.

49 Jackson, A. and van der Horst, C. (2012) New insights in the prevention, diagnosis, and treatment of cryptococcal meningitis. *Curr. HIV/AIDS Rep.*, 9 (3), 267–277.

50 de Ory, F., Avellón, A., Echevarría, J.E. *et al.* (2013) Viral infections of the central nervous system in Spain: a prospective study. *J. Med. Virol.*, 85 (3), 554–562.

51 Ferro, J.M., Canhão, P., Bousser, M.G. *et al.* (2005) Cerebral vein and dural sinus thrombosis in elderly patients. *Stroke*, 36 (9), 1927–1932.

52 Dentali, F., Squizzato, A., Marchesi, C. *et al.* (2012) D-dimer testing in the diagnosis of cerebral vein thrombosis: a systematic review and a meta-analysis of the literature. *J. Thromb. Haemost.*, 10 (4), 582–589.

53 Coutinho, J., de Bruijn, S.F., Deveber, G., and Stam, J. (2011) Anticoagulation for cerebral venous sinus thrombosis. *Cochrane Database Syst. Rev.*, 8, CD002005.

54 Toth, C. (2003) Medications and substances as a cause of headache: a systematic review of the literature. *Clin. Neuropharmacol.*, 26 (3), 122–136.

55 Katsarava, Z. and Obermann, M. (2013) Medication-overuse headache. *Curr. Opin. Neurol.*, 26 (3), 276–281.

56 Feske, S.K. (2011) Posterior reversible encephalopathy syndrome: a review. *Semin. Neurol.*, 31 (2), 202–215.

57 Edmeads, J. (1988) The cervical spine and headache. *Neurology*, 38 (12), 1874–1878.

58 Ringeisen, A.L., Harrison, A.R., and Lee, M.S. (2011) Ocular and orbital pain for the headache specialist. *Curr. Neurol. Neurosci. Rep.*, 11 (2), 156–163.

59 Papademetriou, V. (2004) Cardiovascular risk assessment and triptans. *Headache*, 44 (**Suppl. 1**), S31–S39.

60 Sumamo Schellenberg, E., Dryden, D.M., Pasichnyk, D. *et al.* (2012) *Acute Migraine Treatment in Emergency Settings*. Comparative Effectiveness Review No. 84. (Prepared by the University of Alberta Evidence-based Practice Center under Contract No. 290-2007-10021-I.) AHRQ Publication No. 12(13)-EHC142-EF, Agency for Healthcare Research and Quality, Rockville, MD.

61 Evans, R.W. and Friedman, B.W. (2011) Headache in the emergency department. *Headache*, 51 (8), 1276–1278.

62 Levin, M. (2010) Nerve blocks in the treatment of headache. *Neurotherapeutics*, 7 (2), 197–203.

63 Friedman, B.W., Adewunmi, V., Campbell, C. *et al.* (2013) A randomized trial of intravenous ketorolac versus intravenous metoclopramide plus diphenhydramine for tension-type and All nonmigraine, noncluster recurrent headaches. *Ann. Emerg. Med.*, 62 (4), 311–318.e4.

11 Dyspnea in the elderly

Mercedes Torres & Siamak Moayedi

Department of Emergency Medicine, University of Maryland, Baltimore, MD, USA

Section I: Case presentation

An 80-year-old woman presented to the emergency department (ED) with altered mental status. She was in distress and unable to provide any history. Emergency medical services (EMS) providers had been activated by an out-of-state son who had been unable to reach the patient by telephone for two days. EMS providers reported that they arrived to find the patient disheveled, confused, and with urine-soaked clothing. She lived in subsidized senior housing, apartment which was small and filled with medications which were strewn about on a table by the couch. Her son was reached by telephone to confirm code status which was DNR/DNI. He reported that his mother has progressive dementia and he had been actively working on relocating her to his home out of state.

Her son did not know her medical history and she had no medical records at the hospital. EMS providers collected all the pill bottles they could from the scene prior to transport. Half full bottles at the bedside included: lisinopril, metoprolol, simvastatin, and levothyroxine. There were two empty bottles of aspirin and an unopened bottle of sublingual nitroglycerin pills. Also found were several inhalers including tiotropium.

The vital signs were as follows: temperature of 38 °C, pulse 115 beats/min, respirations of 30 breaths/min, blood pressure of 180/110, and a pulse oximetry of 89% on nonrebreather mask. The cardiac exam was notable for well-healed surgical scar above the sternum and an s3 gallop. The pulmonary exam was notable for increased work of breathing as indicated by deep rapid breaths. Chest was barrel shaped with decreased breath sounds at the bases and a brief end expiratory squeak. She had pitting edema to the knees bilaterally. Bedside ultrasound examination of the inferior vena cava measured 3 cm and did not change with the respiratory cycle.

Section II: Case discussion

Dr. Peter Rosen (PR): This is your typical geriatric patient, the presentation could be any one of 3000 pages of Emergency Medicine text and you have to start somewhere.

What would be the first thing that you would want to accomplish for this patient before actually getting into a specific diagnosis?

Dr. Amal Mattu (AM): Well, it is cliché I am sure, but I think you start with the ABCs.

She is a bit hypoxic with a pulse oximetry of 89%.

I think she is awake and maintaining her airway, so the A, the airway is probably OK, but she needs some oxygen, so I would get her on some supplemental oxygen. Actually, I see her pulse oximetry is 89% already on a non-rebreather mask, so I would probably start getting airway equipment, at least ready, in case we need to start heading in that direction, and I would consider some noninvasive airway ventilation in the mean time.

I would certainly get her a good working IV in place, and get her on a monitor.

Any elderly patient with shortness of breath must be strongly considered for acute coronary syndrome

Geriatric Emergencies: A Discussion-Based Review, First Edition.
Edited by Amal Mattu, Shamai A. Grossman and Peter L. Rosen.
© 2016 John Wiley & Sons, Ltd. Published 2016 by John Wiley & Sons, Ltd.

(ACS), as well, so I would get a quick electrocardiogram (EKG) on her. Once I've got those ABCs done, then I am going obtain the history and perform the physical exam assessment.

If this were a younger patient then I might be somewhat concerned, but in an elderly patient I am very, very concerned, as she is tachypneic, tachycardic, she's got a fever, she is already on a nonrebreather, and hypoxic. This is somebody who deserves the highest level of attention immediately.

PR: I think that is a pretty good summary of where to begin and we are not going to get an awful lot of help from history because the patient is being described as confused and there may not be anyone who can give us much of her past history. It is certainly worth asking the paramedics what they were told at the patient's house, but there may be no one who knows anything about her.

Given the fact she probably was already confused before she became ill, is there anything special you would like to begin with prior to your acting out on some of the concerns that Amal has already articulated?

Dr. Shamai Grossman (SG): I look at this patient as I would any patient who really can't give you a history. You always have to assume as, we should always do in Emergency medicine, that the patient has every horrible disease that you could actually imagine and then kind of work backward after you have checked off things in your list and say "Well, I have ruled out one life threat or another life threat" and then eventually come to your diagnosis rather than looking at what is the most likely diagnosis. The patient can't tell you. Clearly this patient, as Amal said, has abnormal vital signs, with a saturation of 89%, a heart rate of 115. Clearly, the patient needs immediate attention while we are trying to sort out exactly what the etiology is, which means stabilization of the airway.

The patient is 89% on a nonrebreather that is what needs to be addressed first. Once you stabilize the airway, you can start thinking back, to what was the cause of the respiratory compromise, what is the cause of the patient's alteration in mental status, whether it is a single disease process or multiple disease processes, whether it is acute or chronic. That, I do not need to know at the moment. What I need to do right now is to keep the patient alive long enough for us to complete the workup.

PR: Is there anything in this patient's presentation that would trigger you to look for something unusual other than perhaps to focus on perhaps sepsis and new pulmonary embolism (PE)?

SG: We have to have a very broad differential in our geriatric population for possible causes of dyspnea, but common things being common in this patient, I would consider an infectious etiology as well as heart failure or a chronic obstructive pulmonary disease (COPD) exacerbation. She may have some progressive hypercapnia that could be accounting for a worsening mental status that then could have led to aspiration leading to her presentation today. When I think of dyspnea in an elderly person, I think of either primary pulmonary causes or extra-pulmonary causes of their etiology for their symptoms.

As soon as I have secured her airway, I would obtain a chest x-ray as the first step before I consider some more esoteric causes of her symptoms.

PR: Looking at this patient's medications, there are a couple of things that strike me, but what strikes me that we all tend to forget, is blood glucose. Any confused patient should have immediate blood glucose determination by a finger-stick. I have been fooled into thinking that the patient's confusion was long term from the patient's senility as opposed to something acute from hypoglycemia. Even though the patient has a fever and one would expect hypoglycemia to cause a lowering of the patient's temperature, I think it should be part of every workup on every confused patient. The second point was that she is on a thyroid medication. We have an elderly patient who is confused, who has edema, and we all know that is almost impossible to pinpoint a diagnosis of thyroid disease without thyroid hormones, but certainly one of the things I would think about in this patient is myxedema coma and one of the things that might help you early on is to check her reflexes and see if she has a prolonged relaxation phase of her deep tendon reflexes.

To change directions just a little bit, this is a patient who also has the physical appearance of COPD. I think one of the things that we tend to do badly in COPD is to be convinced we need to intubate the patient because they have such terrible blood gases, but in point in fact, most of them live with bad blood gases and it is hard to use that as an indication for intubation. Will you take us through your thought process in approaching a patient such this as to what you would like to start with and when would you consider taking over the patient's airway?

Dr. Scott Wilbur (SW): At this point watching her work of breathing for a few minutes is probably reasonable to see with a respiratory rate of 30, tachycardic, and 89% on a nonrebreather, whether she is going to turn for the worst while we are getting started with lines, monitors and intubation preparations. We know that she is on a long-acting bronchodilator, so beginning bronchodilators along with oxygen immediately would seem to make sense. I think that a blood gas can help, although sometimes you have to make a decision without the benefit of the blood gas. This is somebody that we might want to consider for noninvasive ventilation. As mentioned, she has an increased work of breathing, she is tachypneic, she is obviously in some stress because of tachycardia; being able to take over some of the work of breathing for her may be beneficial. I have noted though that with some patients who have COPD it seems as though the noninvasive ventilation can be problematic because they have a longer recovery period so this may not be as effective as it would be in patients with congestive heart failure (CHF).

It was mentioned that the son was contacted to confirm code status but it was not mentioned what the code status was. I would want to know if this patient would want to have support of her airway and be intubated and placed on the ventilator.

Dr. Rob Anderson (RA): It was not written there, but she had DNR/DNI order.

PR: I think that this is one of those situations, however, in which before we give up on the patient, it would be nice to know whether we have something that is reversible and whatever her code status, we have to assume that if it is readily reversible, it is not our usual choice to just sit back and let someone expire because they have a DNR order.

What I like to do with COPD is to see if I can stimulate the person to breathe better and make them cough, and see if I can wake them up by not only talking to them and asking them to cough and and take a deep breathe but also by tapping their chest. I am not a big fan of noninvasive ventilation for COPD. I think it works for many patients, but I think there is a risk with it and the risk is when it fails, those patients do worse than had they been intubated directly. So my preferred approach is to see if I can stimulate the patient to improve their ventilation while giving them the bronchodilator that Scott prescribed for us.

Could you take us down to what you would like to do next in terms of both management and evaluation.

RA: I would echo your previous comment that a DNR/DNI order does not mean do not treat. And putting this person who is in obvious distress on BIPAP early would be a great move to see if you can get them out of trouble.

SG: I would add one point to that as well. We studied these patients and found out that if you actually talk to patients and give them scenarios of when they would want to be resuscitated, for instance, if they come in with anaphylaxis, or they come in with pneumonia, and up to 25–30% of patients do not want to be DNR. "That is not what I meant, I meant if I have a nonreversible etiology of my respiratory distress, then I do not want to be placed on the ventilator, but otherwise please do whatever you can."

PR: That is a fantastic point. It is such a complicated topic, that it really deserves, a full chapter in this book discussing the resuscitative wishes of people.

RA: One of the teaching points of this case is understanding geriatric physiology and just how really sick she is when she arrived. Her ability to maintain an elevated respiratory rate and her ability to maintain her tachycardia are going to be very limited, thus highlighting the need to act. These vital signs mean something completely different in an 80 year old than they do in a 20 year old, indicating she and her body may be exhausted. On exam, she also has a sternotomy scar, which might mean she has a history of heart failure. Therefore, thinking about her from a heart failure or acute pulmonary edema stand point I think would be important in this case. Regardless, putting her on BIPAP is going to help treat both COPD and heart failure so that is what I would start with here. While working on improving her respiratory status I might add some nitroglycerin for that blood pressure.

PR: This is a patient in whom I would not argue with anyone who said we need immediate intubation, we need to take away her work of respiration. We have a patient who has such a complexity in the potential cause of the failure that in order to sort it out we need to get her back to at least a safer piece of stability. One of the things that you mentioned is that there were two empty bottles of aspirin and we know that salicylate intoxication in an elderly patient can be very difficult to define and that it can certainly produce failure, it certainly can produce a respiratory picture as you have described here. Long before we have a chance to do a tox screen on her, we need to think about aspirin toxicity and start acting on it.

RA: I designed this case to highlight, in some regard, the unsatisfactory feeling you get with these folks who could have anything going on. If you placed this person on BIPAP, gave them nitroglycerin, drew blood cultures, gave them antibiotics, gave them diuretics, gave them bronchodilators, and treated them with a multiprong approach, you would not be faulted. If you treat them for one angle and the patient ends up in the unit and they figure out that she had pneumonia you would be faulted for not initiating all the therapy early on the patient. I am sure that we have all been there with this person where we are treating with multiple therapies at the same time, because we are not entirely sure what is going on.

PR: As we said last week, you have to kind of shot-gun these elderly patients because they have so many different pathologies with all of their concomitant diseases and this patient certainly seems like another example of that.

We have already talked about the ethical problems in managing this patient, but the pragmatic realization for me is that many hospitals have an ICU policy that if the patient is DNR you can't admit the patient to the ICU.

Could you articulate how you would manage that in a patient who you really don't know what their personal wishes are and are unlikely to find out about them?

SW: I think that regardless of whether this patient has a DNR order or not, she is going to require aggressive treatment. There are probably not many hospitals that can provide the level of care that this patient would need outside of an intensive care unit. She is probably going to need some combination of very frequent aerosols, neuro checks, monitoring the heart rate, and monitoring the response to therapy, so she is going to need nursing care in a ratio higher than a regular medical floor. I suppose that it is possible that this patient could be treated in the ED and we could see if a response to therapy might suggest a different level of care. I would look to see in this patient to see a decrease in her pulse and her respiratory rate as an indication that this patient might be able to be managed outside of an intensive care unit.

As this is a patient who certainly could be septic and we are all keyed to aggressive intervention on a septic patient before they crash would you be inclined to place a central line in this patient?

AM: I would say that if you can get good peripheral access with good size IV catheters, I don't think I would necessarily jump right to a central line.

When you look at the resuscitation ability from good peripheral access versus a central line, there is not much of a difference. What is the benefit of putting a central line in? You could use a central line for pressors, as we tend to be a little reluctant to use vasopressors through peripheral lines. In the past, people were using a central line to try to measure a CVP and but recently we have, to some extent, gotten away from using a central line for CVP because they are not quite good at measuring volume status as we had always thought, and the use of ultrasound is probably even better and simpler than using the central lines. In summary, I would not necessarily go straight to a central line at this point if we do have good peripheral access. However, if she is potentially heading downhill or if you are thinking that she is going to end up needing pressors, then I would go ahead and get a central line and not wait until she crashed because it will be tougher to get in a central line at that point.

PR: Personally, I have a great deal of prejudice against central lines in patients such as this, because the last thing she needs is to have an iatrogenic pneumothorax and anything that might keep you away from using a pressor I think it is worth doing, which means if you don't need a central line to give her a pressor then don't put in a central line, because I think we overuse pressors on patients such as this who are already hypertensive.

We have all noted this patient has lots of reasons for us to believe that she is in failure and it does not truly matter whether the failure is from the left heart that comes from arteriosclerosis or whether it is right heart that induced left heart failure from cor pulmonale, but given the fact that she seems to have some acute changes with the failure, how do you feel about medications for that? Would you give her some enalapril, would you give her some morphine? or would you start diuresing her as opposed to trying to give her a volume load?

SG: The first question before you start treating her, although she may have some element of failure, is to address the temperature of 38. I am wondering if her presentation might be more from an infectious etiology. You might get some basic information from a bedside ultrasound and looking at the IVC. You might get some useful information from a quick portable chest X-ray, and then you might get some information as you learn a little bit more about her past medical history, which is often the case. As the patient spends more time in the department, some of the information starts trickling in. I would not run to start diuresis in this patient. If I were to give her any medication at this point, it would probably be broad spectrum antibiotics and then if the chest X-ray doesn't show some infiltrate, but rather a pattern that might be more consistent with CHF I might be starting intravenous nitroglycerin for some afterload reduction and then as things work themselves out a little bit more, then consider diuretics a little bit later in the course.

I think if you give diuretics now, you will likely make the patient volume depleted which could be disastrous if there is an element of sepsis as well.

AM: There are a couple of misconceptions out there that Dr. Grossman alluded to. There is a misconception that everybody who has acute CHF is volume overloaded. In reality, if this patient has CHF, it is probably as a complication of her infectious process and we know that elderly patients can go into CHF

as a result of stressors from other body parts. For example, if you have a bad infection, you can also develop CHF and that might be the case here, but that does not mean she is fluid overloaded. In fact, if she does have an infectious process, there is a good chance that she is fluid depleted and yet has developed acute heart failure. So Shamai's point of not rushing into diuresis is a really important point. If you diurese her, you will make her even more dehydrated and worsen her prognosis, using a medication such as nitroglycerin would be perfect, because it would treat her CHF without depleting her volume. Chances are she probably needs more volume, but she needs more volume in the right place. Right now if she has CHF she has fluid in the wrong place and nitroglycerin rather removing fluid will just redistribute the fluid and probably get her out of CHF without making her further dehydrated.

The other point I would reiterate is that elderly patients can develop CHF or acute heart failure due to infections. But again, that does not mean that the patients are fluid overloaded. They simply have two processes now going on that need to be addressed.

PR: I think those are very important points. It is really important to recognize that you have multiple entities here that are probably additive rather than subtractive. It has been my experience, for every degree of fever you probably have 500 cc of insensible fluid loss and we don't know how long she has in fact been febrile. Would you be interested in putting a foley catheter in this patient?

Not only because you want some accuracy in what she is putting out if you decide to diurese her but also as part of your investigation as to one of the probable causes of her sepsis. We all know that one of the sources of confusion in the elderly is urinary tract infection, and waiting for her to void spontaneously may put some hours between us and having a reasonable explanation in what triggered her decline.

I think in this particular patient, I would be in favor of foley catheter placement. At least in our ED, this probably would have already happened by the nursing staff without me giving a clear order. But in general I am not in favor of foley catheters because they are a nidus of infection. But in this critically ill patient there are multiple benefits from the foley including evaluating for infection, urinary retention and for inpatient folks as well as us in the ED if we decide to diurese her, to have adequate intake and output so we know what her fluid balance is with our ongoing treatment.

Could give us some more information that has evolved in the care of this patient?

RA: Her chest radiograph is suggestive of volume overload, but limited because of the technique. Electrocardiograph shows persistent left bundle branch block pattern. No change from a prior tracing that was tracked down by a good medical student who found an old EKG. She is put on BIPAP 15/7 and given some sublingual nitroglycerin pills and in about 10 min her respiratory status and blood pressure improved somewhat, she is not out of the woods yet but she is looking better. Some labs trickle back. She has an elevated troponin, her BNP is elevated, and blood cultures are collected. Antibiotics are administered and she is admitted to the intensive care unit. Pneumonia on repeat imaging is found in the ICU.

PR: Could you give us some advice on how you would tract down some of the odd things that might have caused this presentation that we already alluded to such as salicylate intoxication, or hypothyroidism or some other things that are going to be very hard to diagnose in the ED. How far should we be pursuing them as we go through the exercise at least described in this patient?

RA: I think from the presentation it is pretty clear that this was some type of pulmonary source of shortness of breath. But we need to think about in patients who do not have hypoxia but rather just present with shortness of breath and tachypnea that there may be other reasons for the shortness of breath and tachypnea. I would think about a metabolic acidosis. You mentioned a hypoglycemia in a confused patient, but hyperglycemia with diabetic ketoacidosis (DKA) can also cause people to have shortness of breath and tachypnea. I would want to know her hemoglobin as severe anemia could be causing the shortness of breath. To evaluate for salicylate toxicity, an ABG would be helpful to look for the mixed pattern of salicylate toxicity. I think a tox screen may be necessary or a salicylate level, but as you alluded, chronic salicylate toxicity might be difficult to determine. If you are in a hospital where you can get a thyroid stimulating hormone (TSH) rapidly, that may be

helpful. Thats depends on whether that is something that turns around in your laboratory quickly. There would really be no way outside of thyroid studies to be able to diagnose that in this patient in the ED.

PR: What we are hearing is the reality that we all live with and that is that many of the diagnoses we would like to pinpoint are not going to be available in our ED, but it does not really alter our approach or our management to think about them and to start the workup and let the final information trickle through to the inpatient service. We talked about the issues where we need to take rapid steps to intervene. If you really thought she was hypothyroid, I would use the deep tendon reflexes as an indication to consider starting thyroxine as part of therapy for what she is facing. Other than that, I think we can wait for some of the results of the laboratory studies as an inpatient.

We could spend an hour talking about the ethics of caring for patients like this, but I prefer to simplify and say that until we know that this isn't an immediately reversible problem, let's stop worrying about what the long-term desires of the patient are and get on to the business of correcting what can be corrected quickly.

Case resolution

The patient was put on BIPAP and a portable chest X-ray suggested volume overload. She was treated with sublingual nitroglycerin with improvement of her hypertension and work of breathing. Blood cultures were drawn. Her troponin and BNP were elevated. She was admitted to the ICU where the working diagnosis was acute heart failure triggered by pneumonia.

Section III: Concepts

Introduction

Dyspnea is one of the most common presenting symptoms in the elderly. In contrast to younger patients, there are three specific considerations that are unique to the elderly. The first is the increased likelihood that multiple physiologic and pathologic processes are at play. The second is the increased urgency to act as a result of an older person's decreased physiologic reserve. And lastly, considerations for end-of-life wishes are critical when endotracheal intubation is a treatment option.

It is easy to understand how pneumonia, for example, might stress an 85 year old differently than a 25 year old. What is more challenging to incorporate into clinical practice, however, is how pneumonia in an 85 year old might contribute to ACS. In other words, it may be difficult to sort out a single unifying cause for acute dyspnea in older ED patients. Thus, evaluating and treating for multiple presumed etiologies while in the ED is acceptable and not unexpected. For example, one may need to initiate antibiotics while ordering a heparin infusion.

Anticipating the tenuous nature of the acutely dyspneic elder is essential. Regardless of underlying health status, increasing age is defined by the loss of reserve to deal with stress. This translates into early and aggressive support whether that is supplemental oxygen, noninvasive or invasive ventilation. This, in turn, translates to either moving the acutely dyspneic elder to a resuscitation room or having advanced airway equipment at the ready.

Finally, unique to geriatric patients is consideration for end-of-life wishes. We have the unique opportunity to alleviate the obvious suffering associated with dyspnea. Interventions such as morphine can provide immediate comfort to the patient and the family. However, establishing a patient's wishes can be a challenging task, even in quiet times. Developing a standard script may be of help such as "Your husband seems very ill. Because I am meeting you both for the first time, I would like to make sure I am respecting his wishes. Has he shared with you his wishes regarding his care if he were to become as ill as he is now?" Learning to provide effective end-of-life comfort will be an evolving role in the ED.

Acute coronary syndrome (ACS)

Coronary artery disease (CAD) is a leading killer in the geriatric population. The incidence of CAD and associated ACS increase with age. In general, patients 65 years and older account for 60–65%

of acute myocardial infarctions (MIs) and 80% of related deaths [1]. Age is an independent risk factor for CAD beyond traditional risk factors including smoking, hypertension, hyperlipidemia, and diabetes. Age-related cardiovascular changes include decreased arterial compliance, increased cardiac afterload, and left ventricular diastolic dysfunction. In addition, elderly patients have been shown to have increased circulating levels of cytokines and inflammatory biomarkers, which have been linked to the development of cardiovascular disease. Comorbidities, poor nutritional status (evidenced by decreased albumin levels and reported weight loss), and impaired renal clearance of cardiac medications can complicate the presentation in geriatric patients [2].

The dominant presenting symptom in over half the patients with ACS without chest pain is dyspnea [3]. Dyspnea accompanied by diaphoresis, nausea, vomiting, or syncope describes the geriatric patient who may be presenting with ACS [2]. ACS presenting with atypical symptoms is associated with worsened prognosis [3–5]. Cognitive impairment, myocardial collateral circulation from chronic progressive CAD, and reduced sensitivity to pain are hypothesized to explain the atypical presentation of MIs in the elderly [4]. In addition, hearing or visual impairments and socioeconomic factors can delay or obscure the presentation of geriatric patients with ACS. Remarkably, while silent MIs occur in 25% of the general population, they account for 60% of patients over 85 years of age [2].

In many cases, ACS may occur as a result of the increased myocardial oxygen demand of a preceding or coexistent pathologic process. Geriatric patients who present after a fall, recent severe infection, or disease process causing physical stress may be experiencing ACS as well. Many of these patients have underlying atherosclerotic disease, which lowers their threshold for cardiac decompensation and increases their myocardial demand at times of stress [2].

The physical examination is not overly useful in the diagnosis. Physical findings including hypotension, rales, and peripheral edema all suggest chronic as well as acute pump failure and connote a grim prognosis [1]. Obtain an EKG in any dyspneic patient. The prevalence of clinically unrecognized MIs detected by routine EKGs in the elderly ranges from 21% to 68% [4]. One normal EKG does not rule out an

ACS. Moreover, the elderly tend to have abnormal baseline EKGs due to the sequelae of prior MIs, left ventricular hypertrophy (LVH), preexisting blocks, and nonspecific ST and T wave abnormalities. Try to obtain a baseline EKG for comparison.

The initial approach to geriatric patients with ACS remains the same as their younger cohorts. In fact, aspirin has been shown to demonstrate an increased benefit for elderly patients. Clopidogrel is also recommended in appropriate cases as its benefits are equivalent in elderly patients. The evidence regarding the use of GIIb/IIIa inhibitors is less clear, with increased bleeding complications in elderly patients reported. When this class of medications is prescribed in the ED, calculation of dosing using creatinine clearance and an accurate weight is of utmost importance to decrease the risk of bleeding complications [2]. Nitrates have been shown to be effective and safe for reducing recurrent ischemia in elderly patients and should be used in the appropriate clinical scenario regardless of age [6].

Geriatric patients presenting with ST-segment-elevation myocardial infarctions (STEMIs) demonstrate improved outcomes after percutaneous coronary intervention (PCI) versus fibrinolytic treatment. Most notably, in elderly patients 6–12 h from symptom onset, PCI is preferred. When prescribing fibrinolytics, reduced dosing of adjunctive heparin can minimize bleeding risks while maintaining efficacy. In studies comparing adjunctive unfractionated heparin to low-molecular-weight heparin, the latter has shown efficacy with decreased bleeding complications when used in a modified dosing scheme for patients older than 75 years or with a creatinine clearance less than 30 ml/min. Geriatric-specific relative contraindications to PCI or fibrinolysis include baseline abnormalities in the EKG of unknown duration, poorly controlled hypertension, presentation to the ED greater than 6 hours after the onset of symptoms, prior stroke, dementia, or chronic anticoagulation therapy. These factors, in addition to patient preferences and social factors, have contributed to historically decreased rates of either reperfusion strategy in otherwise eligible elderly patients. However, geriatric patients who receive reperfusion therapy have a lower risk of death compared with those who do not [6].

Congestive heart failure

CHF is one of the most common causes of dyspnea. Studies indicate that moderate-to-severe diastolic or systolic dysfunction is present in more than 10% of all people over the age of 65 [7]. Decompensated CHF is the most common reason for admission in elderly patients [1]. The high rates of CHF in the elderly population are in part attributable to physiologic changes related to aging. The aorta and other great vessels demonstrate decreased elasticity with age. This increases afterload, causing LVH, increased oxygen demands, and ultimately systolic and/or diastolic heart failure [1]. In addition, the cardiomyocytes increase in size with age, causing increased myocardial thickness, and ultimately reshaping the left ventricle. The more spherical remodeling of the left ventricle results in decreased efficiency of cardiac contractility [8]. This process is then further complicated by decreasing cardiac output, which decreases renal perfusion, leading to fluid retention and worsened symptoms of volume overload with an insufficient pump [1]. Heart failure with a preserved ejection fraction is more common in geriatric patients [9, 10].

The diagnosis of CHF in elderly patients presenting with dyspnea is often delayed due to atypical symptoms and multiple comorbidities. Classic clinical features of CHF such as a third heart sound, pulmonary rales, increased jugular venous distention (JVD), and lower extremity edema are both insensitive and nonspecific in elderly patients [11]. Instead, elderly patients may complain of dyspnea with a variety of vague symptoms such as fatigue, decreased exercise tolerance, decreased activity levels, poor appetite, and confusion. Significant overlap exists between these complaints and the diagnoses of COPD, renal failure, and anemia [10].

The causes of new onset CHF in elderly patients include hypertension (preserved ejection fraction), CAD (systolic heart failure), valvular disease (commonly aortic stenosis or mitral regurgitation), or new onset atrial fibrillation (often with rapid ventricular response (RVR)) [11]. Exacerbations of previously diagnosed CHF can occur due to ACS, uncontrolled hypertension, infection, and other physiologic stressors. In the case of elderly patients with decompensated CHF, medication noncompliance is frequently a factor. Possible reasons for medication noncompliance include polypharmacy, complex dosing regimens, the inability to swallow pills (due to a physiologic decline in swallowing function), cognitive impairment, depression, and financial burden of medication compliance [12].

Once identified, the treatment of elderly patients presenting with CHF may include medications as well as ventilator support depending on the severity of presentation. In patients who are alert and cooperative but experiencing significant respiratory distress, noninvasive ventilation can be a rapid, life-saving intervention, preventing the subsequent need for intubation. In general, medical therapy for CHF in elderly patients is similar to that of the nonelderly. Diuretics, angiotensin-converting-enzyme (ACE) inhibitors, beta-blockers, and digoxin are all recommended for management of heart failure symptoms in elderly patients, with some caveats. In the kidney, age results in a decreased diluting and concentrating capacity as well as an overall decrease in glomerular filtration rate (GFR). As a result, elderly patients on diuretics are predisposed to electrolyte disturbances and hypovolemia. Hypokalemia, hyponatremia, and hypovolemia increase the risk of arrhythmias, falls, cognitive changes, and renal injury in elderly patients [13]. ACE inhibitors and angiotensin II receptor blockers (ARBs) can also contribute to worsening renal function and specifically cause hyperkalemia. Declines in renal function with age can complicate the use of digoxin as well, increasing blood concentrations at lower doses, therefore risking toxicity [14]. While beta-blockers are very effective for management of CHF in elderly patients [10, 14, 15], they are contraindicated in the presence of comorbid pulmonary disease and can cause symptomatic bradycardias and atrioventricular (AV) nodal conduction disorders [14]. Although two thirds of elderly patients are able to tolerate beta-blocker therapy, the tolerated dose is typically 40–70% of the targeted dose [15]. When prescribing any of the aforementioned medication classes for the management of CHF in elderly patients, using lower doses and close monitoring of renal function, electrolyte levels, and volume status is recommended [13].

Atrial fibrillation

Atrial fibrillation is the most common life-threatening dysrhythmia in the elderly with a prevalence of 5% in patients older than 65 years [1]. Comorbidities associated with atrial fibrillation in the elderly include hypertension, heart failure, CAD, diabetes mellitus, obesity, COPD, and obstructive sleep apnea. In the case of comorbid heart failure, the cause of acute decompensation can be elusive as atrial fibrillation with rapid ventricular response (RVR) can cause clinical heart failure, and heart failure itself can increase the propensity for the development of atrial fibrillation. Once present, atrial fibrillation increases the risk for the development of cognitive disorders and dementia in the elderly [16].

Geriatric patients presenting with dyspnea in the setting of chest pain, syncope, frequent falls, or the sensation of anxiety warrant evaluation for atrial fibrillation (with or without RVR) as the etiology. More classic symptoms of palpitations or increased cardiac awareness are less frequent in elderly patients. When present, atrial fibrillation frequently develops in the elderly as a response to a primary stressor, such as infection, cardiac decompensation, respiratory decompensation, or a surgical procedure. As a result, the diagnostic approach to the dyspneic elderly patient with atrial fibrillation should focus on identification of the underlying trigger. Electrolyte abnormalities and medication errors/side effects are other possible contributors [16].

The acute management of atrial fibrillation in the elderly involves the two issues of symptom control and stroke prevention. The optimal management of acute symptoms in the elderly is debated. In the unstable elderly patient with atrial fibrillation and RVR, synchronized electrical cardioversion should be attempted. Chemical cardioversion may be attempted with amiodarone, but overall rhythm control has been shown to be a less effective option in these patients. This strategy is limited by the prevalence of comorbid heart failure, as well as renal dysfunction and hepatic dysfunction, which can alter the metabolism of antiarrhythmics. As a result, rate control, even in the acute setting, is often preferable. Intravenous beta-blockers are generally recommended, especially for patients with CAD or heart failure. For patients with underlying pulmonary disease, nondihydropyridine calcium channel blockers are favored. Caution is advised with the use of digoxin in elderly patients given variable renal clearance rates [16].

The other component of atrial fibrillation management in the acute and chronic setting is stroke prevention. The literature clearly supports the use of vitamin K antagonists over aspirin toward this goal. However, the use of vitamin K antagonists in elderly patients presents increased bleeding risks, especially if the patient is at increased risk of drug–drug interactions, hepatic or renal dysfunction, recurrent falls, noncompliance due to cognitive disorders, or protein–energy malnutrition. Newer oral anticoagulants at lower doses have shown a decreased risk of intracranial hemorrhage compared with vitamin K antagonists. These medications, such as dabigatran and rivaroxaban, can be used in elderly patients but require decreased dosing and careful consideration of creatinine clearance prior to prescription [16].

Pneumonia

Pneumonia should be included in the differential diagnosis of the elderly patient who presents to the ED with dyspnea accompanied by altered mental status, hypoxia, decreased appetite, or generalized weakness. Typical clues to this diagnosis, including fever, cough, myalgias, or chest pain, are more commonly absent from the history in the majority of elderly patients. The presence of tachypnea on physical examination, even without other respiratory complaints or findings, should prompt evaluation for the possibility of pneumonia, among other processes [17].

The incidence of pneumonia in patients over 65 years old is four times that of the general population. Furthermore, the incidence is between 6 and 10 times higher for people in residential care facilities. Elderly patients are more susceptible to pneumonia for a variety of reasons. The physiologic changes of aging, such as decreased elastic recoil of the lungs, decreased chest wall compliance, and decreased respiratory muscle strength, can lead to mechanical difficulties in achieving effective respiration. The workload of basic respiration is further increased by changes that occur in the lung parenchyma, causing enlargement of the alveoli, increased functional residual capacity, and subsequent increased lung volumes. In addition, mucus is not cleared from the respiratory tract as easily given that the mucociliary ladder and ability to cough are both less effective [17].

Aspiration is a significant risk factor for pneumonia in geriatric patients. Elderly patients are more likely to silently aspirate; therefore, there may be a paucity of clues to this etiology on initial presentation. In other cases, underlying comorbidities such as dementia or stroke contribute to the increased risk of aspiration, resulting in pneumonia. Even geriatric patients without a history of stroke demonstrate a loss of swallowing function with age and increased time of swallowing. Medications commonly prescribed to elderly patients to treat comorbid conditions, including antidepressants, anti-Parkinsonian agents, diuretics, antihistamines, and antihypertensives, decrease salivation and place patients at further risk of aspiration. Furthermore, oral bacterial colonization increases with age due to a diverse group of circumstances, such as prolonged exposure to cigarette smoke (first or second hand), malnutrition, poor oral hygiene, antibiotic exposure, or severe illness [17].

Given the aforementioned risk factors, an approach to the dyspneic geriatric patient should be multifaceted and include an assessment of mental status, swallowing function, nutritional status, respiratory muscle strength (the ability to cough), and oral hygiene. Any recent severe illnesses or intubations may prompt an evaluation for pneumonia. In addition, any changes in the patient's overall functional status and ability to care for self can be subtle clues to an otherwise elusive diagnosis of pneumonia [17].

Respiratory fluoroquinolones or a combination of a cephalosporin and macrolide antibiotic are the backbone of antimicrobial therapy for pneumonia for all patients with community-acquired pneumonia. Some elderly patients may require broader coverage because they are at risk for health care acquired pneumonia based on their residence in a long-term care facility, frequent hospitalizations, polypharmacy including antibiotics, and comorbidities, such as renal failure on hemodialysis or chronic wound care management. The spectrum of antimicrobial coverage in these patients requires consideration of methicillin-resistant *Staphylococcus aureus* (MRSA) and multidrug-resistant gram-negative pathogens, not covered with community-acquired regimens. The duration of antimicrobial treatment should be 5–7 days, regardless of the severity of illness, unless they are immunocompromised [18].

Asthma and COPD

COPD is diagnosed in 34 of every 1000 people over the age of 65 and is the fourth leading cause of death in elderly patients [19]. Asthma, importantly, is commonly overlooked and underdiagnosed in the elderly, with an overall prevalence of 7–9% in patients over the age of 70 [20]. Asthma in the aging population carries a remarkably high morbidity and mortality as 80% of deaths from asthma in the United States occur in patients over the age of 55 [20].

The pathophysiology of COPD in the elderly is characterized by decreased elastic recoil of the airways causing air trapping and hyperinflation in the case of emphysema, and hypertrophy of mucus glands causing airflow obstruction and hypercapnia in chronic bronchitis [19, 21]. Degeneration of the elastic fibers around the alveolar ducts is a physiologic change of aging that occurs at ~50 years of age. Subsequently, air spaces expand, the number of alveoli decrease, and the surface area for gas exchange decreases [22]. In asthma, the decreased sympathetic and parasympathetic nerve function that occurs with age can lead to decreased beta receptor function. Atopy and allergy are less prominent in elderly asthmatics as less than 20% of asthmatics over 50 years old have been shown to have atopic triggers [20].

Both asthma and COPD can present with symptoms that overlap with other common diseases in the elderly such as CHF, pneumonia, and gastroesophageal reflux disease (GERD). Furthermore, elderly patients with COPD may have other comorbid diseases, such as cardiovascular disease, malnutrition, obesity, osteoporosis, anemia, obstructive sleep apnea, and depression, which not only complicates their presentations but also increases the likelihood of decompensation due to medication interactions [22, 23]. Patients with both decompensated COPD and CHF commonly present to the ED with similar presentations: dyspnea, audible wheezing, and hypoxemia on examination. Fortunately, early oxygen therapy and noninvasive ventilation are

key components of the initial resuscitation for both disease processes. A chest X-ray can be very helpful in differentiating pulmonary edema/cardiac wheezing from bronchoconstriction due to COPD.

Immediate stabilization of geriatric patients with an asthma or COPD exacerbation can be complicated by a history of CAD, recent MI, or tachydysrhythmia. Inhaled beta-agonists can cause tachycardias or prove less effective in the setting of systemic, nonselective beta blockade. Ipratropium bromide is a reasonable alternative in these patients given its bronchodilatory effects with decreased risk of arrhythmia. Conversely, when searching for the trigger for reactive airways disease exacerbations in the elderly, a review of the medication list should focus on any recent initiation of beta blockade in cardiac patients as well as those with glaucoma [23].

Consideration of the elder's cognitive and functional status in the setting of lung disease is also important. Chronic and acute hypoxemia and hypercapnia are associated with cognitive decline in elderly patients with COPD. The strongest association exists with a resting oxygen saturation of less than 88%. In these patients, cognitive declines are reported in memory, motor, and executive functioning [24]. Questioning family or friends regarding the presence of these symptoms is imperative to determining future risk as well as the need for ongoing home oxygen therapy in COPD patients. Furthermore, motor and executive function declines can create barriers to effective outpatient management of COPD patients as patients lose the coordination required for proper medication delivery via metered-dose inhalers (MDIs). The addition of a spacer to the MDI delivery system or the use of nebulized medications when possible can improve compliance and outpatient outcomes [22, 23].

Pulmonary embolism

Increasing age is one of the most powerful risk factors for venous thrombosis [25]. Attempts to sort out if the risk is attributable to age itself or age-accumulated comorbidities have not been successful. However, it is safe and prudent to consider increasing age plus comorbid conditions to be strongly associated with increased risk. The incidence of venous thrombosis increases fivefold for patients over 75 [26]. CHF has been shown to increase the risk of venous thrombosis by 1.5–2.5 times in patients over age 65. Stroke has been associated with 1.3- to 3.5-fold risk of venous thrombosis in same age group. Finally, COPD in patients over age 60 is associated with 1.2–1.4 times increased risk of PE [25]. To compound the issue, the mortality of PE at 1 year in the elderly is 39% [26].

Appreciating the increased prevalence and high mortality of PE is the first and most important step to making the diagnosis in older patients. As highlighted throughout this text, there are a variety of physiologic reasons why older adults may not have dramatic presentation of disease. This is made worse by comorbidities that can further complicate interpretation of heart rate, blood pressure, and pulse oximetry.

Unfortunately, the utility of PE clinical decision rules (CDRs) to stratify older patients is limited. Siccama *et al.* attempted systematic review on the topic and after reviewing 1538 eligible citations, they could find only nine that met their study criteria. They concluded from those nine studies that CDRs for venous thromboembolism in the elderly may have respectable sensitivity and safety but are not specific or effective (Siccama). Given above limitations of CDRs for elderly patients with suspected PE, the use of D-dimer is also limited. This is despite some evidence that age adjusted cutoff values for older adults may have clinical utility [27].

While research into geriatric-specific CDRs is sorely needed, the workup remains the standard imaging with either ultrasound or computed tomography (CT) angiogram. While there have been trends toward outpatient treatment in younger patients with newly diagnosed PE, this approach is less safe with older patients. For example, the PE Severity Index score reveals increasing mortality risk most associated with age and altered mental status [28].

Section IV: Decision-making

- The elder dyspneic patient is challenging. Due to age-related physiologic changes and age-accumulated disease, they may present with subtle findings or, even worse, late in their disease process.

- The cause for their symptoms is likely to be multi-factorial.
- Initial treatments should be aggressive given the loss of reserve with aging.
- Rapid and aggressive therapy must be tempered by patient and family wishes regarding end-of-life care.

References

1 Gupta, R. and Kaufman, S. (2006) Cardiovascular emergencies in the elderly. *Emerg. Med. Clin. North Am.*, 24, 339–370.
2 Alexander, K.P., Newby, L.K., Cannon, C.P. *et al.* (2007) Acute coronary care in the elderly, part I: Non-ST-segment-elevation acute coronary syndromes: a scientific statement for healthcare professionals from the American Heart Association Council on Clinical Cardiology: in collaboration with the Society of Geriatric Cardiology. *Circulation*, 115 (19), 2549–2569.
3 Brieger, D., Eagle, K.A., Goodman, S.G. *et al.* (2004) Acute coronary syndromes without chest pain: an under-diagnosed and undertreated high-risk group. *Chest*, 126 (6), 461–469.
4 Aronow, W.S. and Silent, M.I. (2003) Prevalence and prognosis in older patients diagnosed by routine electrocardiograms. *Geriatrics*, 58 (1), 24–40.
5 Ritter, D. (2004) Troponin I in patients without chest pain. *Clin. Chem.*, 50 (1), 112–119.
6 Alexander, K.P., Newby, L.K., Armstrong, P.W. *et al.* (2007) Acute coronary care in the elderly, part II: ST-segment-elevation myocardial infarction: a scientific statement for healthcare professionals from the American Heart Association Council on Clinical Cardiology: in collaboration with the Society of Geriatric Cardiology. *Circulation*, 115 (19), 2570–2589.
7 Redfield, M.M., Jacobsen, S.J., Burnett, J.C. *et al.* (2003) Burden of systolic and diastolic ventricular dysfunction in the community. *J. Am. Med. Assoc.*, 289 (2), 194–202.
8 Fleg, J.L. and Strait, J. (2012) Age-associated changes in cardiovascular structure and function: a fertile milieu for future disease. *Heart Fail. Rev.*, 17 (4–5), 545–554.
9 Kaila, K., Haykowsky, M.J., Thompson, R.B., and Paterson, D.I. (2012) Heart failure with preserved ejection fraction in the elderly: scope of the problem. *Heart Fail. Rev.*, 17 (4–5), 555–562.
10 Chan, M. and Tsuyuki, R. (2013) Heart failure in the elderly. *Curr. Opin. Cardiol.*, 28 (2), 234–241.
11 Manzano, L., Escobar, C., Cleland, J.G., and Flather, M. (2012) Diagnosis of elderly patients with heart failure. *Eur. J. Heart Fail.*, 14 (10), 1097–1103.

12 Grady, K.L. (2006) Management of heart failure in older adults. *J. Cardiovasc. Nurs.*, **21** (**5, Suppl. 1**), S10–S14.

13 Wehling, M. (2013) Morbus diuretics in the elderly: epidemic overuse of a widely applied group of drugs. *J. Am. Med. Dir. Assoc.*, **14** (6), 437–442.

14 Rich, M.W. (2012) Pharmacotherapy of heart failure in the elderly: adverse events. *Heart Fail. Rev.*, **17** (4–5), 589–595.

15 Dobre, D., Haaijer-Ruskamp, F.M., Voors, A.A., and van Veldhuisen, D.J. (2007) beta-Adrenoceptor antagonists in elderly patients with heart failure: a critical review of their efficacy and tolerability. *Drugs Aging*, **24** (12), 1031–1044.

16 Hanon, O., Assayag, P., Belmin, J. *et al.* (2013) Expert consensus of the French Society of Geriatrics and Gerontology and the French Society of Cardiology on the management of atrial fibrillation in elderly people. *Arch. Cardiovasc. Dis.*, **106** (5), 303–323.

17 Chong, C.P. and Street, P.R. (2008) Pneumonia in the elderly: a review of the epidemiology, pathogenesis, microbiology, and clinical features. *South. Med. J.*, **101** (11), 1141–1145.

18 Wunderink, R.G. and Waterer, G.W. (2014) Clinical practice. Community-acquired pneumonia. *N. Engl. J. Med.*, **370** (6), 543–551.

19 Imperato, J. and Sanchez, L.D. (2006) Pulmonary emergencies in the elderly. *Emerg. Med. Clin. North Am.*, **24**, 317–338.

20 Braman, S.S. (2003) Asthma in the elderly. *Clin. Geriatr. Med.*, **19**, 57–75.

21 Shiber, J.R. and Santana, J. (2006) Dyspnea. *Med. Clin. North Am.*, **90**, 453–479.

22 McDonald, V.M., Higgins, I., and Gibson, P.G. (2013) Managing older patients with coexistent asthma and chronic obstructive pulmonary disease: diagnostic and therapeutic challenges. *Drugs Aging*, **30** (1), 1–17. doi: 10.1007/s40266-012-0042-z.

23 Kitch, B.T., Levy, B.D., and Fanta, C.H. (2000) Late onset asthma: epidemiology, diagnosis and treatment. *Drugs Aging*, **17** (5), 385–397.

24 Landi, F., Pistelli, R., Abbatecola, A.M. *et al.* (2011) Common geriatric conditions and disabilities in older persons with chronic obstructive pulmonary disease. *Curr. Opin. Pulm. Med.*, **17** (**Suppl. 1**), S29–S34.

25 Engbers, M.J., Van Hylckama Vleig, A., and Rosendaal, F.R. (2010) Venous thrombosis in the elderly: incidence, risk factors, risk groups. *J. Thromb. Haemost.*, **8**, 2105–2112.

26 Siccama, R.N., Janssen, K.J., Verheijden, N.A. *et al.* (2011) Systematic review: diagnostic accuracy of clinical decision rules for venous thromboembolism in elderly. *Ageing Res. Rev.*, **10**, 304–313.

27 Schouten, H.J., Geersing, G.J., Koek, H.L. *et al.* (2013) Diagnostic accuracy of conventional or age-adjusted D-dimer cut-off values in older patients with suspected venous thromboembolism: systematic review and meta-analysis. *Br. Med. J.*, **346**, f2492.

28 Aujesky, D., Obrosky, D.S., Stone, R.A. *et al.* (2005) Derivation and validation of a prognostic model for pulmonary embolism. *Am. J. Respir. Crit. Care Med.*, **172** (8), 1041–1046.

12 Acute chest pain in the geriatric patient

Marianne Haughey

Albert Einstein College of Medicine, Jacobi Medical Center, Program Director Emergency Medicine Residency, St. Barnabas Hospital Bronx, New York, NY, USA

Section I: Case presentation

An 80-year-old man with a history of coronary artery disease (CAD) status post percutaneous transluminal coronary angioplasty (PTCA) × 2, diabetes, and hypertension, complained of sudden onset of sharp anterior chest pain radiating to his back. He stated this felt different from his prior cardiac pain. There were associated nausea, shortness of breath, and mild dizziness. He denied fever, cough, diaphoresis, or chest wall trauma. He took aspirin and nitroglycerin without effect.

The past surgical history was notable for an appendectomy 50 years ago and a hernia repair 10 years ago. The patient drank a glass of wine occasionally, quit smoking more than 20 years ago, and denied illicit drugs.

The patient's current medications included aspirin, atenolol, sublingual nitroglycerin, and glipizide. He had no allergies.

Vital signs were as follows: temperature 37.2° C (98.9° F), heart rate 105 beats/min, blood pressure 170/95 mm/Hg, respiratory rate 20 breaths/min, and oxygen saturation 94% on room air. On examination, he appeared uncomfortable. The heart was regular, tachycardia, with no murmurs or gallops. Pulmonary examination revealed basilar crackles bilaterally without wheezing. The abdomen was soft, nontender, and nondistended. There was no lower extremity edema.

An EKG (electrocardiogram) showed normal sinus rhythm at 105 beats/min with nonspecific ST-T changes.

Laboratory Testing was unremarkable including a normal set of cardiac enzymes. A portable chest X-ray study showed a widened mediastinum. Labetalol was started, and a contrast chest CT (computed tomography) scan was ordered, which revealed a type A aortic dissection.

Section II: Case Discussion

Dr Peter Rosen (PR): Would you comment on what might be helpful in being alert to cardiac problems in the elderly? It has been written that frequently they don't present with chest pain, and when they do present with chest pain, it does not always have the classic character. Is there anything that pushes your cardiac button when you hear it from an elderly patient?

Dr Andrew Chang (AC): If the patient has certain medical problems, such as hypertension, hypercholesterolemia, or diabetes, then I'm more likely to be concerned about cardiac causes. As you mentioned, part of the problem with evaluating older adults with acute coronary syndrome (ACS) is that they don't present with classic chest pain. Instead, they may present with vague symptoms such as generalized weakness, shortness of breath, dizziness, nausea, or syncope. The patient's past medical history may point me toward cardiac problems, such as a history of hypertension, hypercholesteremia, or known CAD.

Geriatric Emergencies: A Discussion-Based Review, First Edition.
Edited by Amal Mattu, Shamai A. Grossman and Peter L. Rosen.
© 2016 John Wiley & Sons, Ltd. Published 2016 by John Wiley & Sons, Ltd.

In addition, certain symptoms and signs such as diaphoresis raise my antenna toward serious cardiac problems.

PR: Are you tuned into particular complaints such as weakness or shortness of breath or anything that might suggest to you the onset of an ischemic coronary event?

Dr Shamai Grossman (SG): Weakness and shortness of breath are good examples of a patient who presents with symptoms that aren't easily explained. In my mind, if you're old the symptoms certainly could be ischemic in nature. The elderly also can present with classic cardiac disease, but when they present with vague symptoms, they need to be assessed for a cardiac etiology as well. Dizziness as the sole complaint, and syncope that can't be explained by the patient are more commonly ominous symptoms in the elderly.

PR: We classically try to distinguish between stable angina and unstable angina. I think that by definition, a new onset of angina is unstable, but here we have a patient who has a past history of CAD, who, of course, has significant risk factors in his diabetes and hypertension, who has had at least two stents placed, who is taking a number of cardiac medications, and who has chest pain. Is there anything you would do to help you to decide if this is new disease, or just a presentation of his chronic disease?

Dr Don Melady (DM): I must say that I was a little stumped by this case. It is a typical geriatric presentation. There is nothing that points one way or the other; and I was a bit surprised when it turned out to be what it was. One part of the history that is helpful is that the man himself says that this is "different" from his other experiences of chest pain. Yet, when I put on my geriatric hat, I must mention that we are now basing all of our approach on this man's own recounted history. Therefore, it would be good to include some assessment of his cognitive status in our physical examination as well. Dementia often goes unnoticed in the emergency department (ED). If we are making decisions based on this man's memory of his recent or past symptoms, it would be helpful to have some assessment of his ability to remember!

PR: I think that is a very a good point. Maybe it was done by observation of the patient, or maybe family was there to give you some notion of his general functioning, but that is certainly something we want to be cognizant of in every geriatric patient. Here is a patient who has a history of hypertension whose blood pressure is elevated; do you find it helpful to find out what this patient's pressures have been running, or do you find that often they don't know?

AC: I work primarily in a poor urban setting, so most of my elderly patients don't routinely check or know their blood pressures. Sometimes, I'll look up the patient's vital signs in our computer system to see what has been recorded in the inpatient setting in the past. In this particular case, I think you could argue that his blood pressure is running high because he is in pain. Lack of medication compliance might be another reason to explain his current blood pressure.

DM: I don't know about your practice setting, but in mine, many of my elderly patients have a home blood pressure monitor. They check it unnecessarily several times a day, and often write things down. I find that lots of people can give me a detailed account of what their blood pressure has been over the last week or month. Now, how helpful that is and how true his blood pressure of 170/95 mm/Hg is, or whether this is a manifestation of his pain or the excitement and worry of being in the ED is also another good question.

PR: I don't know how helpful it has been over the last 6 months, but certainly if he has been running at less than 140, and today he is now this elevated, I think that it helps you in trying to think what is changing here, and if it has something to do with the disease. I was also surprised at the ultimate pathology in this case, and I was trying to think about how I would separate the two pathologies when I initially evaluated the patient. Do you have any clues for us, on what would make you sensitive to a pathology of aortic dissection over coronary artery ischemia in the initial evaluation?

SG: In this particular patient, you have a couple of pieces of information that might make it a little easier. For one, as far as blood pressures go, I don't usually worry about an elevated pressure in the ED, but I would like to find the baseline. The same would be true about a low blood pressure, unless I don't expect it to be a low pressure. Unless you have something out of the ordinary, I don't find the blood pressure particularly helpful, but I find the history often is. In a

153

patient with a history of cardiac disease, the simplest question to ask the patient is whether the acute chest pain is similar to prior pain. If they say no, then I have to worry that there is a process that is going on that they haven't experienced before. That is the first clue I would use in any patient, particularly one who presents with a history of CAD. Next, although chest pain that radiates to the back can be seen in many presentations of cardiac ischemia, it is not the norm and that raises some red flags that this may not be the run-of-the-mill cardiac ischemia. Whether the pain is sharp, dull, or achy, I don't find particularly helpful. The textbooks all say that sharp pain is classic with dissection and that dull pain is typical with acute myocardial infarction (MI), but I don't think this is a reliable distinction. As I talk to these patients, I generally put my hands on their ankles, and I do it for several reasons. First, it enables me to develop a relationship with the patient, but more importantly, it gives me the ability to do a quick vascular examination making sure that they have equal pulses in both lower extremities. With the information that I get within the first 1–2 min of meeting the patient, I know where I am headed.

AC: It is classically taught that patients who have aortic dissection will have interscapular back pain, but the IRAD (International Registry of Aortic Dissection) registry that came out a number of years ago sort of dispelled that dogma and showed that most patients with aortic dissection actually present with anterior chest pain. I, too, think we have to be wary and consider the diagnosis even if the patient does not have the "classic" interscapular back pain.

PR: I have found that in many cases involving the elderly the inability to relieve the pain with conventional pain management, or with what seems to work well with MI pain, is what stands out in my mind. We are somewhat lucky here in that the patient's EKG is not significantly abnormal for CAD, but we could have been further confused if he had persistent ST elevation because of a ventricular aneurysm, or because he had many of the changes that were caused by his previous MI. I think it also helps to trigger some concern about dissection when the EKG doesn't match the patient's symptoms. There are a couple of questions I would ask you to comment on: (1) Are there EKG changes that suggest dissection to you? (2) To change direction a little bit, how would you

manage this patient's pain given the fact that he is 80 years old?

DM: I am unaware of any EKG changes specific for dissection, or findings that would make me think of dissection in an 80-year-old man. I don't know how any particular finding on the EKG would sway my thinking with regards to this rather generic atypical presentation of chest pain in an 80 year old. With regard to managing his pain, the most concerning part of this whole scenario in my mind are his vital signs; the blood pressure we have already talked about, but the heart rate is also not normal. Older people do run at a higher rate normally, but this is someone who is beta blocked. One hundred and five is really not a normal heart rate, so there must be something driving it. Pain itself might cause this, and maybe controlling his pain would be helpful in making a determination there. At this point, I am not thinking that the pain is ischemic so, I would use hydromorphone starting at a low dose such as 0.5 mg IV to see if that makes a difference in his comfort.

PR: I, too, am not aware of any specific EKG changes that suggest dissection other than in a negative fashion that I have already alluded to. Here is a patient who is having chest pain, and who has known CAD, whose EKG is relatively benign, which would make me not think of CAD but something else.

SG: I am also unaware of any specific EKG changes that one might see that might make one think more about aortic dissection. In fact, one of the most confusing scenarios is when a patient has an aortic dissection and concomitantly dissects one of his coronary arteries, and in that case, the EKG looks like an ST-elevation MI. Those cases are even more difficult to evaluate and discern regarding the etiology of their symptoms. On the other hand, a nonspecific EKG may make you want to look one way and another for other etiologies, but up to 50% of EKGs don't show a ST-elevation myocardial infarction (STEMI) on initial presentation.

PR: I noticed that his portable chest X-ray study showed a widened mediastinum. I was surprised this bothered someone, because I can't remember a patient of this age who didn't have a widened mediastinum on a portable chest X-ray study. How would you know that isn't normal for a man of his age?

AC: This is similar to having a comparison EKG when you have an abnormal EKG. If you have a prior portable chest X-ray study, that shows a normal mediastinum, then seeing a widened mediastinum would be concerning, and might move dissection up the list in the differential diagnosis. At the same time, a normal mediastinum does not rule out a diagnosis of aortic dissection.

PR: I compliment the team that diagnosed this patient for getting to the right diagnosis. What would you do if he had ST elevations, but you were also concerned about dissection?

SG: This is not a rare scenario, and I think the ideal way to manage it is to take the patient to the catheterization laboratory, and prior to an intervention obtain a view under fluoroscopy of the aortic arch. You should be able to answer your question very quickly. The problem with a CT angiogram prior to taking them to the catheterization laboratory is that you are subjecting them to a double dye load, and that is less than ideal. More often than not, the managing physicians equivocate and believe this is a just a STEMI. But after the chest X-ray reading comes back, they end up getting the CT angiogram believing that it will be normal. The third option is something of a compromise: do a transthoracic echocardiogram (TTE) in the ED. The problem with that is the delay in care, which is probably similar to obtaining the CT angiogram.

AC: Did you mean to say transesophageal echocardiogram (TEE)?

SG: No, I said specifically transthoracic, because the problem with transesophageal is that it is even more time-consuming, and at most institutions, even more difficult to obtain on an emergent basis.

AC: I agree that it is fairly difficult to obtain even at academic institutions, but I believe the sensitivity and specificity is pretty poor with transthoracic echocardiography in terms of diagnosing aortic dissection. I guess if the transthoracic echo showed wall motion abnormality, then that would lead me more toward ACS as the cause. This situation (STEMI secondary to aortic dissection) has actually been addressed at my institution. Our cardiothoracic surgeons and cardiologists have requested that we should not perform CT angiograms in the ED in patients with STEMI and potential aortic dissection due to the additional dye load that Dr Grossman alluded to earlier. Instead, they want us to let them know that we are concerned about aortic dissection, and when the patient goes to the catheterization lab, they will specifically look for this.

SG: That is the ideal way to manage that and the way we try to manage it at our institution. However, because many of these cases do not go to a tertiary referral center, but are initially evaluated in the community, we find that more often than not, there is a delay for computed tomography angiography (CTA) or some other testing. The transesophageal echo gives you great view, and very good answer as to whether the diagnosis is aortic dissection or not. The problem is the lack of quick availability that often precludes them from being a diagnostic test that you can obtain in the ED.

AC: Do you know how accurate transthoracic echo is in ruling out aortic dissection?

SG: Studies place it in the 60–80% range, not ideal when ruling out life-threatening disease, but if readily available and positive, it could prompt the surgeons to take this patient to the operating room sooner.

PR: Are your CT surgeons doing stents for dissection now as opposed to open surgery?

DM: They certainly are doing them, though I suspect this would not be the appropriate management for this man. Given the acuity of the symptoms, I assume that he was established as a type A dissection, which generally means a surgical approach.

PR: Since he already was on a beta-blocker, why was it that you started him on labetalol to lower his pressure?

AC: We generally have two methods to manage the blood pressure and heart rate in patients with aortic dissection. The first is to give a single agent, typically labetalol. Alternatively, one can give another beta-blocker, such as metoprolol, followed by nitroprusside once they are sufficiently beta blocked. The order is important so that you don't cause a reflex tachycardia that might occur when lowering the blood pressure. In this case, it was just out of convenience that we chose labetalol. But we could have also used a combination of beta-blocker and nitroprusside.

155

PR: Do you have a recommendation for us on how to start therapy for these patients?

SG: Dr Chang alluded to our first order of business, which is to decrease dP/dT, or lower wall stress, and that is the role of beta blockade. In patients that come in hypertensive and tachycardia, you have to wonder if they have been adequately beta blocked, or beta blocked at all. We certainly don't know about the patient's compliance. Starting with a beta-blocker is reasonable, then adding an agent such as nitroprusside, or something similar would be quite appropriate. If you are worried about cardiac ischemia, then you might try IV nitroglycerin instead of nitroprusside, as you may have some concerns for subclavian steal and worsening of the infarction if you employ nitroprusside as your second agent for afterload reduction.

AC: If the diagnosis is aortic dissection, and you've chosen to use dual therapy, I think it's important to use IV nitroprusside as opposed to IV nitroglycerin, the latter of which has often been started on the assumption that the etiology is ACS in nature. IV nitroprusside is a much better arterial vasodilator, and I would recommend taking nitroglycerin down and replacing it with nitroprusside once the diagnosis of aortic dissection is made.

DM: I am a labetalol enthusiast largely for reasons that Dr Chang mentioned. It is quick. It is easy. I know how to dose it. It is readily available. The nurses are familiar with it.

PR: Given that this patient is a diabetic, do you think he now requires some insulin as you manage his other disease process? Should you prevent his diabetes from worsening since we know that many patients with diabetic ketoacidosis (DKA) are actually presenting with DKA secondary to an acute MI?

AC: Intensive insulin therapy was kind of a hot topic a few years ago for intensive care unit (ICU) patients. I don't know if anyone has done a subanalysis for aortic dissection patients.

DM: I think where this man's diabetes is going to be most problematic is in getting the CT angiogram. It's not mentioned anywhere here, but his creatinine is almost certainly not normal. I think that is always a big obstacle to move the investigations forward. I know at our institution, the radiologists don't want

to give contrast dye if the creatinine is elevated at all. At least this man isn't on metformin. Sometimes, you must settle for a noncontrast study, which I think is not going to be helpful in making this diagnosis.

PR: I think that is a terrific point, and I have had that fight for 25 years. The radiologists don't seem to understand that sometimes the patient's criticality trumps their prudence. Without an answer as to whether he is dissecting, why save his kidney function when you can't save his life?

DM: That is a very hard argument to make with a radiologist as we all know.

PR: Sometimes you have to put it in their lap: "Well, are you going to take responsibility for his dissection by refusing to do a study that I need to have you do?" That usually succeeds, but it is always unpleasant. This is a patient who seems to have weathered a normal workup process, in that you had time to obtain some laboratory studies including cardiac enzymes. Is there a time constraint on aortic dissection that makes you want to rush to the operating room (OR)?

AC: I do think we want to get the patient to the OR as fast as we can if it's a type A aortic dissection. That's because we worry about the various complications that can occur especially if the dissection works its way back toward the heart to involve the coronary arteries, as mentioned earlier, or cause other serious complications, such as pericardial tamponade or valve rupture. Most patients with aortic dissection are hypertensive, but if the patient has an aortic dissection and is hypotensive, that can be ominous. I remember a case as a resident where we had a patient with chest pain who was hypotensive. We obtained a portable X-ray study that showed a widened mediastinum and a calcium separation sign, and that patient went immediately to the OR without any further testing, but she unfortunately expired. But for most patients we have more time. Another important point is the need to initiate treatment with beta-blocker and blood pressure control prior to confirming the diagnosis of aortic dissection if the clinical presentation suggests dissection.

PR: I think once they start dropping their blood pressure we may be on the point of the curve we aren't going to be easily able to reverse, even though we must try. My experience with elderly dissection is not favorable, with more dying than surviving, and I think it is a very lethal disease in this age group. The faster you recognize it, the greater your chance to do some good. These patients are so brittle that they don't tolerate the major surgical procedure very well. They have vessels that are hard to deal with and the postop course is often complicated.

PR: Could you summarize the outcome of this case for us?

AC: After the patient had a chest X-ray study that was concerning for a widened mediastinum, labetalol was started, and a chest CTA was obtained, which confirmed a type A aortic dissection. The patient was then taken to the OR by cardiothoracic surgery, where he underwent successful repair of an aortic dissection.

Section III: Concepts

Chest pain is one of the four most common ED complaints in the United States (US) [1, 2]. Etiologies of chest pain range from life-threatening cardiac causes, such as MI and aortic dissection, to more benign causes, such as heartburn and muscle strain. The incidence, acuity, morbidity, and mortality of various causes of chest pain increase with aging.

The emergency physician (EP) needs to develop solid strategies to differentiate worrisome patients from those who are less concerning. Unfortunately, some of the usual strategies used for younger patients may be less helpful when evaluating older adults who, for example, often present with different symptoms as compared to younger adults with the same diagnosis.

Older adults have lived longer and often need to convey more information regarding medical issues or prior surgeries. There are multiple impediments in eliciting a useful history from an older adult. This can include simple physical limitations such as visual loss, hearing loss, cognitive impairment, or mobility limitations. Indeed, the noise and controlled chaos of the ED can make a functional but mildly demented older adult confused enough to prevent an accurate history from being obtained. Providing a relatively quiet and calm space may assist in obtaining a higher quality history from older adults. Supplemental sources of history, such as from family, electronic medical records, and records from a long-term care

facility, can also be valuable when the patient is unable to provide a reliable history. Information should be obtained regarding the baseline, whether that is a baseline EKG, baseline mental status, or usual medications.

The history from even a high functioning older adult can nevertheless be challenging. Older adults often perceive pain differently from younger patients such that their chest pain may be expressed in an "atypical" manner [3–5]. This altered perception, in addition to the decreased pain sensation that occurs with other chronic diseases such as diabetes, may result in a lowered concern for potential seriousness by both patient and EP [6]. For example, older adults may not consider chest tightness or chest pressure as forms of chest pain and hence may answer negatively when asked the question, "Do you have chest pain?" This alteration in perception of pain is identified as one of the causes of delays in diagnosing older adults with serious illnesses, such as MI, aortic dissection, and pneumothorax [4].

Different disease processes, such as CAD, chronic obstructive pulmonary disease (COPD), and cancer, become more prevalent with aging and have often had more time to cause further associated damage. These disease processes can lead to certain sequelae, such MIs and aortic dissections from CAD, spontaneous pneumothoraces from COPD, and pulmonary emboli and cardiac tamponade from cancer.

The goal of this chapter is to provide the information that may allow the EP to carefully weigh the possibilities of diagnostic concerns in older adults presenting to the ED with acute chest pain.

Acute MI/cardiac ischemia

When considering "acute chest pain" as a general complaint in the ED, most EPs will immediately consider ACS in the differential diagnosis. How ironic then that what is often considered first in the younger population with complaints of "chest pain" can be missed so easily in the older population, which has a disproportionate number of cardiac ischemic events. Over 60% of acute MIs occur in patients older than 65 years of age, with one third of the MIs occurring in patients over age 75 [7]. In addition, the morbidity and mortality of MI are higher in older adults, as those over age 65 account for approximately 85% of the deaths due to MI [7–11].

The likelihood of patients having ACS is related to a number of risk factors, many of which increase with aging. The prevalence of hypertension, diabetes, and hyperlipidemia increases with age, and the duration of older adults' exposure to these risk factors is longer than that of younger adults [7, 8]. There are also additional age-related changes in the cardiovascular system, such as increased vascular "stiffness," and alterations in the balance of intrinsic thrombus formation and lysis. These physiologic changes can create more demand for oxygen on the cardiac system while simultaneously decreasing the capability of the cardiac system to provide adequate oxygenation [7, 12–14].

A key fact to consider when caring for older adults is the difference in their disease process, and how it affects their history and physical examination. Because older adults with ACS can present without chest pain, ACS can easily be missed. Missed MI rates in older adults range from 21% to 68% [15–17]. Rittger's study took patients undergoing percutaneous coronary intervention (PCI) and intentionally created ischemia by inflating the balloon in the coronary artery [3]. He then divided patients into two groups based on a cutoff age of 69 years. He found a significant time lag in the perception of angina pain as well as the severity of chest discomfort among the older group compared to the younger group, even though ECG evidence of ischemia was no different between the groups experiencing these ischemic events.

Seventy-five percent of patients aged 70 years and younger who have an MI will have some chest pain or discomfort complaint when asked. By age 80–84, only 50% of patients with documented MI will complain of chest pain, and by age 85, less than 40% of patients with an MI will complain of chest pain [7, 18]. Therefore, it is important to be alert to "atypical" complaints in older adults when ACS is in the differential diagnosis. Since pain perception from cardiac ischemia is often decreased in older adults, they may instead complain of symptoms related to the effects of decreased cardiac performance, such as dyspnea [3]. This complaint increases with age so that by age 85, more patients complain of dyspnea than of chest pain or chest pressure [7, 18]. There is also a steady progression in complaints of "confusion" in those actually having an MI, increasing from 3% in patients less than 70 years to 20% in those aged 85 years [7, 18].

EKGs are often be less helpful in older adults, who are more likely to present with non-ST-elevation myocardial infarctions (NSTEMIs) or nondiagnostic ECGs compared to younger patients [7]. In addition, they are more likely than younger patients to have an abnormal baseline ECG, such as a left bundle branch block, a paced rhythm, or other underlying ECG findings that can cause confusion during the initial assessment.

Cardiac enzymes should be sent more liberally in older patients, including those complaining of dyspnea, confusion, and weakness among other more nonspecific complaints, because of the aforementioned difficulties in diagnosing ACS in older adults.

Older adults with acute MI have a much worse prognosis than younger patients and a higher mortality rate [9, 19]. Those who are diagnosed with MI without chest pain have an even higher mortality than older adults with MI and chest pain as a symptom [17]. Boucher finds that the in-hospital mortality rate among those with acute myocardial infarction (AMI) who are less than 55 years old is 2.1%. This increases to 26.3% for those aged 85 years and older [9]. It is likely that at least part of this increase in mortality is due to delays in making the diagnosis of MI in older adults. Since they present with less typical symptoms, they delay calling paramedics and present later in the process to the ED [19]. Moreover, as mentioned earlier, their histories can be confusing and their ECGs are less diagnostic, which create further delays in definitive care.

Older adults have an increased risk for complications of MI such as heart failure, atrial fibrillation, heart block, myocardial rupture, and cardiogenic shock [7, 20]. In addition, there is both reduced efficacy of thrombolysis in older adults and decreased usage of thrombolytics in otherwise appropriately aged patients with MI [9, 7, 21, 22].

Aortic dissection

Aortic dissection typically results from an intimal tear with subsequent dissection of the medial layer of the arterial wall. "Acute" aortic dissection is defined as up to 14 days after the initial event [23]. Though relatively rare (3 per 100,000), aortic dissection can be devastating [24–27]. The Stanford classification is most commonly used, which divides aortic dissection into one of two categories. Type A dissection includes dissection of the ascending aorta and may include the descending aorta, whereas type B involves the descending aorta alone. Surgery is often the treatment of choice in type A dissections, whereas medical management is the preferred treatment of choice for most type B dissections. The IRAD has provided a large amount of information regarding the history, diagnosis, treatment, and prognosis of aortic dissection [23].

The overall in-hospital mortality is 27% for patients (all age groups) identified in the IRAD registry [23]. For type A patients, surgically treated patients have a mortality rate of 26% compared to 58% mortality for those who are medically managed. For type B patients, medically managed patients have a mortality of 10% compared to 31% mortality for those who undergo surgery. Since the IRAD registry only includes patients who survive to reach the hospital, overall mortality rates are likely even higher. Mortality is higher during the first 7 days after presentation [23].

Not surprisingly, delays occurred in the presentation, identification, and management of aortic dissection in older adults in the IRAD registry. Mehta *et al.* have looked at the data for type A and type B dissections specifically among older adults, using the age cutoff of 70 to distinguish the younger population from the older population [28, 29]. Unlike with ACS, Mehta *et al.* find that although older patients with a type B dissection are about as likely to complain about chest or back pain as younger patients, among those with a type A dissection, older adults are significantly less likely to present with an abrupt onset of chest or back pain (76.5% vs 88.5%, $p = 0.0005$) [28, 29].

The IRAD data has shown that aortic dissection, with a few exceptions, is generally a disease of older adults. The mean age of those identified is 63.1 years, although with a standard deviation of 14 years. A subset of younger patients with connective tissue disorders, such as Marfan's syndrome or Ehlers–Danlos, present with aortic dissection at a mean age of 36 years, with a range of 13–52 years. In the older group (age >70 years), there are no patients with Marfan's syndrome. Factors associated with aortic dissection among those aged more than 70 years are hypertension, iatrogenic dissection from a cardiac procedure, diabetes, and atherosclerotic disease [28–31]. Men are most commonly affected by aortic dissection although at the higher age groups, women make up an increasing percentage of patients, likely due to their longer lifespan.

Diagnostic strategy

In the IRAD registry, the most common presenting complaint is severe pain (95% of patients). Eighty-five percent note abrupt onset and 73% complain specifically of chest pain [23]. Identifying the patient who has aortic dissection is complicated by the fact that one of the most common complaints in patients presenting to the ED is "chest pain." Ideally, a non-invasive study would be used to quickly distinguish the patient with an aortic dissection from one with ACS, especially since the latter is often treated with anticoagulation or antiplatelet agents, which can produce disastrous results when given to the patient with aortic dissection.

Unfortunately, there are significant limitations in the diagnostic studies initially used to evaluate chest pain when considering the diagnosis of aortic dissection. For example, it is typically taught that one should look for a widened mediastinum on a chest radiograph. However, the IRAD study finds that 37.5% of patients with aortic dissection do not have a widened mediastinum and 12.4% have a completely normal chest radiograph [23]. An EKG is neither sensitive nor specific and is found to be normal in 31.3% of patients with dissection, with nonspecific abnormalities being the most common finding [23]. Among older adults with aortic dissection, Mehta *et al.* find that pulmonary effusion on chest radiograph is a more common finding than among the population with the disease as a whole and that ECGs among older adults with type A aortic dissection are more likely to demonstrate new Q waves or ST segment deviations compared to younger patients (9.7% vs 5.2%) [28]. In type B dissections, there are no differences in ECG findings between younger and older patients [29].

Some have proposed that the D-dimer might be a way to screen out patients with aortic dissection, but this is not yet accepted and used routinely [32]. Ruling out the diagnosis of acute dissection requires CT angiography, transesophageal echocardiography, magnetic resonance angiography (MRA), or cardiac angiography.

Type A dissections and type B dissections are treated differently and have different findings. Type A dissections are more likely to be surgically managed and type B medically managed. There are additional concerns for older adults with aortic dissections. Operating on the aorta is always a high-risk procedure and requires consideration of a risk/benefit analysis. Older adults (age over 70) with a type B aortic dissection have a higher likelihood of experiencing in-hospital hypotension or shock compared with younger patients (<70 years old) [29]. Hypotension, branch vessel involvement, and periaortic hematoma are independent predictors of in-hospital mortality in older adults with type B aortic dissection [29]. Older adults without these risk factors with a type B dissection constitute 60% of the older adults in the IRAD registry, and have a very low in-hospital mortality of 1.4% when medically managed [29]. Unsurprisingly, older patients with type B dissection who have hypotension or shock have the highest risk of in-hospital mortality (56%) [29]. In type A dissections, patients older than age 70 are less likely to present with sudden onset chest pain or back pain than patients younger than 70 [28]. These older adults also have increased risk of mortality, with fewer older patients going to surgery because of comorbid conditions [28]. Among type A dissection patients going to surgery, mortality rates increase significantly with increasing age [28].

Pneumothorax

There is a striking difference in the presentation of older patients compared with younger patients when there is a pneumothorax. Although acute chest pain is a common complaint in younger patients, Liston *et al.* find that only 18% of patients aged 65 years and older complain of chest pain compared to 67% of patients aged 20–35 years of age. Instead, 82% of older adults complain of dyspnea. All of the older adults have evidence of prior lung disease, with the majority (82%) having signs of hyperinflation, and the others show abnormalities consistent with prior tuberculosis. Compared to younger patients, there is significant delay among older adults in presentation to the hospital from symptom onset, decreased clinical diagnosis pre-chest X-ray study, increased morbidity in the hospital, and a much longer hospital stay (33.5 days vs 9.3 days) [33].

Pulmonary embolism

Older adults with pulmonary embolism (PE) provide multiple challenges to the EP. Although the incidence increases with age, the usual testing strategies employed with younger patients have significant limitations in older adults. As with other serious diagnoses, older adults do not present with the same symptom complex as younger patients, and this causes delays in identification and subsequent treatment. In one study of older adults 90 years of age and greater, isolated dyspnea or syncope is the most likely presenting symptom in patients with an acute PE [34].

Pulmonary embolism is a continuation of the disease of venous thrombosis (VT). The incidence of VT increases with age [35]. Twenty-five to thirty-year olds have a rate of about 1/10,000 of incidence of VT per year. In the 85-year-old and older age group, the incidence of VT is 80/10,000, showing an 80-fold increase [35, 36].

Older adults with PE tend to present with different complaints compared to younger adults. A retrospective study by Timmons *et al.* looked at patients found to have PE on chest CT and evaluated their initial complaints. They divided subjects into two groups – an "older" and a "younger" group, with a cutoff of 65 years of age. Fewer older adults complain of "pleuritic" chest pain (60% vs 87%, $p < 0.02$) and pain is the primary presenting complaint in fewer older adults as well (45% vs 84%, $p < 0.002$) [37]. Of note, 25% of the older patients present with either syncope or cardiac arrest compared to only one younger patient [37]. Older adults are also more likely to have an oxygen saturation less than 90% (32% vs 5%, $p = 0.04$) and appear cyanotic (14% vs 0%, $p = 0.05$). Similar rates of abnormal vital signs, such as tachycardia, tachypnea, or hypotension, are present in both groups. In addition, similar proportions of patients in both groups complain of dyspnea and palpitations and have clinical signs of deep venous thrombosis (DVT) [37]. Although older adults are more likely to have abnormal ECGs, these are neither specific nor diagnostic of PE.

Unfortunately, there is no one test with a high enough sensitivity and specificity to allow it to be "the" test for PE. Current diagnostic algorithms use highly sensitive but poorly specific tests to screen "out" patients with PE, and then more specific tests to try to screen "in" those with the disease. The particular patient or a subpopulation tested may have limitations compared to the population in general. There are limitations in general for each of these examinations in considering the diagnosis of PE, and the limitations specific to the geriatric population may shift the practice of the physician pursuing a diagnosis in older adults [38].

Clinical evaluation

Patients in whom the diagnosis of PE are being considered are typically divided into low, intermediate, or high probability based on scoring systems or clinical gestalt. The Prospective Investigation of Pulmonary Embolism Diagnosis (PIOPED), which used clinical gestalt, finds a 9% prevalence of PE in the low probability group, 30% prevalence in the intermediate probability group, and 68% prevalence in the high probability group [39]. Wells and the original Geneva scores have been found to perform similarly in the general population [40, 41]. The Wells score does not consider age, but the Geneva score does, with 1 point for ages 60–79 years and 2 points if older than 80 years [42]. Their revised score also considers age and is more easily calculated without blood gases [42]. Of note, the PERC (Pulmonary Embolism Rule-out Criteria) rule is not used in higher risk patients and is invalid to use in patients over the age of 50 years [43].

Righini et al. compared the use of Wells and Geneva scores in younger (age <50 years) and older (age >75 years) patients [41, 44]. The Geneva score used in older patients classifies 37% with a low probability/low risk of PE, with a true prevalence of the disease being 6% in that population. The Geneva score in the younger patients identifies 73% of the population to be at low risk, with an actual prevalence of PE of 5%. The Wells score classifies 52% of the older adults as having low probability of PE, but there is a 15% prevalence of actual PE in that group. The score identifies 71% of the younger patients as being in the low probability group, with an actual prevalence of 7%. Although the scoring systems seem to have similar prevalence of patients accurately identified in the younger age group, there are significant differences between the "false negative" rate in the Wells and the Geneva scores. As this is usually a first-line "test" used to screen out those unlikely to have the disease, the rate of false negatives should be as low as possible, and missing a 15% prevalence of the disease versus missing a 6% prevalence with the Geneva score makes it worth considering the Geneva score instead of the Wells score in older patients [44].

Among older adults, there are significant limitations in using ventilation–perfusion (V/Q) lung scans as well as D-dimer blood tests. The preferred finding with V/Q scans is either high probability, which rules in the diagnosis, or normal, which rules it out. Unfortunately, there are a large percentage of "indeterminate" scans that fall between these two diagnostically helpful zones. The number (and percentage) of nondiagnostic scans increases with age. Righini et al. [45] find that the diagnostic yield of lung scans decreases from 68% in the age group less than 40 years to only 42% in the age group greater than 80 years.

D-dimers have been used early in the decision tree and are considered a highly sensitive test though fairly nonspecific test. Older adults often have more reasons to have a false positive D-dimer. Righini et al. find that a negative D-dimer is able to exclude PE as a diagnosis in two thirds of patients less than 40 years old, but in only 5% of patients 80 years and older [45]. Some suggest raising the D-dimer cutoffs for older adults, which would make the test less sensitive, but also lead to fewer false positives, though others have expressed doubt whether the trade-off in sensitivity is worth it [44, 46].

Venous compression ultrasound and helical chest CT scan have similar test characteristics among older versus younger adults. Ultrasound is noninvasive, and although it is possible that a patient can have a PE without a DVT, it is more likely that patients will have a DVT as well [47]. Advantages of ultrasound studies include no radiation, no contrast dye, and minimal discomfort during the examination. Many EPs now have the ability to do a bedside ultrasound to establish the diagnosis of DVT. If a DVT is found, then the patient with a possible PE does not need any further PE studies, and treatment can be initiated if not already started.

The advantages of chest CT scan are myriad. In addition to making the diagnosis of PE, it may identify other reasons for the patient's symptoms. A CT scan is also generally readily available around the clock to ED patients. Limitations include misdiagnosis of smaller, peripheral PEs. This may not necessarily make them less dangerous in the long term since the patient presumably has clot that is breaking off from somewhere and going to the lung, although subsegmental PEs are generally perceived as less worrisome. This is one reason that some advocate the combination of lower extremity duplex ultrasound with CT scanning. The major limitation of the CT scan in older adults often centers about the issues of contrast-induced nephropathy as many older adults have chronic kidney disease.

Physiological changes in the renal system, including a decreased number of nephrons and decreased blood flow to the glomerulus both due to factors intrinsic and extrinsic to the kidney itself, are an unavoidable fact of aging and contribute to the risk of contrast-induced nephropathy during a CT scan to evaluate for PE [48].

Creatinine is a commonly used measurement of renal function due to its convenience. Creatinine is a muscle breakdown product that is excreted through the kidney, and since older adults often have lower muscle mass, they excrete less creatinine [48]. An apparently normal creatinine in an older adult, however, does not mean that the older adult has a "normal" kidney or one that can tolerate a nephrotoxic insult. An older woman's normal creatinine means that she can filter the lower level of creatinine that her kidneys are being called upon to excrete. Although a younger patient with the same creatinine level might not be at risk from contrast-produced renal toxic drug exposure, an older adult may decompensate and develop renal injury. The risk of contrast-induced nephropathy is 14% in older patients (aged 75 years and older) in a study by Motohiro *et al.* [49].

Although not typically considered a "risk" when we embark upon using a CT scan for evaluation of possible PE, we may find other disease processes that may (or may not) explain the symptoms of the day, but may have significant implications in and of themselves. A finding that fits under this rubric is discovering a cancer that is now causing dyspnea, or is perhaps completely unrelated. It is appropriate to include this point in discussions regarding the risks and benefits of testing [50].

The mainstay of treatment for PE is anticoagulation, and the benefit generally outweighs the risks of bleeding in those without obvious contraindications.

In one study, the proportion of patients aged 90 years and older who have recurrent venous thromboembolism (VTE) despite treatment (4.9%) is similar to the proportion of patients who have bleeding complications (6.2%) after treatment with anticoagulation. The cause of death for 5.9% of patients is a fatal PE, whereas only 2.2% of patients die from fatal bleeding events [34].

Zoster

It would be unfortunate to miss the presentation of herpes zoster (shingles) in a "chest pain" patient since it can be one of the causes most easily defined on physical examination. It is a disease that affects older adults disproportionately worldwide due to their immunosenescence [51]. Pain and skin tenderness in a dermatological distribution may precede the tell-tale lesions. Occasionally, one or two lesions may be identified by looking carefully at the disrobed patient, and the diagnosis can be made. This can relieve much anxiety, especially given that other diagnoses involved in the chest pain differential can have such devastating effects. Prompt diagnosis is also important as antivirals are best started in the first 72 h of the outbreak [52].

A major concern after the acute outbreak of herpes zoster is the high incidence of postherpetic neuralgia in older adults. Early treatment with antivirals has been associated with a lower risk of progressing to this painful complication [51]. Other complications, such as herpes encephalitis or pneumonia, are much rarer [51]. Postherpetic neuralgia can be a devastating problem, with often poor control of the pain with narcotics and significant costs to the healthcare system [53]. The risk of the associated postherpetic neuralgia increases with age, and 20% of those older than 50 years of age will develop it [53, 54]. The 2008 recommendations of the advisory panel on vaccines recommend vaccination of immunocompetent adults aged 60 and above, although the need to vaccinate post outbreak in older adults is controversial [55]. In older adults, the immune system becomes senescent, and, therefore, cannot mount an adequate response to new varicella expression from the original infection of varicella, which typically occurs during childhood. The rate of recurrent herpes zoster after an outbreak in older adults is relatively low, presumably because the immune system has now had a prompting to revamp the response to the appropriate antigens [56]. Although vaccinating patients after an outbreak has been shown to be safe, it is not a suggested practice in the ED as it is probably unnecessary for most patients [56, 57].

Pericarditis

Pericarditis accounts for only 5% of all ED patients presenting with chest pain [58–60]. The underlying causes are multifactorial and can best be divided into infectious, noninfectious, neoplastic, metabolic, idiopathic, and "other" [58]. Certain etiologies should be considered more strongly in older adults simply because older adults are more likely to have an underlying disease process, such as cancer-causing neoplastic pericarditis or hypothyroidism-causing myxedema pericarditis [60, 61]. Symptoms can range from chest pain to weakness to frank syncope. Symptoms of chest pain may be worse with recumbency and improved upon sitting forward. A pericardial friction rub is often heard and is diagnostic.

The EKG also may help in diagnosis and commonly evolves through four stages. Stage 1 shows diffuse ST segment elevation (concave up) with PR segment depression. Stage 2 shows normalization of ST and PR segments. Stage 3 shows widespread T-wave inversion. Stage 4 shows normalization of the T waves [58]. If the patient presents while in phase 2 or phase 4, then the ECG will not be diagnostic for pericarditis.

The most important issue to consider in a patient with pericarditis is pericardial tamponade, which is an emergency. Bedside echocardiography or an ED performed cardiac ultrasound, which is readily available in most EDs, is invaluable in both diagnosis and treatment (via ultrasound-guided pericardiocentesis) [62].

Patients with a subacute onset, a large pericardial effusion, recent trauma, cardiac tamponade, signs of infection (fever >38°C), or immunosuppression, myopericarditis, and those on anticoagulation should all be admitted [58]. Patients at high risk for bacterial infection or development of pericardial tamponade probably should be admitted as well. Patients without these high-risk factors may safely be managed as an outpatient [58].

Myocarditis

Myocarditis is another chest pain syndrome that is the end result of a diverse group of illnesses. Causes include viral infections, autoimmune disease, bacterial infections metal poisoning, and drug reactions [63]. Approximately 32% of myocarditis patients across the age spectrum complain of chest pain, but the diagnosis should be considered in sudden unexplained cardiomyopathy and congestive heart failure [64, 65]. The typical ED studies would include an EKG, a chest radiograph, and an echocardiogram if available. The EKG might show persistent ST segment elevation and inverted T waves [66]. The chest radiograph may show a new cardiomyopathy with acute congestive heart failure, which can also be supported by findings on echocardiogram. Older adults with myocarditis generally should be admitted for further workup and management.

GERD

Healthy older adults with gastroesophageal reflux disease (GERD) have a higher percentage of impaired clearance of reflux and abnormal peristalsis compared to younger patients [67]. Pilotto et al. find that the "elderly" (70–84) and "very elderly" (85 years and older) study groups have less typical presentations of heartburn/acid reflux and pain or indigestion syndromes than the "young" [18–49] or "adult" [50–69] groups in patients with endoscopy proven erosive reflux gastritis. The older patients have comparatively more nonspecific symptoms such as dysphagia, anorexia, anemia, weight loss, or vomiting [68, 69]. The severity of esophagitis in the older patient population group is also more likely to be significantly worse [68].

Section IV: Decision-making

- Older adults with critical diagnoses often present with atypical symptoms.
- Dyspnea can be the sole complaint in older adults presenting with pneumothorax, MI/angina, PE, and myocarditis.
- It is important to appreciate the different yield in older adults compared with younger patients among the typical tests used in patients presenting with "chest pain."
- Delays in care occur in older adults with concerning frequency. The delays begin with the patient or family not recognizing the significance of what may be an atypical presentation for a serious disease.

Unfortunately, first responders, triage nurses, EPs, and inpatient providers may also not identify the seriousness of the disease, allowing further significant delay to occur.

- Older adults are often less physically resilient to the medical insults that result from these serious illnesses, as well as the treatments, especially if invasive. Risks and benefits of treatment and diagnostic strategy choices should be clearly explained to patients and families.

Simplified Wells Score

	Points
Alternative diagnosis less likely than PE	+3
Tachycardia	+1.5
Immobilization in the last 4 weeks (including surgery)	+1.5
Clinical signs of DVT	+3
Previous PE or DVT	+1.5
Malignancy	+1
Hemoptysis	+1
Clinical probability	
Low	0–1
Medium	2–6
High	7 or more

The Revised Geneva Score [42]

	Points
Previous PE or DVT	+3
Tachycardia	+1
Recent surgery or lower limb fracture (in the last 4 weeks)	+3
Malignancy	+2
Unilateral lower limb pain	+3
Hemoptysis	+2
Heart rate 75–94	+3
Heart rate 95 or higher	+5
Clinical signs of DVT	+4
Clinical probability	
Low	0–3
Intermediate	4–10
High	11 or more

The Geneva Score (Wicki)

Previous PE or DVT	+2
Tachycardia	+1
Recent surgery (last month)	+3
Age	
60–79	+1
80 or older	+2
Partial pressure of arterial CO_2	
<4.8 kPa	+2
4.8–5.19 kPa	+1
Partial pressure of arterial O_2	
<6.5 kPa	+4
6.5–7.99 kPa	+3
8–9.49 kPa	+2
9.5–10.99 kPa	+1
Atelectasis	+1
Elevated hemidiaphragm	+1
Clinical probability	
Low	0–4
Intermediate	5–8
High	More than 9

References

1 Bohrn, M., Mattu, A., and Browne, B. (2011) Chest pain, in *Cardiovascular Problems in Emergency Medicine: A Discussion-based Review* (eds S.A. Grossman, W.J. Brady, D.F. Browne *et al.*), Wiley-Blackwell.

2 Merrill, C.T., Owens, P.L., and Stocks, C. (2005) *Emergency Department Visits for Adults in Community Hospitals from Selected States.* Statistical Brief #47, Agency for Healthcare Research and Quality (AHRQ), Rockville, MD.

3 Rittger, H., Rieber, J., Breithardt, O.A. *et al.* (2011) Influence of age on pain perception in acute myocardial ischemia: a possible cause for delayed treatment in elderly patients. *Int. J. Cardiol.*, **149**, 63–67.

4 Hung, C.L., Hou, C.J., Yeh, H.I., and Chang, W.H. (2010) Atypical chest pain in the elderly: prevalence, possible mechanisms and prognosis. *Int. J. Gerontol.*, **4**, 1–8.

5 Cole, L.J., Farrell, M.J., Gibson, S.J., and Egan, G.F. (2010) Age-related differences in pain sensitivity and regional brain activity evoked by noxious pressure. *Neurobiol. Aging*, **31**, 494–503.

6 Wandner, L.D., Scipio, C.D., Hirsh, A.T. *et al.* (2012) The perception of pain in others: how gender, race, and age influence pain expectations. *J. Pain*, **13**, 220–227.

7 Rich, M.W. (2006) Epidemiology, clinical features and prognosis of acute myocardial infarction in the elderly. *Am. J. Geriatr. Cardiol.*, **15**, 7–11.

8 American Heart Association (2005) *Heart Disease and Stroke Statistics-2005 update*, American Heart Association, Dallas, TX.

9 Boucher, J.M., Racine, N., Thanh, T.H. *et al.* (2001) Age-related differences in in-hospital mortality and the use of thrombolytic therapy for acute myocardial infarction. *Can. Med. Assoc. J.*, **164**, 1285–1290.

10 Udvarhelyi, I.S., Gatsonis, C., Epstein, A.M. *et al.* (1992) Acute myocardial infarction in the medicare population: process of care and clinical outcomes. *J. Am. Med. Assoc.*, **268**, 2530–2536.

11 Maggioni, A.P., Mascri, A., Fresco, C. *et al.* (1993) Age-related increase in mortality among patients with first myocardial infarctions treated with thrombolysis. The investigators of the Gruppo Italiano por lo Studio della Sopravvivenza nell'Infarco Miocardico (GISSI-2). *N. Engl. J. Med.*, **329**, 1442–1448.

12 Lakatta, E.G. and Levy, D. (2003) Arterial and cardiac aging: major shareholders in Cardiovascular disease enterprises, Part I: aging arteries: a "set-up" for vascular disease. *Circulation*, **107**, 139–146.

13 Lakatta, E.G. and Levy, D. (2003) Arterial and cardiac aging: major shareholders in Cardiovascular disease enterprises, Part II: the aging heart in health: links to heart disease. *Circulation*, **107**, 346–354.

14 Lakatta, E.G. and Levy, D. (2003) Arterial and cardiac aging: major shareholders in Cardiovascular disease enterprises, Part III: cellular and molecular clues to heart and arterial aging. *Circulation*, **107**, 490–497.

15 Aronow, W.S. (1987) Prevalence of presenting symptoms of recognized acute myocardial infarction and of unrecognized healed myocardial infarction in elderly patients. *Am. J. Cardiol.*, **60**, 1182.

16 Rodstein, M. (1956) The characteristics of non-fatal myocardial infarction in the elderly. *Arch. Intern. Med.*, **98**, 84–90.

17 Canto, J.G., Shlipak, M.G., Rogers, W.J. *et al.* (2000) Prevalence, clinical characteristics, and mortality among patients with myocardial infarction presenting without chest pain. *J. Am. Med. Assoc.*, **283**, 3223–3229.

18 Bayer, A.J., Chadha, J.S., Farag, R.R., and Pathy, M.S. (1986) Changing presentation of myocardial infarction with increasing old age. *J. Am. Geriatr. Soc.*, **34**, 263–266.

19 Tresch, D.D., Brady, W.J., Aufderheide, T.P. *et al.* (1996) Comparison of elderly and younger patients with out-of-hospital chest pain. *Arch. Intern. Med.*, **156** (10), 1089–1093.

20 Foreman, D.E. and Rich, M.W. (1996) Management of acute myocardial infarction in the elderly. *Drugs Aging*, **8**, 358–377.

21 Thiemann, D.R., Coresh, J., Shulman, S.P. *et al.* (2000) Lack of benefit for intravenous thrombolysis in patients with myocardial infarction who are older than 75 years. *Circulation*, **101**, 2239–2246.

22 Soumerai, S.B., McLaughlin, T.J., Ross-Degnan, D. *et al.* (2002) Effectiveness of thrombolytic therapy for acute myocardial infarction in the elderly: cause for concern in the old-old. *Arch. Intern. Med.*, **162**, 561–568.

23 Hagan, P.G., Nienaber, C.A., Isselbacher, E.M. *et al.* (2000) The international registry if acute aortic dissection: new insights into an old disease. *J. Am. Med. Assoc.*, **283**, 897–903.

24 Golledge, J. and Eagle, K.A. (2008) Acute aortic dissection. *Lancet*, **372**, 55–66.

25 Clouse, W.D., Hallett, J.W. Jr.,, Schaff, H.V. *et al.* (2004) Acute aortic dissection: population-based incidence compared with degenerative aortic aneurysm rupture. *Mayo Clin. Proc.*, **79**, 176–180.

26 Meszaros, I., Meszaros, I., Morocz, J. *et al.* (2000) Epidemiology and clinicopathology of aortic dissection. *Chest*, **117**, 1271–1278.

27 Olsson, C., Thelin, S., Stahle, E. *et al.* (2006) Thoracic aortic aneurysm and dissection: increasing prevalence and improved outcomes reported in a nationwide population-based study of more than 14 000 cases from 1987 to 2002. *Circulation*, **114**, 2611–2618.

28 Mehta, R.H., O'Gara, P.T., Bossone, E. *et al.* (2002) Acute type A aortic dissection in the elderly: clinical characteristics, management, and outcomes in the current era. *J. Am. Coll. Cardiol.*, **40**, 685–692.

29 Mehta, R.H., Bossone, E., Evangelista, A. *et al.* (2004) Acute type B aortic dissection in elderly patients: clinical features, outcomes, and simple risk stratification rule. *Ann. Thorac. Surg.*, **77**, 1622–1629.

30 Howard, D.P., Banerjee, A., Fairhead, J.F. *et al.* (2013) Population-based study of incidence and outcome of acute aortic dissection and premorbid risk factor control: 10 year results from the oxford vascular study. *Circulation*, **127**, 2031–2037.

31 Leontyev, S., Borger, M.A., Legare, J.F. *et al.* (2012) Iatrogenic type A aortic dissection during cardiac procedures: early and late outcomes in 48 patients. *Eur. J. Cardiothorac. Surg.*, **41**, 641–646.

32 Shimony, A., Filion, K.B., Mottillo, S., and Eisenberg, M.J. (2011) Meta-analysis of usefulness of D-dimer to diagnose acute aortic dissection. *Am. J. Cardiol.*, **107**, 1227–1234.

33 Liston, R., McLoughlin, R., and Clinch, D. (1994) Acute pneumothorax: a comparison of elderly with younger patients. *Age Ageing*, **23**, 393–395.

34 Monreal, M. (2010) lopez-Jimenez L. Pulmonary embolism in patients over 90 years of age. *Curr. Opin. Pulm. Med.*, **16**, 432–436.

35 Engbers, M.J., Van Hylckama Vlieg, A., and Rosendaal, F.R. (2010) Venous thrombosis in the elderly: incidence, risk factors and risk groups. *J. Thromb. Haemost.*, 8, 2105–2112.

36 Naess, I.A., Christiansen, S.C., Romundstad, P. *et al.* (2007) Incidence and mortality of venous thrombosis: a population based study. *J. Thromb. Haemost.*, 5, 692–699.

37 Timmons, S., Kingston, M., Hussain, M. *et al.* (2003) Pulmonary embolism: differences in presentation between older and younger patients. *Age Ageing*, 32, 601–605.

38 Robert-Ebadi, H. and Righini, M. (2014) Diagnosis and management of pulmonary embolism in the elderly. *Eur. J. Intern. Med.*, 25, 343–349.

39 The Pioped Investigators. Value of the ventilation/perfusion scan in acute pulmonary embolism. Results of the prospective investigation of pulmonary embolism diagnosis (PIOPED). *J. Am. Med. Assoc.* 1990; 263(20):2753–2759.

40 Wicki, J., Perneger, T.V., Junod, A.F. *et al.* (2001) Assessing clinical probability of pulmonary embolism in the emergency ward: a simple score. *Arch. Inern. Med.*, 161, 92–97.

41 Righini, M., Le Gal, G., Perrier, A., and Bounameaux, H. (2004) Effect of age on the assessment of clinical probability of pulmonary embolism byprediction rules. *J. Thromb. Haemost.*, 2, 1206–1208.

42 Le Gal, G., Righini, M., Roy, P.M. *et al.* (2006) Prediction of pulmonary embolism in the emergency department: the revised Geneva score. *Ann. Intern. Med.*, 144, 165–171.

43 Hugli, O., Righini, M., Le Gal, G. *et al.* (2011) The pulmonary embolism rule-out criteria (PERC) rule does not safely exclude pulmonary embolism. *J. Thromb. Haemost.*, 9, 300–304.

44 Righini, M., Le Gal, G., Perrier, A., and Bounameaux, H. (2005) The challenge of diagnosing pulmonary embolism in elderly patients: influence of on commonly used diagnostic tests and strategies. *J. Am. Geriatr. Soc.*, 53, 1039–1045.

45 Righini, M., Goehring, C., Bounameaux, H., and Perrier, A. (2000) Effects of age on the performance of common diagnostic tests for pulmonary embolism. *Am. J. Med.*, 109, 357–361.

46 Schouten, H.J., Geersing, G.J., Koek, H.L. *et al.* (2013) Diagnostic accuracy of conventional or age adjusted D-dimer cutoff values in older patients with suspected venous thromboembolism: a systematic review and meta-analysis. *Br. Med. J.*, 346, f2492(13 pgs).

47 Murin, S., Romano, P.S., and White, R.H. (2002) Comparison of outcomes after hospitalization for deep venous thrombosis or pulmonary embolism. *Thromb. Haemost.*, 88, 407–414.

48 Wiggins, J. and Patel, S.R. (2009) Changes in kidney function, in *Hazzard's Geriatric Medicine and Gerontology*, Chapter 85, 6th edn (ed W.R. Hazzard), McGraw-Hill Medical Publishing Division.

49 Motohiro, M., Kamihata, H., Suwa, Y. *et al.* (2013) Incidence and clinical outcome of contrast-induced nephropathy in the elderly patients. *Jpn. J. Geriatr.*, 50, 227–232.

50 Hoffman, J.R. and Cooper, R. (2012) Overdiagnosis of disease: a modern epidemic. *Arch. Intern. Med.*, 172 (15), 1123–1124.

51 Schmader, K. (1999) Herpes zoster in the elderly. *Clin. Infect. Dis.*, 28, 736–739.

52 Gan, E.Y., Tian, E.A., and Tey, H.L. (2013) Management of herpes zoster and post-herpetic neuralgia. *Am. J. Clin. Dermatol.*, 14, 77–85.

53 Gauthier, A., Breuer, J., Carrington, D. *et al.* (2009) Epidemiology and cost of herpes zoster and post-herpetic neuralgia in the United Kingdom. *Epidemiol. Infect.*, 137 (1), 38–47.

54 Bowsher, D. (1999) The lifetime occurrence of herpes zoster and prevalence of postherpetic neuralgia: a retrospective survey in an elderly population. *Eur. J. Pain*, 3, 335–342.

55 Harpaz, R., Ortega-Sanchez, I.R., Seward, J.F., and Advisory Committee on Immunization Practices (ACIP) Centers for Disease Control and Prevention (CDC) (2008) Prevention of herpes zoster: recommendations of the Advisory Committee on Immunization Practices (ACIP). *MMWR Reccomm. Rep.*, 57 (RR-5), 1–30.

56 Morrison Morrison, V.A., Oxman, M.N., Levin, M.J. *et al.* (2013) Safety of Zoster vaccine in elderly adults following documented herpes zoster. *J. Infect. Dis.*, 208, 559–563.

57 Tseng, H.F., Chi, M., Marcy, S.M. *et al.* (2012) Herpes zoster vaccine and the incidence of recurrent herpes in an immunocompetent elderly population. *J. Infect. Dis.*, 206, 190–196.

58 Imazio, M. and Trinchero, R. (2007) Triage and management of acute pericarditis. *Int. J. Cardiol.*, 118, 286–294.

59 Launberg, J., Fruengaard, P., Hesse, B. *et al.* (1996) Long term risk of death, cardiac events and recurrent chest pain in patients with acute chest pain of different origin. *Cardiology*, 87, 60–66.

60 Otero, R.M. and Chandra, A. (2006) Pericarditis, in *Cardiac Emergencies*, Chapter 35 (eds W.F. Peacock and B.R. Tiffany), McGraw-Hill, New York.

61 Cuitlhuac, G.F.L., Guadalupe, A.L., and Ulises, P.Z.M. (2010) Elderly woman with massive pericardial effusion, cardiac tamponade and hypothyroidism. *J. Am. Geriatr. Soc.*, 58, 2234.

62 Seferovic, P.M., Ristic, A.D., Imanzio, M. *et al.* (2006) Management strategies in pericardial emergencies. *HERZ*, **31**, 891–900.

63 Gupta, S., Markham, D.W., Drazner, M.H., and Mammen, P.P. (2008) Fulminant myocarditis. *Nat. Clin. Pract. Cardiovasc. Med.*, **5**, 693–706.

64 Cooper, L.T. (2009) Myocarditis. *N. Engl. J. Med.*, **360**, 1526–1538.

65 Hufnagel, G., Pankuweit, S., Richter, A. *et al.* (2000) The European study of epidemiology and treatment of cardiac inflammatory diseases (ESETCID): first epidemiological results. *HERZ*, **25** (3), 279–285.

66 Chida, K., Ohkawa, S.I., and Esaki, Y. (1995) Clinicopathologic characteristics of elderly patients with persistent ST segment elevation and inverted T waves: evidence of insidious or healed myocarditis? *J. Am. Coll. Cardiol.*, **25**, 1641–1649.

67 Feriolli, E., Oliveira, R.B., Matsuda, N.M. *et al.* (1998) Aging, esophageal motility, and gastroesophageal reflux. *J. Am. Geriatr. Soc.*, **46**, 1534–1537.

68 Pilotto, A., Francesschi, M., Leandro, G. *et al.* (2006) Clinical features of reflux esophagitis in older people: a study of 840 consecutive patients. *J. Am. Geriatr. Soc.*, **54**, 1537–1542.

69 Furuta, K., Kushiyama, Y., Kawashima, K. *et al.* (2012) Comparisons of symptoms reported by elderly and non-elderly patients with GERD. *J. Gastroenterol.*, **47**, 144–149.

13 Acute cardiac disease in elder patients

Susanne DeMeester

Emergency Observation Center, Saint Joseph Mercy Hospital
Department of Emergency Medicine, University of Michigan, Ann Arbor, MI

Section I: Case presentation

A 70-year-old man complained of worsening dyspnea on exertion for 3 weeks. He stated he was unable to climb a flight of stairs without stopping to catch his breath. This was preceded by 2–3 months of fatigue while walking to the subway to get to work. He also frequently had associated exertional chest pain, which he described as pressure like and substernal without radiation. He denied nausea and diaphoresis but occasionally got dizzy. On arrival to the emergency department (ED), he was symptom free.

The patient denied prior medical problems, but also stated he hadn't seen a physician in "many years." He was an active smoker and was overweight. Vital signs included temperature 37.2°C (98.9°F), blood pressure 200/110 mm Hg, heart rate 85 beats/min, and respiratory rate 14 breaths/min. Physical examination was unrevealing, with no murmurs or gallops, clear lungs, and no peripheral edema.

Section II: Case discussion

Dr Shamai Grossman (SG): Is there any reason why you would not require an EKG on this patient?

Dr Jon Mark Hirshon (JMH): Someone who comes in at his age with his complaint constellation and particularly over this time frame, needs an EKG along with a chest X-ray study, and basic laboratory tests. I'd also make an effort to see if I could find an old EKG to compare it to.

SG: Now, if his EKG was normal, would that change your management?

JMH: No, but were there to be an abnormality, management would vary depending on the nature of the abnormality. If I see an ST elevation, I'll send him directly to the catheterization laboratory, but in general the answer is I'm going to work him up for cardiac chest pain and consider a broad differential to start with, including whether there is some other vascular reason for his presentation.

Dr Amal Mattu (AM): Some people might even suggest that the whole purpose of getting the EKG in suspected acute coronary syndrome (ACS) is really to do nothing more than to identify an ST-segment elevation myocardial infarction (STEMI). Everything else is all based on the history of the present illness (HPI), so with this HPI, he is definitely going to be worked up for an ACS, and if there is no STEMI, he will stay in the ED for the initial part of that workup.

JMH: Clearly, we are looking for a STEMI, but assuming it's not, I want to screen to see how aggressive I'm going to be. If there are EKG abnormalities, then I'm more likely to be more aggressive. In this case, unfortunately we don't have an old EKG, but we have to presume these are new changes.

Geriatric Emergencies: A Discussion-Based Review, First Edition.
Edited by Amal Mattu, Shamai A. Grossman and Peter L. Rosen.
© 2016 John Wiley & Sons, Ltd. Published 2016 by John Wiley & Sons, Ltd.

Dr Scott Wilber (SW): I think it helps with risk stratification. If you have an abnormal EKG, it pushes the patient into a higher risk category.

SG: What did the EKG show?

Dr Andrew Chang (AC): It showed downsloping ST segments with some T-wave inversions in the inferior leads and in V5, and V6, similar to a strain pattern from left ventricular hypertrophy. This was his first visit to our ED, so unfortunately there was no prior EKG to compare with.

SG: Given this EKG, what would you do next in regard to further testing in this patient?

AM: The workup is going to include getting the basic laboratory studies including a complete blood count (CBC) – largely you want to take a look at his hematocrit and see if he has demand ischemia from severe anemia. I would also want to check electrolytes and correct any significant electrolyte abnormalities as those can be associated with dysrhythmias in the setting of ACS.

SG: What if this patient had presented with just the latter part of his story, where, "I just had a couple months of fatigue while walking to the subway to get to work, and I decided it was time to see a doctor, because I don't see doctors." Where would you have gone with him at that point? Would you work him up in the same way? Would you have the same concerns? Or would you have thought about it a little differently?

AC: Does he deny chest pain in this hypothetical scenario?

SG: Yes, at this point, his only complaint is fatigue for 2–3 months while getting to the subway to get to work.

AC: I would at least do screening tests, such as labs to make sure he wasn't anemic, in renal failure, or hypoglycemic. A chest X-ray would look for congestive heart failure (CHF), cardiomegaly, and obvious lung cancer in this chronic smoker. An EKG would still be important to rule out a dysrhythmia or ischemia as a possible cause of his fatigue. In his case, the previously undiagnosed diabetes would make me more concerned that maybe he has atypical symptoms of ACS.

JMH: I think this raises another interesting question, which is the difference between ED presentation versus a primary care physician's perspective. I know that in the ED, I would aggressively work this patient up, but had the patient presented to his primary care provider, especially one who saw him on a regular basis, their workup might have been slower.

SG: Does it make a difference whether this patient was 70 years old or 35 years old?

AM: In terms of deciding whether to work this patient up for ACS, I don't think it makes much of a difference with the history that's provided here. This is a really concerning history with two factors that are provided in the history that markedly increase the risk that this patient will rule in for ACS, and that is the presence of diaphoresis with the chest pain and also the presence of exertional chest pain.

SG: If that is true, is ACS really any different in the elderly? Should we have any specific concerns for the elderly when they develop an ACS or presentations that are concerning for ACS?

AM: In terms of treating this patient, regardless of age you are probably going to head down a very similar pathway. You might need to adjust certain medication dosages based on the higher probability of renal insufficiency in an elderly patient, and there might be some greater concerns about bleeding risk. But really age is not so much of a contraindication anymore for any of the aggressive medications that we typically use in younger patients. Elderly patients need to be treated as aggressively as younger patients, and, in terms of the presentation, you need to lower your threshold for what you might consider ACS in an elderly patient because we know so many of them don't present with what you would consider a classic ischemic chest pain – although with this case, the way it's written, it really does scream ACS to you.

SG: Realizing that our patient is 70 years old, is there really any reason to try and encourage him modify his lifestyle on ED discharge? Is it really going to make him live longer?

AC: I do think modifying his lifestyle is important in order to decrease further risk of ACS or other complications, such as stent failure, in the future. One would also try to get his blood pressure and blood sugars under control, stop smoking, and hopefully have him lose some weight. Although these are more the responsibilities of the PCP or cardiologist, I still think it is important that we, as emergency physicians, take a minute to emphasize these points to him while he is in the ED.

SG: I think that the data would bear that out as well in at least every risk factor with perhaps the exception of smoking.

AC: Many of the large cardiac studies specifically exclude elderly patients, and most elderly patients have a lot of comorbidities that the 35 year old wouldn't – so you have to take that into consideration. In addition, one has to also consider the functional status of elderly patients. If the patient were nonambulatory, nonverbal, or living in a nursing home, you might not be as aggressive as somebody of the same age but who plays piano and is active with his grandchildren.

SG: I agree, there are 70 year olds who are the equivalent of 40 year olds, and there are 70 year olds who are the equivalent of 90 year olds, and care is often dependent on how functional they are. That said, there is a fair amount of data out there that looks at the physiology of atherosclerosis in the elderly, it's very clear that the older you get the more at risk you are for atherosclerosis, fibrosis of the vessels, valvular thickening, and even decreased cardiac output. That said, as emergency physicians we don't often think of pathophysiology. Instead we think of the patient presenting in front of us, and more of the story and the EKG, which prompts us to act so that it really doesn't matter so much what their prior history and risk factors were, but what their presentation is today in the ED.

SG: Can you tell us what happened next to the patient?

AC: A chest X-ray study was unremarkable, his initial creatine phosphokinase (CPK) was 89, his troponin was less than 0.01, and the rest of his blood work was unremarkable except for a blood glucose of 240. He was given 325 mg of acetylsalicylic acid (ASA), and cardiology was consulted.

SG: If this were your patient, what would be your disposition?

SW: In my institution, the disposition could be the observation unit, although with his EKG changes he may actually meet criteria for inpatient management, and so he would probably go to telemetry. I don't think any other disposition would be likely given the EKG changes.

SG: Without an old EKG, we can't really say if it's changed or not.

JMH: I would admit this patient. I might talk to cardiology, but they are a very busy unit, and without more, I would be doubtful that they would accept the patient. Still, I would try to put this patient on the cardiology service.

SG: Why put him on your cardiology service instead of drawing two sets of serial enzymes and EKGs and performing a treadmill test in your observation unit?

JMH: He's an individual without a lot of past interactions with the healthcare system, who probably has new onset diabetes, an abnormal EKG, abnormal blood pressure, and a likelihood of low compliance. So I would prefer not to put him in my observation unit but to admit him to the hospital since there is more potential for involvement within the healthcare system. Whether it's medicine or cardiology – his story is concerning enough for me that I would prefer cardiology even though his enzymes were negative- but most likely he would end up on medicine in a monitored bed.

SW: Looking at my InterQual book under ACS inpatient versus observation criteria, I realized that my ED transitional care coordinators would come to me and say that this patient does not meet inpatient criteria. Therefore, I could either put him as observation on the floor or in our clinical decision unit (CDU) in the ED, but he doesn't meet inpatient, which requires more significant EKG abnormalities or abnormal enzymes.

SG: If in fact our healthcare system is going to push us to care for this patient beyond the few hours that we regularly care for patients in the ED, we must ask what our role is in the ED in preventative care or in risk modification. When we get saddled with a patient who needs a cardiac workup, we can do so in an observation unit – if he has a positive stress test we can consult cardiology and determine if he needs a catheterization or not, but if the stress test isn't positive, we are going to have to figure out how to get this patient into the system, which is not always so simple.

SW: We have two options for observation. The more high-risk patients can go to an inpatient observation unit while the lower risk patients can go to the ED CDU. Either way I would get a cardiology consult on this patient. If the patient was in the ED observation unit (CDU), I would probably have cardiology see him prior to ordering a stress test. My guess is that given his history and EKG, our cardiologists would probably take him to have a catheterization rather than try to do a provocative test, though the decision is cardiologist dependent. He could return to the CDU if he had a normal angiogram and be discharged home from the CDU. This does put a lot of pressure on the emergency physician to get him connected. Typically, if we are discharging patients home from our CDU, they have a primary care appointment scheduled prior to leaving.

SG: I don't think a primary care appointment would have been enough for this patient. In my mind, this patient with new-onset diabetes, obesity, presumably with hyperlipidemia, as well as coronary artery disease (CAD) in some form, also needs some more impetus at least from case management to try and figure out how to get this patient to see a doctor on a regular basis and start intervening positively in his health care, which clearly he hasn't done thus far.

SG: Is there another method in your institution or some other resources that you might employ in helping take care of this patient if he didn't end up with a full admission on an inpatient service?

JMH: Our social work infrastructure and case management service has improved over the past several years so we do have resources. I think that even if the InterQual guidelines may not admit him for the cardiac purposes, in this case, I would still try to figure out a way to admit him. But if by chance he wound up in our observation unit, and let us say his stress test was negative, I would try to make sure that I either get him follow up with family practice or someone else.

One advantage you can say is that as a 70 year old he should have access to Medicare.

SG: Is there anything else in your differential or other tests you might have ordered on him before you said, "alright, well, this is clearly a cardiac case and we need to deal with it as such"?

AM: When somebody comes in with chest pain, the other killers that you want to think about include pulmonary embolism (PE), aortic dissection, and pericarditis with tamponade. But I think the way the history is, it really does point much more toward ACS than any of the alternatives. If I saw this patient, I would not do any other tests looking for PE, dissection, or tamponade. It would be easy enough of course to just do a bedside ultrasound and take a look at the chambers of his heart to make sure that there is normal left ventricular function and no right ventricular distention from a PE. The one other test that could be considered would be a formal echo, but again, I'm not sure that I would do this unless there was concern for CHF or concern for a valvular abnormality or some type of complication of ACS. I don't feel strongly that any other path of workup was really indicated.

SG: I would tend to agree. Sometimes we do miss things in the ED, but when patients come in with very clear histories I think it behooves us to care for the primary issue that his history suggests rather than looking for zebras. Should his workup turn out to be negative after he is admitted, then I think it becomes the responsibility of the inpatient staff to steer the patient in the correct direction for other etiologies of the patient's symptoms or presentation, but given that we don't think that is going to be the case, then I too would stop here.

JMH: Based on the story I would agree, but one needs to be cautious not to have diagnostic myopathy. If there is anything in the story that changes, or something happens, then it behooves us to always be aware of other potential diagnoses in the differential.

SG: What finally happened to this patient?

AC: Because of a high probability of CAD by history and his comorbidities, he preceded directly to angiography about 2 h after he arrived in the ED. The cath showed several ostial and mid-left anterior descending coronary artery (LAD) stenoses. He had two stents placed in his LAD and had balloon percutaneous coronary intervention (PCI) of his ostial left circumflex. He was discharged 2 days later on aspirin, clopidogrel, carvedilol, atorvastatin, and lisinopril and metformin. What distinguished this case is that he was chest pain free and had a negative troponin, and the cardiologist still skipped all the usual serial enzymes and stress tests, and went directly to cardiac catheterization. This doesn't happen as often as I think it should, but he was so high risk that I think the cardiologists realized that it was kind of pointless to do all those other tests.

SG: Yet, I don't believe the literature supports emergent cardiac catheterization in this patient. The literature suggests that if this patient was medically managed, he would do just as well. This reflects what we call the "Oculostenotic reflex" where you see a lesion, you open it up, because that's the way to cure someone. Cardiac catheterization isn't always the cure. Dr Mattu, would you have wanted this patient to go emergently to angiography?

AM: No, I agree with you. Although it's important to be aggressive about working up patients that have ACS, and his history is suggestive of ACS, we haven't really proved that he does have ACS, and the literature that you're referring to suggests that in the absence of true ACS, there is no significant benefit to aggressively revascularizing these patients versus aggressive medical, noninterventional therapy.

AC: What's your feeling on the use of a thrombolysis in myocardial infarction (TIMI) score on somebody like him?

SG: TIMI scores, like other scores, can have some utility, although ultimately I believe one needs to make medical decisions based on the clinical history and their own gestalt when seeing a patient. This I find more useful than using a scoring system, and that's because the scoring systems have not been shown to be more useful than our own clinical gestalt. But, if you're forced to try to risk stratify patients because your stress laboratory or catheterization laboratory will only take patients who have a TIMI score of x

or y, then obviously it would be useful. But beyond that, I don't think that in my day-to-day practice of emergency medicine, TIMI scores, or any other scores like that are particularly useful.

AC: For me, his chest pain and his story sounded like ACS, he had risk factors for ACS, and he had a good clinical story. His EKG had T-wave inversions and we didn't have an old one. I rarely use TIMI scores. However, I advocated for him to go to the cath lab, and speaking in the cardiologist's native language (i.e. TIMI is elevated at 4) helped in this particular case.

SG: Clearly, this is one of those cases where using your TIMI score got you what you thought was appropriate for the patient, and for that reason, it might be a reasonable indication. Again, it's more case dependent than that in my mind, and I would not put a hard and fast rule on it to say that we need to use TIMI scores to care for patients in the ED.

Dr Peter Rosen (PR): Obviously, were he to have more chest pain, he would go to angiography. Unfortunately, there is no way to know how long he would have prior to having an infarction. I think one has to individualize every patient, and I don't think the studies suggesting medical management equals surgical are based on a population of diabetic, obese, and no healthcare patients. It also depends on what endpoints you care about: the mortality may be equal in the two modalities of treatment, but the patient will have a lower risk for CHF, and incapacitating angina if he has reperfusion, and he might feel better enough to be motivated to take the other health steps discussed initially.

SG: We see lots of patients who come in with various risk factors, and come in with health changes that today we have the ability to modify. I was wondering what you think our role should be in the ED in preventative medicine, or in trying to initiate risk modification? This is not necessarily for this patient, but in general.

SW: This question is one that will probably be debated for as long as we have EDs. We do some public health activities that clearly we embrace, such as updating people's tetanus shots and HIV screening, but then there are other places where we tend to feel it's not really our role. In this patient a few things jump out. First, regardless of his symptoms, he is an active smoker at age 70 and many people would argue that even a brief intervention would be beneficial to help plant the seed of quitting smoking. As we know, most adults who are active smokers would actually like to quit. Sometimes, the ED might offer a teachable moment to have a patient stop smoking. For instance, his untreated hyperglycemia and his elevated blood pressure to me are clearly comorbidities that we need to be thinking about and be making at a minimum, outpatient followup. A lot of the controversy here is in regard to the difficulty in various places in getting patients established with primary care doctors or into clinics. We have places where that may be very easy and we can get a lot of help so you don't have to do as many of those things yourself. For example, I can have a transitional care coordinator arrange an appointment and get in touch with that doctor and maybe start some medicines out of the ED if he didn't need to be admitted, and then have him seen relatively quickly in the outpatient setting. In other institutions, this process may take a month or two, and that increases the rates of noncompliance. Overall I think that we need to do more than we are currently.

SG: I know that there have been studies looking at the utility of the ED in preventative care, and there clearly are initiatives that we are able to take, and the question is whether we should be taking them? Part of this falls into the rubric of what our role is as ED doctors. As physicians, we are obligated to take care of patients and to do the most we can for our patients. But if we try and intervene on each patient and do everything for each patient we wouldn't be taking care of anyone else in the ED. Sometimes, we are stuck between a rock and a hard place and for that reason I agree, I don't know that we'll ever find the right answer, or get to the right mix of where we should be in terms of initiating preventative care or focusing only on what's clear emergency management.

SG: Do you want to summarize the case for us?

AM: This was a case of a 70-year-old male who presented with a few weeks of possible anginal type of symptoms, and by the time he presented he had much more concerning and even classic type of symptoms of exertional chest pain. He was noted to have a handful of cardiac risk factors aside from his age including smoking, obesity, hypertension, and he was identified as having new diabetes in the ED. During his workup, he had an abnormal EKG, but no old EKGs were obtained for comparison. Despite negative cardiac enzymes, he was admitted and worked up aggressively and found to have significant atherosclerotic lesions for which he received a percutaneous intervention, and was discharged fortunately in good condition a couple of days later on aspirin, beta-blockers, statins, and medications for diabetes and hypertension. I think this case gave us an opportunity to discuss some atypical features of elderly patient's presentations and the importance of an aggressive workup based on HPI, and a little bit less based on a patient's age. We talked about cardiac biomarkers and EKG utility as aggressive interventional versus medical therapies in patients that have cardiac complaints.

Section III: Concepts

With life expectancies continuing to increase and with the aging of the baby boomer population, elderly patients account for more and more of the patients seen in the ED. In addition to comprising a growing patient base, these patients carry with them a unique set of special needs. Therapies require modifications due to changing physiology, and cognitive and social issues require special consideration, as they will influence a patient's response or ability to participate in or comply with treatment.

Expertise in the management of cardiac emergencies in this population is especially important because these conditions require time-sensitive identification and treatment. Due to its prevalence and associated high morbidity and mortality, this chapter focuses primarily on ischemic heart disease. Other topics to be discussed include atrial fibrillation (AF) and CHF.

Acute coronary syndrome

Background

ACS encompasses a spectrum of cardiac ischemia, which includes unstable angina (UA), non-ST segment elevation myocardial infarction (NSTEMI), and STEMI, and each will be discussed individually later. Death from cardiac ischemia is the leading cause of mortality worldwide, and disproportionately affects the geriatric population, in particular, those greater than 75 years of age especially elderly women. This group of elderly patients accounts for greater than 60% of mortality related to acute myocardial infarction (AMI) [1]. Despite these population statistics, the vast majority of clinical trials exclude elderly patients, leading to difficultly extrapolating conclusions and recommendations for their care. Less than half of all studies examining ACS even enroll patients older than 75 years of age [2]. This lack of evidence-based data for the elderly population translates into reluctance and avoidance of both pharmacologic and medical interventions. This is unfortunate because, compared with younger age groups, the elderly with ACS appear to benefit the most from treatment [1].

STEMI is defined by electrocardiogram (ECG) criteria in the setting of elevated cardiac biomarkers, whereas NSTEMI typically refers to nonspecific ECG changes with elevated cardiac biomarkers. In the case of UA, both biomarkers and ECG may not be diagnostic, nevertheless, the patient's history suggests incomplete coronary artery occlusion. Rapid PCI is the cornerstone of therapy for STEMI, whereas, NSTEMI and UA may be treated either medically or invasively, depending on risk. The elderly are much less likely to present to the ED with a STEMI, while the other two entities comprise anywhere from 60% to 90% of patients with ACS [2].

Presentation

The geriatric patient with ACS poses a great diagnostic and treatment challenge for a myriad of reasons. According to the National Registry of Myocardial Infarction (NRMI), over half of patients over the age of 85 with a discharge diagnosis of ACS lacked this as the admission diagnosis. Though chest pain is the most common symptom regardless of age, many elderly patients present without this complaint. Associated symptoms, such as diaphoresis and nausea, may also be absent. Dyspnea (49%), diaphoresis (26%), nausea (24%), and syncope (19%) without chest discomfort are common chief complaints of patients greater than 65 years of age [3]. Decreased pain perception and comorbid conditions, particularly diabetes, contribute to these less typical presentations of ACS. Unrecognized or silent myocardial infarction

occurs most commonly in the very elderly (>85 years) population, accounting for 60% of myocardial infarction in this age group [3]. Altered mental status is the primary presentation of ACS in the very elderly, and these patients often present because they are brought in by concerned family members [4]. In addition to atypical or minimal symptoms, unique psychosocial factors also contribute to delays in the diagnosis of an ACS in the elderly. Even in the setting of chest pain, it is not unusual for elderly patients to delay seeking attention for hours [5, 6]. Issues with cognitive decline, fear of presenting to the hospital, and even a patient's inability to identify their own atypical symptoms make a timely diagnosis more challenging. Unfortunately, these delays in presentation and diagnosis all contribute to an increased morbidity and mortality in the geriatric population.

Diagnosis

History

In the absence of a clear STEMI, it is the patient's history that stimulates a clinician's concern for possible ACS. In the elderly patient, often with vague and atypical symptoms, a broad differential diagnosis encompassing far more than the usual "big three" of chest pain must be considered. Casting a large net, while necessary, also adds to delays in diagnosis.

Attempts to gather a complete history may be hampered by cognitive decline, memory issues, and dementia. Therefore, one must utilize supplemental information from outside nursing facilities, emergency medical services (EMS), and family members. The evaluation of chest pain typically includes a review of past medical, family, and social history to identify cardiac risk factors. Moreover, risk factors for the elderly are different than for younger populations. Neither family and social histories nor a history of hyperlipidemia places the elderly at higher risk for an acute event. However, both diabetes and hypertension are considered major risk factors for ACS in this population [7, 4].

Electrocardiogram (ECG)

ECG is the most readily available tool for initial diagnostic testing in ACS [5]. ECG interpretation in the aging patient, as with history, also tends to carry with it significant limitations. Baseline ECG abnormalities are often present, and, unless a previous ECG is available for comparison, initial interpretation may prove difficult. Not only are the elderly less likely to present with STEMI, they often lack the associated classical ECG findings and are more likely to manifest with a new left bundle branch block (LBBB), again emphasizing the importance of obtaining old ECGs [2]. All of these factors contribute to delays in efficient diagnosis of ACS in this population.

Unclear presentations frequently lead to delays in obtaining an initial ECG. The CRUSADE Registry in 2005, which provided guidelines for the timely recognition and treatment of AMI, finds significant differences in door to ECG time in the geriatric group. Again, two particular groups, the very old and elderly women, bear the brunt of these delays, with an average of 45 min after presentation. These two subgroups of patients were also least likely to present with typical symptoms and chest pain [8].

Biomarkers

Because history and ECGs may not provide a clear diagnosis of ACS, cardiac biomarkers guide further therapy in the geriatric population. Yet this laboratory test should not be used in isolation, as elevated troponin levels may also be seen in other conditions, including renal failure, intracranial hemorrhage, PE, and severe sepsis [6]. Furthermore, biomarkers may not be elevated in the setting of UA.

Treatment of STEMI

In contrast to NSTEMI and UA treatment, the treatment of a STEMI is time sensitive, with goals for reperfusion of 90 min for PCI, and 30 min for thrombolytics when PCI is unavailable. PCI for STEMI is more beneficial than both thrombolysis and medical management in all age subgroups. Current evidence suggests that the elderly gain the greatest benefit from invasive therapy despite the comorbidities associated with advancing age [2]. The higher risk the patient, the more beneficial PCI will be over medical management. Therefore, rapid PCI is recommended over thrombolysis in the elderly as coronary revascularization results in overall fewer complications. Paradoxically, this group of patients receives invasive care only 20–40% of the time, with fewer interventions associated with the very elderly [9].

While the elderly may benefit the most from rapid reperfusion with PCI, advancing age carries with it overall higher risks of mortality and complications [10]. This is somewhat related to the expected physiologic changes associated with aging, including worsening CAD and diminished cardiac reserve and collateral flow. Elderly patients are also more likely to carry with them more comorbid conditions, especially diabetes, renal insufficiency, cerebrovascular disease, and heart failure (HF). This further complicates treatment decisions, as well as increasing morbidity and mortality [2]. Delays in presentation, and failure by both patients and providers to recognize symptoms, also contribute to higher procedure-related morbidity rates.

PCI is associated with higher rates of site-related and gastrointestinal hemorrhage, but has a lower risk of intracranial hemorrhage compared to thrombolysis. Patients undergoing PCI should be monitored for serious complications, including stroke, major bleeding, mechanical complication, and contrast nephropathy. These occur at significantly higher rates in very elderly and elderly female patients [10]. This proves to be somewhat of a therapeutic challenge as this is precisely the patient population that demonstrates the largest survival benefit with PCI versus medical management alone [11].

While PCI is preferred in all age groups, in the absence of availability, thrombolytics, compared to medical management alone, has been shown to be more beneficial in the elderly [2]. Nevertheless, compared with younger age groups, elderly patients carry higher risks of serious complications associated with this medication, including intracranial hemorrhage (1.4%), ventricular free wall rupture (17%), compared to 7.9% of patients who do not receive thrombolysis and 4.9% who undergo PCI. Exclusion criteria may significantly limit which patients can receive thrombolysis. Furthermore, provider reluctance to administer this therapy to the geriatric population results in very few patients who actually receive thrombolytics [7].

Treatment of NSTEMI and UA

While patients with STEMI are constrained by time-sensitive therapies, those suffering from UA or NSTEMI receive therapy based on two strategies. With the early invasive approach, patients receive

PCI within 48 h of presentation [9]. However, with elderly patients, ischemia-guided medical management is often preferred. In this later method, the decision to proceed with invasive intervention is based on a period of observation and monitoring of the patient's symptoms. Reasoning for this approach is multifactorial, and factors such as comorbidities, increased complication rates associated with PCI, psychosocial issues, as well as practitioner fear often result in utilization of this less invasive approach. The CRUSADE initiative finds that even in the setting of elevated troponin and diagnosis of NSTEMI, only 11.2% of patients over the age of 85 and less than 50% of patients over the age of 75 receive early invasive care [9].

However, current evidence supports that, in the absence of contraindications, early invasive intervention benefits higher risk subgroups of the elderly population with NSTEMI/UA the most. Moreover, the ACC and AHA recommend that elderly patients with high-risk features and concerning history undergo early invasive treatment over medical management alone. High-risk patients include those with recurrent angina, ischemia with low level of activity, elevated cardiac markers, ST segment depression, CHF or depressed ejection fraction (EF), and prior coronary artery bypass grafting (CABG) or PCI within the past 6 months [8, 12]. Still, these high-risk features often lead to provide apprehension with delivering more invasive and aggressive therapies, and less than half of patients over the age of 65, and only 10% over the age of 85, receive this management [9]. The ischemia-guided approach, while more popular, can be problematic given the frequency of atypical symptoms and silent ischemia in the geriatric population. Nevertheless, in the TACTICS-TIMI 18 study, a randomized control study of 2220 patients, the early invasive strategy demonstrates significant morbidity and mortality risk reductions (over 50%) compared to younger patients [13].

Pharmacotherapy

ACC/AHA guidelines regarding medication administration in ACS is the same across all age groups. Nonetheless, as seen with invasive interventions, elderly patients often do not receive the same therapy as their younger counterparts [9]. Despite support by ACC/AHA, pharmacologic therapy, even aspirin, is often withheld in the elderly again, due to apprehension and fear of adverse effects. According to the CRUSADE National Quality Improvement Initiative, which compared national guidelines across four age groups in over 56,000 patients, clopidogrel and glycoprotein IIb/IIIA inhibitors are much less likely to be used in the elderly populations [9]. Differences with aspirin and beta-blocker adherence are less profound. Paradoxical undertreatment in this high-risk population has been demonstrated in numerous other studies and registries [14].

Certainly, emergency providers need to recognize additional precautions with pharmacotherapy in the elderly. The elderly typically suffer from other comorbid conditions, such as diabetes and hypertension. These diseases mandate a separate host of medications, which may interact with new medications initiated after ACS, and can contribute to further adverse effects. Physiologic changes related to aging can lead to increased rates of adverse reactions and drug complications. Autonomic dysfunction may lead to difficulty tolerating beta-blockers and ACE inhibitors. Therefore, patients should receive education to expect common symptoms, including lightheadedness and extreme fatigue, and also anticipatory guidance to expect improvement after a few weeks. In addition to altered vascular responsiveness, diminished renal function is prevalent. The emergency physician should modify medication doses appropriately, with particular attention to the novel oral anticoagulants (NOACs). These medications also require further dose modifications in patients greater than 75 years of age and those less than 60 kg [9].

Aspirin should be given to all patients with ACS as long as no clear contraindications are present. This medication reduces the risk of myocardial infarction in all ages and offers more risk reduction with increasing age [8, 9]. Providers should also use clopidogrel in elderly patients undergoing PCI. Those with high TIMI scores appear to benefit the most and have similar, though not significant greater, reductions in 1 year cardiovascular morbidity and mortality compared to younger patients. Because of an associated high risk of bleeding, clopidogrel should be withheld in elderly patients receiving thrombolytics [2].

No clear consensus exists for the use of glycoprotein IIb/IIIa inhibitors in elderly patients. Some studies suggest benefit in certain subgroups, while others find equivocal or no improved outcomes. These medications are also associated with an increased risk of bleeding in older subgroups and patients on multiple other anticoagulants. Furthermore, there is a need for dose modification in patients with depressed creatinine clearance.

The elderly with suspected or confirmed ACS should receive unfractionated or low-molecular-weight heparin (LMWH). All patients should be evaluated for any contraindications to anticoagulation. The very old appear to be at greater risk for bleeding complications after invasive therapy, but also benefit the most from this approach [10, 11, 13]. Though weight-based dosing is employed for all ages, do not "overdose" the elderly patient. For many reasons, including altered body composition and diminished renal clearance, the elderly may have higher blood levels of heparin. Despite the cautions associated with anticoagulants, these patients do benefit from these medications, and extra consideration by the practitioner can minimize adverse effects [9, 5]. Multiple patient registries, such as global registry of acute coronary event (GRACE), find that elderly patients are less likely to receive anticoagulation with heparin, mainly due to provider concerning regarding bleeding risk [14].

Symptom control with nitrate therapy is a cornerstone of ACS therapy in all ages. In the elderly, in particular, nitrates actually decrease mortality and incidence of new HF [2]. Because of lower cardiac reserve in this population, providers should consider lower starting doses. Providers should also be vigilant for developing hypotension in patients with posterior ischemia.

Hemodynamically stable elderly patients should receive oral beta blockade within 24 h of presentation. Given the often unclear and evolving clinical picture, it is not necessary that this medication be administered in the ED. Similarly, patients suffering from myocardial infarction often benefit from ACE inhibitors, but also do not need this to be started in the ED.

Surgery

There is a growing volume of evidence supporting CABG on elderly patients despite earlier findings showing overall poor prognosis in patients greater than 70 years of age. Patients require careful selection, based on both medical and psychosocial factors, to deem them appropriate for CABG. Overall, elderly patients undergoing surgery are sicker than younger patients and have higher intra- and postoperative mortality rates [11].

A retrospective review of over 25,000 patients, with over 6000 older than the age of 70, finds that patients undergoing CABG and PCI for ischemic heart disease have improved survival rates when compared to medical management alone. Survival differences are most notable in patients greater than 80 years old with a 77.4% 4-year survival rate for the CABG group, 71.6% for PCI and 60.3% for those receiving medical therapy alone.

Prognosis

The elderly comprise a growing majority suffering from ACS and mortality increases with increasing age. This population demonstrates significantly greater mortality and morbidity rates, largely attributed to atypical presentations, comorbidities, and expected age-related diminished cardiac reserve [3]. "Frailty," advanced age, hypotension, and tachycardia all indicate poor prognosis, regardless of even initially aggressive therapy [15]. The elderly are also at high risk for complications, such as CHF, AF, heart block, cardiogenic shock, and ventricular free wall rupture following an acute event. Even so, established evidence shows that elderly patients reap the greatest benefits from early interventions.

Atrial fibrillation

Background

AF is the most common cardiac dysrhythmia in the United States, and prevalence increases with age, with 5% and 9% of the population over the ages of 65 and 80, respectively, being affected [16]. A diagnosis of AF carries with it exponentially higher mortality and morbidity rates when compared to similar populations in normal sinus rhythm. The risk of subsequent stroke is the most ominous complication, and patients may present with this diagnosis in the setting of previously undiscovered AF. While AF is typically a chronic disease with waxing and waning presence, symptomatic patients seek emergency care. A first documented episode of AF is termed first-detected AF, paroxysmal if lasting for less than 7 days, "persistent" if greater than 7 days, and permanent if greater than 1 year.

AF affects elderly to a disproportionate degree and for a variety of reasons. In the young, AF is most often associated with family history, cardiomyopathy, stimulant use, obesity, and physical activity. In contrast, cardiac disease is responsible for the majority of AF in the elderly. Major risk factors in this population include age, hypertension, CHF, and valve disorders [17]. While the etiology of most cases of AF is related to these factors, there are other potential causes, including alcohol abuse, PE, emphysema, hyperthyroidism, electrolyte abnormalities, obesity, and obstructive sleep apnea [18].

Diagnosis

As with ACS, elderly patients with AF may present with vague and nonspecific symptoms. They may complain of dizziness or fatigue, but often do not provide a history of palpitations. The dysrhythmia may, in fact, be incidentally discovered. It is not unusual for AF to secondarily reveal itself during times of stress, such as infection, trauma, or surgery [18]. Identification of AF, in addition to ACS, is yet another reason to liberally obtain ECGs in elderly patients with nonspecific symptoms. Review the ECG for evidence of ischemia, which, even if rate-related, should be identified early. If the initial ECG is unrevealing, continuous monitoring should be utilized. Laboratory testing can identify underlying etiologies of new-onset AF, such as hyperthyroidism or hypokalemia, but cardiac biomarkers have limited utility in the diagnosis of an ACS. Biomarker elevation may occur in the setting of accelerated heart rate, and may not indicate need for aggressive intervention, once rate or rhythm control has been achieved. Nonetheless, troponin elevations have been found to be an indicator of short-term morbidity in patients presenting with AF [19]. Enzyme elevations may be used, especially in patients destined for an inpatient unit, as prognostic markers for coexistent cardiovascular and cerebrovascular disease.

Imaging

Transthoracic echocardiography is recommended in all patients with AF to evaluate for structural abnormalities. However, if concern exists for intracardiac thrombus, transesophageal echo is indicated. Echocardiography is not to be performed in the ED, but transesophageal echocardiography (TEE) is particularly useful prior to cardioversion and also in the evaluation of a patient with stroke of unclear etiology [18].

Stroke and anticoagulation

By far the largest and most feared complication of AF is embolic stroke. AF carries with it a significant annual risk of stroke, which ranges from 5% overall to over 20% in octogenarians. Rates of cerebrovascular accident (CVA) are similar in both paroxysmal and permanent AF. The presence of certain comorbid conditions, such as diabetes and HF, greatly increases stroke risk in the setting of AF. Anticoagulant medications can reduce stroke risk by 60–70% [20]. Scoring systems, such as CHADS2 and, more recently, CHA2DS2-VASc, can be used to calculate stroke risk

Table 13.1 CHA2DS2-VASc scoring system.

Text	Comorbidity	Points
C	CHF	1
H	Hypertension (> 140/90 mmHg)	1
A2	Age ≥ 75	2
D	Diabetes	1
S2	Prior stroke or TIA or thromboembolism	2
V	Vascular disease (i.e., peripheral vascular disease, coronary artery disease, myocardial infarction)	1
A	Age 65–74 years	1
Sc	Sex category (female)	1

Adapted from Sankaranarayanan *et al.*

Table 13.2 CHA2DS2-VASc score and stroke rate.

0	0
1	1.3
2	2.2
3	3.2
4	4.0
5	6.7
6	9.8
7	9.6
8	6.7
9	15.2

Adapted from Nantsupawatv *et al.*

and need for anticoagulation (Tables 13.1 and 13.2). CHA2DS2-VASc places extra weight on advanced age and is useful in further identifying the truly low stroke risk patient [21, 22]. With a CHADS2 score of zero or one before initiation of anticoagulation, recompute with the CHA2DS2-VASc scale. With a CHA2DS2-VASc of zero, patients do not require anticoagulation. With a score of one, anticoagulation with warfarin or NOACs should be undertaken [22].

Just over half of elderly patients who are at very high risk for stroke are anticoagulated. The etiology of underutilization of thromboprophylaxis is myriad and includes factors such as physician practice habits, declining renal function, presence of comorbid conditions, and psychosocial factors. Fall risk is perhaps the most common reason for avoiding warfarin or NOACs. However, current evidence suggests that, even in patients at risk of falls, protective benefit against stroke outweighs risk of fall-induced intracranial hemorrhage [22]. As with scoring to calculate stroke risk, scoring systems can be utilized to calculate bleeding risk. Physician perceptions of bleeding risk can be minimized by well-established scoring systems, such as the HAS-BLED. The HAS-BLED score is simple and assigns points based on hypertension, abnormal renal/hepatic function (1–2), stroke, bleeding, labile international normalized ratios (INRs), elderly (>65), and drugs/EtOH (Tables 13.3 and 13.4). For example, patients with a score of 3 carry a 5% chance of bleeding.

Pharmacotherapy

Warfarin, with LMWH bridging, is the current cornerstone of anticoagulation and emergency practitioners will often face initiating or monitoring anticoagulant therapy. Elderly patients typically require lower doses of warfarin than the general population. These patients often experience supra-therapeutic INR

Table 13.4 Risk of spontaneous major bleeding (%/year).

HAS-BLED score	Major bleeding event (%/year)
0	0
1	0.83
2	1.88
3	5.72
4	5.61
5 or more	16.48

Adapted from Nantsupawatv *et al.*

Table 13.3 HASBLED scoring system.

H	Hypertension	1
A	Abnormal renal and liver function (1 point each)	1 or 2
S	Stroke	1
B	Bleeding (predispostion to bleeding or previous major bleed)	1
L	Labile INR (unstable, high; <60% time in the therapeutic range)	1
E	Elderly (Age ≥ 65)	1
D	Drugs (antiplatelet or NSAIDS) or alcohol	1 or 2

Adapted from Nantsupawatv *et al.*

levels, which are associated with higher risk and incidence of serious bleeding [22]. Therefore, clear education about the medication, diet, as well as reasons for immediate ED return, should be discussed with the patient and caregivers. Careful monitoring of INR as an outpatient must be emphasized to a departing ED patient as supra-therapeutic INRs are associated with an increased risk of intracranial bleeding.

Aspirin can be considered in low-risk patients who are not candidates for anticoagulation; however, it is not an equivalent substitute for warfarin [23]. The BAFTA study of patients greater than 75 years of age finds that warfarin provides a 52% reduction in risk of embolism compared to aspirin [18]. Clopidogrel monotherapy is also not protective, and, when combined with aspirin, results in a higher risk of serious bleeding without much benefit.

NOACs have recently gained great popularity as alternatives to warfarin. These medications offer the benefit of rapid onset, carry less dietary restrictions, and do not require monitoring. Bleeding risk is equivocal, if not lower than with warfarin, probably related to the issue of supra-therapeutic dosing. Unlike warfarin, there is no rapid reversal agent currently available for NOACs. Moreover, they are very expensive compared to warfarin.

The randomized evaluation of long-term anti-coagulation therapy (RE-LY) trial evaluated more than 18,000 elderly patients and finds a 34% stroke reduction in patients taking twice a day dabigatran compared to warfarin, and also a lower chance of intracranial bleeding [18]. Dabigatran is an oral direct thrombin inhibitor, without an approved reversal agent, which is cleared renally. A patient with a creatinine clearance of less 30 mg/min should not receive this medication. Other studies, such as ROCKET (for rivaroxaban) and ARISTOTLE (for apixaban), support the findings of the RE-LY trial, demonstrating reduction in thromboembolic events compared to aspirin and warfarin, as well as lower rates of intracranial hemorrhage.

Rate control

Strategies of rate versus rhythm control are therapeutic options to control symptoms and instability. Numerous trials have compared these drugs for use in elderly patients, finding improved outcomes with rate control. Patients receiving antidysrhythmic therapy demonstrate increased morbidity and mortality rates. Especially in the geriatric patients, these drugs carry a high propensity for metabolic abnormalities, bradycardia, and interactions with other medications [18]. Therefore, current guidelines recommend lenient rate control over rhythm control for the geriatric patient. Rate-control goals of less than 110–115 beats/min have replaced previous recommendations of 80 beats/min [20].

Based on current evidence, beta-blockers are considered first-line treatment of AF in the elderly, especially those with a history of heart disease or failure [18]. Beta-blockers should be avoided in patients with a significant history of reactive airway disease. Calcium channel blockers are also acceptable agents for rate control. In the cases of intolerance to these medications, digoxin can also achieve satisfactory rate control. Nevertheless, digoxin dosing and monitoring are complicated in the elderly. Adverse effects and unintentional overdoses are commonplace, especially in the setting of declining renal function.

"Unstable" patients should be treated with intravenous beta-blockers, calcium channel blockers, or digoxin. Elderly patients often require a smaller bolus (or even no bolus) of these medications before initiating the intravenous infusion. Monitor closely for developing bradycardia and associated hypotension. Stable patients may receive oral medications for rate control.

Elderly patients are more sensitive to medication side effects and may return to the ED for related evaluations. An aging electrical system contributes to blocks and bradycardias. Complaints of "dizziness" and "weakness" are common with the use of beta and calcium channel blockers, which may lead to falls. These factors require careful consideration in the anticoagulated patient. Patients starting on these medications should receive clear education regarding adverse effects, many of which are temporary.

Rhythm control

As an alternative to rate control, patients may receive pharmacologic or electrical cardioversion. Pharmacologic rate control is preferred to rhythm control in the geriatric population for several reasons.

Agents used for rhythm control are often not tolerated or dangerous for this population. Maintenance on these drugs requires frequent ECGs, as well as close monitoring of potassium and renal function. Sotalol, sometimes used in the setting of heart disease, is poorly tolerated by the elderly and also carries with it a risk of Torsades. Patients taking amiodarone require testing of thyroid and liver function, as well as regular chest X-rays. Dronedarone, which exhibits properties of all four classes of antidysrhythmics, requires regular liver panels in addition to surveillance chest X-ray studies [18].

Immediate cardioversion can be considered for unstable patients. In these cases, heparin should be started concurrently, and patients should receive postprocedural anticoagulation for at least 3 weeks. In more stable patients, it is recommended by AHA/ACC that patients receive 3 weeks of anticoagulation prior to cardioversion. Patients typically require anticoagulation for 4 weeks after cardioversion. Rate control over cardioversion is usually preferred in the elderly population, given the associated procedural complications and the temporary success of the procedure. ED cardioversion with subsequent discharge has gained popularity in recent years. This model hinges on an onset of symptoms within 48 h of presentation and often involves pretreatment with pharmacologic antidysrhythmic therapy [24]. Patients being considered for immediate cardioversion should demonstrate structurally "normal" hearts on transthoracic echo (TTE) and have no history of heart disease [24]. It is unlikely that a significant proportion of elderly patients will be considered suitable candidates for this rapid protocol. As mentioned previously, it is quite common for elderly patients to present with nonspecific and vague symptoms rather than complaining of a clear onset of palpitations. Therefore, it is difficult to identify a time of onset. Patients with underlying cardiac disease are not candidates for ED cardioversion and discharge, thus eliminating the majority of geriatric patients with this condition.

Catheter ablation

Ablation should be considered in elderly patients with symptomatic AF who have failed a trial of antidysrhythmic therapy. Most randomized control trials, thus far, have excluded elderly patients [16].

No randomized control studies exist comparing antidysrhythmic drug therapy to ablation for the treatment of AF in the elderly population [25]. Extrapolation from other patient populations, as well as optimistic findings in case series, observational and retrospective studies indicate ablation may be a reasonable option for the aging population. A prospective observation study examined 400 elderly patients with symptomatic persistent AF, who themselves chose pharmacotherapy (259) versus ablation (153), found catheter ablation to be more successful at maintaining sinus rhythm (76% vs 46% at mean 60 months). While the patients undergoing ablation report an improved quality of life, they also demonstrate a higher postprocedural stroke risk (i.e., cerebral thromboembolism). Procedure-related stroke risk is highest in patients with a previous history of transient ischemic attack (TIA) or CVA. Ideal candidates for ablation are otherwise active patients with significant impairment of function by the dysrhythmia [18]. Regardless of treatment, therapy should be symptom driven for elderly patients. Until randomized control studies are completed in this population, catheter ablation remains a therapeutic option only after pharmacology rate control proves unsuccessful.

Summary

AF is common in the elderly, who may present with or without symptoms. Once identified, treatment is required as AF carries with it significant increases in morbidity and mortality. In addition to CVA, patients with AF are more likely to develop HF and ischemic heart disease. In addition to a significant impact on the quality of life in the elderly patient, a diagnosis of AF has also been linked to accelerated cognitive decline, frailty, and dementia [21].

Lenient rate control with anticoagulation is the optimal treatment in this age group. Use the CHA2DS2-VASc and the HAS-BLED scores to develop a treatment plan that balances stroke risk with potential bleeding risk. Utilizing a comprehensive geriatric assessment is critical to providing safe and effective treatment for AF [18]. Nursing or social work typically assist in this time-intensive evaluation, which assesses patients for "frailty," ability to perform activities of daily living (ADLs), cognitive function, nutrition, mood disorders, living conditions, social isolation, and risk of falls.

Heart failure

Background

HF is, for the most part, a disease of the elderly and is the number one admission diagnosis in Medicare [26]. In patients older than 65, HF is the number one reason for 30-day readmission regardless of original admission diagnosis. Over 5 million people in the United States are affected annually, and HF is the only cardiovascular disease with increasing annual incidence [3]. With increasing age, patients are also more likely to present with acute HF in the setting of ACS, with rates increasing exponentially with increasing age [8, 9].

HF is defined by the ACC and AHA as "a complex clinical syndrome that can result from any structural or functional cardiac disorder that impairs the ability of the ventricle to fill with or eject blood." These societies, as well as ACEP, define acute HF syndrome as the "gradual or rapid deterioration in heart failure signs and symptoms resulting in a need for urgent therapy" [27].

Unlike ACS and AF, there is a large amount of literature regarding the treatment and outcomes of elderly patients with HF. However, where the literature falls short is in the ED. Most studies come from the cardiology arena, with a data starting point after inpatient admission, and are lacking the initial valuable data from the ED. Therefore, current guidelines for the ED treatment of acute HF syndrome, as defined above, are based on expert consensus from the arenas of cardiology rather than clinical trials. The staggering statistics offered in the introduction underscore the importance of nurturing further ED-based research [26].

Diagnosis

History
There is a 20% misdiagnosis rate in ED patients presenting with HF [28]. Diagnosis of acute HF syndrome begins with a careful history and physical examination. This may sometimes be more difficult in the elderly population, due to issues such as hearing loss, cognitive decline, and dementia. Involvement of the family, therefore, is often essential and may help identify issues with medication and dietary compliance. Patient and families should be questioned regarding weight gain and medication changes or missed doses. Family involvement is also a significant factor at the time of discharge and can assist with avoiding admission and readmission.

As with ACS and AF, elderly patients may have trouble identifying or clarifying reason for presentation to the ED. Dyspnea is, by far, the most common symptom [29]. Question the patient with dyspnea regarding positional component and paroxysmal nocturnal dyspnea.

Investigation into triggering factors is also an important component of the diagnostic process. The most common inciting factors include noncompliance with medications or diet, acute ischemia, and dysrhythmia (AF being a common offender). Anemia is also a common cause of exacerbation, with a 40% prevalence in the elderly HF population [3]. With increasing age, patients more often present with acute HF in the setting of ACS, and rates increase exponentially with increasing age [8, 9]. Often, it may be difficult to determine whether dysrhythmia provoked the ischemia or vice versa.

Physical

Physical examination can provide important clues into the diagnosis of AHFS. Physicians should evaluate for signs of vascular congestion, including elevated jugular venous pressure (JVP), S3, and congestion on pulmonary examination. Patients may also demonstrate hepatomegaly and increased lower extremity edema. Look for other potential cause of dyspnea, such as unilateral edema or calf tenderness for PE, or findings suggestive of pulmonary infection.

ECG

As emphasized earlier, ECG should be obtained in elderly patients presenting with vague complaints. In the setting of limited history, the ECG can be reviewed for strain patterns or an inciting dysrhythmia. Of utmost importance is the identification of acute ischemia or dysrhythmia. A normal ECG is very unlikely in the setting of AHFS and should prompt a search for other possible etiologies of dyspnea [30].

Imaging

A chest X-ray study may support the clinical diagnosis of AHFS with findings such as congestion and cardiomegaly. However, nearly 20% of radiographs may not reveal signs of congestion; this occurs most commonly in chronic HF patients, but also in the very early stages of acute decompensation [31].

Bedside ultrasound has recently gained popularity in the evaluation of patients presenting to the ED with acute dyspnea. The inferior vena cava (IVC) may be imaged as a marker of elevated filling pressures, or collapsibility. Ultrasound of the anterior chest may reveal comet tails, which supports cardiogenic pulmonary edema [32]. Bedside ultrasound can also provide insights into immediately life-threatening causes of HF, including acute mitral regurgitation (MR) or LV rupture with tamponade. It can also provide an estimate of LV function.

In the case of an unstable patient or concern exists for acute structural abnormality, cardiology should be consulted to perform bedside echo (either TTE or TEE). Such an imaging may identify or exclude other life-threatening etiologies, such as PE, tamponade, acute valvular dysfunction, LV rupture, or aortic dissection. Early involvement of the cardiac surgeon will be useful.

More advanced imaging studies, such as computerized tomography (CT), ventilation–perfusion (VQ), or MR, play a limited role in the acute evaluation, especially in unstable patients. These imaging modalities, however, may be helpful in ruling out other etiologies of dyspnea in these patients, that is, PE.

Labs

In addition to ECG and imaging, patients with AHFS will undergo laboratory studies. Electrolytes may reveal imbalances related to HF (i.e., hyponatremia) or the patients' medications (i.e., hypo- or hyperkalemia). A CBC may help identify symptomatic anemia as the etiology of patient's acute dyspnea. Cardiac biomarkers can provide insights into potential underlying ischemia and should be repeated during the patient's hospital course.

Measurement of brain natriuretic peptide (BNP) provides useful information in both the diagnosis and treatment of AHFS. BNP is generated by cardiac myocytes in response to ventricular dilatation and pressure overload. Typically, the magnitude of elevation is correlated with disease severity. Though levels increase with increasing age, BNP may still be helpful in the care of the elderly patient. The Breathing Not Properly Trial (2002) was a prospective multicenter observational study evaluating 1586 patients [26]. The study finds that a low BNP, less than 100 pg/ml, or high BNP, greater than 400 pg/ml, effectively ruled out or in the diagnosis of AHF. In addition to being highly sensitive and specific, BNP is the strongest independent predictor of CHF compared to history, physical examination, and chest X-ray study [26]. Other conditions such as renal failure, and those causing right heart strain (such as PE), and severe sepsis also elevate the BNP making a negative level more useful than a positive one. For patients with chronic HF or chronic BNP elevations, comparison to previous values may be useful. Studies show a rise of between 50% and 70% may be indicative of HF exacerbation [26].

Treatment

Current standard therapy for AHFS involves inpatient admission, and 80% of patients presenting to the ED are admitted [27]. As previously mentioned, there is little evidence and virtually no large good quality studies guiding ED treatment and disposition. What is clear, however, is that patients with HF are significantly undertreated, with a significant gap between practice and evidence [33].

Treatment of patients should begin with categorizing them into one of three groups. Those with acute ischemia require immediate identification and treatment. Particular attention should be initially given to life-threatening mechanical complications, such as acute MR and LV rupture, as these patients can quickly deteriorate into cardiogenic shock.

The remaining patients should receive treatment based on presenting blood pressure: either hypertensive or normotensive. About half of patients will demonstrate significantly elevated blood pressures. Left ventricular function is usually preserved. ED presentation is dramatic and often includes tripoding, agitation, and severe dyspnea. Patients with blood pressures over 140 mm Hg typically respond quickly to medical therapy and the therapy should focus on rapid blood pressure reduction. These patients also carry with them a better prognosis, which is a combination of several factors, including reversible cause, often preserved EF and greater cardiac reserve [34, 26].

Nitrates provide benefit with both preload and afterload reduction and are first line in the ED treatment of AHFS in the setting of hypertension. Sublingual therapy should be followed by high-dose intravenous therapy to achieve blood pressure and symptom control. Each sublingual nitroglycerin provides 400 µg of nitroglycerin; therefore, when switching to an intravenous infusion, rapid up-titration is often required [30]. Evidence supports the use of high-dose nitrate therapy in the treatment of AHFS. A prospective randomized study of 104 elderly patients finds a lower incidence of mechanical ventilation and AMI in patients with "congestive symptoms" receiving the high-dose nitrate therapy [35].

ACE inhibitors provide preload and afterload reduction and are considered second line for the reduction of blood pressure in the setting of AHFS. Patients can receive an intravenous dose and should be monitored for first-dose hypotension. This potential side effect is usually not a significant concern in patients presenting with severe hypertension and HF.

Despite lack of clear evidence, hydralazine may be employed for further blood pressure control.

Patients presenting with normal blood pressure pose a greater challenge and carry with them higher morbidity and mortality rates. In addition, about 5% of these patients will actually be hypotensive and portend an even worse prognosis. These patients usually have depressed cardiac function and reserve and are often unable to tolerate nitrate or ACE inhibitor therapy. Pharmacotherapy may involve simultaneous use of pressors and nitrates to achieve respiratory and cardiovascular stability [29]. Care of hypotensive patients should involve consultation with a cardiologist and, depending on the etiology, a cardiac surgeon.

Diuretics are often perceived as the cornerstone of therapy for AHFS. Despite a lack of evidence, their early administration is often recommended in HF task force goals. While daily diuretic therapy is well established for the outpatient treatment of HF, clinical studies give a mixed picture of the benefit of diuretics in the setting of AHFS. Loop diuretics have a delayed onset, 45–120 min, and, therefore, do not serve to stabilize the acutely decompensating patient. Patient response to diuretics also depends on underlying pathophysiology, and it is useful to again categorize patients based on blood pressure. In patients who are normo- or hypotensive, exacerbation often results from increased afterload, and not fluid overload. For these patients, diuretic therapy may actually prove deleterious in the acute phase and has been associated with higher levels of acute renal dysfunction and, subsequently, higher mortality [30, 26]. Patients with initially elevated blood pressures are typically volume overloaded and will benefit from diuresis [34]. The AHA/ACC recommends that patients receive an intravenous dose at least equal to their oral home dose [26].

Noninvasive ventilation (NIV)

In addition to aggressive pharmacotherapy, patients may require further respiratory support. While some patients may require endotracheal intubation, NIV can be considered in alert patients with significant respiratory workload. Numerous meta-analyses, retrospective studies, and anecdotal evidence support the use of NIV in high-resistance hypertensive pulmonary edema. [36]. Stronger studies, such as the 3-CPO trial, show less clear benefits [29]. This multicenter, prospective, randomized control trial evaluated 1000 patients (mean age 78) with severe pulmonary edema and found no significant differences in intubation rates or short-term mortality. However, patients did report improved symptoms and were found to have decreased heart rates, less acidosis, and decreased hypercapnia. It is important to note that patients in the 3-CPO study also received aggressive nitrate therapy. The use of NIV is supplemental to but not replacing first-line treatment with nitrate pharmacotherapy.

Other therapeutic options

In the rapidly decompensating HF patient, intra-aortic balloon pump (IABP) may provide temporary support. This therapy is most effective for those with acute ischemia and associated mechanical complications (acute MR) as a bridge to surgical intervention.

Patients with AF with a rapid ventricular response (RVR) deserve special mention, as the two entities often present together. In patients without a history of HF, the rapid rate may itself be responsible for the patient's decompensation. However, patients with a standing history of HF are predisposed to the development of AF, and rate may not be the direct cause of symptoms. Unstable patients with a rapid rate should be cardioverted, whereas pharmacotherapy can be employed for more stable patients. Digoxin may be favored over beta and calcium channel blockers in elderly patients with acute HF [29].

Disposition

As mentioned earlier, the vast majority of patients presenting to the ED with AHFS are eventually admitted [26]. Renal dysfunction, hyponatremia, ischemia on the ECG, elevated BNP, elevated troponin, and low blood pressures are all features associated with higher short- and long-term mortality [26, 32]. While high-risk features are a known entity, identification of lower risk, potentially dischargeable patients continues to pose challenges and further underlines the need for ED-based studies. Several existing decision rules have not been validated, and, while they may be useful in identification of high-risk features, they do not reliably characterize low-risk patients [31].

Several studies demonstrate the use of the ED observation unit for monitoring and treating patients who may be at lower risk [37]. However, most patients currently admitted for AHFS have over a 48-h length of stay, and, therefore, would not be an ideal observation unit candidate. The success of such use requires an integrated "HF team," comprised of emergency providers, cardiologists, nursing, and social workers. Clear communication with the primary care provider also reduces the rate of short-term readmission.

Conclusion

The elderly comprise a growing proportion of patients seen in the ED. Those patients who are suffering from cardiac emergencies have disproportionally higher complication and death rates than younger patients. Presentations of acute cardiac processes in the elderly often manifest atypically, and these patients may delay their presentation for many reasons, including failure to recognize symptoms, psychosocial factors, and apprehension regarding entry in the hospital. Thoughtful conversations regarding diagnosis, treatment options, and patient goals are required. The emergency provider must consider comorbid conditions, frailty, and cognitive state when developing a treatment plan for the patient that, ideally, involves family, nursing, and social work.

Current evidence encourages an aggressive, time-sensitive treatment approach across *all* age groups. Patients with STEMI should receive emergent PCI, whereas those with UA and NSTEMI will benefit from pharmacotherapy and early revascularization rather than the "wait-and-see" approach. In the case of AF, elderly patients benefit from rate control over rhythm control. ED cardioversion can be considered in unstable patients; however, it is not recommended for the treatment of most geriatric patients due to unclear onset of symptoms and frequency of associated underlying heart disease. Rather than relying upon their own perceptions of bleeding risk, providers should employ validated scoring to evaluate for both stroke and bleeding risk. HF has reached epidemic proportions and these patients are commonly encountered in the ED. Presenting blood pressure should guide treatment, with significant caution and concern for those who present normotensive or hypotensive.

The current standard therapy for elderly patients suffering from ACS, AF, and AHFS generally involves inpatient admission. Further ED-based research is needed to facilitate our understanding of this growing patient population and identify low-risk patients, who can be discharged home. Stronger evidence will lead to improved care for elderly patients, who require specialized attention from emergency providers.

Section IV: Decision-making

- Consider a cardiac etiology in older adults presenting to the ED with vague complaints.
- Liberal obtaining of ECGs is advised in older adults. ECGs may be especially helpful in identification of ischemia and AF.

- Early intervention with PCI, while carrying a higher risk of procedure-related complications, is associated with improved outcomes in older patients presenting with ACS.
- Rate control, with allowance for mild tachycardia and avoidance of bradycardia, is recommended for older patients presenting with AF with RVR.
- Initial decision-making in patients presenting with AHFS should be based on presenting blood pressure.
- Patients and families should be involved in decision-making with special consideration for aging-related concerns.

References

1 Berg, J., Björck, L., Dudas, K. *et al.* (2009) Symptoms of a first acute myocardial infarction in women and men. *Gend. Med.*, **6** (3), 454–462.

2 Jokhadar, M. and Wenger, N.K. (2009) Review of the treatment of acute coronary syndrome in elderly patients. *Clin. Interv. Aging*, **4**, 435–444. 1.

3 Cheng, J.W. and Nayar, M. (2009) A review of heart failure management in the elderly population. *Am. J. Geriatr. Pharmacother.*, **7** (5), 233–249.

4 Goch, A., Misiewicz, P., Rysz, J., and Banach, M. (2009) The clinical manifestation of myocardial infarction in elderly patients. *Clin. Cardiol.*, **32** (6), E46–E51.

5 Alexander, K.P., Roe, M.T., Chen, A.Y. *et al.* (2005) Evolution in cardiovascular care for elderly patients with non-ST-segment elevation acute coronary syndromes: results from the CRUSADE National Quality Improvement Initiative. *J. Am. Coll. Cardiol.*, **46** (8), 1479–1487.

6 Schrock, J.W. and Emerman, C.L. (2009) Observation unit management of acute decompensated heart failure. *Heart Fail. Clin.*, **5**, 85–100.

7 Bhatia, L.C. and Naik, R.H. (2013) Clinical profile of acute myocardial infarction in elderly patients. *J. Cardiovasc. Dis. Res.*, **4** (2), 107–111. doi: 10.1016/j.jcdr.2012.07.003

8 Goldberg, R., Goff, D., Cooper, L. *et al.* (2000) Age and sex differences in presentation of symptoms among patients with acute coronary disease: the REACT Trial. Rapid Early Action for Coronary Treatment. *Coron. Artery Dis.*, **11** (5), 399–407.

9 Alexander, K.P., Newby, L.K., Cannon, C.P. *et al.* (2007) Acute coronary care in the elderly, part I: Non-ST-segment-elevation acute coronary syndromes: a scientific statement for healthcare professionals from the American Heart Association Council on Clinical Cardiology: in collaboration with the Society of Geriatric Cardiology. *Circulation*, **115** (19), 2549–2569 (Review).

10 Oduncu, V., Erkol, A., Tanalp, A.C. *et al.* (2013) Comparison of early and late clinical outcomes in greater than or equal to 80 versus less than 80 years of age after successful primary angioplasty for ST segment elevation myocardial infarction. *Turk Kardiyol. Dern. Ars.*, **41** (4), 319–328.

11 Bach, R.G., Cannon, C.P., Weintraub, W.S. *et al.* (2004) The effect of routine, early invasive management on outcome for elderly patients with non-ST-segment elevation acute coronary syndromes. *Ann. Intern. Med.*, **141** (3), 186–195.

12 Savonitto, S., Cavallini, C., Petronio, A.S. *et al.* (2012) Early aggressive versus initially conservative treatment in elderly patients with non-ST-segment elevation acute coronary syndrome: a randomized controlled trial. *JACC Cardiovasc. Interv.*, **5** (9), 906–916.

13 Rich, M.W., Mensah, G.A., and PRICE-V Investigators (2010, Winter) Fifth pivotal research in cardiology in the elderly (PRICE-V) symposium: preventive cardiology in the elderly – executive summary. Part II: afternoon session. *Prev. Cardiol.*, **13** (1), 42–47.

14 Avezum, A., Makdisse, M., Spencer, F. *et al.* (2005) Impact of age on management and outcome of acute coronary syndrome: observations from the Global Registry of Acute Coronary Events (GRACE). *Am. Heart J.*, **149** (1), 67–73.

15 Austruy, J., El Bayomy, M., Baixas, C. *et al.* (2008) Are there specific prognostic factors for acute coronary syndrome in patients over 80 years of age? *Arch. Cardiovasc. Dis.*, **101** (7–8), 449–458.

16 Stepanyan, G. and Gerstenfeld, E.P. (2013) Atrial fibrillation ablation in octogenarians: where do we stand? *Curr. Cardiol. Rep.*, **15** (10), 406.

17 Heck, P.M., Lee, J.M., and Kistler, P.M. (2013) Atrial fibrillation in heart failure in the older population. *Heart Fail. Clin.*, **9** (4), 451–459.

18 Hanon, O., Assayag, P., Belmin, J. *et al.* (2013) Expert consensus of the French Society of Geriatrics and Gerontology and the French Society of Cardiology on the management of atrial fibrillation in elderly people. *Arch. Cardiovasc. Dis.*, **106** (5), 303–323.

19 Conti, A., Mariannini, Y., Viviani, G. *et al.* (2013) Abnormal troponin level as short-term predictor of poor outcome in acute atrial fibrillation. *Am. J. Emerg. Med.*, **31** (4), 699–704.

20 Sankaranarayanan, R., Kirkwood, G., Dibb, K., and Garratt, C.J. (2013) Comparison of atrial fibrillation in the young versus that in the elderly: a review. *Cardiol. Res. Pract.*, **2013**, 976976.

21 Yates, S.W. (2013) Novel oral anticoagulants for stroke prevention in atrial fibrillation: a focus on the older patient. *Int. J. Gen. Med.*, **6**, 167–8028.

22 Nantsupawat, T., Nugent, K., and Phrommintikul, A. (2013) Atrial fibrillation in the elderly. *Drugs Aging*, **30** (8), 593–601.

23 Graham, M.M., Ghali, W.A., Faris, P.D. *et al.* (2002) Survival after coronary revascularization in the elderly. *Circulation*, **105** (20), 2378–2384.

24 Stiell, I.G., Macle, L., and CCS Atrial Fibrillation Guidelines Committee (2011) Canadian Cardiovascular Society atrial fibrillation guidelines 2010: management of recent-onset atrial fibrillation and flutter in the emergency department. *Can. J. Cardiol.*, **27** (1), 38–46.

25 Laish-Farkash, A., Khalameizer, V., and Katz, A. (2013) Atrial fibrillation in the elderly: to ablate or not to ablate. *J. Cardiovasc. Electrophysiol.*, **24** (7), 739–741.

26 Weintraub, N., Collins, S., Pang, P. *et al.* (2010) Acute heart failure syndromes: emergency department presentation, treatment, and disposition: current approaches and future aims: a scientific statement from the AHA. *Circulation*, **122**, 1975–1996.

27 Silvers, S.M., Howell, J.M., Kosowsky, J.M. *et al.* (2007) Clinical policy: critical issues in the evaluation and management of adult patients presenting to the emergency department with acute heart failure syndromes. *Ann. Emerg. Med.*, **49** (5), 627–669.

28 Peacock, W.F. (2002) Rapid optimization: strategies for optimal care of decompensated congestive heart failure patients in the emergency department. *Rev. Card. Med.*, **3** (4), S41–S48.

29 Pang, P.S. (2011) Acute heart failure syndromes: initial management. *Emerg. Med. Clin. North Am.*, **29**, 675–688.

30 Collins, S., Storrow, A.B., Kirk, J.D. *et al.* (2008) Beyond pulmonary edema: diagnostic, risk stratification and treatment challenges of acute heart failure management in the emergency department. *Ann. Emerg. Med.*, **51** (1), 45–57.

31 Collins, S.P., Lindsell, C.J., Storrow, A.B. *et al.* (2006) Prevalence of negative chest radiography results in the emergency department patient with decompensated heart failure. *Ann. Emerg. Med.*, **47** (1), 13–18.

32 Strehlow, M. (2009) Acute heart failure: advances in diagnosis and treatment, ACEP lecture, June 10 2009.

33 Michota, F.A. Jr., and Amin, A. (2008) Bridging the gap between evidence and practice in acute decompensated heart failure management. *J. Hosp. Med.*, **3** (Suppl. 6), S7–S15.

34 Salem, R., Sibellas, F., Socrates, T. *et al.* (2010) Novelties in the early management of acute heart failure syndromes. *Swiss Med. Wkly.*, **140**, w13031, 1–7 (Early online pub).

35 Cotter, G., Metzkor, E., Kaluski, E. *et al.* (1998) Randomized trial of high-dose isosorbide dinitrate plus low-dose furosemide versus high-dose fuorsemide plus low-dose isosorbide dinitrate in severe pulmonary oedema. *Lancet*, **351**, 389–393.

36 Sacchetti, A., Ramoska, E., Moakes, M.E. *et al.* (1999) Effect of ED management on ICU use in acute pulmonary edema. *Am. J. Emerg. Med.*, **17** (6), 571–574.

37 Peacock, W.F. and Emerman, C.L. (2004) Emergency department management of patients with acute decompensated heart failure. *Heart Fail. Rev.*, **9**, 187–193.

38 Chan, P.S., Nallamothu, B.K., Krumholz, H.M. *et al.* (2013) American Heart Association Get with the Guidelines – Resuscitation Investigators. Long-term outcomes in elderly survivors of in-hospital cardiac arrest. *N. Engl. J. Med.*, **368** (11), 1019–1026.

39 Eggers, K.M., Al-Shakarchi, J., Berglund, L. *et al.* (2013) High-sensitive cardiac troponin T and its relations to cardiovascular risk factors, morbidity, and mortality in elderly men. *Am. Heart J.*, **166** (3), 541–548.

40 Bauduceau, B., Doucet, J., Le Floch, J.P., and Verny, C. (2013) Cardiovascular events and geriatric scale scores in elderly (70 years old and above) type 2 diabetic patients at inclusion in the Gerodiab cohort. *Diabetes Care*.

41 Roe, M.T., Goodman, S.G., Ohman, E.M. *et al.* (2013) Elderly patients with acute coronary syndromes managed without revascularization: insights into the safety of long-term dual antiplatelet therapy with reduced-dose prasugrel versus standard-dose clopidogrel. *Circulation*, **128** (8), 823–833 (Epub 12 July 2013).

42 Bogomolov, A.N., Kozlov, K.L., Kurochkina, O.N., and Ole-Siuk, I.B. (2013) Coronary stenting in elderly patients with acute myocardial infarction (review). *Adv. Gerontol.*, **26** (1), 151–160. Russian.

43 Bally, K.W. and Nickel, C. (2013) Acute hospital admissions among nursing home residents – benefits and potential harms. *Prax. (Bern 1994)*, **102** (16), 987–991.

44 Scherff, F., Vassalli, G., Sürder, D. *et al.* (2011) The SYNTAX score predicts early mortality risk in the elderly with acute coronary syndrome having primary PCI. *Invasive Cardiol.*, **23** (12), 505–510.

45 Saab, F.A., Steg, P.G., Avezum, A. *et al.* (2010) Can an elderly woman's heart be too strong? Increased mortality with high versus normal ejection fraction after an acute coronary syndrome. The Global Registry

of Acute Coronary Events. *Am. Heart J.*, **160** (5), 849–854.

46 Hsieh, T.H., Wang, J.D., and Tsai, L.M. (2012) Improving in-hospital mortality in elderly patients after acute coronary syndrome – a nationwide analysis of 97,220 patients in Taiwan during 2004–2008. *Int. J. Cardiol.*, **155** (1), 149–154.

47 Li, R., Yan, B.P., Dong, M. *et al.* (2012) Quality of life after percutaneous coronary intervention in the elderly with acute coronary syndrome. *Int. J. Cardiol.*, **155** (1), 90–96.

48 Bahrmann, P., Bertsch, T., Christ, M., and Sieber, C.C. (2012) Diagnosis of acute coronary syndrome in elderly patients in the emergency department. *Dtsch. Med. Wochenschr.*, **137** (5), 177–180.

49 Shanmugasundaram, M. and Alpert, J.S. (2009) Acute coronary syndrome in the elderly. *Clin. Cardiol.*, **32** (11), 608–613.

50 Yan, R.T., Yan, A.T., Tan, M. *et al.* (2006) Age-related differences in the management and outcome of patients with acute coronary syndromes. *Am. Heart J.*, **151** (2), 352–359.

51 Woon, V.C. and Lim, K.H. (2003) Acute myocardial infarction in the elderly – the differences compared with the young. *Singapore Med. J.*, **44** (8), 414–418.

52 Harpaz, D., Rozenman, Y., Behar, S. *et al.* (2007) Coronary angiography in the elderly with acute myocardial infarction. *Int. J. Cardiol.*, **116** (2), 249–256.

53 Ramos, A.M., Pellanda, L.C., Vieira, P.L. *et al.* (2012) Prognostic value of fasting glucose levels in elderly patients with acute coronary syndrome. *Arq. Bras. Cardiol.*, **98** (3), 203–210.

54 Wajnberg, A., Hwang, U., Torres, L., and Yang, S. (2012) Characteristics of frequent geriatric users of an urban emergency department. *J. Emerg. Med.*, **43** (2), 376–381.

55 Martin, A.C. and Monsegu, J. (2010) ST-elevation myocardial infarction in octogerians. *Ann. Cardiol. Angeiol. (Paris)*, **59** (6), 349–355.

56 Madsen, T.E., Bledsoe, J., and Bossart, P. (2008) Appropriately screened geriatric chest pain patients in an observation unit are not admitted at a higher rate than nongeriatric patients. *Crit. Pathw. Cardiol.*, **7** (4), 245–247.

57 Gori, T. and Parker, J.D. (2008) Nitrate-induced toxicity and preconditioning: a rationale for reconsidering the use of these drugs. *J. Am. Coll. Cardiol.*, **52** (4), 251–254.

58 Cichocka-Radwan, A. and Lelonek, M. (2014) Atrial fibrillation and prognosis in patients 80+ years old with chronic heart failure. *Aging Clin. Exp. Res.*, **26** (1), 53–60.

59 Aronow, W.S. (1995) A review of the pathophysiology, diagnosis, and treatment of aortic valve stenosis in elderly patients. *Hosp. Pract.*, **41** (4), 66–77.

60 Roig, T., Márquez, M.A., Hernández, E. *et al.* (2013) Geriatric assessment and factors associated with mortality in elderly patients with heart failure admitted to an acute geriatric unit. *Rev. Esp. Geriatr. Gerontol.*, **48**, 254–258.

61 Formiga, F., Chivite, D., Solé, A. *et al.* (2006) Functional outcomes of elderly patients after the first hospital admission for decompensated heart failure (HF). A prospective study. *Arch. Gerontol. Geriatr.*, **43** (2), 175–185.

62 Mant, J., Hobbs, F.D., Fletcher, K. *et al.* (2007) Warfarin versus aspirin for stroke prevention in an elderly community population with atrial fibrillation (the Birmingham Atrial Fibrillation Treatment of the Aged Study, BAFTA): a randomised controlled trial. *Lancet*, **370** (9586), 493–503.

63 Yiin, G.S., Howard, D.P., Paul, N.L. *et al.* (2013) Incidence, outcome and future projections of atrial fibrillation-related stroke and systemic embolism at age >=80 years: 10-year results of a population-based study. *J. Neurol. Neurosurg. Psychiatry*, **84** (11), e2.

64 Lubitz, S.A., Bauer, K.A., Benjamin, E.J. *et al.* (2013) Stroke prevention in atrial fibrillation in older adults: existing knowledge gaps and areas for innovation: a summary of an American federation for aging research seminar. *J. Am. Geriatr. Soc.*, **61** (10), 1798–1803.

65 Marcucci, M., Nobili, A., Tettamanti, M. *et al.* (2013) Joint use of cardio-embolic and bleeding risk scores in elderly patients with atrial fibrillation. *Eur. J. Intern. Med.*, **24**, 800–806.

66 Ruwald, M.H., Hansen, M.L., Lamberts, M. *et al.* (2013) Comparison of incidence, predictors, and the impact of co-morbidity and polypharmacy on the risk of recurrent syncope in patients <85 versus ≥85 years of age. *Am. J. Cardiol.*, **112**, 1610–1615.

67 Barco, S., Cheung, Y.W., Eikelboom, J.W., and Coppens, M. (2013) New oral anticoagulants in elderly patients. *Best Pract. Res. Clin. Haematol.*, **26** (2), 215–224.

68 Ganga, H.V., Nair, S.U., Puppala, V.K., and Miller, W.L. (2013) Risk of new-onset atrial fibrillation in elderly patients with the overlap syndrome: a retrospective cohort study. *J. Geriatr. Cardiol.*, **10** (2), 129–134.

69 Hess, P.L., Kim, S., Piccini, J.P. *et al.* (2013) Use of evidence-based cardiac prevention therapy among outpatients with atrial fibrillation. *Am. J. Med.*, **126** (7), 625–632. e1.

70 Ogbonna, K.C. and Clifford, K.M. (2013) Moving beyond warfarin-are we ready? A Review of the efficacy and safety of novel anticoagulant agents

compared to warfarin for the management of atrial fibrillation in older adults. *J. Gerontol. Nurs.*, **39** (7), 8–17.

71 Chiong, J.R. and Cheung, R.J. (2013) Long-term anticoagulation in the extreme elderly with the newer antithrombotics: safe or sorry? *Korean Circ. J.*, **43** (5), 287–292.

72 Forman, D.E. and Goyette, R.E. (2014) Oral anticoagulation therapy for elderly patients with atrial fibrillation: utility of bleeding risk covariates to better understand and moderate risks. *Clin. Appl. Thromb. Hemost.*, **20** (1), 5–15.

73 Poulin, F., Khairy, P., Roy, D. *et al.* (2013) Atrial fibrillation and congestive heart failure trial investigators. Atrial fibrillation and congestive heart failure: a cost analysis of rhythm-control vs rate-control strategies. *Can. J. Cardiol.*, **29** (10), 1256–1262.

74 Kennedy, R. and Oral, H. (2013) Catheter ablation of atrial fibrillation in the elderly: does the benefit outweigh the risk? *Expert Rev. Cardiovasc. Ther.*, **11** (6), 697–704.

75 Thacker, E.L., McKnight, B., Psaty, B.M. *et al.* (2013) Atrial fibrillation and cognitive decline: a longitudinal cohort study. *Neurology*, **81** (2), 119–125.

76 Polidoro, A., Stefanelli, F., Ciacciarelli, M. *et al.* (2013) Frailty in patients affected by atrial fibrillation. *Arch. Gerontol. Geriatr.*, **57** (3), 325–327.

77 Ertas, F., Oylumlu, M., Akil, M.A. *et al.* (2013) Non-valvular atrial fibrillation in the elderly; preliminary results from the National AFTER (Atrial Fibrillation in Turkey: Epidemiologic Registry) Study. *Eur. Rev. Med. Pharmacol. Sci.*, **17** (8), 1012–1016.

78 Ruiz Ortiz, M., Ogayar, C., Romo, E. *et al.* (2013) Long-term survival in elderly patients with stable coronary disease. *Eur. J. Clin. Invest.*, **43** (8), 774–782.

79 Zhang, Y., Protogerou, A.D., Iaria, P. *et al.* (2013) Prognosis in the hospitalized very elderly: the PROTEGER study. *Int. J. Cardiol.*, **168** (3), 2714–2719.

80 Blandino, A., Toso, E., Scaglione, M. *et al.* (2013) Long-term efficacy and safety of two different rhythm control strategies in elderly patients with symptomatic persistent atrial fibrillation. *J. Cardiovasc. Electrophysiol.*, **24** (7), 731–738.

81 Harrington, A.R., Armstrong, E.P., Nolan, P.E. Jr., and Malone, D.C. (2013) Cost-effectiveness of apixaban, dabigatran, rivaroxaban, and warfarin for stroke prevention in atrial fibrillation. *Stroke*, **44** (6), 1676–1681.

82 Atzema, C.L., Austin, P.C., Chong, A.S., and Dorian, P. (2013) Factors associated with 90-day death after emergency department discharge for atrial fibrillation. *Ann. Emerg. Med.*, **61** (5), 539–548. e1.

83 Frewen, J., Finucane, C., Cronin, H. *et al.* (2013) Factors that influence awareness and treatment of atrial fibrillation in older adults. *Q. J. Med.*, **106** (5), 415–424.

84 Arowolaju, A. II, and Gillum, R.F. (2013) A new decline in hospitalization with atrial fibrillation among the elderly. *Am. J. Med.*, **126** (5), 455–457.

85 Deedwania, P.C. (2013) New oral anticoagulants in elderly patients with atrial fibrillation. *Am. J. Med.*, **126** (4), 289–296.

86 Hsiao, J., Motta, M., and Wyer, P. (2012) Validating the acute heart failure index for patients presenting to the emergency department with decompensated heart failure. *Emerg. Med. J.*, **29** (12), E5.

87 Matsuo, S., Yamane, T., Hioki, M. *et al.* (2010) Acute progression of congestive heart failure during paroxysmal supraventricular tachycardia in a patient without structural heart disease. *J. Cardiol. Cases*, **1** (3), e133–e136.

88 O'Donnell, S., McKee, G., O'Brien, F. *et al.* (2012) Gendered symptom presentation in acute coronary syndrome: a cross sectional analysis. *Int. J. Nurs. Stud.*, **49**, 1325–1332.

89 Michota, F.A. Jr., and Amin, A. (2008) Bridging the gap between evidence and practice in acute decompensated heart failure management. *J. Hosp. Med.*, **3** (6), S7–S18.

90 Rogers, R. (2009) Managing complication of acute myocardial infarction and acute heart failure: advances in diagnosis and treatment. Lectures from Boston Scientific Assembly.

91 Tresch, D.D. (1996) Signs and symptoms of heart failure in elderly patients. *Am. J. Geriatr. Cardiol.*, **5** (1), 27–33.

92 Phang, R. and Olshanksy, B. (2013) Management of New Onset Atrial Fibrillation, Uptodate.com. November 2013.

93 Gregoratos, G. (2001) Clinical manifestations of acute myocardial infarction in older patients. *Am. J. Geriatr. Cardiol.*, **10** (6), 345–347. Review.

94 Kelly, B.S. (2007) Evaluation of the elderly patient with acute chest pain. *Clin. Geriatr. Med.*, **23** (2), 327–349, vi. Review.

95 Rich, M.W. (2006) Epidemiology, clinical features, and prognosis of acute myocardial infarction in the elderly. *Am. J. Geriatr. Cardiol.*, **15** (1), 7–11; quiz 12. Review.

96 Albarran, J.W., Clarke, B.A., and Crawford, J. (2007) "It was not chest pain really, I can't explain it!" An exploratory study on the nature of symptoms experienced by women during their myocardial infarction. *J. Clin. Nurs.*, **16** (7), 1292–1301.

97 Zimetbaum, P.J., Josephson, M.E., McDonald, M.J. *et al.* (2000) Incidence and predictors of myocardial

infarction among patients with atrial fibrillation. *J. Am. Coll. Cardiol.*, **36** (4), 1223–1227.

98 Alpert, J.S. (2010) Managing myocardial infarction in the elderly: what should the clinician do? *Am. J. Med.*, **123** (11), 969–970.

99 Humphries, K.H., Izadnegahdar, M., and Mackay, M.H. (2012) Sex differences in presentation of myocardial infarction. *J. Am. Med. Assoc.*, **307** (23), 2486–2487; author reply 2487.

100 Løvlien, M., Johansson, I., Hole, T., and Schei, B. (2009) Early warning signs of an acute myocardial infarction and their influence on symptoms during the acute phase, with comparisons by gender. *Gend. Med.*, **6** (3), 444.

101 Rich, M.W., Mensah, G.A., and PRICE-V Investigators (2009, Fall) Fifth pivotal research in cardiology in the elderly (PRICE-V) symposium: preventive cardiology in the elderly-executive summary. Part I: morning session. *Prev. Cardiol.*, **12** (4), 198–204.

102 Pfisterer, M., Buser, P., Osswald, S. *et al.* (2003) Outcome of elderly patients with chronic symptomatic coronary artery disease with an invasive vs optimized medical treatment strategy: one-year results of the randomized TIME trial. *J. Am. Med. Assoc.*, **289** (9), 1117–1123.

103 Anderson, J.L., Halperin, J.L., Albert, N.M. *et al.* (2013) Management of patients with atrial fibrillation (compilation of 2006 ACCF/AHA/ESC and 2011 ACCF/AHA/HRS recommendations): a report of the American College of Cardiology/American Heart Association Task Force on practice guidelines. *Circulation*, **127**, 1916–1926.

Syncope in Geriatrics

14

Timothy C Peck, Nissa J Ali & Shamai A Grossman

Department of Emergency Medicine, Harvard Medical School, Beth Israel Deaconess Medical Center, Harvard Affiliated Emergency Medicine Residency, Boston, MA, USA

Section I: Case presentation

A 76-year-old man was brought to the emergency department (ED) from a restaurant after he fainted while dining with his family. He initially complained of nausea, and then when he stood up to go to the restroom, immediately fell backward and was helped to a chair. His son stated that he was unconscious for approximately 1 min, following which he recovered completely. He denied any palpitations before the event.

The past medical history was notable for hypertension, hyperlipidemia, and depression. Three years ago, he was briefly admitted to a hospital for chest pain but was told that he did not have a heart problem. His medications were lisinopril, simvastatin, and fluoxetine.

On arrival at the ED, he stated that he felt like his usual self with no symptoms to report; blood pressure was 127/63 mm Hg, heart rate 78 beats/min, and respiratory rate 14 breaths/min. The physical examination was unremarkable. One liter of intravenous fluids was administered, and he felt even better. Laboratory evaluations including hematocrit and troponin were unremarkable.

Section II: Case discussion

Dr Peter Rosen (PR): Can you give us some generic geriatric principles in syncope that perhaps differ from a younger patient? Are there specific features that we need to be aware of unusual diseases that we should be thinking of that might point us in a different direction then had our patient been a 25 year old?

Dr Amal Mattu (AM): There are a couple of disease processes that I would be more concerned about in an elderly patient, especially with this patient's past medical history. I would worry more about cardiac problems, in particular, dysrhythmias, and I would be more concerned about the potential for medication side effects or interactions than I would be in a young person. I might also be more concerned about an abdominal aortic aneurysm and aortic dissection, so I'd focus my history and examination, asking more questions pertaining to those things. Nevertheless, if there is nothing in the history and physical examination, that makes me concerned about any of these disease processes, I wouldn't necessarily do a significantly different workup than I would in a younger person. The workup really starts after the history and physical examination. This workup starts with an electrocardiogram (EKG), yet there are really no other mandatory tests that are automatic, unless the history or physical examination suggests them.

PR: Dr Grossman, you've taught us that syncope is a dangerous diagnosis, when there is a potential cardiac component. How often is there a potential neurologic component, without neurologic symptoms or signs?

Dr Shamai Grossman (SG): Neurologic etiologies of syncope without concomitant neurologic symptoms suggestive of a neurologic cause are exceedingly rare. Nevertheless, syncope is often a symptom that makes people very worried and concerned, especially

Geriatric Emergencies: A Discussion-Based Review, First Edition.
Edited by Amal Mattu, Shamai A. Grossman and Peter L. Rosen.
© 2016 John Wiley & Sons, Ltd. Published 2016 by John Wiley & Sons, Ltd.

in the elderly. People perceive that it's a near-death experience, yet most etiologies of syncope, even in the elderly, are benign. Echoing Dr Mattu's comments, the most important concern here is obtaining an adequate history and looking at elements of the past medical history, to be able to assess the patient's risks of an adverse outcome with this episode of syncope. We have previously shown that a patient who is otherwise healthy, despite being 76-year-old, and has no risk factors for a cardiac event is at no greater risk than any other population for adverse outcome following a syncopal event, despite their age [1].

PR: In the absence of symptoms, we don't have to be quite as worried about a syncopal episode. Nevertheless, when we are discussing geriatric physiology, blood pressure is often confusing. This patient had a history of hypertension, but his blood pressure was normal, and he just had a syncopal episode. Would that be of concern to you?

Dr Maura Kennedy (MK): The absence of symptoms can be a little misleading in the geriatric population because they are less likely to have the prodrome of nausea, flushing and sweating that you expect with a vasovagal or neurocardiogenic mechanism. Sometimes, they can present with none of those symptoms, even though more benign etiologies are the cause of their syncope. Approximately 8% of all syncope in geriatric populations is from orthostatic hypotension [2]. Although we routinely do EKGs for our patients with syncope, we don't routinely test orthostatic blood pressure for a number of reasons, including difficulty in interpreting them. I would say a blood pressure of 127/63 mm Hg in a patient with a history of hypertension might actually be hypotensive for him. I would want to check past medical records, if that's available, and see what his baseline blood pressures are, and see if this is low for him when compliant with his medications. As he takes an angiotensin converting enzyme inhibitor, he is at increased risk for orthostatic hypotension. Standing up and then having syncope again suggests that orthostasis might be a contributor to his syncopal episode.

PR: We have a patient who is eating dinner, but we must still be worried about aortic aneurysm as a cause of syncope. He is an elderly man who seems to be in good health until he eats dinner and then he passes out. What about other vascular problems such as superior mesenteric steal syndrome? How far would you pursue your investigation of a vascular cause from the abdomen in a patient like this?

Dr Vaishal Tolia (VT): Vascular causes of syncope in this age group do need to be evaluated further as they are a higher risk population. The determination of how aggressively to pursue a less common diagnosis needs to be based on the presenting history, as well as the medication history, and any sort of prior events that this person has had. When the elderly have mesenteric steal, abdominal aneurysm or pulmonary embolism, and present with syncope, they do not necessarily present with the typical pain or shortness of breath that we see in other age groups. Therefore, it is critical to obtain a good history from these people and history from bystanders or family members, as well as a medication history. Then, based on your concerns and the clinical history, you can do risk stratification and potentially imaging looking for signs of structural heart disease or dysrhythmic cause. As most of the causes will be benign, we can't do advanced imaging on all elderly people who have syncope, but after risk stratification, if there is a high clinical suggestion of a specific disease, one needs to pursue these diagnoses further.

PR: We seem to have zeroed in on the cardiac potential causes for this particular patient. Yet, we have a blood pressure that is probably in the hypotensive range for this patient. We mentioned that one of the major problems is drug interaction and that certainly is a possible cause of hypotension and syncope. But another possibility is sepsis. Sepsis certainly can produce syncope and certainly can produce low blood pressure. How far would you try to track sepsis in a patient like this?

AM: In a patient like this, where I don't have a clear-cut diagnosis from the history and physical examination, as is often the case, we would routinely screen the patient with a urinalysis and probably a chest X-ray study. If there is nothing on the history or physical examination to make us suspect sepsis and urinalysis and chest X-ray study are normal, I would not pursue sepsis any further. For example, I would not routinely check lactate, send off blood cultures or urine cultures in this type of patient unless there were elements in the history, physical examination and in those basic laboratory studies that made me suspicious for infection.

PR: I agree with Dr Mattu. Routine cultures will not help in the evaluation of this patient, or at least not until later in the patient's course. What about the hypotension? Should this be an indication for drawing a lactate as we would anytime we are screening a potentially septic patient?

MK: I think that I would take it in context of the history. If he had no symptoms suggestive of an infection, no fever, or hypothermia, I would not send a lactate. I think that a lactate might be a little difficult to interpret in this scenario. Certainly, if I was concerned about mesenteric ischemia or sepsis, then I would be inclined to send it. But in our patient's situation, where he was eating, had no abdominal pain, had a prodrome of nausea, then had syncope while standing, and had a history and physical examination that didn't point toward an infectious etiology, I would not have sent a lactate.

PR: What would you do to eliminate the drug agents as a cause of the syncope? I believe he's on a beta-blocker, which when accompanied by a change in positions acutely is a well-known cause of syncope.

VT: It would be useful to know what the patient's prior vital signs were either at home or in clinic settings. Is this a patient who is recurrently coming in to the ED because of syncope, or has he been on these medications for a long time? Have any of these medications been recently titrated? That would make me more concerned for a medication-related event. If I had an electronic medical record (EMR) where I could look at the vital signs for recent clinic visits over the last several months, where the person's blood pressure was higher, that is, 140–150 mm Hg perhaps, then I would be more concerned about a medication-related event.

PR: We seem to have gone down the pathway of ischemic coronary syndrome in this man. Do you think that this man should have a cardiac echocardiogram? We haven't heard anything worrisome about his valves, but it's not always possible to hear a murmur. Dr Tolia suggested that pulmonary embolus is a possibility in a patient like this, but we really haven't done anything to investigate this. We immediately started taking care of him as if he were having chest pain or dysrhythmia. Could you comment on what else we should be doing?

SG: There are no gold standards for testing in syncope. Each test that we do has a yield that is truly very small. At best, an EKG will give you a diagnosis 5% of the time [2]. At best, any laboratory test will give you a diagnosis 2% of the time. An echocardiogram, out of all the other cardiac testing we might do, may be more likely to give you an etiology; still, its sensitivity ranges between 2% and 22% [3, 4]. The real answer here, given the limitations of testing in finding a diagnosis, is it needs to be tailored to your clinical suspicion. Although we are not very good at hearing murmurs in the ED, if we do hear a murmur in that patient, then that patient would warrant an echocardiogram. If one can hear a murmur in noisy environments like the ED, then it's loud enough that it might be significant. If you don't hear a murmur, then my practice is to not routinely get an echocardiogram on these patients. We have some data that bears this out as well. It suggests that patients who don't have a history of a murmur or an audible murmur on examination in the ED are very unlikely to have a valvular etiology of their syncopal event [5].

PR: Would you consider doing a D-dimer on these patients since we're not going to get an echocardiogram, but we were properly concerned about a possible pulmonary embolus?

Dr Scott Wilber (SW): The problem with a D-dimer in someone this age is that the specificity for D-dimer, which is already low, becomes even lower as we age [6]. Once we get to be about 80, the D-dimer is routinely positive [7]. Since we don't have a clear breakdown of normal D-dimers by age, I would assume that it would be positive. Then you have to make decision, are you automatically going to go forward with advanced imaging for pulmonary embolism? As with many other diagnoses, I think that the key here is a good history and physical examination. In the absence of any other evidence for pulmonary embolism, I would not pursue this diagnosis.

PR: No one seems to think that this person has an abdominal problem. Yet a rectal examination was not done on this patient. Would you think that one was indicated before excluding an abdominal cause?

MK: I think that in a patient with syncope, a rectal examination can be informative, particularly if you see melena. Trace hemoccult positive stools would not necessarily be informative and with a normal hematocrit and hemoglobin, I would be reassured. With a geriatric population, they are often mildly anemic at baseline. So if the patient were anemic, I think that a rectal examination would be warranted. It is, after all, an inexpensive test. But with a normal hemoglobin and hematocrit, unless we find significant dehydration, which could cause hemoconcentration, it may be more difficult to interpret than informative.

PR: From what we've been told, this patient has had an ischemic coronary workup that was negative. He was admitted to an observation unit (obs unit), and that is a useful thing to have for geriatric patients. What would you do, if you were working in an ED that didn't have an obs unit?

SG: When we tried to discern which patients actually needed admission for syncope, we tried to be blinded to age. We said age in itself should not be an independent risk factor for syncope. If you're 76 year old, you're otherwise healthy, don't have cardiac risk factors, and you've had a normal evaluation in the ED, then your likelihood of having an adverse outcome should be very small. Our data confirms that this is true [1]. Regardless of age, these patients do very well at 30 day follow-up. Given that, if this patient's workup in the ED was completely negative, I would probably allow this patient go home with follow-up with his physician, avoiding an admission and even avoiding an observation stay.

PR: Is there anything else that you would want to do as part of your workup on this patient?

SW: I think that we have touched on all the important things, and I would emphasize the point that the physical examination and the history are the most important parts of the syncope workup. A thorough examination including some often overlooked parts, such as a rectal examination, is imperative. When considering sepsis, remember to look at all of the patient's skin areas as well as skin infections can also be a source of sepsis. They can be missed easily if we don't take the socks off or fully undress the patient.

PR: Even in the absence of neurologic findings, carotid insufficiency is also a cause of syncope and it's well worth putting your stethoscope on both carotid arteries and vertebral arteries to see if you can hear a bruit. Any patient who has had a syncopal episode, in whom you hear a bruit, requires investigation.

PR: Could you tell us what evolved with this patient?

AM: The patient was admitted to ED observation, where he was given more intravenous fluids and antiemetics. Due to his advanced age, his care team obtained three serial negative cardiac enzymes and EKGs; he was placed on telemetry monitoring and had a transthoracic echocardiogram that was unrevealing aside from mild aortic valve sclerosis. He felt better after about 16 h, tolerated a meal and an ambulation trial. He was diagnosed with a vasovagal syncope (preceded by nausea after the meal) or orthostatic syncope (event preceded by standing). He had no history or signs of structural heart disease. An outpatient stress test was arranged with his primary care physician (PCP) as there was concern that he had no recent ischemic evaluation. No neuroimaging was done as his neuroexamination was normal throughout his stay.

PR: I think in many EDs, this patient would not have gotten as complete a cardiac workup, and probably would have gotten sent home, as the EKG and septic workup were negative. Would you have handled it any differently?

SW: I think the key here is that a patient in this age group needs a period of time of observation with cardiac monitoring. Now whether that could be done in ED observation or inpatient observation probably depends on the hospital. But because of the risk of dysrhythmic syncope in this age group, I think that observation on telemetry is important.

PR: I think that's an interesting observation; these patients deserve a period of watching, yet, we're not very good at this in emergency medicine. Whether they are old or young it doesn't hurt us to have a period of observation in virtually all patients. Today, most of our EDs automatically provide observation because we're not very efficient at getting patients out of the department quickly.

PR: We seem to all share an underlying anxiety about geriatric syncope, and we are surprised when we don't find a serious cause, and we don't feel totally comfortable about letting the patient go as a syncopal episode that was vasovagal. Do you think that there is anything we need to do sociologically with these patients that would make us reassured? For example, I try to make sure that the older person is not living alone after a syncopal episode. If he or she is, I look to a family member to stay with them for a day or two.

AM: Our angst about discharging the geriatric patient largely relates to the fact that most of what we've learned in medicine is based on younger patients. Most of the textbooks were based on studies, where elderly patients were excluded from these studies. We know that elderly patients don't necessarily follow the rules that we've been taught in many aspects of medicine. Thus, just because of our ignorance about the appropriate care of the elderly, we tend to be very conservative. A great example is a computed tomography (CT) scan of the head. Up until 5 years ago, I think it was routine that any elderly patient who came into our department with syncope would automatically get a CT scan of the head. That wasn't because we had any bad experiences, but just because we didn't trust the fact that a normal neurologic examination portends a good brain prognosis. There are now some good studies that have come out on the elderly patient saying that if a patient has syncope, wakes up, and has a normal neurologic examination, a CT scan has an extremely low yield [8, 9]. What would be most helpful in getting over our unnecessary angst would be to get some more good studies published. I think if we can get more studies published that show that a negative simple ED workup on an elderly patient portends a very good prognosis, we'll all start feeling better about doing just a simple workup and then discharging these patients home, rather than routinely admitting every elderly patient with syncope.

SG: As mentioned, the workup of syncope, again, needs to be tailored to the patient's presentation. For instance, Dr Mattu mentioned the utility of CT scan; the patients who ultimately will be found to have abnormal CT scans in syncope are those who present with abnormal neurologic findings or those who have some persistent neurologic symptoms such as headaches or patients who are anticoagulated [9]. Outside of these populations, the benefit of head CT scan has been found to be nil. Similarly, the utility of cardiac enzymes specifically in elderly populations has been studied and found to be useful only in those patients who present with syncope and concomitant cardiac symptoms such as chest discomfort or dyspnea [10]. Those patients who have a normal EKG, in whom you can elicit a complete history, and have no associated symptoms that are concerning for cardiac ischemia beyond their syncopal event are not having a myocardial infarction with syncope. There is growing literature that also suggests that use of echocardiography, telemetry, and ambulatory monitoring also need to be tailored to the population based on presenting complaint, past medical history, physical examination, and ED EKG. I think the workup in this case was largely extraneous and not evidence based.

PR: Assuming we've done everything that was indicated for the patient, how would you arrange follow-up for this patient?

MK: I think it's important to make sure he has close follow-up with his PCP. If feasible, it would be useful to have that follow-up scheduled before he departs, or have some sort of communication with his PCP, though that is often challenging in the emergency setting. I think we need to recognize that syncope is a risk factor for falls, and falls can result in serious morbidity and mortality in the geriatric population. Even though the workup in this example was consistent with a non-dangerous cause of the patient's syncope, the syncope alone puts him at an increased risk of falls. Falls in geriatric patients can cause serious complications or a decrease in the patient's independence. Therefore, when feasible, it is useful to arrange follow-up with the PCP. This is especially true in this patient who takes lisinopril, which may be contributing to his hypotension, and he may need the PCP to make adjustments in his medication. At a minimum, we need to make sure that the patient is instructed to follow up within a few days. Moreover, one needs to make sure that the patient understands the recommendations or that a family member is present and understands the recommendations. We often don't screen for cognitive impairment in the ED, and if there is cognitive impairment, it can affect the understanding of the discharge instructions and may affect long-term outcome.

PR: How far out from the ED visit can we stop worrying about that particular episode?

AM: First, we must make sure that these patients have social support when they go home. Do they have good caretakers or family members who are going to take care of them? We must be careful to explain how long they have to be observed or accompanied by family members. Nevertheless, I don't really have a good sense of the appropriate length of time. I would just be picking an arbitrary number if I said 1 week or 72 h. If we had studies saying the 1 week risk of adverse outcomes is low, then maybe we can call it 1 week or 72 h.

SG: I agree that as far as what to do with syncopal patents when they go home and how far you need to worry, those questions are not completely answered. I applaud efforts, like Dr Rosen's, at making sure they have someone at home with them when they get discharged at least for the first night, because they often had a fall with their syncopal event, and that certainly could happen again. There is clearly an area for study here in how long after the current episode do you need to worry about these patients. When we studied the elderly, we looked at 30-day adverse outcomes, which is generally the length of outcomes for most studies from the ED. The assumption is that if you're okay 30 days later, it's not our problem. But that's not necessarily the right time cutoff.

PR: Dr Grossman, do you have any special recommendations concerning this patient?

SG: Another issue we often gloss over, but shouldn't, is driving after a syncopal event. These patients, if they do have another episode of syncope while driving, could potentially do much damage to themselves or other people on the road. Although this is somewhat arbitrary and not data driven, we routinely tell postsyncope patients and family not to drive at least for a week, until the patient follows up with a PCP.

PR: Do you have any summarizing thoughts for us in regard to this?

MK: I think it's reassuring that the vast majority of the causes of syncope in the elderly are not serious. However, the potential for injury related to syncope is significant. In the geriatric population, given increased risk of ischemic cardiac disease, we have to be much more concerned about cardiac etiologies as well as other illnesses contributing to a syncopal event, and the key is a good history and physical examination and a workup that is guided by the history and physical examination. With a history that is very suggestive of vasovagal or orthostatic etiologies, and without other abnormalities found on EKG, physical examination or results of routine laboratory testing, it is reasonable to discharge a patient without a prolonged workup.

Indeed, there are several European studies that suggest that an abbreviated workup in the ED can successfully identify the cause of syncope in the majority of geriatric patients [11–13]. But we have to be cognizant of ensuring safe follow-up and safe discharge planning.

Section III: Concepts

Introduction

Although syncope is one of the most common symptoms of elderly patients presenting to the ED, the underlying etiology of syncope is frequently difficult to discern [14–16]. Unfortunately, syncope is also associated with a higher level of morbidity and mortality in the elderly as they are more likely to have associated comorbidities and are more prone to trauma associated with falls following syncope events [17–19].

The diagnosis of syncope is particularly challenging as the causes are complex and often multifactorial in the elderly [20]. The elderly often have multiple medical conditions requiring numerous medications, many of which can cause syncope. Moreover, age alone may predispose one to syncope as many of the physiologic changes associated with the aging process can result in decreased cerebral perfusion [20]. As one grows older physiologically, there may be a decrease in the body's ability to respond to hypotensive challenges causing syncope [16].

Background and epidemiology

Syncope, by definition, is a transient loss of consciousness, producing a brief period of unresponsiveness and a loss of postural tone, ultimately resulting in spontaneous recovery requiring no resuscitation measures [21]. Syncope is caused by a brief loss in generalized cerebral blood flow.

Syncope is very common in the elderly as well as in the general population, accounting for nearly 3% of all ED visits in the United States and 1–6% of all hospital admissions [18, 22]. Syncope is more frequently found in the elderly than in any other age group [19]. Age-related degeneration causing impairment of the heart rate, blood pressure, baroreflex sensitivity, and cerebral blood flow, combined with a higher prevalence of comorbidities and utilization of multiple medications, likely accounts for this increased incidence of syncope [19]. Atypical presentations of conditions are also more likely in the elderly than in younger patients [23].

It has been estimated that 30–50% of all cases of syncope are not given a definable etiology despite extensive medical evaluation [16, 24–26]. Many of the conditions that may be responsible for producing this symptom in the elderly, such as cardiac electroconduction system disease and myocardial ischemia, may go undiscovered and have potentially life-threatening consequences. This concern may be a factor influencing ED physicians to pursue extensive evaluations and hospital admission for most elderly patients who present to the ED with syncope. The value and success of such evaluations has been incompletely studied, and the rationale for inpatient versus outpatient evaluation of elderly patients with syncope remains unproven [5].

Elderly women with syncope are less likely to have concomitant coronary artery disease or diabetes, yet are significantly more likely to present to an ED with syncope [27]. Given that large number of patients presenting to EDs with syncope may remain without diagnosed etiologies, elderly women are even less likely to be discharged with a defined etiology [27].

There is also limited information related to near syncope in the elderly. It's been shown that patients with near syncope are as likely as those with syncope to have adverse outcomes or critical interventions [28]. However, near-syncope patients are less likely to be admitted [28]. Although further studies on near syncope in the elderly are warranted, a workup similar to that of syncope should be considered.

Etiologies

The causes of syncope are diverse, ranging from the benign to the life threatening. Syncope is often incapacitating in patients of all age groups. Syncope in the elderly may be grouped into cardiac and noncardiac etiologies. In those younger than 65 years of age, noncardiac causes clearly make up approximately 40% of syncope cases, whereas 20% may be attributed to cardiac abnormalities. In contrast, cardiac causes may claim up to 40% of cases in patients aged 65 or more, whereas noncardiac causes involve only 20% [26].

Cardiac syncope is characterized by an absent or brief prodrome of less than 5 s, palpitations and a brief loss of consciousness. Syncope of cardiac etiology can be classified into mechanical causes, such as aortic stenosis or cardiac tamponade, and dysrhythmic causes, such as paroxysmal ventricular tachycardia and conduction system disease.

The most commonly identified etiology of syncope in all patients combined is vasovagal or, sometimes called, neurocardiogenic syncope. Vasovagal syncope is characterized by a prodrome lasting more than 5 s and is associated with precipitating events or stresses [29–31]. However, the elderly may be less likely to have the usual prodrome of nausea, flushing, and sweating that one may expect in a younger patient with a vasovagal mechanism. Older individuals are also less likely than younger to report provoking causes such as prolonged standing, warm environment, or change in posture [32]. Thus, the absence of these symptoms can make diagnosing this etiology particularly difficult in the geriatric population. In addition, in younger individuals, syncope is most often associated with a single, isolated disease process [20]. Neurally mediated hypotension is often the lone culprit in this patient population [33]. In contrast, it is often difficult to find a single etiology of syncope in the geriatric population. The neuroreflex forms of syncope, such as situational syncope and carotid sinus syndrome, are also more frequent in younger than in older patients, 62.3% versus 36.2% [34]. However, carotid sinus hypersensitivity should be considered if syncope follows neck turning in the elderly or in older patients with recurrent syncope after negative diagnostic evaluation [26]. The clinical presentation of vasovagal syncope in the elderly may also be more likely to be reported as an unexplained fall and less likely as a complete or near loss of consciousness [32].

Orthostatic hypotension is commonly seen in patients presenting with recurrent episodes of syncope or light-headedness. However, orthostatic hypotension is present in up to 40% of asymptomatic patients older than 70 years and 23% of patients who are younger than 60 years [35].

Geriatric patients, who often take multiple medications, are especially at risk for medication-induced syncope [36]. This must be considered in assessing the etiology of geriatric syncope and in risk/benefit analysis when considering adding new medications to an elderly patient's regimen. Medications causing syncope include most antihypertensive and cardiovascular agents such as diuretics and vasodilators. This has been attributed to the pharmacokinetic and pharmacodynamic changes that occur with aging, which in turn may cause a delay in elimination and increased bioavailability of these drugs in the elderly [37]. Most worrisome are drugs that can prolong the QT intervals; these are associated with life-threatening dysrhythmias such as torsades de pointes. A QT_c over 500 ms heightens the probability of dangerous dysrhythmias. Antidysrhythmics are paradoxically a frequent cause of QT prolongation. Antipsychotics, often prescribed for dementia in the elderly, may also cause dysrhythmias, leading to syncope.

Vascular causes of syncope should also be considered more closely in the elderly than in younger populations. Pulmonary embolism (PE) may present with syncope or other atypical symptoms in geriatric patients [38]. PE should be considered in older populations with risk factors, hypoxia or dyspnea. Less common causes of syncope, such as mesenteric steal, carotid insufficiency, and abdominal aortic aneurysm or aortic dissection, are also important to consider in the elderly. Here again, the patient's risk factors, presenting history, medications, past medical history, and prior events must be taken into account when determining how aggressively to pursue these causes. Yet, once more, the elderly may not present with the typical pain or dyspnea that is seen in younger groups. One retrospective study with a mean age of 66 years finds that 17% of patients with an aortic dissection have no pain on presentation, but 25% of these patients present with syncope [39]. Another retrospective study with a mean age of 73.5 years shows 23% of patients admitted with a ruptured abdominal aortic aneurysm have syncope as a symptom [40].

Sepsis is another life-threatening illness that may manifest as syncope. Realizing that the elderly may be less likely to mount a fever or express a leukocytosis, syncope may be one of the few signs of impending sepsis or severe infection developing in a geriatric patient.

Evaluation

Determining the etiology of a syncopal event, particularly in the elderly, can be challenging. Syncope is often transient and can resolve independently, without recurrence. Often the event is not witnessed and not remembered by the patient, making it difficult to find the specific circumstances that led up to and occurred during the syncopal episode [16]. Therefore, one must first determine whether the patient had a syncopal event. Second, one must determine if this syncopal event is dangerous. If the syncopal event potentially had a worrisome etiology, one must decide what evaluation and what immediate therapy is appropriate. Lastly, if this event does not appear to be dangerous, one must determine whether the patient can be discharged home and define the appropriate follow-up.

The history, physical examination, and EKG have the greatest utility in evaluating syncope in the elderly [2, 41]. To sort out the etiology, the physician must obtain the best history from the greatest number of witnesses. Similarly, all syncope patients need a thorough physical examination. The patient's medication list should be reviewed for drugs that increase the risk for syncope, including antihypertensive, cardiovascular agents, and antipsychotics, as well as recent changes to these medications that may have influenced the event.

The initial task in syncope, as with all ED patients, is to obtain vital signs and determine the need for immediate stabilization. The utility of orthostatic vital signs is controversial, but may be helpful in the elderly or any patient thought to be volume depleted [42]. Again, review of the patient's medication list and careful physical examination may help determine risk of volume depletion. If a patient's syncopal event directly follows standing up, orthostasis may be a contributor. It may be useful to compare the patient's current blood pressure to the baseline blood pressure, as patients who appear normotensive may actually be relatively hypotensive if there is a history of hypertension. Measurements of blood pressure in both arms may be useful to help screen for aortic dissection. Most syncope patients who are otherwise asymptomatic should have normal or near normal vital signs within minutes following resolution of their syncopal event.

Physical examination should include a neurologic examination, careful auscultation of the carotid arteries, heart and lungs, as well as palpation of the peripheral arteries. There is no clear evidence to support routine stool sampling in syncope. However, if there is concern for gastrointestinal bleeding based on history, vital signs, or a low hemoglobin/hematocrit, then an examination should be performed. A history of melena may be more informative than trace hemoccult positive stools in patients with syncope. It is also important to look at all skin areas to evaluate for trauma or skin infections that may be easily missed, particularly if considering a source for sepsis.

Evidence of trauma such as lacerations from tongue biting, contusions or fractures, should be meticulously noted. In determining whether the patient experienced a seizure, stroke, or a syncopal episode, several factors should be considered. While lateral tongue lacerations tend to support the existence of tonic–clonic seizures, anterior lacerations can be the result of a fall from syncope [43]. Generalized seizures will often have postictal confusion, whereas loss of consciousness from a stroke is generally not transient.

Testing

There is no gold standard against which the results of diagnostic tests can be measured in syncope [2, 41]. All patients with syncope should likely have basic tests such as an EKG and a finger stick glucose test. Blood tests such as electrolytes, complete blood count, cardiac enzymes, lactate, blood cultures, and imaging modalities such as head CT and echocardiography should be guided by history and physical examination [44]. Routine blood tests typically only confirm clinical suspicion in syncope patients [2]. Specifically, cardiac enzymes are of little value if drawn routinely on elderly patients who are admitted with syncope. Cardiac enzymes should only be drawn if the patient has other signs or symptoms suggestive of myocardial ischemia by history such as chest pain or dyspnea, or by ECG such as new STTW abnormalities, ST elevation, or an ECG that is uninterpretable for ischemia [10]. Similarly, it's suggested that lactate only be sent if there's concern for sepsis or mesenteric ischemia based on the history and physical examination. Urine and blood cultures should only be sent if there's concern for sepsis. A D-dimer for pulmonary embolus is of limited value as D-dimers often become elevated with age, and there is no clear breakdown of normal D-dimers by age [6, 7].

Head CT scans should be limited to those with signs of trauma, neurologic deficit, or neurologic complaints [8, 9]. All other patients presenting with syncope have a low likelihood of having abnormal findings on head CT and do not require a scan [44].

In one pilot study, limiting CT scans to patients with signs or symptoms of neurologic disease including headache, trauma above the clavicles or medicating with warfarin, would have reduced scans by 56% [44].

If a new murmur is heard on examination, then an echocardiogram may be obtained. However, if a patient doesn't have a history of a murmur or an audible murmur on examination, they are unlikely to have a valvular etiology of their syncope [5]. An echocardiogram may give a diagnosis 2–22% of the time, and most often from aortic stenosis [3, 4].

Additional studies should be used sparingly and based on the initial data, as many tests for syncope have a low diagnostic yield. For example, an EKG will determine the cause of syncope in only 5% of patients [2]. Studies have shown that telemetry may help determine the etiology of syncope in only 3–5% of patients, from causes such as atrial fibrillation or bradycardia [3, 4]. Choosing tests based on history and examination and prioritizing less expensive and higher yield tests may enable a more informed and cost-effective approach to evaluating syncope in the elderly [44].

Disposition

Successful response to treatment is difficult to predict in the elderly [18]. With concern that potentially life-threatening diseases might be the etiology, elderly patients are frequently admitted to the hospital regardless of the likely etiology, comorbidities or lack thereof and regardless of response to therapies such as fluid resuscitation. Potential for transient dysrhythmia is likely the most significant issue influencing physicians to pursue inpatient evaluations for those patients presenting with syncope of unknown origin. However, recommendations for hospital admission should be based on the potential for adverse outcomes if further evaluation and workup is delayed or thought to be unnecessary [1].

One study used four predictors of adverse outcomes in 72 h including a history of ventricular dysrhythmia, an abnormal EKG in the ED, age older than 45 years and a history of congestive heart failure [45]. In patients with none of these risk factors, there was no 72 h cardiac mortality, but a 0.7% risk of dysrhythmia [45]. One-year cardiac mortality and dysrhythmia rates range from 7% in those with no risk factors to 57% in those with three and 80% in those with four risk factors [45].

The San Francisco Syncope Rule (SFSR) was thought to be a promising tool to predict serious outcome of patients with syncope [46]. However, multiple recent studies have been unable to validate this rule [47–49]. Schladenhaufen looked specifically at the utility of the SFSR in the elderly and finds particularly low sensitivities and specificities [50]. Thus, SFSR may not be applicable to the elderly ED population.

The Boston Syncope Criteria accurately identifies ED patients at risk for adverse outcomes at 30 days [5]. Utilizing risk factors to screen syncope patients yields a sensitivity of 97%, specificity of 62% with a negative predictive value of 99% [51]. Risk factors for adverse outcome include signs and symptoms of acute coronary syndrome, a cardiac or valvular disease history, family history of sudden death, signs of conduction disease, persistent abnormal vital sign in the ED, or profound volume depletion such as with gastrointestinal bleeding [5, 51]. In this population, admitting only those patients identified by risk factors would reduce hospital admissions by 11–48% [5, 51].

Another study demonstrates that of high-risk patients who presented with a benign etiology of syncope (vasovagal or dehydration) with a normal ED workup, none would benefit from hospitalization based on risk factors alone [52]. If these patients with a benign etiology and negative workup were sent home, an additional 19% reduction in hospital admissions would have occurred [52]. Similarly, although near-syncope patients may have risk factors for adverse outcomes similar to syncope [28], if the etiology of near syncope is vasovagal or dehydration with a normal workup, these patients may be discharged [53].

The Boston study did not use age as a criterion for admission; although geriatric patients with syncope have a higher incidence of adverse outcome, they find this to be related to other comorbidities. Thus, if an otherwise historically and currently healthy, elderly patient has a lone syncopal event, that event should be considered benign [5]. Roussanov similarly finds that new-onset syncope is not an independent predictor of mortality in elderly patients [54]. As age over 65 without risk factors does not appear to be an independent predictor of an adverse outcome following a syncopal event, it is safe to discharge

geriatric patients with syncope but without other risk factors, regardless of age, without further risk stratification [1].

If a patient is discharged from the ED, regardless of etiology, he should have close follow-up with his PCP, ideally scheduled prior to discharge. Direct communication between the PCP and emergency team can be particularly useful. The social and home situation must be considered prior to discharging elderly with syncope. An elderly patient may need social support at home, particularly if there is concern for recurrent syncope and falls. Although there is no data to suggest an appropriate length of time, our practice is to advise the patient not to drive at least until PCP follow-up occurs. As with any patient, discharge instructions are useless if the patient lacks the cognitive ability to understand the discharge instructions.

Conclusion

Assessing and managing syncope in the elderly patient is a daunting task. The presentations are myriad, the histories are often limited, and the spectrum of disease is considerable. Successful interventions center primarily on the cardiovascular disorders that cause syncope in the elderly. Disposition should be predicated on the results of the initial evaluation as well as risk factors for adverse outcomes with syncope. With a growing geriatric population worldwide, the future rests in creating more directed and expeditious protocols for evaluation and testing of syncope patients and increasing public awareness to the nuance of worrisome concurrent symptomatology [55].

Section IV: Decision-making

- Syncope causes in geriatric patients may present differently than in younger populations.
- Obtain a detailed history of present illness, medication list, and past medical history to assess the risk of an adverse outcome.
- Causes of syncope in the elderly that should be considered include cardiac dysrhythmias, vasovagal, orthostatic hypotension, neurologic, pulmonary embolism, abdominal aortic aneurysm, aortic dissection, sepsis, and medication side effects.

- The most common etiology is vasovagal or neuro-cardiogenic syncope. However, the elderly may not have the prodromes of nausea, flushing, and sweating that one may expect in a younger patient.
- The syncope workup should be tailored to the patient's presentation. History, medications, physical examination, EKG, and fingerstick glucose determination will help define the appropriate workup.
- Neurologic etiologies of syncope typically have concomitant neurologic symptoms or abnormal neurological findings on examination. Head CT scans should be limited to those with signs of trauma, neurologic deficit, or complaints.
- Disposition should be predicated on the results of the initial evaluation and risk factors for adverse outcomes. Age alone does not appear to be an independent predictor of an adverse outcome.
- If discharging, social support should be considered and the patient should have close follow-up with their PCP, ideally with communication between the PCP and emergency team.

References

1 Grossman, S.A., Chiu, D., Lipsitz, L. et al. (2014) Can elderly patients without risk factors be discharged home when presenting to the emergency department with syncope? Arch. Gerontol. Geriatr., 58, 110–114.

2 Linzer, M., Yang, E.H., Estes, N.A. III, et al. (1997) Diagnosing syncope. Part 1: Value of history, physical examination, and electrocardiography. Clinical Efficacy Assessment Project of the American College of Physicians. Ann. Intern. Med., 126, 989–996.

3 Mendu, M.L., McAvay, G., Lampert, R. et al. (2009) Yield of diagnostic tests in evaluating syncopal episodes in older patients. Arch. Intern. Med., 169, 1299–1305.

4 Chiu, D.T., Shapiro, N.I., Sun, B.C. et al. (2014) Are echocardiography, telemetry, ambulatory electrocardiography monitoring and cardiac enzymes in emergency department patients presenting with syncope useful tests? A preliminary investigation. J. Emerg. Med., 47 (1), 113–118. doi: 10.1016/j.jemermed.2014.01.018. Epub 2014 Mar 31.

5 Grossman, S.A., Fischer, C., Lipsitz, L. et al. (2007) Predicting adverse outcomes in syncope. J. Emerg. Med., 33, 233–239.

6 Tita-Nwa, F., Bos, A., Adjei, A. et al. (2010) Correlates of D-dimer in older persons. Aging Clin. Exp. Res., 22 (1), 20–23.

7 Harper, P.L., Theakston, E., Ahmed, J., and Ockelford, P. (2007) D-dimer concentration increases with age reducing the clinical value of the D-dimer assay in the elderly. Intern. Med. J., 37, 607–613.

8 Goyal, N., Donnino, M.W., Vachhani, R. et al. (2006) The utility of head computed tomography in the emergency department evaluation of syncope. Intern. Emerg. Med., 1, 148–150.

9 Grossman, S.A., Fischer, C., Bar, J.L. et al. (2007) The yield of head CT in syncope: a pilot study. Intern. Emerg. Med., 2, 46–49.

10 Grossman, S.A., Van Epp, S., Arnold, R. et al. (2003) The value of cardiac enzymes in elderly patients presenting to the emergency department with syncope. J. Gerontol. A Biol. Sci. Med. Sci., 58, 1055–1059.

11 Sarasin, F.P., Pruvot, E., Louis-Simonet, M. et al. (2008) Stepwise evaluation of syncope: a prospective population-based controlled study. Int. J. Cardiol., 127, 103–111.

12 Brignole, M., Menozzi, C., Bartoletti, A. et al. (2006) A new management of syncope: prospective systematic guideline-based evaluation of patients referred urgently to general hospitals. Eur. Heart J., 27, 76–82.

13 Baron-Esquivias, G., Martinez-Alday, J., Martin, A. et al. (2010) Epidemiological characteristics and diagnostic approach in patients admitted to the emergency room for transient loss of consciousness: Group for Syncope Study in the Emergency Room (GESINUR) study. Europace, 12, 869–876.

14 Lipsitz, L.A. (1983) Syncope in the elderly. Ann. Intern. Med., 99, 92–105.

15 Kapoor, W., Snustad, D., Peterson, J. et al. (1998) Syncope in the elderly. Am. J. Med., 80, 419–428.

16 Lipsitz, L.A., Pluchino, F.C., Wei, J.Y., and Rowe, J.W. (1986) Syncope in institutionalized elderly: the impact of multiple pathological conditions and situational stress. J. Chronic Dis., 39, 619–630.

17 Kapoor, W.N. (1991) Diagnostic evaluation of syncope. Am. J. Med., 90, 91–106.

18 Kapoor, W.N. (1990) Evaluation and outcome of patients with syncope. Medicine, 69 (3), 160–175.

19 Kenny, R.A. (2003) Syncope in the elderly: diagnosis, evaluation, and treatment. J. Cardiovasc. Electrophysiol., 14 (Suppl. 9), S74–S77.

20 Kapoor, W.N. (1987) Evaluation of syncope in the elderly. J. Am. Geriatr. Soc., 35, 826–828.

21 Kapoor, W.N., Karpf, M., Wieand, S. et al. (1983) A prospective evaluation and follow-up of patients with syncope. N. Engl. J. Med., 309, 197–204.

22 Sun, B.C., Emond, J.A., and Camargo, C.A. Jr. (2005) Direct medical costs of syncope-related hospitalizations in the United States. Am. J. Cardiol., 1 (95), 668–671.

23 Hood, R. (2007) Syncope in the elderly. Clin. Geriatr. Med., 23, 351–361.

24 Getchell, W.S., Larsen, G.C., Morris, C.D., and McAnulty, J.H. (1999) Epidemiology of syncope in hospitalized patients. *J. Gen. Intern. Med.*, **14**, 677–687.

25 Kapoor, W. and Hanusa, B. (1996) Is syncope a risk factor for poor outcomes? Comparison of patients with and without syncope. *Am. J. Med.*, **100**, 647–655.

26 Kapoor, W.N. (1992) Evaluation and management of the patient with syncope. *J. Am. Med. Assoc.*, **268**, 2553–2560.

27 Grossman, S.A., Shapiro, N.I., Van Epp, S. *et al.* (2005) Sex differences in the emergency department evaluation of elderly patients with syncope. *J. Gerontol. A Biol. Sci. Med. Sci.*, **60**, 1202–1205.

28 Grossman, S.A., Babineau, M., Burke, L. *et al.* (2012) Do outcomes of near syncope parallel syncope? *Am. J. Emerg. Med.*, **30**, 203–206.

29 Martin, G., Adams, S., Martin, H. *et al.* (1984) Prospective evaluation of syncope. *Ann. Emerg. Med.*, **13**, 499–504.

30 Calkins, H., Shyr, Y., Frumin, H. *et al.* (1995) The value of the clinical history in the differentiation of syncope due to ventricular tachycardia, atrioventricular block, and neurocardiogenic syncope. *Am. J. Med.*, **98**, 365–373.

31 Day, S.C., Cook, E.F., Funkenstein, H., and Goldman, L. (1982) Evaluation and outcome of emergency room patients with transient loss of consciousness. *Am. J. Med.*, **73**, 15–23.

32 Duncan, G.W., Tan, M.P., Newton, J.L. *et al.* (2010) Vasovagal syncope in the older person: differences in presentation between older and younger patients. *Age Ageing*, **39**, 470–475.

33 Braunwald, E. (ed) (1997) *Heart Disease: A Textbook of Cardiovascular Medicine*, 5th edn, WB Saunders, Philadelphia, PA, pp. 868–935.

34 Ungar, A., Mussi, C., Del Rosso, A. *et al.* (2006) A diagnosis and characteristics of syncope in older patients referred to geriatric department. *J. Am. Geriatr. Soc.*, **54** (**10**), 1531–1536.

35 Atkins, D., Hanusa, B., Sefcik, T., and Kapoor, W. (1990) Syncope and orthostatic hypotension. *Am. J. Med.*, **91**, 179–185.

36 Hanlon, J., Linzer, M., MacMillan, J. *et al.* (1990) Syncope and presyncope associated with probable adverse drug reactions. *Arch. Intern. Med.*, **150**, 2309–2312.

37 Verhaeverbeke, H. and Mets, T. (1997) Drug-induced orthostatic hypotension in the elderly: avoiding its onset. *Drug Saf.*, **17** (**2**), 105–118.

38 Kokturk, N., Oguzulgen, I.K., Demir, N. *et al.* (2005) Differences in clinical presentation of pulmonary embolism in older vs younger patients. *Circ. J.*, **69**, 981–986.

39 Imamura, H., Sekiguchi, Y., Iwashita, T. *et al.* (2011) Painless acute aortic dissection. *Circ. J.*, **75** (**1**), 59–66.

40 Akkersdijk, G.J. and van Bockel, J.H. (1998) Ruptured abdominal aortic aneurysm: initial misdiagnosis and the effect on treatment. *Eur. J. Surg.*, **164**, 29–34.

41 Linzer, M., Yang, E.H., Estes, N.A. III *et al.* (1997) Diagnosing syncope. Part 2: Unexplained syncope: clinical efficacy assessment project of the American College of Physicians. *Ann. Intern. Med.*, **127**, 76–86.

42 Ooi, W.L., Hossain, M., and Lipsitz, L.A. (2000) The association between orthostatic hypotension and recurrent falls in nursing home residents. *Am. J. Med.*, **108**, 106–111.

43 Benbadis, S., Wolgamuth, B., Goren, H. *et al.* (1995) Value of tongue biting in the diagnosis of seizures. *Arch. Intern. Med.*, **155**, 2346–2349.

44 Grossman, S.A. (2006) Testing in syncope. *Intern. Emerg. Med.*, **1**, 135–136.

45 Martin, T.P., Hanusa, B.H., and Kapoor, W.N. (1997) Risk stratification of patients with syncope. *Ann. Emerg. Med.*, **29**, 459–466.

46 Quinn, J.G., Stiell, I.G., Seller, K.A. *et al.* (2002) The San Francisco Syncope Rule to predict patients with serious outcomes. *Acad. Emerg. Med.*, **9**, 358.

47 Fischer, C.M., Shapiro, N.I., Lipsitz, L. *et al.* (2005) External validation of the San Francisco Syncope Rule. *Acad. Emerg. Med.*, **12**, S127.

48 Sun, B.C., Mangione, C.M., Merchant, G. *et al.* (2007) External validation of the San Francisco Syncope Rule. *Ann. Emerg. Med.*, **49**, 420–427.

49 Birnbaum, A., Esses, D., Biju, P. *et al.* (2008) Failure to validate the San Francisco Syncope Rule in elderly ED patients. *Am. J. Emerg. Med.*, **26**, 773–778.

50 Schladenhaufen, R., Feilinger, S., Pollack, M. *et al.* (2008) Application of San Francisco Syncope Rule in elderly ED patients. *Am. J. Emerg. Med.*, **26**, 773–778.

51 Grossman, S.A., Bar, J., Fischer, C. *et al.* (2012) Reducing admissions utilizing the Boston Syncope Criteria. *J. Emerg. Med.*, **42** (**3**), 345–352.

52 Grossman, S.A., Fischer, C., Kancharla, A. *et al.* (2011) Can benign etiologies predict benign outcomes in high-risk syncope patients? *J. Emerg. Med.*, **40** (**5**), 592–597.

53 Grossman, S.A., Babineau, M., Burke, L. *et al.* (2012) Applying the Boston syncope criteria to near syncope. *J. Emerg. Med.*, **43** (**6**), 958–963.

54 Roussanov, O., Estacio, G., Capuno, M. *et al.* (2007) Outcomes of unexplained syncope in the elderly. *Am. J. Geriatr. Cardiol.*, **16**, 249–254.

55 Grossman, S.A. (2009) Assessing and managing syncope in older subjects. *J. Gene Med.*, **21** (**4**), 19–22.

15 Stroke

Julie Watkins-Torrey, Roxanna Sadri & Kama Guluma

Department of Emergency Medicine, Timaru Public Hospital, South Canterbury District Health Board, Department of Hyperbaric Medicine, Christchurch Public Hospital, Canterbury Health Board, New Zealand

Section I: Case presentation

A 70-year-old man presents unresponsive to the emergency department (ED) with pinpoint pupils and irregular respirations. Two hours prior he had told his wife that his chronic low back pain was worse than usual and that he took a few extra pills of his sustained release morphine sulfate. He expressed to her that he was feeling ill with a severe headache; he vomited more than 10 times, had slurred speech, blurry vision, and was having difficulty ambulating, reportedly falling in all directions. He denied abdominal pain, diarrhea, or fever. His wife also noted that his eyes were twitching abnormally. He crawled from the kitchen to his room to take a nap. When his wife went to check on him an hour later, she was unable to wake him. Emergency medical services (EMS) found the patient to have pinpoint pupils and that he was unresponsive to naloxone.

Past medical history was significant for hypertension, hyperlipidemia, atrial fibrillation, coronary artery disease, carotid artery atherosclerosis, and a 40-pack-year history of cigarette smoking. He was status post right carotid endarterectomy 10 years prior for a 70% stenosis. There was no known history of a cerebrovascular accident (CVA). He had not been taking his lipid-lowering agent for 1 year due to expense. He had been lost to follow-up at the Coumadin clinic. The family history was significant for stroke, diabetes, and myocardial infarction (MI).

On physical examination, the vital signs were as follows: temperature 37°C, pulse 60 beats/min, respirations 20 breaths/min and irregular, blood pressure 190/110 mm Hg, and pulse oximetry 98%. There was a significant left carotid bruit. The pupils were fixed and pinpoint. Additional doses of naloxone were given with no change in the mental status. The patient exhibited extensor posturing when the nurse attempted to obtain additional intravenous access. The Glasgow Coma Score was 4. When doll's eye maneuver was performed, the patient's eyes remained in a fixed position mid-orbit, not moving when the head was turned. Cardiac, pulmonary, and abdominal examinations were normal. No skin lesions were seen. The patient was intubated with rapid sequence intubation with fentanyl, etomidate, and rocuronium. A noncontrast head computed tomography (CT) scan was negative for intracranial hemorrhage or mass lesion. An electrocardiogram (EKG) showed atrial fibrillation with a rate of 80 beats/min. Comprehensive metabolic panel and complete blood count with differential were within normal limits.

Section II: Case discussion

Dr Peter Rosen (PR): We have here a typical geriatric infinite possibility patient. I can see why they were concerned about a morphine overdose. However, have you ever experienced a morphine overdose with rapid respirations?

Dr Maura Kennedy (MK): That would be atypical. I was expecting him to be bradypneic. In someone who is tolerant of morphine, I wouldn't expect this severity of vomiting. Certainly, a decreased level of

Geriatric Emergencies: A Discussion-Based Review, First Edition.
Edited by Amal Mattu, Shamai A. Grossman and Peter L. Rosen.

arousal, pinpoint pupils, bradypnea would be more consistent. However, certain features including the posturing, the irregularity of respirations and the vomiting, don't seem consistent with a morphine overdose.

PR: The blood sugar was normal. Have you ever encountered the need for obtaining more than one blood sugar to make sure you aren't dealing with hypoglycemia?

Dr Scott Wilber (SW): Typically, when I see that the patient's symptoms are due to hypoglycemia, but that the blood sugar is normal, the patient has had prolonged hypoglycemia, which has been corrected. I haven't seen a lot of errors with blood sugars that are reportedly normal, and the patients are actually hypoglycemic.

PR: I've seen a couple of patients with reasons for being hypoglycemic, and while the blood sugar corrected with a bolus, the blood sugar then rapidly decreased, and the patient needed more sugar. There are many times where I thought the patient had a midbrain stroke, and the patient was actually hypoglycemic. We oftentimes listen for a bruit over the carotid artery, but we forget to listen for bruit over the vertebral artery, which is always a good thing to do in a patient with known vascular disease because you can often hear more than one bruit. To me, this sounds like a brainstem stroke and clearly the team was moving toward a CT scan and intubated the patient first, which was very appropriate. Do you have any other suggestions for other things that might be done prior to the CT scan?

Dr Don Melady (DM): One thing that needs to come up early in geriatric critical care management is the "goals of care discussion." Ultimately as we see later, that ended up happening. However, it might be reasonable to start talking about what the goals of care would be much earlier on. When this man rolls through the door and his wife is present, given he is 70 and has a number of comorbidities and there is a lot that we don't know about him, *that* is the time to start the discussion. I think likely in such a situation with such a rapid decrease from a functional baseline, the approach would be a "go ahead and do everything." But you can turn up a lot of interesting things, with a 2-min quick talk, such as "he was diagnosed last week with metastatic cancer,

and he turned down chemotherapy." Initiating that conversation, in a patient with such a calamitous decline can important to do early on.

Dr Shamai Grosman (SG): This may be even more important in this case where there are dangerous but powerful transforming therapies that may be offered, such as thrombolytics, and there may be a substantial transformation in quality of life, on the other hand you may substantially shorten the quantity of life with a bad outcome.

PR: One of the surprising things given the history, in this case, is that he didn't turn out to have an intracerebral hemorrhage. We know that the posterior fossa is not a good place to image on CT scan. Sometimes, if we are concerned about this, we can ask the radiologist to do a more focused posterior fossa scan and not have to go to a magnetic resonance imaging (MRI). At any rate, this patient did not appear to have a major brainstem hemorrhage, which I would have predicted given he was lost to follow-up at the Coumadin clinic. We didn't know what the status of his prothrombin time was initially, although ultimately it proved to be normal. Would you briefly discuss what your indications would be for reperfusion in a patient like this?

DM: I think that most academic centers now have collaboration with the neurologic stroke service. I'm guessing this patient came in with a "stroke code" type alert from the field. I think the role that we have is oftentimes to put in perspective for the neurologist what the family's wishes are, and oftentimes we think a little bit long term and a little more practically about fibrinolytic agents. In my experience, I've seen a lot of aggressive neurologists who give fibrinolytic agents even to patients in their 80–90s, with many comorbidities, and, in general, have poor expected outcome based on their initial presentation. I don't know if it's for litigious reasons or otherwise. One of the roles that emergency physicians can play is to step back and understand the likelihood of recovery for a patient of this age and these comorbidities and to stop and analyze whether lytic agents would be of benefit or harm.

SG: Remember it's not the family's wishes that are important, but the patient's or the family's perception of the patient's wishes. Our job in emergency medicine (EM) is primarily to care for the sick patient before us.

Dr Jon Mark Hirshon (JMH): This is a very interesting topic, because there are times when there are people that I've evaluated in the ED, in whom I feel that their outcomes are poor, but the stroke team wishes to be more aggressive in their management. Thus, there is an ethical quandary. Within our medical cultural paradigm, I tend not to disagree with them even though personally, I would not agree with their management.

PR: I think reperfusion gives you a greater risk of hemorrhage at the price for a greater chance of functional recovery. That being the case, you are in an ethical dilemma that probably should be resolved by the family and the patient's wishes, rather than the physician and his wishes. What does the family think is a likely outcome of the prospective treatment, and if there is a chance to recover brain function, would the patient be willing to risk an increased risk of hemorrhage. If they are willing, I don't see any problem with reperfusion.

DM: I think there is a big role for the emergency physician here. Family and patient decisions need to be guided by information that they don't have. To make decisions in this situation, family members look to somebody who may not have evidence-based knowledge but certainly has more experience. Emergency physicians are naturally optimistic, or we wouldn't be doing this job. Moreover, trainees and junior physicians, in particular, feel impelled to bring a great aura of optimism and hope to situations like this. I think it's best to speak frankly and give one's best opinion for the likely possibilities are here – and even make a recommendation. When I see a 70-year-old man with a precipitous decline to a Glasgow Coma Scale (GCS) of 4, and I see a big bleed or big infarction in the brainstem, I'm not filled with optimism for a meaningful recovery. A family needs to know what "meaningful recovery" means: "he may perk up a bit and we may be able to get the tube out," "it seems very unlikely that he will ever live independently again," "I think it's unlikely that he will be going home," and "I think that if this were my brother or my father, I would not want this for them." I don't know how comfortable others are in saying these things, but it would it be part of my conversation in this situation.

PR: For many young EM physicians, death is the worst possible outcome, but for the older physician who has

to face his own impending demise, it's not the worst outcome. I think our discussion is different depending on our own individual circumstances. Sometimes, I think we get caught up in our own definitions of life quality and what we would want for ourselves rather than what the patient would want or what the patient's family would want. That is an easy trap to fall into.

SG: Any time we approach a patient and say "I would or would not want an intervention done," we are expressing our own belief rather taking into account the patient's or the family's personal belief. First and foremost, our job is to take care of the patient, but at the same time we need to try to figure out where the patient is coming from, and what is his or her ethical belief system. There are ethical belief systems that believe that any form of life is better than no life. Still, there are others who believe that the only life worth living is one that has quality that is similar to prior the event. It's critical to try to understand from the family through our conversation with them what direction they are coming from before we can make recommendations that is biased by our own belief system. Sometimes, this is very tricky because the family has no idea that even if we are actually very aggressive and do everything possible for the patient, the outcome may be abysmal, whereas if we don't do anything, their outcome will probably be death, and that may or may not be what they are hoping and willing to settle for.

JMH: Once the family has made a decision with consultation and guidance of the physician, I'm obligated to the family to help them to complete that process, whether through thrombolytics or other things. In this instance, I would want to make sure that an adequate workup has been performed, as shown, and there is not an alternative diagnosis. But in the end, if ultimately it's a pontine or cerebellar stroke, and we've made a decision to give thrombolytics, we would aggressively pursue that to try to get the best outcome from that course of action.

PR: I would take it that from your institution, that reperfusion goes to the ICU?

JMH: Correct, in this instance, we would engage our neurosurgical and neurology colleagues depending on whether it's a bleed or stroke. We would get the CT scan to see if it was an ischemic stroke and get our neurology colleagues involved. Neurology would likely be involved from the very beginning because we have a brain attack team that we engage early on when we suspect an ischemic stroke and the patient may need thrombolytics. It would be a smooth transition from us to them as they begin managing the patient along with the thrombolytic administration. They would expect to admit to the Neuro ICU, albeit how quickly that would occur would depend on the space in the hospital.

PR: I worked in Jackson Hole, where there is no neurology and we could call the neurology service in Denver, and they would help us initiate reperfusion with phone consultation. Have you ever been in the situation where you wanted to reperfuse the patient but the neurology service didn't?

MK: I've been in that situation previously. I think that one of the challenges is determining the time of onset. Sometimes, the stroke consultant wants a certainty of onset, and in this case, there seems to be a clear certainty of onset. When there is confusion or disagreement about the certainty of onset, I have seen disagreements about the appropriateness of reperfusion. I have also seen disagreements with respect to the improvement of symptomatology, that is, particularly in a young individual who had a pretty dense left-side hemiparesis who seemed to be having a very mild return of function, but was classified as non-tPA (tissue plasminogen activator) eligible, and I had some disagreement with that. I've also been in the situation many times where via telemedicine at one of our community affiliates I can assist them in making the decision to give tPA. I think another challenging situation, from the community perspective, is that oftentimes it's hard to get a good neurologic examination when you're at the bedside and even more so when you're communicating via television and telephone.

PR: If you're at a tertiary care hospital and you got a call from a rural hospital concerning a patient like this, would you have any problems in accepting the patient in transfer.

SW: I wouldn't have any problem accepting this patient. I've actually been on the other side as well, because we do staff a rural hospital, and we have neurology available by telephone. I've actually found that neurologists are even more aggressive about giving

TPA over the phone than I feel comfortable with. I would have no problem in accepting the patient.

PR: Would you begin therapy in the community?

SW: I would have no problem beginning therapy. One of the arguments is the patient should be brought to the community hospital to save about 25 or 30 min in drive time, to get the CT scan and tPA started there, and then transferred as protocol. I think that we are wasting a lot of time in driving to a stroke tertiary care center when we have a community hospital that may be able to start tPA. I don't think we want to keep the patient and do all the Neuro ICU care, but we should be able to start care in the community and then transfer. I think that's the best thing for the patient's brain.

PR: I think that functionally, what we have to decide as a tertiary care center is that we are not there to be a barrier to transfer even though we end up accepting a patient who we ultimately can't help. If we are going to produce a network of hospitals, we need to make it easy for the transferring hospital to transfer. Don't permit a junior house officer to make the transfer decision. If you make it easy to transfer, you'll get the patients who should be transferred. The price tag will be a few patients who could have been cared for and pronounced locally, but I think it's worth the cost. As Dr Wilber pointed out, if you're going to save some patients by adopting a system-wide approach, you have to pay the price for it. I sense that this is a patient who initially looks confusing but ultimately reveals the vascular pathway that you know he is going to be on. Does it help you to know that he had a successful carotid endarterectomy 10 years ago? How long are those operations good for?

Dr Vaishal Tolia (VT): It seems like he was fairly noncompliant with his medications. The carotid vessels are larger vessels than coronary vessels, with therapies that are often very similar to that with antiplatelets, anticoagulation for a period of time, as well as lipid-lowering and blood pressure management therapies. With this patient being non-compliant, particularly with his antilipid agents, as well as the finding of the left-side bruits, makes it concerning this therapy 10 years ago was somewhat compromised and that he has some disease reaccumulation. A lot of times now, there are different interventional procedures with stenting as well as endarterectomies that 10 years ago might not have been available. I would be more concerned that with his noncompliance, the time that the vessel should have actually remained fairly open for flow may have been compromised in this case.

PR: I think that we always assume that it's not compliance rather than intolerance. A lot of antilipid agents are not well tolerated, and we prescribe them blindly. There are many patients who simply can't take them, and won't. They aren't able to describe why because they often don't know that it's a side effect of the agent. The fact was concluded that supposedly he wasn't compliant, yet his international normalized ratio (INR) was therapeutic, and he stayed stroke free for 10 years. So something was working, and maybe we just reached the end of the vascular cycle for this patient. He went out in magnificent fashion, but at least for a while he had pretty good control.

SG: I might add that to some extent this highlights some of the failures of our healthcare system. Here we have a patient who we could have potentially better emphasized the need for compliance, anticoagulant therapy, cholesterol-lowering therapies, or another therapy that may have been better tolerated. Yet, somehow he fell through the cracks, and he wasn't as compliant as we would have liked him to be. While it's possible that this was the natural progression of his disease, on the other hand, he might have avoided this natural progression, and he might not have been in this situation in the first place. The cost of ensuring that a patient is compliant with medication and lifestyle changes, which would have been necessary in this patient's case, would have been substantially lower than the cost of the terminal ED and hospital course and possibly the care attempted to salvage what's left.

PR: Don, what do you do with a patient who triages himself incorrectly and comes into your facility with these symptoms by personal car rather than by ambulance?

DM: We have developed quite a robust protocol. The door to the other hospital is 400 ft from our door. So we have developed a protocol wherein these patients are identified at triage by an EM physician, a code stroke is called, and the EMS system drives them the 400 ft from one door to the other. This works quite well for the most part. We also have access to an underground tunnel between the two hospitals for the stroke team to come over and manage the patient in our ED.

PR: I imagine there are parts of our country where there is not easy access to a stroke team, and probably those folks don't fare as well as when there is quick easy access. Do you have any suggestions on how to make this a little easier in more remote parts of rural America?

JM: You highlight the fact that the key for this is organization and that you want to have a preplanned course of action so that if you do get someone like this you are able to rapidly respond. In a rural setting, you have to depend on telemedicine and telephone consultation, so you need to have the design in advance so that you are able to access the appropriate consultation services. It's a little problematic to get adequate evaluation and management when your resources are limited.

PR: I was asked a question about telemedicine. It seems to me that it's not necessary, and what is necessary is easy transferability. There are not all that many cases where it helps you to see the films and to see the patient. What you really need is access to the facility that has tertiary care. That can be a lot harder to arrange, and probably is a lot cheaper than trying to set up telemedicine in remote places in rural parts of our country.

JM: The advantage of setting up telemedicine is that you develop these lines of bidirectional communication, which is what is required for these rapid transfers. The amount of infrastructure required for some of the telemedicine is relatively limited and particularly necessary if you look outside of the country to resource-limited settings such as parts of Africa, where telemedicine might be the only option. Again, it doesn't have to be a robust, high-speed Internet connection. What is necessary is the ability to be able to transmit information, which I think is critical.

VT: I'm involved in telemedicine research at our UC hospitals. We use telemedicine for a variety of reasons, stroke being the initial one, which has prompted other groups at UC Davis to use it for pediatric transfers. They've published some fairly interesting data on the appropriateness of transfers, and being able to intervene early on sicker kids, and even avoiding transfers for kids who might otherwise have been unnecessarily transferred long distances. Telemedicine has its origin in stroke, and having the ability to use an expert neurologist to help make the treatment decisions. Unlike acute MI where a catheterization laboratory is needed, the emergency physician still has the ability to initiate treatment that can sometimes be the most important intervention in acute stroke. Having that access to initiate therapy is probably the biggest utility for telemedicine in this case.

PR: Do you have any summarizing thoughts about the case?

VT: Having a process in place in any community to deal with acute stroke patients is vitally important. In this case, though the outcome was poor, care went very smoothly. There was discussion between the wife and the emergency physician, as well as with the neurocritical care stroke team. The wife wanted to proceed, and the patient was taken to MRI immediately. This revealed the pontine infarction and the vertebral artery stenosis. We were able to eventually lower the blood pressure using the nipride drip, and to give fibrinolytic therapy, and admit the patient to the neurocritical care unit. We could anticipate from the initial presentation that he would not improve, and subsequently several discussions with the wife took place regarding long-term morbidity and mortality, eventually a comfort care decision was made. The question always remains whether the decision and discussion should have been made earlier in the ED on the initial presentation, which could have guided us to how aggressive our approach would have been. In a patient who we know is likely going to have a devastating outcome, having the discussion initially with the wife, any family members, emergency physicians, and neurostroke team, to really paint a realistic picture with the information we have, may save time, effort, and bring peace to the family.

PR: I agree with Dr Melady, we need to have these discussions early. When we recognize there is likely going to be a bad outcome, it's easy for us to duck the responsibility as emergency physicians, but we really need to hold up our end of the game, and get those conversations started.

Section III: Concepts

Introduction to geriatric strokes

CVAs, broadly defined as disruption of blood flow to the brain, are in the vast majority a geriatric illness. The terms *CVA* and *stroke* will be used interchangeably throughout this chapter. As life expectancy increases, the very old are expected to become a growing proportion of stroke victims [1, 2]. Comorbidities that commonly develop with age, such as hypertension, diabetes mellitus, atrial fibrillation, vascular disease atherosclerosis, and renal dysfunction, are risk factors for CVA. Prior stroke is the strongest risk factor for having a stroke. In addition, a recent case crossover study by Shin *et al.* finds that the use of atypical antipsychotics, risperidone and quetiapine, in the elderly is a risk factor for CVA [3]. Stroke has long been recognized as an important cause of functional dependence among the elderly (over 80 years of age) [4, 5]. Initial evaluation should include evaluation for possible mimics such as hypoglycemia, hypoxia, confusion, seizures, toxins, neoplasms, subdural hematomas, as well as possible contributing factors, such as atrial fibrillation, recent MI, recent neck manipulation, valvular surgery, and polycythemia among others. Therefore, point of care glucose and hemoglobin, as well as EKG and pulse oximetry measurement, should be performed immediately [6]. Symptoms of CVA range from obvious focal weakness, facial droop, dysarthria, to more vague concerns of weakness, imbalance, and paresthesia. It was previously thought that women are less likely to experience typical symptoms; recent studies have not shown this to be true. Women have been found to have three times the delay in treatment when compared to men, which may be related to the fact that they are more likely to experience somatic symptoms in addition to the classic stroke symptoms, thus confusing the clinical picture [7].

Hemorrhagic versus ischemic stroke

While the clinical presentation of hemorrhagic versus ischemic stroke may be quite similar and is based on the cerebral distribution of inadequate blood flow, differentiating between the two is imperative to tailor appropriate, time-sensitive management. Approximately 80% of all strokes are ischemic secondary to thrombotic, embolic or hypoperfusion etiologies. Hemorrhagic strokes represent approximately 20% of strokes and can be traumatic or atraumatic, such as with a subarachnoid hemorrhage [8]. Hemorrhagic strokes are more often associated with headache than ischemic strokes [9]. A head CT scan and an MRI without contrast are generally the first imaging modalities if a supratentorial CVA is suspected, whereas an MRI is the appropriate imaging modality for suspected posterior fossa CVA. The cerebellum and brainstem are suboptimally visualized on CT, and this is therefore neither a sensitive nor a specific study to identify and rule out posterior circulation CVAs [10].

NIH stroke scale

The NIH stroke scale (NIHSS) is a preferred diagnostic tool used to identify evidence of stroke and predict prognosis. It involves evaluation for level of consciousness, orientation, ability to follow commands, gaze palsy, visual field deficits, facial palsy, upper and lower extremity weakness, ataxia, sensory deficit, aphasia, dysarthria, and neglect [11]. A score of zero indicates no stroke present. A score of 1–4 suggests a mild stroke; 5–15 is considered a moderate stroke; 16–20 is a moderate to severe stroke, whereas 21–42 is considered a severe stroke. NIHSS is a preferred stroke scale as it has been shown to predict 3-month outcomes, and scores have been shown to correlate fairly well with the volume of brain affected by stroke [12, 13]. Studies show that thrombolysis in patients with NIHSS scores of 5–24 confers improved outcomes. While extremes of NIHSS scores may benefit from thrombolysis, the data is less conclusive for these patients [14]. When considering thrombolysis, extremes of the NIHSS score should not be used as the sole contraindication to administering tPA, as it was found in a 2002 study to inconsistently correlate with severity/volume of brain involved in right hemispheric stroke. In such cases, MRI more accurately demonstrates the severity of stroke. Obtaining an emergent MRI, if available, can help guide management in this situation [15]. In addition, the NIHSS score may be elevated in patients with prior stroke whose acute presentation is attributable to toxic or metabolic etiology [6].

Types of strokes

Anterior cerebral artery (ACA) infarction

Anterior cerebral artery (ACA) infarction results in contralateral sensory and motor deficit in the contralateral lower extremity, sparing the hand and face. Right-sided ACA occlusion results in confusion and motor hemineglect, whereas left-sided lesions result in akinetic mutism and transcortical motor aphasia [16].

Lacunar infarction

Hypertension and increasing age are associated with lacunar infarcts, which cause purely sensory or purely motor symptoms. The prognosis is considered better than other stroke syndromes, and the presentation may be subtle and subacute [17]. This is also a common incidental finding on neuroimaging in the geriatric population.

Cervical artery dissection

More common in younger and middle-aged people, this condition is associated with unilateral neck or head/face pain, a neurologic deficit that is either transient or persistent, a partial Horner's syndrome with miosis and ptosis, neck manipulation or trauma, connective tissue disease, or history of migraine headaches. Dissection occurs due to trauma to a vessel or an intrinsic defect. Carotid artery dissection and vertebral artery dissection have distinct presentations with associated neurologic deficits representing disruption of anterior and posterior circulation, respectively. Diagnostic imaging including MRI/MRA (magnetic resonance imaging/magnetic resonance angiogram) and CT/CTA (computed tomography/computed tomography angiography) are radiologic studies of choice [18].

Middle cerebral artery stroke

This includes both Broca's and Wernicke's areas, the centers for expressive and receptive speech, respectively. Aphasia is a common finding in middle cerebral artery (MCA) disruption if the dominant hemisphere is affected. Motor regions are also commonly involved, resulting in hemiparesis, sensory loss, and facial plegia in the contralateral side. This is the most common vessel implicated in stroke. Presentation varies based on hemisphere affected. Right-hand-dominant and 80% of left-hand-dominant people have a dominant left hemisphere. Findings common in nondominant MCA disruption include hemineglect, dysarthria, and inattention. Homonymous hemianopsia and gaze preference toward the affected side can be seen with either dominant or nondominant infarcted MCA [19]. The mortality is 41–79% without intervention [20].

Posterior cerebral artery stroke

Posterior cerebral artery (PCA) infarct, representing 5–10% of ischemic strokes, classically presents with unilateral headache, visual field deficits, such as unilateral cortical blindness or contralateral homonymous hemianopsia. Left PCA disruption may cause difficulty reading, whereas right PCA infarct may cause visual neglect and disorientation for place. Amnesia may result from bilateral PCA infarcts. Motor function is minimally affected [21].

Posterior circulation stroke

Posterior circulation strokes in the elderly can present as mimics of benign disease with vague nonspecific symptoms that can easily lead to misdiagnosis in the ED [22–24]. Elderly patients may present with sudden onset of "dizziness" that may be attributed to nonspecific symptoms or peripheral vertigo, vomiting that may be attributed to gastroenteritis, hearing loss that may be attributed to a nonvascular cochlear issue, or "blurred vision" that may be attributed to aging eyes or nonspecific visual changes. These patients should be carefully screened for posterior circulation strokes and examined accordingly.

Strokes are found at the same rate among patients who use the nonspecific term of *dizziness* as in those who use the more specific term of *vertigo* [25]. Caution has to be exercised in elderly patients presenting with what appears to be isolated vertigo. As many as 25% of elderly patients with risk factors for stroke who present to an emergency medical setting with isolated, severe vertigo, nystagmus, and postural instability have an infarction of the inferior cerebellum [26]. The abrupt onset of isolated vertigo lasting for minutes in a person with risk factors for stroke suggests a transient ischemic attack (TIA) in the vertebrobasilar system, including transient ischemia of the vestibular labyrinth [27–29]. Isolated sudden

hearing loss in an elderly patient may represent an isolated stroke to the labyrinth and should not be immediately discounted as a nonemergent otological phenomenon. It may be an anterior inferior cerebellar artery stroke and may herald a catastrophic posterior circulation event [30–32]. Key physical examination elements include gait testing (an ambulation trial), visual field testing to confrontation, and a complete cerebellar examination [33]. Acute unilateral disorders of the peripheral vestibular labyrinth or nerve produce a tendency to lean or fall in one direction, with a tendency to veer to one side during gait testing; whereas patients with acute cerebellar stroke are often unable to walk without falling and direction of leaning or falling on the Romberg test may be variable [34].

Cerebellar infarction

Cerebellar infarction presents with nausea, vomiting, vertigo, ataxia, headache, gait disturbance, drowsiness, and dysarthria. If presentation is delayed, it can present with coma secondary to cerebellar edema [35]. CT has poor sensitivity for this diagnosis but is usually more readily available and therefore the first imaging modality used. MRI is the most sensitive and specific diagnostic tool and should be obtained early in suspected cases [36]. Additional risk factors for hemorrhagic cerebellar infarct include cervical spinal surgery [37].

Vertebrobasilar infarction

Vertigo, cranial nerve palsies, ataxia, weakness, visual disturbances, nausea, limb weakness, and sensory disturbances are common symptoms of vertebrobasilar infarction. Deficits involving ipsilateral cranial nerves and contralateral motor nerves are classic findings [21]. Cervical spondylosis may increase the risk of vertebrobasilar insufficiency [38].

Basilar artery occlusion

Basilar artery infarct, accounting for 20% of ischemic strokes, results in *locked-in syndrome* (when pontine tectum is affected), quadriplegia, and possibly coma. Upward gaze is preserved. Poor outcomes and high mortality of 85–95% are associated with basilar artery infarcts.

Transient ischemic attack

TIAs are neurologic deficits suggestive of cerebral artery occlusion that lasts less than 24 h. Symptoms usually last less than 2 h. Risk factors are similar as those described for stroke. TIAs are a risk factor for stroke, and studies indicate that the 90-day stroke risk after TIA is ≥9.5%, 50% of which may present within 48 h after the TIA. Stroke risk increases with a history of DM, weakness, speech disturbance, hypertension, and symptom duration ≥10 min [39]. Patients with a history of TIA should be managed by their primary care physician on risk reduction medications including clopidogrel and statins. The geriatric patient with TIA should be managed aggressively, if comorbid conditions don't create a contraindication, due to the often devastating quality of life issues from subsequent stroke.

Recognizing a stroke in the elderly patient – the clinical approach to the "stealth stroke"

Elderly patients with stroke tend to present atypically, compared with their younger counterparts. The elderly are more likely to be confused and to have altered mental status or be in a coma, swallowing difficulty, urinary incontinence, language deficits, or paralysis [40, 41]. These symptoms may easily be misattributed to nonneurological clinical entities such as "urosepsis," "over medication," or other common geriatric emergency conditions. If the patient presents in a coma, certain key signs and symptoms may suggest stroke as the etiology of coma. *Pupils*: Absence or abnormality in pupillary reaction suggests an ischemic etiology to coma, whereas normal pupillary reactivity suggests a metabolic (e.g., pharmacological and toxicological) etiology to coma [42–44]. *Posturing*: The presence of posturing and the absence of doll's-eye movements implies an ischemic etiology to the coma, as opposed to a metabolic (e.g., pharmacological and toxicological) etiology to coma [44]. Delirium is frequently an underappreciated abnormality in emergency patients and should be actively screened for in an elderly patient presenting with undifferentiated illness [45, 46]. Delirium is also a frequent presentation of stroke in elderly patients, especially those with preexisting dementia, and is associated with increased mortality [47–49]. Three percent of patients with stroke present with delirium, a delusional state, acute onset of dementia,

or mania mimicking a psychiatric illness. Delirium is seen in patients with right-sided (nondominant) focal strokes in the frontal and parietal regions and in patients with subcortical and limbic involvement. In addition, an inability to perceive or express the appropriate emotional inflection (aprosodia), leading to monotonous speech, may be misdiagnosed as a flat affect [50, 22, 24]. A stroke should be in the differential diagnosis of an elderly patient with delirium or an acute behavioral disturbance, along with the many other causes of delirium and behavioral disturbance.

Treatment

Intravenous thrombolysis

Intravenous thrombolysis, if given appropriately, has been shown to confer benefit. The literature has shown that thrombolysis is less effective in the elderly than in their younger counterparts [51–53]. With regard to hemorrhage risk, data from the ECASS II trial suggests that advanced age is a risk factor for postthrombolysis tPA symptomatic intracranial hemorrhage (although it is noted that this might be related to a correlation with age-related aspirin use) [54]. In addition, a pooled analysis of the seminal ATLANTIS, ECASS, and NINDS rt-PA stroke trials suggests that age is an independent risk factor for postthrombolysis tPA symptomatic intracranial hemorrhage [55]. However, more recent literature and a meta-analysis suggest that the elderly are not prone to higher rates of post-tPA symptomatic intracranial hemorrhage than their younger counterparts [56–60, 53]. Finally, while the elderly have a worse prognosis with stroke in general, literature suggests that elderly stroke patients treated with tPA have a better outcome than those who are not [58]. The severity of the presenting symptoms along with patient and family wishes should be considered when administering thrombolytics. It is often the role of the emergency physician to be a patient and family advocate when communicating with our stroke neurology colleagues to determine which will be the best course of action from a patient-centered perspective.

Intra-arterial and interventional measures

In addition to IV tPA, there is also the option of mechanical embolectomy at certain stroke centers.

211

However, while it is effective for recanalization of an occluded vessel, it has not been shown to have an effect on overall outcome [61–63]. Data specific to the efficacy and safety of mechanical embolectomy in the elderly is conflicting. A smaller review containing 49 elderly patients suggested that the elderly fare worse [64]. On the other hand, a significantly larger review with 1182 elderly patients from a consortium of stroke centers suggests that the elderly do not fare worse [65]. Careful selection for intra-arterial/intervention therapy is indicated, but it appears that the elderly are not inherently at higher risk [66].

Ethical considerations and heroic care in the elderly

While the treatment decision in elderly patients with strokes of moderate intensity is relatively clear, there are still considerations in patients in whom a stroke is considered too minor to be worth the risk of intracranial hemorrhage, or so severe that the potential resultant hemorrhage would be catastrophic. It is important to discuss both of these points with the patient and family early in the care process and communicate this to the involved consulting services and care team.

Minor strokes

Even mild strokes have measurable and significant effects on outcome, especially when cognitive outcome is considered. Ischemic stroke is associated with significant morbidity and an overall 90-day mortality rate of 20–40% depending on the population being studied, and the terms "mild" stroke and "better" outcome are relative to this. About 5% of untreated stroke patients with an NIHSS of 0–3 will have a poor outcome (unable to follow commands, unable to live independently, in a vegetative state, or dead) at 90 days, with about 1% mortality; in patients with NIHSS scores of 4–6 these proportions rise to approximately 12% and 2%, respectively [67]. In absolute terms, a "mild" stroke with an NIHSS of 0–4 points is therefore not inconsequential. It is now established that even patients with mild stroke or rapidly improving deficits, typically excluded from standard reperfusion therapies because of the risks associated with those therapies, do not have a completely benign prognosis [68–70]. Furthermore, when deficits beyond simple motor ability and activities of daily living are evaluated, the sequelae of mild strokes

become even more significant. Edwards prospectively and specifically assessed the impact of mild stroke (defined as a NIHSS score ≤5) at 6 months, with standard assessments of function, health-related well-being, and activity participation, and found an 87% prevalence of dysfunction (including impaired executive function and impaired attention) despite full independence in basic activities of daily living [71], a theme echoed from prior studies [72, 73].

The correlation between NIHSS score and post-tPA symptomatic intracranial hemorrhage has been an established connection since the seminal NINDS. Mild strokes are less likely to bleed with thrombolytic therapy [74]. However, the above are primarily considerations in younger, high-functioning patients, and many elderly patients present with poor premorbid function (e.g., advanced dementia and relative immobility) in which the decision to treat with thrombolytics has to be a carefully considered one that takes into account the potential gain in the context of potential risk.

Severe strokes

Severe strokes are more likely to bleed with thrombolytic therapy and with intra-arterial therapy [75]. A meta-analysis of neurointerventional therapy trials shows that interventional therapy is significantly more likely to be futile in patients with advanced age [76]. However, catheter-based thrombolytic or mechanical therapy can be considered on a compassionate basis [66]. An example of this would be a vertebrobasilar/basilar occlusion (VBO). Untreated VBOs have a high mortality (40–80%) and typically leave patients with a profound debility, especially if they are elderly [77]. Interventional therapy can have a significant impact on recanalization and outcome [78, 79] although intravenous tPA may also be effective [80].

Prognosis

Important in the outcome of elderly stroke patients is the consideration of transfer to a stroke center. There are two types: Primary Stroke Centers (PSCs) and Comprehensive Stroke Centers (CSCs). PSCs are sites with acute stroke teams, stroke units, written care protocols, and an integrated emergency response system, as well as the availability and interpretation of cranial CT scans around the clock [81], and have been shown to decrease door to needle times and rapidity of treatment [82]. CSCs, in addition, have (1) specific expertise in neurosurgery and vascular neurology, (2) advanced neuroimaging capabilities such as MRI and cerebral angiography, (3) surgical and endovascular capability, and (4) other stroke-specific infrastructure such as an intensive care unit [83]. They have been shown to neutralize irregularities in care related to weekend coverage [84], to reduce length of stay, and to improve clinical outcomes related to critical care [85–87]. They also provide dedicated neurorehabilitation services, and as a whole are recommended for patients with large strokes and significant comorbidity, a consideration that naturally extends to the elderly [82]. Elderly patients with large strokes may benefit from a transfer to a CSC if indicated.

Unfortunately, the elderly fare worse with a stroke than their younger counterparts [88–90]. There are reports indicating that 50% of elderly stroke patients are either dependent or dead 6 months after stroke [91]. The poorer prognosis seen in elderly patients may be influenced by the fact that they are worked up and treated less aggressively (*significantly* less likely to have MRIs, ECHOs, angiograms, and neurosurgery) resulting in a self-fulfilling prophecy [40]. A striking prospective cohort study by Bell *et al.* finds that in older women, prestroke obesity is associated with a better outcome. Factors associated with worse poststroke mortality include diabetes mellitus, active smoking, low physical activity, and the lowest physical function quartile [92]. Guo *et al.* also find that renal dysfunction and prior stroke are associated with increased mortality [93]. Weiss *et al.* find that worse mortality is seen with advanced age (>75), female gender, comorbidity of congestive heart failure, and average systolic blood pressure of >160 mm Hg within the first 24 h after stroke onset [94]. Outcome is directly related to the time of onset to intervention, and, therefore, early recognition of stroke symptoms is key to prognosis.

Conclusion

Stroke care in the elderly requires an organized and collaborative effort. Outcomes in higher risk patients can be very poor, and the known interventions can do more harm than good. Communication with consultants and family is of utmost important when stroke is suspected. Stroke mimics need to be carefully evaluated and considered, and geriatric patients can often present with vague symptoms. Community awareness, access to primary care, and public health education are therefore imperative to improving stroke outcomes in all age groups, especially the elderly.

Section IV: Decision-making

- The presentation of stroke in the geriatric population is varied.
- Obtaining a detailed and rapid history, last known normal time, and patient/family wishes can help guide in management.
- Stroke prevention in TIA and atrial fibrillation patients should be managed closely by primary care physicians and necessary specialists.
- Stroke centers can provide a multidisciplinary approach to stroke care for the elderly, but community hospitals can initiate care.
- Lytic therapy is controversial and should be discussed on a case-by-case basis.
- Stroke mimics should be carefully evaluated in the elderly, along with nonspecific symptoms that could be suggestive of acute stroke.

References

1 Feigin, V.L., Lawes, C.M.M., Bennett, D.A., and Anderson, C.S. (2003) Stroke epidemiology: a review of population-based studies of incidence, prevalence, and case-fatality in the late 20th century. *Lancet Neurol.*, **2** (1), 43–53.

2 Rothwell, P.M., Coull, A.J., Silver, L.E. *et al.* (2005) Population-based study of event-rate, incidence, case fatality, and mortality for all acute vascular events in all arterial territories (Oxford Vascular Study). *Lancet*, **366** (9499), 1773–1783.

3 Shin, J.Y., Choi, N.K., Jung, S.Y. *et al.* (2013) Risk of ischemic stroke with the use of risperidone, quetiapine and olanzapine in elderly patients: a population-based, case-crossover study. *J. Psychopharmacol.*, **27** (7), 638–644.

4 Silliman, R.A., Wagner, E.H., and Fletcher, R.H. (1987) The social and functional consequences of stroke for elderly patients. *Stroke*, **18** (1), 200–203.

5 Marini, C., Baldassarre, M., Russo, T. *et al.* (2004) Burden of first-ever ischemic stroke in the oldest old: evidence from a population-based study. *Neurology*, **62** (1), 77–81.

6 Hand, P.J., Kwan, J., Lindsey, R.I. *et al.* (2006) Distinguishing between stroke and mimic at the bedside: the brain attack study. *Stroke*, 37, 769–775.

7 Stuart-Shor, E.M., Wellenius, G.A., DelloIacono, D.M., and Mittleman, M.A. (2009) Gender differences in presenting and prodromal stroke symptoms. *Stroke*, 40, 1121–1126.

8 Van der Worp, H.B. and Van Gijn, J. (2007) Acute ischemic stroke. *N. Engl. J. Med.*, 357, 572–579.

9 Goddeau, R.P. and Alhazzani, A. (2013) Headache in stroke: a review. *Headache: J. Head Face Pain*, 53 (6), 1019–1022.

10 Hwang, D.Y., Silva, G.S., Furie, K.L., and Greer, D.M. (2012) Comparative sensitivity of computed tomography vs. magnetic resonance imaging for detecting acute posterior fossa infarct. *J. Emerg. Med.*, 42 (5), 559–565.

11 National Institute of Health *National Institute of Neurological Disorders and Stroke. Stroke Scale*, http://www.ninds.nih.gov/doctors/NIH_Stroke_Scale.pdf (accessed 25 August 2015).

12 Weimar, C., Konig, I., Kraywinkel, K. *et al.* (2012) Age and national institutes of health stroke scale score within 6 hours after onset are accurate predictors of outcome after cerebral ischemia – Development and external validation of prognostic models. *Stroke*, 35 (1), 158–162.

13 Glymour, M., Berkman, L., Ertel, K. *et al.* (2007) Lesion characteristics, NIH stroke scale, and functional recovery after stroke. *Am. J. Phys. Med. Rehabil.*, 86 (9), 725–733.

14 Mishra, N.K., Lyden, P., Grotta, J.C., and Lees, K.R. (2010) Thrombolysis is associated with consistent functional improvement across baseline stroke severity: a comparison of outcomes in patients from the virtual international stroke trials archive (VISTA). *Stroke*, 41, 2612–2617.

15 Fink, J.N., Selim, M.H., Kumar, S. *et al* (2002) Is the association of National Institutes of Health Stroke Scale scores and acute magnetic resonance imaging stroke volume equal for patients with right and left hemisphere ischemic stroke? *Stroke*, 33, 954–958.

16 Barnett, H.J. and Vinuela, F. (1983) Occurrence and mechanisms of occlusion of the anterior cerebral artery. *Stroke*, 14, 952–959.

17 Pantoni, L., Fierini, F., and Poggesi, A. (2014) Thrombolysis in acute stroke patients with cerebral small vessel disease. *Cerebrovasc. Dis.*, 37, 5–13.

18 Shea, K. and Stahmer, S. (2012) Carotid and vertebral arterial dissections in the emergency department. *Emerg. Med. Pract.*, 14 (4), 1–23.

19 Lewandowski, C.A., Rao, C.P., and Silver, B. (2008) Transient ischemic attack: definitions and clinical presentations. *Ann. Emerg. Med.*, 52 (2), S7–S16.

20 Park, B.S., Kang, C.W., Kwon, H.J. *et al.* (2013) Endovascular mechanical thrombectomy in basilar artery occlusion: initial experience. *J. Cerebrovasc. Endovasc. Neurosurg.*, 15 (3), 137–144.

21 Cereda, C. and Carrera, E. (2012) Posterior cerebral artery territory infarctions. *Front. Neurol. Neurosci.*, 30, 128–131.

22 Huff, J.S. (2002) Stroke mimics and chameleons. *Emerg. Med. Clin. North Am.*, 20 (3), 583–595.

23 Savitz, S.I., Caplan, L.R., and Edlow, J.A. (2007) Pitfalls in the diagnosis of cerebellar infarction. *Acad. Emerg. Med.*, 14 (1), 63–68.

24 Edlow, J.A. and Selim, M.H. (2011) Atypical presentations of acute cerebrovascular syndromes. *Lancet Neurol.*, 10 (6), 550–560.

25 Kerber, K.A., Brown, D.L., Lisabeth, L.D. *et al.* (2006) Stroke among patients with dizziness, vertigo, and imbalance in the emergency department: a population-based study. *Stroke*, 37 (10), 2484–2487.

26 Norrving, B., Nagnusson, M., and Holtas, S. (1995) Isolated acute vertigo in the elderly; vestibular or vascular disease? *Acta Neurol. Scand.*, 91, 43–48.

27 Grad, A. and Baloh, R.W. (1989) Vertigo of vascular origin. Clinical and electronystagmographic features in 84 cases. *Arch. Neurol.*, 46, 281–284.

28 Fisher, C.M. (1967) Vertigo in cerebrovascular diseases. *Arch. Otolaryngol.*, 85, 529–534.

29 Gomez, C.R., Cruz-Flores, S., Malkoff, M.D. *et al.* (1996) Isolated vertigo as a manifestation of vertebrobasilar ischemia. *Neurology*, 47, 94–97.

30 Lee, H., Whitman, G.T., Lim, J.G. *et al.* (2001) Bilateral sudden deafness as a prodrome of anterior inferior cerebellar artery infarction. *Arch. Neurol.*, 58 (8), 1287–1289.

31 Lee, H., Sohn, S.I., Jung, D.K. *et al.* (2002) Sudden deafness and anterior inferior cerebellar artery infarction. *Stroke*, 33 (12), 2807–2812.

32 Lee, H. (2008) Sudden deafness related to posterior circulation infarction in the territory of the nonanterior inferior cerebellar artery: frequency, origin, and vascular topographical pattern. *Eur. Neurol.*, 59 (6), 302–306.

33 Chase, M., Joyce, N.R., Carney, E. *et al.* (2012) ED patients with vertigo: can we identify clinical factors associated with acute stroke? *Am. J. Emerg. Med.*, 30 (4), 587–591.

34 Hotson, J.R. and Baloh, R.W. (1998) Acute vestibular syndrome. *N. Engl. J. Med.*, 339 (10), 680–685.

35 Searls, D.E., Pazdera, L., Korbel, E. *et al.* (2012) Symptoms and signs of posterior circulation ischemia in the New England medical center posterior circulation registry. *Arch. Neurol.*, 69 (3), 346–351.

36 Mostofi, K. (2013) Neurosurgical management of massive cerebellar infarct outcome in 53 patients. *Surg. Neurol. Int.*, **4**, 28.

37 Huang, P.H., Wu, J.C., Cheng, H. *et al.* (2013) Remote cerebellar hemorrhage after cervical spinal surgery. *J. Chin. Med. Assoc.*, **76** (10), 593–598.

38 Denis, D.J., Shedid, D., Shehadeh, M. *et al.* (2013) Cervical spondylosis: a rare and curable cause of vertebrobasilar insufficiency. *Eur. Spine J.*

39 Siket, M.S. and Edlow, J.A. (2012) Transient ischemic attack: reviewing the evolution of the definition, diagnosis, risk stratification, and management for the emergency physician. *Emerg. Med. Clin. North Am.*, **30** (3), 745–770.

40 Di Carlo, A., Lamassa, M., Pracucci, G. *et al.* (1999) Stroke in the very old: clinical presentation and determinants of 3-month functional outcome: a European perspective. European BIOMED Study of Stroke Care Group. *Stroke*, **30** (11), 2313–2319.

41 Carlberg, B., Sundström, G., and Asplund, K. (1992) Stroke in the elderly observations in a population-based sample of hospitalized patients. *Cerebrovasc. Dis.*, **2** (3), 152–157.

42 Malik, K. and Hess, D.C. (2002) Evaluating the comatose patient. Rapid neurologic assessment is key to appropriate management. *Postgrad. Med.*, **111** (2), 38–40.

43 Tokuda, Y., Nakazato, N., and Stein, G. (2003) Pupillary evaluation for differential diagnosis of coma. *Postgrad. Med. J.*, **79** (927), 49–51.

44 Bateman, D. (2001) Neurologic assessment of coma. *J. Neurol. Neurosurg. Psychiatry*, **71** (**Suppl. 1**), i13–i17.

45 Han, J.H. and Wilber, S.T. (2013) Altered mental status in older patients in the emergency department. *Clin. Geriatr. Med.*, **29** (1), 101–136.

46 Han, J.H., Zimmerman, E.E., Cutler, N. *et al.* (2009) Delirium in older emergency department patients: recognition, risk factors, and psychomotor subtypes. *Acad. Emerg. Med.*, **16** (3), 193–200.

47 Sheng, A.Z., Shen, Q., Cordato, D. *et al.* (2006) Delirium within three days of stroke in a cohort of elderly patients. *J. Am. Geriatr. Soc.*, **54** (8), 1192–1198.

48 Oldenbeuving, A.W., de Kort, P.L., Jansen, B.P. *et al.* (2011) Delirium in the acute phase after stroke: incidence, risk factors, and outcome. *Neurology*, **76** (11), 993–999.

49 McManus, J., Pathansali, R., Hassan, H. *et al.* (2009) The course of delirium in acute stroke. *Age Ageing*, **38** (4), 385–389.

50 Huffman, J. and Stern, T.A. (2003) Acute psychiatric manifestations of stroke: a clinical case conference. *Psychosomatics*, **44** (1), 65–75.

51 Heuschmann, P.U., Kolominsky-Rabas, P.L., Roether, J. *et al.* (2004) Predictors of in-hospital mortality in patients with acute ischemic stroke treated with thrombolytic therapy. *J. Am. Med. Assoc.*, **292** (15), 1831–1838.

52 Mouradian, M.S., Senthilselvan, A., Jickling, G. *et al.* (2005) Intravenous rt-PA for acute stroke: comparing its effectiveness in younger and older patients. *J. Neurol. Neurosurg. Psychiatry*, **76** (9), 1234–1237.

53 Bhatnagar, P., Sinha, D., Parker, R.A. *et al.* (2011) Intravenous thrombolysis in acute ischaemic stroke: a systematic review and meta-analysis to aid decision making in patients over 80 years of age. *J. Neurol. Neurosurg. Psychiatry*, **82** (7), 712–717.

54 Larrue, V., von Kummer, R.R., Müller, A., and Bluhmki, E. (2001) Risk factors for severe hemorrhagic transformation in ischemic stroke patients treated with recombinant tissue plasminogen activator: a secondary analysis of the European-Australasian Acute Stroke Study (ECASS II). *Stroke*, **32** (2), 438–441.

55 Hacke, W., Donnan, G., Fieschi, C. *et al.* (2004) Association of outcome with early stroke treatment: pooled analysis of ATLANTIS, ECASS, and NINDS rt-PA stroke trials. *Lancet*, **363** (**9411**), 768–774.

56 Berrouschot, J., Röther, J., Glahn, J. *et al.* (2005) Outcome and severe hemorrhagic complications of intravenous thrombolysis with tissue plasminogen activator in very old (> or =80 years) stroke patients. *Stroke*, **36** (11), 2421–2425.

57 Engelter, S.T., Bonati, L.H., and Lyrer, P.A. (2006) Intravenous thrombolysis in stroke patients of > or =80 versus <80 years of age--a systematic review across cohort studies. *Age Ageing*, **35** (6), 572–580.

58 Zeevi, N., Chhabra, J., Silverman, I.E. *et al.* (2007) Acute stroke management in the elderly. *Cerebrovasc. Dis.*, **23** (4), 304–308.

59 Lansberg, M.G., Albers, G.W., and Wijman, C.A. (2007) Symptomatic intracerebral hemorrhage following thrombolytic therapy for acute ischemic stroke: a review of the risk factors. *Cerebrovasc. Dis.*, **24** (1), 1–10.

60 Pundik, S., McWilliams-Dunnigan, L., Blackham, K.L. *et al.* (2008) Older age does not increase risk of hemorrhagic complications after intravenous and/or intra-arterial thrombolysis for acute stroke. *J. Stroke Cerebrovasc. Dis.*, **17** (5), 266–272.

61 Smith, W.S., Sung, G., Saver, J. *et al.* (2008) Mechanical thrombectomy for acute ischemic stroke: final results of the Multi MERCI trial. *Stroke*, **39** (4), 1205–1212.

62 Mishra, N.K., Ahmed, N., Andersen, G. *et al.* (2010) Thrombolysis in very elderly people: controlled comparison of SITS International Stroke Thrombolysis Registry and Virtual International Stroke Trials Archive. *BMJ*, **341**, c6046.

63 de Weerd, L., Luijckx, G.J.R., Groenier, K.H., and van der Meer, K. (2012) Quality of life of elderly ischaemic

stroke patients one year after thrombolytic therapy. A comparison between patients with and without thrombolytic therapy. *BMC Neurol.*, **12**, 61.

64 Chandra, R.V., Leslie-Mazwi, T.M., Oh, D.C. *et al.* (2012) Elderly patients are at higher risk for poor outcomes after intra-arterial therapy. *Stroke*, **43** (9), 2356–2361.

65 Willey, J.Z., Ortega-Gutierrez, S., Petersen, N. *et al.* (2012) Impact of acute ischemic stroke treatment in patients >80 years of age: the specialized program of translational research in acute stroke (SPOTRIAS) consortium experience. *Stroke*, **43** (9), 2369–2375.

66 Kim, D., Ford, G.A., Kidwell, C.S. *et al.* (2007) Intra-arterial thrombolysis for acute stroke in patients 80 and older: a comparison of results in patients younger than 80 years. *Am. J. Neuroradiol.*, **28** (1), 159–163.

67 Adams, H.P. Jr., Davis, P.H., Leira, E.C. *et al.* (1999) Baseline NIH stroke scale score strongly predicts outcome after stroke: a report of the Trial of Org 10172 in Acute Stroke Treatment (TOAST). *Neurology*, **53** (1), 126–131.

68 Smith, E.E., Abdullah, A.R., Iva, P. *et al.* (2005) Poor outcomes in patients who do not receive intravenous tissue plasminogen activator because of mild or improving ischemic stroke. *Stroke*, **36**, 2497–2499.

69 Rajajee, V., Kidwell, C., Starkman, S. *et al.* (2006) Early MRI and outcomes of untreated patients with mild or improving ischemic stroke. *Neurology*, **67** (6), 980–984.

70 Nedeltchev, K., Schwegler, B., Haefeli, T. *et al.* (2007) Outcome of stroke with mild or rapidly improving symptoms. *Stroke*, **38**, 2531–2535.

71 Edwards, D.F., Hahn, M., Baum, C., and Dromerick, A.W. (2006) The impact of mild stroke on meaningful activity and life satisfaction. *J. Stroke Cerebrovasc. Dis.*, **15** (4), 151–157.

72 Clarke, P.J., Black, S.E., Badley, E.M. *et al.* (1999) Handicap in stroke survivors. *Disabil. Rehabil.*, **21** (3), 116–123.

73 Carlsson, G.E., Möller, A., and Blomstrand, C. (2003) Consequences of mild stroke in persons <75 years – A 1-year follow-up. *Cerebrovasc. Dis.*, **16**, 383–388.

74 Mazya, M., Egido, J.A., Ford, G.A. *et al.* (2012) Predicting the risk of symptomatic intracerebral hemorrhage in ischemic stroke treated with intravenous alteplase: Safe Implementation of Treatments in Stroke (SITS) symptomatic intracerebral hemorrhage risk score. *Stroke*, **43** (6), 1524–1531.

75 Kidwell, C.S., Saver, J.L., Carneado, J. *et al.* (2002) Predictors of hemorrhagic transformation in patients receiving intra-arterial thrombolysis. *Stroke*, **33** (3), 717–724.

76 Hussein, H.M., Georgiadis, A.L., Vazquez, G. *et al.* (2010) Occurrence and predictors of futile recanalization following endovascular treatment among patients

with acute ischemic stroke: a multicenter study. *Am. J. Neuroradiol.*, **31** (3), 454–458.

77 Schonewille, W.J., Algra, A., Serena, J. *et al.* (2005) Outcome in patients with basilar artery occlusion treated conventionally. *J. Neurol. Neurosurg. Psychiatry*, **76** (9), 1238–1241.

78 Hacke, W., Zeumer, H., Ferbert, A. *et al.* (1988) Intra-arterial thrombolytic therapy improves outcome in patients with acute vertebrobasilar occlusive disease. *Stroke*, **19** (10), 1216–1222.

79 Lutsep, H.L., Rymer, M.M., and Nesbit, G.M. (2008) Vertebrobasilar revascularization rates and outcomes in the MERCI and multi-MERCI trials. *J. Stroke Cerebrovasc. Dis.*, **17** (2), 55–57.

80 Schonewille, W.J., Wijman, C.A., Michel, P. *et al.* (2009) Treatment and outcomes of acute basilar artery occlusion in the Basilar Artery International Cooperation Study (BASICS): a prospective registry study. *Lancet Neurol.*, **8** (8), 724–730.

81 Alberts, M.J., Hademenos, G., Latchaw, R.E. *et al.* (2000) Recommendations for the establishment of primary stroke centers. Brain attack coalition. *J. Am. Med. Assoc.*, **283** (23), 3102–3109.

82 Jauch, E.C., Saver, J.L., Adams, H.P. Jr. *et al.* (2013) Guidelines for the early management of patients with acute ischemic stroke: a guideline for healthcare professionals from the American Heart Association/American Stroke Association. *Stroke*, **44** (3), 870–947.

83 Alberts, M.J., Latchaw, R.E., Selman, W.R. *et al.* (2005) Recommendations for comprehensive stroke centers: a consensus statement from the Brain Attack Coalition. *Stroke*, **36** (7), 1597–1616.

84 McKinney, J.S., Deng, Y., Kasner, S.E., and Kostis, J.B. (2011) Comprehensive stroke centers overcome the weekend versus weekday gap in stroke treatment and mortality. *Stroke*, **42**, 2403–2409.

85 Suarez, J.I. (2006) Outcome in neurocritical care: advances in monitoring and treatment and effect of a specialized neurocritical care team. *Crit. Care Med.*, **34**, S232–S238.

86 Rincon, F. and Mayer, S.A. (2007) Neurocritical care: a distinct discipline? *Curr. Opin. Crit. Care*, **13**, 115–121.

87 Suarez, J.I., Zaidat, O.O., Suri, M.F. *et al.* (2004) Length of stay and mortality in neurocritically ill patients: impact of a specialized neurocritical care team. *Crit. Care Med.*, **32**, 2311–2317.

88 Pohjasvaara, T., Erkinjuntti, T., Vataja, R., and Kaste, M. (1997) Comparison of stroke features and disability in daily life in patients with ischemic stroke aged 55 to 70 and 71 to 85 years. *Stroke*, **28** (4), 729–735.

89 Sharma, J.C., Fletcher, S., and Vassallo, M. (1999) Strokes in the elderly – higher acute and 3-month mortality – an explanation. *Cerebrovasc. Dis.*, **9** (1), 2–9.

90 Kammersgaard, L.P., Jorgensen, H.S., Reith, J. *et al.* (2004) Short- and long-term prognosis for very old stroke patients. The Copenhagen Stroke Study. *Age Ageing*, **33** (2), 149–154.

91 Soares, I., Abecasis, P., and Ferro, J.M. (2011) Outcome of first-ever acute ischemic stroke in the elderly. *Arch. Gerontol. Geriatr.*, **53** (2), e81–e87.

92 Bell, C.L., Lacroix, A., Masaki, K. *et al.* (2013) Prestroke factors associated with poststroke mortality and recovery in older women in the women's health initiative. *J. Am. Geriatr. Soc.*, **61**, 1324–1330.

93 Guo, Y., Wang, H., Zhao, X. *et al.* (2013) Relation of renal dysfunction to the increased risk of stroke and death in female patients with atrial fibrillation. *Int. J. Cardiol.*, **168** (2), 1502–1508; S0167-5273(13)00010-7.

94 Weiss, A., Beloosesky, Y., Kenett, R.S., and Grossman, E. (2013) Systolic blood pressure during acute stroke is associated with functional status and long-term mortality in the elderly. *Stroke*, **44**, 2434–2440.

16 Infections

Jason Ondrejka & Scott Wilber

Department of Emergency Medicine, Summa-Akron City Hospital, Akron, OH, USA

Section I: Case presentation

An 81-year-old man presents from a skilled nursing facility (SNF) to the Emergency Department (ED) with a report of low blood pressure. His baseline mental status is alert and oriented to person and place. Today he seems to be more confused, and nurses recorded a blood pressure of 82/50 torr. The patient has no other complaints upon arrival to the ED and was given 500 ml of normal saline by paramedics.

He has a history of Parkinson's disease, prostate cancer requiring prostatectomy, dementia, and coronary artery disease. He has a no cardiopulmonary resuscitation order on his chart.

Upon arrival his vital signs were as follows: temperature 36.7°C pulse 88 beats/min, blood pressure 101/52 torr, respirations 18 breaths/min, and pulse oximetry 96%. He was in mild distress and agitated requiring verbal redirection. The mucous membranes were slightly dry. The cardiopulmonary examination was normal. His abdomen was tender and mildly distended in the suprapubic region. Pulses were 2+ and symmetric. His neurological examination was nonfocal, and he was moving all extremities equally without slurred speech or facial droop. He was oriented to person but not time or place, and had impaired three-item recall. The remainder of his examination was unremarkable.

Two 18-gauge intravenous catheters were placed, and blood cultures drawn. He was incontinent of urine, so catheterization was performed and elicited 550 ml of cloudy urine. He had one episode of hypotension in the ED with a systolic blood pressure

of 90 torr and a mean arterial pressure (MAP) of 60 torr, and was given an additional 1500 ml normal saline bolus. He had stable chronic kidney disease with a serum creatinine of 1.84. His serum lactate was 2.7 mmol/l. White blood cell (WBC) count was 13.8 with 21% bands. Urinalysis showed 2+ leukocyte esterase, positive nitrates, and was "grossly loaded" with WBCs on microscopic analysis. Two hours after presentation, his systolic blood pressure remained above 110 torr with a MAP above 65 torr. A repeat ("delta") serum lactate improved to 2.1 mmol/l, and he was admitted to the medical floor after receiving broad-spectrum antibiotics.

Approximately 16 h after being transferred to the medical floor, the hypotension recurred, and he required further normal saline boluses. Repeat laboratory testing showed a serum lactate of 4.2 mmol/l. His mental status deteriorated, and the physician contacted his family. They requested the patient be kept comfortable rather than have invasive monitoring or mechanical ventilation. The patient died later that night. Urine cultures confirmed Proteus and Enterococcus infections. Blood cultures were negative.

Section II: Case Discussion

Dr. Shamai Grossman (SG): Going back to the case presentation, were there other tests you should have performed prior to the patient going upstairs? Should the patient have had a more robust workup in the ED?

Geriatric Emergencies: A Discussion-Based Review, First Edition.
Edited by Amal Mattu, Shamai A. Grossman and Peter L. Rosen.
© 2016 John Wiley & Sons, Ltd. Published 2016 by John Wiley & Sons, Ltd.

Dr. Amal Mattu (AM): With an elderly patient with signs of infection, one should use a shotgun approach. The key laboratory studies obtained in this case are a lactate level, a metabolic panel, and broad cultures. The rest of the laboratory tests are fairly routine, including the complete blood count (CBC), chemistries, along with a chest X-ray study. Also, if there is altered mental status, I would also obtain a noncontrast computerized tomography (CT) scan of the head. I don't think there would be anything else I would have otherwise added.

SG: What about an electrocardiogram (EKG)?

AM: Yes, I would have obtained an EKG as well to look for potential stress-induced ischemia.

SG: One of the points that Dr Rosen would emphasize is that we should have obtained a fingerstick blood sugar level. This is one of the first labs that should be obtained, which is usually overlooked. Dr Wolfe, what are your concerns when an elderly patient such as this presents to the ED?

Dr. Richard Wolfe (RW): There are two main issues: the first is the hypotension that immediately catches your attention. The approach should be to determine the underlying cause of the hypotension. Certainly, there are a lot of findings that would place sepsis high on your differential. Nevertheless, you should always approach any case on a step-by-step basis to verify this is the case. What we do to verify this is to obtain a rapid ultrasound on arrival to assess the hemodynamics. Do the ultrasound findings suggest a hypovolemic state versus a hyperdynamic state that one would see with sepsis due to the distributive shock, versus pump failure? With a systolic blood pressure of 82 torr, it is evident that there is a component of shock. The first order of business is to understand which type of shock. Once you determine if it's a distributive shock, then one can start moving down the sepsis pathway. The ultrasound study, in this case, would be hyperdynamic, concomitant with a physical examination, looking specifically for jugular venous distension, feeling the extremities to see if they're warm and flushed, which you would also see in this patient with sepsis. This is the first check to make sure that your physical findings are consistent with your working diagnosis. The other issue is the altered mental status. Although the patient has an underlying history of dementia, one has to start wondering about delirium. What we don't do enough of, although there is a trend moving in this direction, is to obtain a delirium screen on these patients. Doing these tests and determining the patient is delirious is a poor prognostic indicator. The mortality is going to be higher, and therefore suggests that you should admit the patient to an intensive care unit (ICU). The question from the testing then is "how far do we work up the delirium especially since you have a source." I agree, I would also obtain a head CT scan. The other question is when would you perform a lumbar puncture on this patient along with the initial workup? Finally, it's reasonable to obtain testing that will allow you to count the number of organs affected, including liver function tests (LFTs), and chemistries for renal function. One of the values that we look at the least that should matter the most is the platelet count. One of the independent predictors of severe sepsis early on is a platelet count of less than 100,000. Finally, a low platelet count is 1 point on the multiorgan failure scale, which gives you an initial assessment of the severity of the patient's condition, underscoring the importance of admission to an ICU, aggressive goal-directed therapy approach as opposed to something more relaxed.

SG: would you have scanned the patient's abdomen?

Dr. Jon Mark Hirshon (JMH): This would be entirely based on how the patient appears from a clinical perspective and palpation of the abdomen. If it's clear, we have a source in the pelvis with a urinary tract infection (UTI), obtaining a scan would depend on the overall patient's response to therapy, their repeat lactate level, and overall clinical course. I would scan the abdomen if I felt that what I saw was not consistent with a UTI.

SG: What would be the key differences in how you would approach a younger patient?

Dr. Michael Winters (MW): One should certainly be more cautious with elderly patients given the increased risk of severe sepsis compared to younger patients. I agree with this management, including the need for adequate vascular access. I would draw focus on the bandemia and the drop in systolic blood pressure, with a MAP below 60 torr. Even a single drop in blood pressure in the elderly is associated with an increase in hospital morbidity and mortality. I agree that after

219

the saline bolus, serial lactate tests and serial ultrasound studies would be fantastic to obtain an overall assessment of his left ventricular (LV) function and the inferior vena cava (IVC). With his history of coronary artery disease, one should combine the cardiac and IVC window with the lung window to look for pulmonary edema. In my approach, I would commence vasoactive agents.

Dr. Ula Hwang (UH): I would have a different approach with this patient. I would not be as aggressive to obtain CT images in this patient. I agree we have to investigate potential cardiac causes of his hypotension. However, infection is usually a sufficient cause. Those are the things that we definitely want to stabilize in the patent when he comes in. This was a very well-managed case, as he was hemodynamically stabilized in the ED. I would also be more aggressive once realizing this is delirium, and that there probably was urosepsis, and that this was driving the patient's delirium. I would be more aggressive in determining what his advanced directives were. I would reach out to the family to determine whether there were any preestablished goals of care. As the population is aging, are we going to be doing a full body scan on everyone who comes in with hypotension, and send everyone to the unit? These are issues that as a group, healthcare clinicians have to resolve. What can we do early on in the ED that will ultimately change how the patient is going to be managed upstairs? If one would be able to stabilize the hypotension and sepsis to see if the mental status improves, do we necessarily need to go down the route of a body scan and ICU? This patient was stabilized in the ED and did not have to go to the ICU. The family was later brought in to discuss the goals of care. Could this have been done earlier in the ED setting? These are things we need to consider.

SG: Daniel Callahan, who is now emeritus director of the Hastings Center for Ethics, published an editorial last week in the New York Times in which he said that we are not obligated to help older people become older. In fact, our duty might even be the reverse, to allow death to have its day. What do you think? Is there merit in what he says? Should we really be doing all this for this patient, after all he is 81 years old.

RW: The reason why it's a complex problem is that, first of all, there is no question we are already doing too much for the elderly population. And if one looks at the cost of health care delivered in this country, and tries to find out what we are doing differently and where are we using most of these expenses, the largest proportion is in the last months of care. The issue is "how do we stop" and figure out where we draw the line. From an ethical standpoint, if the person has a quality of life you can preserve, and you are going to restore them to a point where they still have life to enjoy, then it's our duty to look out for the patient more than to look out for society. Second of all, there are obviously legal ramifications if you fail to perform standard of care, and if you have a delayed diagnosis or an incorrect one, there is a high probability of becoming the plaintiff in a malpractice law suit. The other issue is communication and thresholds. We need to be better able to allow the patient's wishes to be expressed, and be held to it. How many times have we worked a shift where a patient who was a do not resuscitate (DNR) has their DNR reversed by family, requiring absolutely everything. When are we going to reach a point the patient is a Do Not Scan, because we are not going to act on the findings of a chronic subdural or a small bleed. Where is the real danger in terms of the test itself, radiation which is itself hard to quantify, or similarly that of intravenous contrast? It would be helpful to have pretemplated rules to guide the providers when to say yes and how much should be done. After the fact, it's easy to criticize what was done, or worse, what wasn't done.

In this case, you have a cause that could potentially explain the delirium. You are going to be keeping this patient in a supervised environment. Therefore, it is a judgment call how far you go. It depends on who you hand your patient off to and how much you trust your downstream care. How much further investigation can be moved to the inpatient setting given our EDs tend to be crowded? The workup can take place in the inpatient setting just as well.

Dr. Peter Rosen (PR): The crux of the problem whether or not you accept the recommendations of the ethicists, who are never at risk for carrying out the policy they advise, is that the physicians by themselves cannot be the ones to decide what is an acceptable amount of care to be delivered.

In most societies, the relatives of the patient have to assume some of the financial burden of "all out" care, as well as some of the work of delivering it. In our society, we can demand that others provide the work and the financing of our relative's care. The other difficult issue is to try to define an acceptable quality of life, without knowing what the patient is perceiving or whether the patient is capable of enjoying. Nevertheless, it does appear that much of our ICU overcrowding is produced by trying to do everything for patients whose quality of life is not capable of being improved by any amount of very expensive care.

SG: Would you consider placing the patient in the ICU?

Dr. Scott Wilbur (SW): That was the reason for repeating the lactate levels and keeping the patient down in the ED longer. The idea was that if the lactate did not improve, he would have been admitted to the unit. At the time of the ED visit, we did not have the family available to discuss goals of care. Sixteen hours later, it became clear that the patient would not have wanted aggressive intervention.

RW: A lot of factors need to be considered to make that decision. If you think the patient may benefit from treatment, I think it's reasonable and prudent to be aggressive initially. More than the lactate level, I would look at the platelets and other markers of organ dysfunction, and assess the delirium. Any findings showing multiorgan system failure or if the patient is delirious would show you the patient needs the ICU initially. From there, you can always move patients to a step-down unit. But on the floor, recognition that the patient is worsening is often delayed. We don't have a lot of time to put out the fire of the inflammatory cascade.

SG: The family decided that they wanted to withhold invasive monitoring and ventilation. Do the two seem synonymous to you, or can you differentiate those who need vasoactive agents alone as resuscitation and not intubation?

AM: Oftentimes, people look at things as "all or nothing." DNR is sometimes interpreted as "Do Not Be Aggressive." There is a difference in how far you go in terms of airway management and also in terms of other aggressive interventions. It really should be based largely on the discussion with the family before the patient crashes and needs those interventions. We've all been in a scenario where the patient or family wishes full resuscitation, including chest compressions but not intubation and vice versa.

SG: In this case, given the family wasn't available, would you have intubated, and placed on intensive hemodynamic monitoring including a central line?

AM: It's a tough call. If this patient has severe peritoneal dialysis (PD) and dementia, and a terminal illness, you would be justified if you were to treat with antibiotics and fluids, and not be overly aggressive with mechanical ventilation and the placement of central lines. Practically speaking, if there is no DNR on the chart, and the family cannot be contacted, 90% of the time in my center, we would go all the way and place an arterial line, and central line, and intubate. In our society and our culture because of medical–legal concerns, people have done that. In a more rational society, this patient has a terrible prognosis from which he will not regain full neurological recovery, and we should then try to make this patient as comfortable as possible.

PR: I think we make a mistake when we dictate individual procedures that are no longer allowed, and don't allow the physician any judgment about what may be acute and reversible. I believe it would be a better idea to promise no futile treatment, but concerned, useful, and comforting care.

SG: Do you think this is a terminal illness? Sepsis in the elderly? Where would this fall in the spectrum?

MW: I don't think this is a terminal illness. I think he certainly has a high inpatient mortality. However, I don't think he is terminal. We certainly get patients like this, who may or may not have episodes of transient hypotension, who have evidence of a pneumonia or a UTI, whose lactates are marginal, and who receive broad-spectrum antibiotics, and who do just fine. Where is he in terms of the spectrum of illness? He certainly has a source of infection, transient episodes of hypotension, and with an elevated lactate level that improves with IV fluids. I don't think he's in septic shock yet.

RW: If you had a little more data, you could do a multiorgan failure score, and I suspect his mortality is probably 20–30% in-house. The other issue is that he is going to take a permanent hit. Every time you have septic shock, you don't bounce back completely. He will be worse off once he emerges compared to before he entered. That said, this episode is probably completely survivable with a reasonable quality of life.

SG: Would anyone check with the family and discuss with the family that the patient is on antibiotics, which are going to take 48–72 hours to have full effect and to see if the patient responds, and we should go ahead with the invasive approach for that period? Would this approach be reasonable?

UH: Communication and threshold are important. When we are able to reach family members who are able to represent the patient's and the family wishes, we need to respect and follow those preferences. If the family requests comfort care only, we can't then be aggressive with care. We can advise, but the priority is to respect the family's decision. The counterpart is where the family wishes to reverse the DNR directive. In that situation, our role is to advise and advocate for the patient. We as clinicians can only advise. It's the patient's wish, or the legally appointed healthcare proxy, if the patient is unable to express his or her wishes.

PR: We often forget that relatives cannot legally refuse lifesaving care for a patient unless they have been a court-appointed guardian or legal decision-maker.

SW: I agree that sepsis is not going to be the terminal condition in this patient; with some patients, their underlying comorbidities are the terminal illness. In this case, dementia is a potentially terminal illness. You can look at that and try to determine how severe their underlying illness is, and the likelihood they are going to recover a reasonable quality of life after surviving the current episode. Each time a patient presents with an exacerbation of an underlying disease, their quality of life tends to go down after each acute event.

SG: We are operating under the assumption that deterioration of the current quality of life is going to make a difference to the patient or their family. We assume, if they are not going to be quite the way they were previously, then this should push us to be not as aggressive. We cannot make this assumption on the basis of what we deem is an acceptable quality of life rather than what the patient or family believes acceptable.

JMH: When I approach a case like this, my first approach is to evaluate the patient on a medical basis and to stabilize them. So I start off with a relatively assertive rather than aggressive clinical management perspective. In the process of gathering data, I am going to gather information about the desires and wishes as voiced by them in their paperwork or by the family members. Initially, if the person comes in with urosepsis, I am going to try to treat what is likely going to be a temporary condition but could be fatal, and go forward from there.

UH: We certainly don't impose our values on what we believe the patient should be receiving or what the family should be doing. Our role is to advise and provide accurate facts. I think a lot is based on expectations. We cannot tell the family that aggressive treatment is going to result in complete recovery. The family should be made aware that once any patient is in the ICU, they are at an increased risk of dementia down the line. In addition, mental and cognitive functions will actually decline after an ICU stay. Even after non-ICU hospitalization, older adults will have functional decline.

SG: In addition, I also wanted to mention certain key features endemic to this patient population. First of all, the patient doesn't meet systemic inflammatory response syndrome (SIRS) criteria, which is common in this patient population. Temperature and heart rate (HR) are normal; however, the blood pressure is low. Another factor that I always consider in this patient population is to investigate all possible sources of infection. We frequently look at pulmonary sources and UTIs. However, we also have to look closely at the skin and inside the abdomen. Frequently, we are quick to move to a UTI as the sole etiology.

MW: I would wholeheartedly agree to casting a broad net in a patient presenting with obtundation and delirium. Regarding sepsis, pneumonia is the most frequent cause, so be sure to look in the chest of these patients. Following pneumonia, urinary tract, intra-abdominal, skin and soft tissue, and indwelling catheters round out the top five causes of sepsis. Unfortunately, the blood cultures were negative in this case, as they are in typically one third of the cases. Patients with positive cultures are more likely to have gram-negative infections, with *Escherichia coli*, Klebsiella, and Pseudomonas being the most common isolates. Other important things to note are the thrombocytopenia, the bandemia, a low white count, a low temperature, tachypnea, as well as elevations in bilirubin. These are some other findings that can indicate someone is sicker than they initially appear to be.

Section III: Concepts

Clinical features of early systemic infection/bacteremia

Bacteremia tends to result from disseminated local infection and commonly leads to systemic inflammatory sepsis. Bacteremia in the elderly often presents subtly with fewer clinical signs than in the young, a recurring theme in the evaluation of geriatric infection [1]. We will use the available observational data on bacteremic elderly patients as a framework to discuss the clinical features of infections in adults older than 65.

The most common source of bacteremia in the elderly is genitourinary (GU) infection closely followed by lower respiratory tract infections [2, 3]. *E. coli* followed by staphylococcal species (frequently methicillin-resistant *Staphylococcus aureus* (MRSA)), *Streptococcus pneumoniae*, Enterococcus species, Pseudomonas species, Klebsiella species, and anaerobes are the most common isolates [1]. The risk of multidrug-resistant organisms increases if the patient presents from an extended care facility (ECF) [4].

Bacteremic patients 65–84 years old present with atypical symptoms in 54% of cases and those ≥85 years old in 64%, compared to 36% in those younger than 65 [5]. Atypical symptoms can include malaise, weakness, fall, dizziness, syncope, unsteadiness, immobility, acute incontinence of urine or feces, stroke-like symptoms, and delirium [5, 6]. Ascertaining baseline cognitive function and assessing for an acute change can be a diagnostic clue of delirium from bacteremia, which increases the likelihood of a poor prognosis [1, 2]. Fever tends to be one of the more reliable clinical features, yet is only present in 70% of bacteremic older adults [1]. Fever in bacteremia tends to be protective against mortality in those older than 65, likely resulting from more expeditious treatment [5]. Conversely, lack of fever with bacteremia is associated with increased mortality [7]. Ultimately, the emergency physician must include early systemic infection and bacteremia in a differential diagnosis in those older than 65 with nonspecific symptoms of illness.

The diagnosis of suspected bacteremia in the ED is primarily clinical. Blood culture results are infrequently available to the emergency physician. Promising new technologies are being developed and have the potential to make blood pathogen data available to the emergency physician for a faster diagnosis and more specific initial treatment [8]. Ancillary testing in the ED for systemic infection will be discussed further in the setting of sepsis below.

Patients older than 65 with suspected bacteremia should be started on intravenous antibiotics pending results of blood cultures. Broad-spectrum coverage against both gram-negative organisms (including Pseudomonas species) and gram-positive organisms (including MRSA) is required when treating the elderly patient with suspected bacteremia. Inappropriate empiric antibiotics for bacteremia are more often administered in the elderly leading to increased mortality [9, 10]. Patients older than 65 with suspected bacteremia who are immunosuppressed or have evidence of hypoperfusion (i.e., systemic sepsis) are at high risk of a complicated hospital course, and should have early and aggressive critical care management [11].

Sepsis in the elderly

Sepsis has an overall estimated incidence of 751,000 patients per year preferentially targeting those older than 65 with an overall mortality of 28.6% that increases with age [12]. The number of elderly patients presenting with sepsis is increasing [13]. Those older than 65 have a higher morbidity and need for placement after hospitalization in extended care facilities compared to younger patients [14]. Older adults are thought to have a higher propensity for developing sepsis from the aging of the immune system known as immunosenescence [15]. The most common causes of sepsis in older adults are GU infections and pneumonia infections [16]. Gram-negative organisms are more likely in the elderly as compared to those less than 65 [14].

Table 16.1 Traditional systemic inflammatory response variables and effect of aging.

Parameter	Criteria	Effect of Aging
Temperature	>38°C (100.4°F) or <36°C (96.8°F)	Blunted fever response with more hypothermia
Heart rate	>90 beats/min	Blunted response
White blood cells (WBCs)	>12,000/mm³, <4000/mm³, or >10% bands	Blunted total WBC response, band count more helpful
Respiratory rate	Rate > 20 or $PaCO_2 < 32$ mmHg	More prevalent

From Ref. [22].

Sepsis is defined as the presence of infection together with systemic manifestations of infection [21]. The systemic inflammatory response syndrome (SIRS) is typically how sepsis is first suspected in the emergency department while investigation for a source of infection is conducted. Components of the traditional SIRS such as fever and tachycardia can be blunted in those older than 65, whereas tachypnea and hypothermia are more common (Table 16.1) [5, 17, 18]. Of the traditional SIRS criteria, hypothermia may be the most ominous sign as it has been independently associated with mortality in older adults with sepsis [19]. SIRS has been frequently criticized for lack of specificity in all ages; however, the lack of sensitivity in the elderly, particularly those ≥85 is of particular concern [20]. In 2012, updated sepsis diagnostic guidelines included a broader list of criteria that when present in a patient with suspected infection are used to diagnose sepsis [21]. More clinical criteria will make the diagnosis of sepsis easier in those who present atypically. Concurrent evaluation for end-organ dysfunction is crucial in the evaluation of sepsis. If sepsis is accompanied by evidence of organ dysfunction, the patient has severe sepsis (Table 16.2). Severe sepsis with hypotension despite adequate fluid administration is defined as septic shock [22].

Evaluation for infection and possible sources

Identification of the source of sepsis is frequently possible based on physical examination alone. This examination should include a complete skin examination (including the back, sacrum, and feet), identification of all indwelling medical devices, and careful palpation of the abdomen. In our experience, the most common reason for missing a source of infection not identified by routine diagnostic testing is a failure to perform a complete physical examination. A CBC should always be accompanied with a differential count. Total white blood count is insensitive in the elderly compared to an elevated band count [17, 23, 24]. Newer evidence suggests that elevations of mean cell volumes of neutrophils and monocytes are associated with early sepsis in those greater than 65; however, these values are currently not routinely reported on the CBC differential analysis [25]. Elevated procalcitonin has better sensitivity than total WBC count in the infected older adults, but cannot be used to rule out the diagnosis of infection [3, 26–28]. Chest radiographs and urinalysis with culture will be the highest yield tests. Blood cultures should be obtained peripherally and from indwelling vascular catheters unless placed ≤48 h prior to presentation. Infections requiring source control (i.e., operative removal, debridement, percutaneous drains, and device removal) must be considered in every septic patient such as intra-abdominal infections, soft tissue/bone infections including decubitus ulcers and preexisting vascular devices.

Evaluation of organ dysfunction

In addition to the CBC discussed above, if early sepsis is a consideration, the clinician should also obtain a basic metabolic panel, platelet counts, hepatic function panel, prothrombin time/partial thromboplastin time, and whole blood lactate level to assess for organ dysfunction (Table 16.2). Strict urine output should be monitored, which may necessitate temporary indwelling bladder catheter in those with severe sepsis or septic shock. An arterial blood gas analysis may be useful if concern for acute lung injury exists. Lastly, an EKG is necessary as the septic elderly patient may often have concomitant stress-induced cardiac ischemia or new-onset atrial fibrillation leading to increased risk of organ failure, stroke, and in-hospital mortality [5, 29].

Quantitative resuscitation

The treatment of early sepsis in the elderly should be aggressive [21]. Protocolized sepsis "bundles" may be beneficial in the elderly both in increasing the diagnosis of sepsis and decreasing mortality [30]. Bundles do

Table 16.2 Clinical variables of sepsis, severe sepsis, and septic shock.

Sepsis: Infection, Documented or Suspected, and Some of the Following	Creatinine level increase >0.5 mg/dl
General Variables	Coagulation abnormalities (INR > 1.5 or aPTT > 60 s)
Fever (temperature > 38.3 °C)	Ileus (absent bowel sounds)
Hypothermia (core temperature < 36 °C)	Thrombocytopenia (platelet count <100,000 µl)
Pulse rate >90/min or more than 2 SDs above the normal value of age	Hyperbilirubinemia (plasma total bilirubin >4 mg/dl)
Tachypnea	**Tissue Perfusion Variables**
Altered mental status	Hyperlactatemia (>1 mmol/l)
Significant edema or positive fluid balance (>20 ml/kg during 24 h)	Decreased capillary refill or mottling
Hyperglycemia (plasma glucose >140 mg/dl or 7.7 mmol/l) in the absence of diabetes	**Severe Sepsis: Sepsis-Induced Tissue Hypoperfusion or Organ Dysfunction (Any of the Following Thought to be Due to Infection)**
	Sepsis-induced hypotension
Inflammatory Variables	Lactate level above upper limits of normal
Leukocytosis (WBC > 12,000 µl)	Urine output of <0.5 ml/kg/h for more than 2 h despite adequate fluid resuscitation
Leukopenia (WBC < 4000 µl)	Acute lung injury with PaO_2/FiO_2 <250 in absence of pneumonia or <200 in presence of pneumonia
Normal WBC with >10% immature forms	
	Creatinine level >2.0 mg/dl
Plasma C-reactive protein more than 2 SDs above the normal value	Bilirubin level >2 mg/dl
Plasma procalcitonin more than 2 SDs above the normal value	Platelet count <100,000 µl
Hemodynamic Variables	Coagulopathy (INR > 1.5)
Arterial hypotension (SBP <90 mmHg, MAP <70 mmHg, or an SBP decrease >40 mmHg in adults or less than 2 SDs below normal for age)	
Organ Dysfunction Variables	**Septic Shock: Persistent sepsis-Induced Hypoperfusion Despite Adequate (≥30 ml/kg Fluid Bolus)**
Arterial hypoxemia (PaO_2/FiO_2 < 300)	*SBP*, systolic blood pressure; *MAP*, mean arterial pressure; *INR*, international normalized ratio; *aPTT*, activated partial thromboplastin time; *SD*, standard deviation.
Acute oliguria (urine output <0.5 ml/kg/h for at least 2 h despite adequate fluid resuscitation)	

Adapted from Ref. [22].

lead to higher volume fluid resuscitation and lower vasopressor use [31]. All too often, aggressive therapy such as large volume fluid resuscitation and critical care management are withheld from patients who are very old. Unless patients have advanced directives against aggressive resuscitation, the elderly benefit *more* than the young from such interventions given the increased mortality of the elderly when developing severe sepsis [32, 33].

Septic patients with hypotension after an initial 30 ml/kg bolus of isotonic intravenous fluids or a serum lactate of ≥4.0 mmol/l should receive quantitative resuscitation beginning in the ED. Frequently used goals include central venous pressure 8–12 mmHg, MAP level greater than or equal to 65 mmHg, urine output greater than or equal to 0.5 ml/kg/h, or ScvO2 or mixed Svo2 of 70% or 65% [21]. Serial lactate monitoring in the first 6 hours of treatment is also advocated as an additional tool to quantitative resuscitation.

Broad-spectrum antibiotics should be started within 1 hour of severe sepsis or septic shock [21, 34]. Isotonic intravenous fluids remain the initial fluid of choice; however, the newest guidelines suggest albumin might have a role in sepsis [21]. The elderly commonly have low albumin, and in the face of bacteremia with low albumin, have increased mortality [35–37]. Norepinephrine should be the vasopressor of choice to achieve a MAP of ≥65 mmHg [38]. There is no more important step to the treatment of systemic sepsis than its early recognition.

Lower respiratory infections

Pneumonia is the leading infection in the elderly that accounts for hospital admissions and is the third leading cause of all hospitalizations in those greater than 85 behind heart disease and injuries [39]. It is the eighth leading cause of death in the United States and is on the rise [40]. Those older than 65 are at increased risk of congestive heart failure and cardiac complications when diagnosed with pneumonia compared to younger patients [41, 42]. The pathogenesis of pneumonia typically results from microorganisms in the nasopharynx propagating in the lower respiratory tract causing community-acquired pneumonia (CAP) or healthcare-associated pneumonia (HCAP). Controversy exists regarding the third classification of pneumonia, aspiration pneumonia, and the relationship between microaspiration from physiologic changes of aging in the development of CAP and HCAP [43]. Risk factors for aspiration pneumonia include age, male gender, lung diseases, dysphagia, diabetes mellitus, severe dementia, poor oral health, malnutrition, Parkinson's disease, and the use of antipsychotic drugs, proton pump inhibitors, and angiotensin-converting enzyme inhibitors [44]. Differentiation of aspiration pneumonia is important as it tends to carry a higher mortality rate in the elderly compared to CAP [45].

The elderly less frequently demonstrate specific symptoms such as productive cough, pleuritic chest pain, and shortness of breath; therefore, evaluation for pneumonia in those with isolated delirium, fever, and generalized weakness should be conducted [46, 47]. Nonspecific symptoms both increase the time to diagnosis and mortality in older patients with pneumonia [48, 49]. Part of the evaluation of these patients should be with a posterior–anterior and lateral chest X-ray series. As discussed previously, laboratory diagnostic criteria should be interpreted with caution. Blood cultures should not be routinely obtained in nonsevere CAP [50]. Once the patient is diagnosed with pneumonia, the clinician often translates physical examination and diagnostic data into a prognostic tool for disposition planning.

Debate currently exists between clinical severity scores; however, it seems that in the elderly, the CURB-65 provides adequate prognostication and is easier to use than the pneumonia severity index (PSI) [51–54]. The CURB-65 and PSI should be avoided in the setting of aspiration pneumonia as they are poorly predictive [55].

Community-acquired pneumonia

CAP of bacterial causes in the elderly are most commonly due to *S. pneumoniae* followed by *Haemophilus influenzae*, *Moraxella catarrhalis*, *Mycoplasma pneumoniae*, *S. aureus*, Legionella species, and *Chlamydophila pneumoniae* [56]. The most notable viral cause of CAP is influenza. Hospitalized patients should be tested for influenza, and it is often prudent to initiate oseltamivir treatment with droplet precautions. In those with suspected or confirmed influenza, pneumonia treatment for coinfection with *S. pneumoniae* and *S. aureus* (including MRSA) should be commenced particularly in the patient with a clinical history of respiratory infection that temporarily improved and subsequently worsened [57].

The development of multidrug-resistant *S. pneumoniae* and MRSA largely dictates the antibiotic recommendations of the Infectious Disease Society of America (IDSA): Resistance profiles of *S. pneumoniae* have shown increasing resistance to both macrolides and fluoroquinolones. Macrolide-only treatment of CAP in the elderly is inappropriate for first-line treatment in patients with chronic heart, lung, liver, and renal diseases, diabetes mellitus, alcoholism, malignancies, asplenia, use of antimicrobials within the previous 3 months, immunosuppressing conditions or use of immunosuppressing drugs (risk factors for macrolide-resistant *S. pneumoniae*). Furthermore, severe CAP or in settings where there is suspected fluoroquinolone-resistant *S. pneumoniae*, combination β-lactam and macrolide are appropriate [57].

Increasing prevalence of community-acquired MRSA led to the recommendation to empirically treat hospitalized patients with severe CAP as defined by any one of the following: (1) a requirement for ICU admission, (2) necrotizing or cavitary infiltrates, or (3) empyema pending sputum or blood culture results, with appropriate MRSA agents (vancomycin, linezolid, clindamycin) [58].

Healthcare-associated pneumonia

HCAP is defined as hospitalization for 2 days or more in the preceding 90 days, residence in a nursing home or ECF, home infusion therapy (including antibiotics), chronic dialysis within 30 days, home wound care, and having a family member with a multidrug-resistant pathogen [59]. HCAP therapy is widely debated as controversies exist primarily in the selection of appropriate antibiotic use in these individuals. While there is clear evidence that empiric antibiotic coverage that fails to cover the responsible organism worsens outcomes, there are also a large proportion of patients with HCAP that are not due to a multidrug-resistant organisms [60, 61]. Empiric treatment is aimed at resistant pathogens including MRSA, *Pseudomonas aeruginosa*, Acinetobacter species, and *Klebsiella pneumoniae*. Hospital formularies should have clear options for empiric antibiotic coverage for HCAP patients to initiate in the ED.

Aspiration pneumonia

Aspiration pneumonia is defined as pneumonia from the inhalation of oropharyngeal contents. This is distinct from aspiration pneumonitis in the sense that pneumonitis is noninfectious from the inhalation of sterile gastric contents and is more common in younger patients. Aspiration pneumonia is frequently caused by *S. aureus*, *S. pneumoniae*, gram-negative bacilli, and rarely anaerobes. Anaerobes should be considered more likely in those with poor dentition, or in the setting of necrotizing pneumonia, abscess or empyema [62]. Due to the paucity of literature on aspiration pneumonia, treatment options are less well defined. Options include clindamycin, piperacillin/tazobactam, ampicillin/sulbactam, amoxicillin/clavulanate, or as an alternative carbapenem [57].

Regardless of pneumonia classification, the principles of treatment in the ED include administration of antibiotics as soon as the diagnosis is made after blood cultures have been obtained (if indicated); however, no clear time guideline is recommended in nonseptic patients [50, 63].

Genitourinary infections

Infections of the urinary tract account for nearly 1 million ED visits per year in patients aged 65 or older

[64]. Community-acquired urinary infections are predominantly caused by *E. coli* in the elderly followed by Proteus spp., Klebsiella spp., Enterococcus spp., Enterobacter spp., Pseudomonas spp., and Staphylococcus spp. [65]. Organisms are similar in ECF environments, but differ dramatically in their resistance patterns. While *E. coli* has 11% resistance to fluoroquinolones in the community in the above study, that rate increases to 50–60% resistance in ECF patients [66]. Similarly, resistance to trimethoprim/sulfamethoxazole commonly exceeds 20%, limiting the use of the most commonly prescribed antibiotics for GU infections [67, 68].

The diagnosis of GU infections is challenging in the elderly as they more often lack specific symptoms, and are more likely to have asymptomatic bacteriuria complicating interpretation of commonly available tests [69]. Asymptomatic bacteriuria is present in 20–50% of elderly in ECFs without catheters, and overtreatment is common and associated with development of resistant organisms [70, 71]. Testing begins with a urinalysis that has poor specificity with 48% false positives when compared to urine culture results in a "clean-catch" specimen [72]. Similar poor results are found when using microscopic urinalysis in a general adult population [73]. In a comparison of older adults presenting with and without symptoms potentially related to GU infections, urine reagent strips are not strongly predictive of having a positive urine culture in either group. Even more striking, 14% of asymptomatic patients have a positive urine culture, calling into question the use of the urine culture as a "gold standard" in a patient without a clinical course consistent with GU infection [74].

Catheter-associated UTIs are the leading cause of nosocomial infection in all ages with over 1 million cases every year [75]. Four percent of elderly patients who receive an indwelling urinary catheter (IUC) in the ED without preexisting urinary infection will develop a catheter-associated urinary infection prior to discharge [76]. An approximate 28% of IUCs are probably not needed, and appropriate discontinuation protocols can dramatically decrease this number while shortening duration of hospital admission and development of nosocomial infections [77–80]. Catheter-associated urinary infections are challenging to diagnose given the frequent coexistence of chronic bacteriuria. Diagnosis should be based on urine culture with $\geq 10^3$ cfu/ml, pyuria, plus signs and symptoms of urinary infection. If the catheter has been in place for more than 2 weeks, it should be changed and culture taken from new catheter.

Culture data supersedes any empiric treatment recommendations. For uncomplicated cystitis, first-line treatment includes trimethoprim-sulfamethoxazole if local resistance is no greater than 20%, and nitrofurantoin [68]. Nitrofurantoin is to be used with caution in older patients with a creatinine clearance less than 60 ml/min [80–82]. First-line fluoroquinolone use for cystitis is discouraged except in unique situations [68]. We prefer using a β-lactam such as cephalexin as second-line treatment. In older adults with pyelonephritis, a dose of intravenous antibiotics, preferably ceftriaxone or an aminoglycoside, may be administered as ciprofloxacin is to be avoided when resistance rates exceed 10% [68]. Guidelines are less clear for patients with a catheter-associated UTI. The recommended duration of treatment is 7–14 days depending on clinical response. Empiric treatment should be based on the clinical condition of the patient pending culture results. If a fluoroquinolone is deemed best and the patient is considered "mildly" ill, then levofloxacin is superior to ciprofloxacin [83].

In summary, the diagnosis of GU infections in the elderly must be made based on the combination of diagnostic testing and clinical symptoms. Overtreatment is common in the elderly and better means of testing and defining true infection are needed going forward.

Skin/soft tissue infections

The aging effects to the skin are less important than the comorbid illnesses that lead to peripheral edema and immobility when discussing skin and soft tissue infections (SSTIs) in the elderly. Population data show the highest incidence of SSTIs are in those greater than 65 in direct correlation with their increased prevalence of diabetes [84]. The two most commonly faced clinical presentations of elderly SSTIs are extremity infections and decubitus wound infections.

Extremity skin/soft tissue infections

SSTIs of the extremity include cellulitis/erysipelas, and necrotizing infections [85]. Very little evidence is available specific to the elderly with an

SSTI [86]. *Streptococcus pyogenes* classically is the leading cause of cellulitis; however, culture data shows that β hemolytic streptococci, *S. aureus*, and gram negative species make up 50% of cases in all ages [87]. Furthermore, MRSA is much more common particularly when associated with an abscess or other portal of entry [88]. When considering elderly patients from extended care facilities, the rates of SSTIs from MRSA appear similar to the community [89]. Necrotizing skin infections can be due to one or many gram-positive, gram-negative, or anaerobic organisms [90].

A mindful emergency physician must be aware of the cellulitis-mimics since conditions such as stasis dermatitis and lymphedema are prevalent in this population [91]. Classically, erysipelas is differentiated from cellulitis based on the fiery red, well-demarcated, and edematous appearance. Cellulitis typically is of acute onset of mainly unilateral extremity redness, with tenderness, swelling, and fever [92]. Blood cultures are costly and rarely change treatment even in complicated cellulitis (defined as cellulitis with underlying comorbidities) and therefore should not be routinely ordered [93, 94]. Necrotizing infections include necrotizing fasciitis, pyomyositis, Fournier's gangrene, and clostridial myonecrosis. Due to the life-threatening nature of these infections with an initial presentation that can appear as cellulitis, look for the following: (1) severe, constant pain; (2) bullae, related to occlusion of deep blood vessels that traverse the fascia or muscle compartments; (3) skin necrosis or ecchymosis (bruising) that precedes skin necrosis; (4) gas in the soft tissues, detected by palpation or imaging; (5) edema that extends beyond the margin of erythema; (6) cutaneous anesthesia; (7) systemic toxicity; and (8) rapid spread, especially during antibiotic therapy [88].

Treatment for cellulitis/erysipelas includes antibiotic administration with or without a local incision and drainage. Antibiotic coverage should include MRSA coverage if the portal of entry is suspected, the patient is clinically toxic, or the patient has a history of MRSA. Emergent surgical consultation and broad-spectrum antibiotics are necessary when necrotizing infection is suspected.

Decubitus ulcers/wounds

Decubitus ulcerations are known as a disease of the elderly or those with spinal cord injury. The challenge to emergency physicians is (1) to examine the entire skin when infection is suspected to evaluate for wounds and (2) determine when a decubitus wound infection is clinically significant. Decubitus wounds are frequently colonized with skin flora. Acute infections can include *P. aeruginosa*, Providencia species, and anaerobes [95].

Wounds can be classified as stage 1 (nonblanchable erythema of intact skin), stage 2 (erosion into epidermis/dermis), stage 3 (full thickness skin wound into subcutaneous tissue), and stage 4 (extension into fascia often involving bone and muscle) [95]. Clinically, acute infection is difficult to diagnose. The most reliable indicator of acute wound infection is increased pain at the wound site, nevertheless lack of pain does not rule out infection [96]. While wound cultures are often obtained, they will not aid in the emergent treatment and are frequently difficult to interpret due to high rate of contamination. Blood cultures should be obtained if evidence of systemic toxicity is present. Imaging may be necessary if there is concern for osteomyelitis.

Intravenous antibiotics should be administered if there is suspected systemic infection from an infected decubitus wound [95]. Wound care or surgical consultations should be obtained for evaluation and possible debridement of the wound.

Central nervous system infections

Acute central nervous system infections such as meningitis and encephalitis are challenging to differentiate from delirium due to non-CNS infection in the elderly. The incidence of bacterial meningitis is highest in those older than 65. The median age of bacterial meningitis has been steadily increasing secondary to lifesaving pediatric/adolescent immunizations against pneumococcus, *Haemophilus meningitis*, *Neisseria meningitidis*, and universal Group B strep screening in pregnancy [97]. The most likely pathogens in order of likelihood are *Staphylococcal meningitis*, Listeria species, *N. meningitidis*, gram-negative bacilli with perhaps 25% of cases from unknown pathogens [98]. *Listeria meningitis* is becoming more common in the elderly as pneumococcal meningitis appears to be decreasing in the elderly since the introduction of the pediatric heptavalent pneumococcal conjugate

vaccine (PCV7) in 2000. As expected, cases from pneumococcal strains not included in the PCV7 vaccine, which are increasingly penicillin-resistant, are on the rise [99].

Older adults with meningitis less often have fever, neck stiffness, or rash but more commonly have altered mental status and seizures. One study found that all patients have at least one of the "classic triad" of fever, headache, and altered mental status, whereas only 39% have all three criteria present [100]. Markers of poor prognosis are stupor, seizure, increased age, and inappropriate initial antibiotics [100]. Cerebrospinal fluid (CSF) evaluation is mandatory but should not delay treatment. Since seizures and altered mental status are more prevalent in the elderly with bacterial meningitis, a head CT scan may commonly be performed. Blood cultures have varying utility in bacterial meningitis but may be helpful in determining causative organisms [101].

Empiric treatment is with vancomycin plus a third-generation cephalosporin and ampicillin as soon as possible [102]. Differentiating meningitis versus encephalitis can initially be difficult; therefore, we also recommend acyclovir as soon as possible for the possibility of herpes simplex virus. Steroid administration in pneumococcal meningitis appears useful and may be beneficial in the elderly [103]. Prompt treatment is necessary as patients older than 65 have increased mortality compared to the young [98, 104, 105].

Section IV: Decision-making

- Atypical symptoms such as delirium, falls, weakness, and dizziness are more common presenting symptoms of infections in the elderly than the young.
- Lung and urinary infections are the most common sources of infection in the elderly.
- Careful examination of the skin, abdomen, back, external GU, and any artificial indwelling medical devices may detect infection source not routinely screened by diagnostic testing.
- Early detection and evidence-based, early resuscitation for systemic sepsis in adults older than 65 combined with aggressive therapy may be lifesaving.

- Antibiotic selection should be based on the source of infection, local resistance patterns, and culture data when possible.

References

1 Chassagne, P., Perol, M.B., Doucet, J. *et al.* (1996) Is presentation of bacteremia in the elderly the same as in younger patients? *Am. J. Med.*, **100** (1), 65–70.

2 Rebelo, M., Pereira, B., Lima, J. *et al.* (2011) Predictors of in-hospital mortality in elderly patients with bacteraemia admitted to an Internal Medicine ward. *Int. Arch. Med.*, **4** (1), 33.

3 Caterino, J.M., Scheatzle, M.D., Forbes, M.L., and D'Antonio, J.A. (2004) Bacteremic elder emergency department patients: procalcitonin and white count. *Acad. Emerg. Med.*, **11** (4), 393–396.

4 Gruber, I., Heudorf, U., Werner, G. *et al.* (2013) Multidrug-resistant bacteria in geriatric clinics, nursing homes, and ambulant care-prevalence and risk factors. *Int. J. Med. Microbiol.*, **303** (8), 405–409.

5 Wester, A.L., Dunlop, O., Melby, K.K. *et al.* (2013) Age-related differences in symptoms, diagnosis and prognosis of bacteremia. *BMC Infect. Dis.*, **13** (1), 346.

6 Han, J.H. and Wilber, S.T. (2013) Altered mental status in older patients in the emergency department. *Clin. Geriatr. Med.*, **29** (1), 101–136.

7 Deulofeu, F., Cervelló, B., Capell, S. *et al.* (1998) Predictors of mortality in patients with bacteremia: the importance of functional status. *J. Am. Geriatr. Soc.*, **46** (1), 14–18.

8 Klouche, M. and Schröder, U. (2008) Rapid methods for diagnosis of bloodstream infections. *Clin. Chem. Lab. Med.*, **46** (7), 888–908.

9 Payeras, A., García-Gasalla, M., Garau, M. *et al.* (2007) Bacteremia in very elderly patients: risk factors, clinical characteristics and mortality. *Enferm. Infecc. Microbiol. Clin.*, **25** (10), 612–618.

10 Lee, C.-C., Chang, C.-M., Hong, M.-Y. *et al.* (2013) Different impact of the appropriateness of empirical antibiotics for bacteremia among younger adults and the elderly in the ED. *Am. J. Emerg. Med.*, **31** (2), 282–290.

11 Caterino, J.M., Murden, R.A., and Stevenson, K.B. (2012) Functional status does not predict complicated clinical course in older adults in the emergency department with infection. *J. Am. Geriatr. Soc.*, **60** (2), 304–309.

12 Angus, D.C., Linde-Zwirble, W.T., Lidicker, J. *et al.* (2001) Epidemiology of severe sepsis in the United States: analysis of incidence, outcome, and associated costs of care. *Crit. Care Med.*, **29** (7), 1303–1310.

13 Baine, W.B., Yu, W., and Summe, J.P. (2001) The epidemiology of hospitalization of elderly Americans for septicemia or bacteremia in 1991–1998. Application of Medicare claims data. *Ann. Epidemiol.*, **11** (2), 118–126.

14 Martin, G.S., Mannino, D.M., and Moss, M. (2006) The effect of age on the development and outcome of adult sepsis. *Crit. Care Med.*, **34** (1), 15–21.

15 Opal, S.M., Girard, T.D., and Ely, E.W. (2005) The immunopathogenesis of sepsis in elderly patients. *Clin. Infect. Dis.*, **41** (Suppl. 7), S504–S512.

16 Strehlow, M.C., Emond, S.D., Shapiro, N.I. *et al.* (2006) National study of emergency department visits for sepsis, 1992 to 2001. *Ann. Emerg. Med.*, **48** (3), 326–331, 331.e1–3.

17 Seigel, T.A., Cocchi, M.N., Salciccioli, J. *et al.* (2012) Inadequacy of temperature and white blood cell count in predicting bacteremia in patients with suspected infection. *J. Emerg. Med.*, **42** (3), 254–259.

18 Girard, T.D., Opal, S.M., and Ely, E.W. (2005) Insights into severe sepsis in older patients: from epidemiology to evidence-based management. *Clin. Infect. Dis.*, **40** (5), 719–727.

19 Tiruvoipati, R., Ong, K., Gangopadhyay, H. *et al.* (2010) Hypothermia predicts mortality in critically ill elderly patients with sepsis. *BMC Geriatr.*, **10**, 70.

20 Lee, C.-C., Chen, S.-Y., Chang, I.-J. *et al.* (2007) Comparison of clinical manifestations and outcome of community-acquired bloodstream infections among the oldest old, elderly, and adult patients. *Medicine (Baltimore)*, **86** (3), 138–144.

21 Dellinger, R.P., Levy, M.M., Rhodes, A. *et al.* (2013) Surviving sepsis campaign: international guidelines for management of severe sepsis and septic shock, 2012. *Intensive Care Med.*, **39** (2), 165–228.

22 Jones, A.E. and Puskarich, M.A. (2014) The Surviving Sepsis Campaign guidelines 2012: update for emergency physicians. *Ann. Emerg. Med.*, **63** (1), 35–47.

23 Drees, M., Kanapathippillai, N., and Zubrow, M.T. (2012) Bandemia with normal white blood cell counts associated with infection. *Am. J. Med.*, **125** (11), 1124.e9–1124.e15.

24 Fontanarosa, P.B., Kaeberlein, F.J., Gerson, L.W., and Thomson, R.B. (1992) Difficulty in predicting bacteremia in elderly emergency patients. *Ann. Emerg. Med.*, **21** (7), 842–848.

25 Lee, A.-J. and Kim, S.-G. (2013) Mean cell volumes of neutrophils and monocytes are promising markers of sepsis in elderly patients. *Blood Res.*, **48** (3), 193–197.

26 Stucker, F., Herrmann, F., Graf, J.-D. *et al.* (2005) Procalcitonin and infection in elderly patients. *J. Am. Geriatr. Soc.*, **53** (8), 1392–1395.

27 Lai, C.-C., Chen, S.-Y., Wang, C.-Y. *et al.* (2010) Diagnostic value of procalcitonin for bacterial infection in

elderly patients in the emergency department. *J. Am. Geriatr. Soc.*, **58** (3), 518–522.

28 De Kruif, M.D., Limper, M., Gerritsen, H. *et al.* (2010) Additional value of procalcitonin for diagnosis of infection in patients with fever at the emergency department. *Crit. Care Med.*, **38** (2), 457–463.

29 Walkey, A.J., Wiener, R., Ghobrial, J.M. *et al.* (2011) INcident stroke and mortality associated with new-onset atrial fibrillation in patients hospitalized with severe sepsis. *J. Am. Med. Assoc.*, **306** (20), 2248–2254.

30 Heppner, H.J., Singler, K., Kwetkat, A. *et al.* (2012) Do clinical guidelines improve management of sepsis in critically ill elderly patients? A before-and-after study of the implementation of a sepsis protocol. *Wien. Klin. Wochenschr.*, **124** (19–20), 692–698.

31 El Solh, A.A., Akinnusi, M.E., Alsawalha, L.N., and Pineda, L.A. (2008) Outcome of septic shock in older adults after implementation of the sepsis "bundle". *J. Am. Geriatr. Soc.*, **56** (2), 272–278.

32 Nasa, P., Juneja, D., Singh, O. *et al.* (2012) Severe sepsis and its impact on outcome in elderly and very elderly patients admitted in intensive care unit. *J. Intensive Care Med.*, **27** (3), 179–183.

33 Caterino, J.M. (2008) Evaluation and management of geriatric infections in the emergency department. *Emerg. Med. Clin. North Am.*, **26** (2), 319–343, viii.

34 Puskarich, M.A., Trzeciak, S., Shapiro, N.I. *et al.* (2011) Association between timing of antibiotic administration and mortality from septic shock in patients treated with a quantitative resuscitation protocol. *Crit. Care Med.*, **39** (9), 2066–2071.

35 Greenberg, B.M., Atmar, R.L., Stager, C.E., and Greenberg, S.B. (2005) Bacteraemia in the elderly: predictors of outcome in an urban teaching hospital. *J. Infect.*, **50** (4), 288–295.

36 Tal, S., Guller, V., Levi, S. *et al.* (2005) Profile and prognosis of febrile elderly patients with bacteremic urinary tract infection. *J. Infect.*, **50** (4), 296–305.

37 Burlaud, A., Mathieu, D., Falissard, B., and Trivalle, C. (2010) Mortality and bloodstream infections in geriatrics units. *Arch. Gerontol. Geriatr.*, **51** (3), e106–e109.

38 De Backer, D., Biston, P., Devriendt, J. *et al.* (2010) Comparison of dopamine and norepinephrine in the treatment of shock. *N. Engl. J. Med.*, **362** (9), 779–789.

39 CDC *Products – Health United States – Older Population* [Internet], [cited 2013 Nov 22], http://www.cdc .gov/nchs/hus/older.htm (accessed 2 September 2015).

40 Miniño, A.M. (2013) *Death in the United States, 2011.* NCHS Data Brief No. 115, pp. 1–8.

41 Aliberti, S., Amir, A., Peyrani, P. *et al.* (2008) Incidence, etiology, timing, and risk factors for clinical failure in hospitalized patients with community-acquired pneumonia. *Chest*, **134** (5), 955–962.

42 Corrales-Medina, V.F., Musher, D.M., Wells, G.A. *et al.* (2012) Cardiac complications in patients with community-acquired pneumonia: incidence, timing, risk factors, and association with short-term mortality. *Circulation*, **125** (6), 773–781.

43 Marik, P.E. and Kaplan, D. (2003) Aspiration pneumonia and dysphagia in the elderly. *Chest*, **124** (1), 328–336.

44 Van der Maarel-Wierink, C.D., Vanobbergen, J.N.O., Bronkhorst, E.M. *et al.* (2011) Risk factors for aspiration pneumonia in frail older people: a systematic literature review. *J. Am. Med. Dir. Assoc.*, **12** (5), 344–354.

45 Komiya, K., Ishii, H., Umeki, K. *et al.* (2013) Impact of aspiration pneumonia in patients with community-acquired pneumonia and healthcare-associated pneumonia: a multicenter retrospective cohort study. *Respirology*, **18** (3), 514–521.

46 Riquelme, R., Torres, A., el-Ebiary, M. *et al.* (1997) Community-acquired pneumonia in the elderly. Clinical and nutritional aspects. *Am. J. Respir. Crit. Care Med.*, **156** (6), 1908–1914.

47 Metlay, J.P., Schulz, R., Li, Y.H. *et al.* (1997) Influence of age on symptoms at presentation in patients with community-acquired pneumonia. *Arch. Intern. Med.*, **157** (13), 1453–1459.

48 Marrie, T.J. and Blanchard, W. (1997) A comparison of nursing home-acquired pneumonia patients with patients with community-acquired pneumonia and nursing home patients without pneumonia. *J. Am. Geriatr. Soc.*, **45** (1), 50–55.

49 Ding, Y.Y., Abisheganaden, J., Chong, W.F. *et al.* (2012) Short-term mortality among older persons hospitalized for pneumonia: influence of baseline patient characteristics beyond severity of illness. *J. Hosp. Med.*, **7** (3), 211–217.

50 Nazarian, D.J., Eddy, O.L., Lukens, T.W. *et al.* (2009) Clinical policy: critical issues in the management of adult patients presenting to the emergency department with community-acquired pneumonia. *Ann. Emerg. Med.*, **54** (5), 704–731.

51 Abisheganaden, J., Ding, Y.Y., Chong, W.-F. *et al.* (2012) Predicting mortality among older adults hospitalized for community-acquired pneumonia: an enhanced confusion, urea, respiratory rate and blood pressure score compared with pneumonia severity index. *Respirology*, **17** (6), 969–975.

52 Yandiola, P.P.E., Capelastegui, A., Quintana, J. *et al.* (2009) Prospective comparison of severity scores for predicting clinically relevant outcomes for patients hospitalized with community-acquired pneumonia. *Chest*, **135** (6), 1572–1579.

53 Ochoa-Gondar, O., Vila-Corcoles, A., Rodriguez-Blanco, T. *et al.* (2011) Comparison of three predictive rules for assessing severity in elderly patients with CAP. *Int. J. Clin. Pract.*, **65** (**11**), 1165–1172.

54 Ma, H.M., Tang, W.H., and Woo, J. (2011) Predictors of in-hospital mortality of older patients admitted for community-acquired pneumonia. *Age Ageing*, **40** (**6**), 736–741.

55 Heppner, H.J., Sehlhoff, B., Niklaus, D. *et al.* (2011) Pneumonia Severity Index (PSI), CURB-65, and mortality in hospitalized elderly patients with aspiration pneumonia. *Z. Gerontol. Geriatr.*, **44** (**4**), 229–234.

56 Thiem, U., Heppner, H.-J., and Pientka, L. (2011) Elderly patients with community-acquired pneumonia: optimal treatment strategies. *Drugs Aging*, **28** (**7**), 519–537.

57 Mandell, L.A., Wunderink, R.G., Anzueto, A. *et al.* (2007) Infectious Diseases Society of America/American Thoracic Society consensus guidelines on the management of community-acquired pneumonia in adults. *Clin. Infect. Dis.*, **44** (**Suppl. 2**), S27–S72.

58 Liu, C., Bayer, A., Cosgrove, S.E. *et al.* (2011) Clinical practice guidelines by the infectious diseases society of america for the treatment of methicillin-resistant *Staphylococcus aureus* infections in adults and children. *Clin. Infect. Dis.*, **52** (**3**), e18–e55.

59 American Thoracic Society and Infectious Diseases Society of America (2005) Guidelines for the management of adults with hospital-acquired, ventilator-associated, and healthcare-associated pneumonia. *Am. J. Respir. Crit. Care Med.*, **171** (**4**), 388–416.

60 Brito, V. and Niederman, M.S. (2009) Healthcare-associated pneumonia is a heterogeneous disease, and all patients do not need the same broad-spectrum antibiotic therapy as complex nosocomial pneumonia. *Curr. Opin. Infect. Dis.*, **22** (**3**), 316–325.

61 Falcone, M., Venditti, M., Shindo, Y., and Kollef, M.H. (2011) Healthcare-associated pneumonia: diagnostic criteria and distinction from community-acquired pneumonia. *Int. J. Infect. Dis.*, **15** (**8**), e545–e550.

62 Kikawada, M., Iwamoto, T., and Takasaki, M. (2005) Aspiration and infection in the elderly: epidemiology, diagnosis and management. *Drugs Aging*, **22** (**2**), 115–130.

63 Quattromani, E., Powell, E.S., Khare, R.K. *et al.* (2011) Hospital-reported data on the pneumonia quality measure "Time to First Antibiotic Dose" are not associated with inpatient mortality: results of a nationwide cross-sectional analysis. *Acad. Emerg. Med.*, **18** (**5**), 496–503.

64 Caterino, J.M., Ting, S.A., Sisbarro, S.G. *et al.* (2012) Age, nursing home residence, and presentation of urinary tract infection in U.S. emergency departments, 2001–2008. *Acad. Emerg. Med.*, **19** (**10**), 1173–1180.

65 Katsarolis, I., Poulakou, G., Athanasia, S. *et al.* (2010) Acute uncomplicated cystitis: from surveillance data to a rationale for empirical treatment. *Int. J. Antimicrob. Agents*, **35** (**1**), 62–67.

66 Parish, A. and Holliday, K. (2012) Long-term care acquired urinary tract infections' antibiotic resistance patterns and empiric therapy: a pilot study. *Geriatr. Nurs.*, **33** (**6**), 473–478.

67 Das, R., Perrelli, E., Towle, V. *et al.* (2009) Antimicrobial susceptibility of bacteria isolated from urine samples obtained from nursing home residents. *Infect. Control Hosp. Epidemiol.*, **30** (**11**), 1116–1119.

68 Gupta, K., Hooton, T.M., Naber, K.G. *et al.* (2011) International clinical practice guidelines for the treatment of acute uncomplicated cystitis and pyelonephritis in women: a 2010 update by the Infectious Diseases Society of America and the European Society for Microbiology and Infectious Diseases. *Clin. Infect. Dis.*, **52** (**5**), e103–e120.

69 Matthews, S.J. and Lancaster, J.W. (2011) Urinary tract infections in the elderly population. *Am. J. Geriatr. Pharmacother.*, **9** (**5**), 286–309.

70 Phillips, C.D., Adepoju, O., Stone, N. *et al.* (2012) Asymptomatic bacteriuria, antibiotic use, and suspected urinary tract infections in four nursing homes. *BMC Geriatr.*, **12**, 73.

71 O'Donnell, J.A. and Hofmann, M.T. (2002) Urinary tract infections. How to manage nursing home patients with or without chronic catheterization. *Geriatrics*, **57** (**5**), 45, 49–52, 55–56 passim.

72 Gordon, L.B., Waxman, M.J., Ragsdale, L., and Mermel, L.A. (2013) Overtreatment of presumed urinary tract infection in older women presenting to the emergency department. *J. Am. Geriatr. Soc.*, **61** (**5**), 788–792.

73 Lammers, R.L., Gibson, S., Kovacs, D. *et al.* (2001) Comparison of test characteristics of urine dipstick and urinalysis at various test cutoff points. *Ann. Emerg. Med.*, **38** (**5**), 505–512.

74 Ducharme, J., Neilson, S., and Ginn, J.L. (2007) Can urine cultures and reagent test strips be used to diagnose urinary tract infection in elderly emergency department patients without focal urinary symptoms? *Can. J. Emerg. Med.*, **9** (**2**), 87–92.

75 Foxman, B. (2002) Epidemiology of urinary tract infections: incidence, morbidity, and economic costs. *Am. J. Med.*, **113** (**Suppl. 1A**), 5S–13S.

76 Hazelett, S.E., Tsai, M., Gareri, M., and Allen, K. (2006) The association between indwelling urinary catheter use in the elderly and urinary tract infection in acute care. *BMC Geriatr.*, **6**, 15.

77 Apisarnthanarak, A., Rutjanawech, S., Wichansawakun, S. *et al.* (2007) Initial inappropriate urinary catheters use in a tertiary-care center: incidence, risk

factors, and outcomes. *Am. J. Infect. Control*, **35** (9), 594–599.

78 Shimoni, Z., Rodrig, J., Kamma, N., and Froom, P. (2012) Will more restrictive indications decrease rates of urinary catheterisation? An historical comparative study. *BMJ Open*, **2** (2), e000473.

79 Janzen, J., Buurman, B.M., Spanjaard, L. *et al.* (2013) Reduction of unnecessary use of indwelling urinary catheters. *BMJ Qual. Saf.*, **22** (12), 984–988.

80 Krein, S.L., Kowalski, C.P., Harrod, M. *et al.* (2013) Barriers to reducing urinary catheter use: a qualitative assessment of a statewide initiative. *J. Am. Med. Assoc. Intern. Med.*, **173** (10), 881–886.

81 American Geriatrics Society 2012 Beers Criteria Update Expert Panel (2012) American Geriatrics Society updated Beers Criteria for potentially inappropriate medication use in older adults. *J. Am. Geriatr. Soc.*, **60** (4), 616–631.

82 Oplinger, M. and Andrews, C.O. (2013) Nitrofurantoin contraindication in patients with a creatinine clearance below 60 mL/min: looking for the evidence. *Ann. Pharmacother.*, **47** (1), 106–111.

83 Hooton, T.M., Bradley, S.F., Cardenas, D.D. *et al.* (2010) Diagnosis, prevention, and treatment of catheter-associated urinary tract infection in adults: 2009 International Clinical Practice Guidelines from the Infectious Diseases Society of America. *Clin. Infect. Dis.*, **50** (5), 625–663.

84 Ray, G.T., Suaya, J.A., and Baxter, R. (2013) Incidence, microbiology, and patient characteristics of skin and soft-tissue infections in a U.S. population: a retrospective population-based study. *BMC Infect. Dis.*, **13** (1), 252.

85 Compton, G.A. (2013) Bacterial skin and soft tissue infections in older adults. *Clin. Geriatr. Med.*, **29** (2), 443–459.

86 Kish, T.D., Chang, M.H., and Fung, H.B. (2010) Treatment of skin and soft tissue infections in the elderly: a review. *Am. J. Geriatr. Pharmacother.*, **8** (6), 485–513.

87 Gunderson, C.G. and Martinello, R.A. (2012) A systematic review of bacteremias in cellulitis and erysipelas. *J. Infect.*, **64** (2), 148–155.

88 Stevens, D.L., Bisno, A.L., Chambers, H.F. *et al.* (2005) Practice guidelines for the diagnosis and management of skin and soft-tissue infections. *Clin. Infect. Dis.*, **41** (10), 1373–1406.

89 Zervos, M.J., Freeman, K., Vo, L. *et al.* (2012) Epidemiology and outcomes of complicated skin and soft tissue infections in hospitalized patients. *J. Clin. Microbiol.*, **50** (2), 238–245.

90 Kihiczak, G.G., Schwartz, R.A., and Kapila, R. (2006) Necrotizing fasciitis: a deadly infection. *J. Eur. Acad. Dermatol. Venereol.*, **20** (4), 365–369.

91 Keller, E.C., Tomecki, K.J., and Alraies, M.C. (2012) Distinguishing cellulitis from its mimics. *Cleve. Clin. J. Med.*, **79** (8), 547–552.

92 Bailey, E. and Kroshinsky, D. (2011) Cellulitis: diagnosis and management. *Dermatol. Ther.*, **24** (2), 229–239.

93 Perl, B., Gottehrer, N.P., Raveh, D. *et al.* (1999) Cost-effectiveness of blood cultures for adult patients with cellulitis. *Clin. Infect. Dis.*, **29** (6), 1483–1488.

94 Paolo, W.F., Poreda, A.R., Grant, W. *et al.* (2013) Blood culture results do not affect treatment in complicated cellulitis. *J. Emerg. Med.*, **45** (2), 163–167.

95 Thomas, D.R. (2001) Prevention and treatment of pressure ulcers: what works? what doesn't? *Cleve. Clin. J. Med.*, **68** (8), 704–707, 710–714, 717–722.

96 Reddy, M., Gill, S.S., Wu, W. *et al.* (2012) Does this patient have an infection of a chronic wound? *J. Am. Med. Assoc.*, **307** (6), 605–611.

97 Thigpen, M.C., Whitney, C.G., Messonnier, N.E. *et al.* (2011) Bacterial meningitis in the United States, 1998–2007. *N. Engl. J. Med.*, **364** (21), 2016–2025.

98 Domingo, P., Pomar, V., De Benito, N., and Coll, P. (2013) The spectrum of acute bacterial meningitis in elderly patients. *BMC Infect. Dis.*, **13**, 108.

99 Hsu, H.E., Shutt, K.A., Moore, M.R. *et al.* (2009) Effect of pneumococcal conjugate vaccine on pneumococcal meningitis. *N. Engl. J. Med.*, **360** (3), 244–256.

100 Erdem, H., Kilic, S., Coskun, O. *et al.* (2010) Community-acquired acute bacterial meningitis in the elderly in Turkey. *Clin. Microbiol. Infect.*, **16** (8), 1223–1229.

101 Brouwer, M.C., Thwaites, G.E., Tunkel, A.R., and Van de Beek, D. (2012) Dilemmas in the diagnosis of acute community-acquired bacterial meningitis. *Lancet*, **380** (9854), 1684–1692.

102 Tunkel, A.R., Hartman, B.J., Kaplan, S.L. *et al.* (2004) Practice guidelines for the management of bacterial meningitis. *Clin. Infect. Dis.*, **39** (9), 1267–1284.

103 Borchorst, S. and Møller, K. (2012) The role of dexamethasone in the treatment of bacterial meningitis – a systematic review. *Acta Anaesthesiol. Scand.*, **56** (10), 1210–1221.

104 Cabellos, C., Verdaguer, R., Olmo, M. *et al.* (2009) Community-acquired bacterial meningitis in elderly patients: experience over 30 years. *Medicine (Baltimore)*, **88** (2), 115–119.

105 Lai, W.-A., Chen, S.-F., Tsai, N.-W. *et al.* (2011) Clinical characteristics and prognosis of acute bacterial meningitis in elderly patients over 65: a hospital-based study. *BMC Geriatr.*, **11**, 91.

17 Dizziness and vertigo in the geriatric population

Jonathan Edlow[1] & Alessandro Cancelliere[2]

[1]*Department of Emergency Medicine, Beth Israel Deaconess Medical Center, Harvard Medical School, Boston, MA, USA*
[2]*Department of Emergency Medicine, University of Massachusetts Medical School, Worcester, MA, USA*

Section I: Case presentation

A 75-year-old woman, with a history of hypertension and hypercholesterolemia, presented to the emergency department (ED) with several episodes of dizziness over the past week. She had a history of benign positional vertigo (BPV) that was successfully treated with the modified Epley maneuver. She stated that her current vertigo was different from her prior episodes of dizziness and was also now associated with generalized weakness and blurry vision. Her symptoms lasted several minutes at a time with associated nausea but no vomiting.

Her physical examination was unremarkable, including a negative Dix–Hallpike test and normal fundi. She was able to walk but stated that her legs were weak and that she felt unsteady. Basic laboratory work was unremarkable and an electrocardiogram showed normal sinus rhythm.

Section II: Case discussion

Dr Peter Rosen (PR): When I hear a history like this in an elderly patient, BPV is not the first diagnosis that comes to my mind. Can you give us an idea of the age at which you should start thinking about other diseases than the most benign and what other diseases you should consider?

Dr Andrew Chang (AC): With older adults, we have to be more concerned about central causes of vertigo, such as vertebrobasilar insufficiency, as opposed to the more benign peripheral causes. Although central causes are more common in the elderly, using age alone is not sufficient to distinguish benign causes of vertigo from central causes. A good example is BPV. This is probably the most common cause of vertigo but at the same time its incidence increases with age. I tend to use comorbidities in conjunction with age – if the patient has diabetes, hypertension, atrial fibrillation, and hypercholesterolemia, then I'm obviously more concerned about a central cause of dizziness. Compared to younger patients, one needs to have a broader differential for elderly patients.

PR: Was there anything on the physical examination that might be of assistance in distinguishing between the different diagnoses?

AC: The neurological examination was relatively unremarkable. I did walk her, and she said her legs felt a little weak. The fundi were normal, and a Dix–Hallpike test was negative as well.

PR: One of the elements we frequently omit on our examination in the elderly and perhaps on most, if not all patients, is auscultation of the carotid and vertebral arteries. The presence of a bruit over the vertebral artery might help place

Geriatric Emergencies: A Discussion-Based Review, First Edition.
Edited by Amal Mattu, Shamai A. Grossman and Peter L. Rosen.
© 2016 John Wiley & Sons, Ltd. Published 2016 by John Wiley & Sons, Ltd.

the diagnosis of vertebrobasilar insufficiency in the differential. Bruits are more common than we expect, but we don't find them because we don't listen for them.

Dr Shamai Grossman (SG): We are missing some essential elements to help with the diagnosis. We need to go through her past medical problems as well as her list of medications. We don't know whether there has been any recent blood loss, so the patient should be queried regarding melanotic or bloody stools. It would be helpful to get not only a full history but also a complete physical examination, including what her conjunctivae and skin color look like. Ambulating the patient is extremely important. All too often, we end up getting ready to send patients home with a normal neurological examination, and when we finally get them up to walk we realize they are very ataxic and thus likely have a central process that was dangerously overlooked. After obtaining a more thorough history and physical examination, I would start with some basic laboratory work including a complete blood count and electrolytes. Anemia and dehydration are particularly common in the elderly and this can cause dizziness from hypoperfusion. We also have to decide whether this patient needs imaging and if so, what type of imaging, whether a computed tomography (CT) scan or magnetic resonance imaging (MRI), as well as whether these studies need to be obtained emergently or nonemergently. In the interim, I would obtain a formal evaluation by a neurologist.

PR: What drugs may have precipitated her symptoms, and assuming these were not the explanation for her symptoms, where would you go next?

Dr Jon Mark Hirshon (JMH): A very broad spectrum of diseases can cause dizziness, lightheadedness, or altered mental status, particularly in the elderly. The list of medications that could be potential culprits is as long as the PDR. Common ones include oxycodone while more serious ones include antiepileptic drugs. I, too, would want to perform a very careful and detailed neurological examination. I remember a case of a patient who was getting ready to sign out, but I noticed he had a very clumsy hand and subtle dysarthria. This patient ended up having a lacunar infarct. For this current patient, the history makes me uncomfortable given the interval change. Since the

laboratory studies are unremarkable, I would have my neurologist see the patient, though if I weren't at an academic center, I would have to consider when a neurologist would need to evaluate the patient in the ED. Given that a vertebrobasilar syndrome would be high on my differential, I would start with a magnetic resonance imaging/magnetic resonance angiogram (MRI/MRA).

PR: The drugs that I would be most concerned about are beta-blockers and calcium channel blockers, and a combination of drugs including both digitalis and calcium channel blockers might have induced symptomatic bradycardia, which we would have seen on her vital signs.

PR: If you thought this was a vascular problem, would you start with an MRI or would you start with angiography?

Dr Vaisha Tolia (VT): It depends what I can access at my institution. At an academic center, you can get an MRI and conventional CT angiography. Although conventional angiography is the gold standard to evaluate vertebrobasilar insufficiency and posterior fossa mass, I would prefer to start with an MRI. However, many of these patients may have implanted devices that would preclude them from obtaining an MRI. If we have to start with a CT scan, I would perform CT angiogram of the head and neck. The vast majority of these patients are going to require advanced imaging of their vasculature as well as their posterior fossa since a normal noncontrast CT scan does not preclude additional workup. If there is a suspicion of central vertigo, then you have to image the central fossa as well as the vertebrobasilar system.

PR: It is my understanding that CT is a poor imaging modality to evaluate the posterior fossa, even if special protocols and cuts are performed. Are there some imaging studies that are more immediately helpful, or would you be more content in the ED with a normal physical examination, including normal gait, to give you more time to evaluate the patient more completely, and would this change if you had an abnormal gait and push you toward emergent angiography?

AC: MRI/MRA is far more sensitive than CT scanning because the latter is inadequate to image posterior

235

fossa ischemia and (especially early on) infarction. Clearly a detailed neurological examination is crucial. Testing gait is important, and if the patient is ataxic or has such severe vertigo that he cannot stand and walk, then this would make me more concerned for a central process and push me toward an MRI/MRA.

PR: I grew up in those years where we were without CT scan and MRI, and where angiography studies were difficult to obtain. We were taught to be worried about vertebrobasilar syndrome by a neurologist at the Mayo Clinic by the name of Merkin Milikin. At that time, he recommended managing these patients with anticoagulants, and he had a large series of patients that he treated with warfarin. His data was reanalyzed years later, and what was found was that although strokes weren't prevented, anticoagulation appeared to have prevented a lot of heart attacks. Back then, if we thought this was vertebrobasilar syndrome, we would have started warfarin. Nowadays, would you cover this patient on any anticoagulant while waiting for definitive imaging?

SG: This would depend on how strong my clinical suspicion was after obtaining a thorough history and physical examination. If I'm left with a real concern that this is a posterior circulation problem, I probably would start the patient on anticoagulation. In many institutions, this patient would get admitted to the hospital as MRI/MRA isn't readily available in the ED. Given the history and physical examination so far I probably would consider anticoagulating this patient, and admitting for further workup.

PR: Is there any cardiac condition short of third-degree block that would give you these symptoms?

SG: One of the more basic tests in working up a dizzy patient is the EKG. I would be looking for bradydysrhythmia. This patient should be on telemetry in the ED and on the floor, given that the EKG is only a snapshot. This presentation would be less likely from ischemia or ventricular dysrhythmias, even though cardiac ischemia can sometimes present with nonspecific findings, including weakness and dizziness.

PR: We know that endocrinopathies can produce rather strange signs and symptoms. Both hypoglycemia and hyperglycemia can produce virtually any neurological deficit. Besides obtaining a chemistry panel or fingerstick blood glucose to rule out neuroglycopenia, what other endocrinopathies would you be concerned about?

JMH: SIADH (the syndrome of inappropriate antidiuretic hormone), and severe hyponatremia, as well as other severe electrolyte abnormalities, could potentially have an impact upon the heart rate and mental status. Other additional culprits that impact electrolytes would include pituitary or thyroid diseases. The underlying systems that could be involved include cardiac, endocrine, and neurologic systems. You have to develop a very broad differential and work your way through it.

PR: It is tempting to achieve a diagnosis by just looking into the central nervous system (CNS) for potential causes, but we have to be concerned about other systems as well. For example, adrenal insufficiency could present like this but not give you much proof in terms of her general electrolyte panel. I also think thyrotoxicosis can be very obscure in the elderly patient population, and not give you much of a tachycardia, but just a dysrhythmia like atrial fibrillation. While I do not think this is the cause here, I just want to emphasize that you cannot zero in too early to the CNS as the potential cause.

AC: Yes, those are very good points. In this particular case, the fact that she had BPV in the past might lead one to prematurely conclude that this is what she is having again. I think with any elderly dizzy patient, the minimum that should be done includes an EKG to rule out a dysrhythmia, and basic screening laboratory studies to rule out anemia, hypoglycemia, dehydration, and electrolyte abnormalities. Since those tests were unremarkable, this particular patient was seen by our neurology colleagues, and they were appropriately concerned for potential vertebrobasilar insufficiency. She was admitted to the neurology service, received an aspirin, and then had an MRI.

PR: I see aspirin used as a general anticoagulant. It could have benefit for a general cardiac condition, but I find it insufficient for someone with an impending stroke. I would not be comfortable watching this patient with aspirin alone and would like to see her on a stronger platelet inhibitor or combination of platelet inhibitor and true anticoagulant such as heparin or warfarin. What did her MRI reveal?

AC: The MRI did show vertebrobasilar stenosis and insufficiency, without evidence of an acute stroke. She was managed conservatively with antihypertensives, antihyperlipidemic agents, and she was discharged with aspirin and clopidogrel but not with warfarin.

PR: This is a situation in which it is hard to justify surgery on the vertebral system given the patient's age. You can achieve a marked protection with anticoagulation. As much as I hate to introduce warfarin into someone's life routine, this is a place where the cure's cost is worth the payment, and I would hate to see this women develop a complete vertebrobasilar stroke. I personally would be less comfortable seeing this patient managed on aspirin and clopidogrel, but I know that's very common today.

VT: I, too, would consider the approach that has been outlined above. Most of these patients at our institution would also get a neurology consult, an expedited MRI/MRA, and would be admitted. Until knowing exactly what the lesion is, starting them on heparin would not be unreasonable while they are making the transition to warfarin. Given concomitant coronary disease, and if she had already been on aspirin and clopidogrel, then warfarin would then be the ideal drug. I think rehabilitation too is underutilized, but that could help this patient regain some of her function and ability to continue her activities of daily living.

PR: Are these patients being managed with some of the novel anticoagulants that do not require frequent lab monitoring, such as enoxaparin?

JMH: These agents are so new on the market that they are being used for cardiac conditions but not for CNS events, but I'm sure that's coming in the future.

PR: The Italian literature does suggest that these novel agents are being used for stroke patients, though I don't know whether they have been used prophylactically for vertebrobasilar syndrome. I believe it would be worth trying these agents if warfarin could not be used for social or lifestyle reasons. I have no information about the substitution of Lovenox for heparin. The advantage is once-a-day administration, and it is not associated with as many dramatic bleeds.

PR: Do you think it would have helped your original diagnosis if this patient would have responded to an Epley maneuver?

AC: If her dizziness had been purely positional, and she had a classic history where the vertigo was brought on by head movement, lasted a couple of seconds, and had a classic upbeat and torsional nystagmus during the Dix–Hallpike test, then I'm pretty confident that her symptoms would have been related to another episode of her BPV, which is a disease process that tends to be recurrent. However, there are several red flags in her presentation. First, her vertigo this time was spontaneous, and not position induced. Although vertebrobasilar insufficiency can worsen with head movement, it doesn't generally require head movement. She also tells you that the dizziness felt different this time, and she had concerning associated symptoms with it, such as leg weakness and change in vision.

AC: In an elderly patient who has multiple risk factors for atherosclerosis, we need to aggressively search for a central cause, or in this case, for posterior circulation ischemia or infarction. Because the head CT scan is not ideal for examining the posterior cranial fossa, MRI/MRA would be the ideal imaging modality. If the clinical presentation is strongly suggestive of vascular disease, it would be important to start anticoagulation, usually with heparin, to prevent complications while awaiting more advanced imaging. These patients will often be admitted for further evaluation and observation.

SG: In conclusion, there is a tendency for premature diagnostic anchoring, especially in patients with a long standing history of vertigo. Thankfully, in this case, the physician caring for this patient didn't stop after hearing what this patient had on prior visits to the ED and didn't assume this was just a benign etiology. Instead, he took a fresh approach, and this patient was investigated further. Clearly, as with every case seen in emergency medicine, we need to approach every case patient as though they are presenting with their disease for the very first time and to take each element of the history in context.

Section III: Concepts

Background – The unique challenges of dizziness and vertigo in older adults

Multiple physiological processes support balance. Various sensory inputs from the peripheral nervous system (PNS), the special senses, and the cerebellum are processed centrally to maintain normal balance. Not surprisingly, all of the functions that are responsible for maintaining balance (vision, hearing, various components of the sensory system, and the peripheral vestibular apparatus along with its central connections and cardiovascular tone and reflexes) degrade with age [1–4].

Dizziness and vertigo are common problems in the community [5], especially in older adults [6]. A recent study has shown that the complaint of dizziness is as high as 45% in adults aged 65 and older and increases significantly with age [7, 8]. In ED studies, these chief complaints are among the most common presenting symptoms, and misdiagnosis is common, even when patients are evaluated by neurologists [9]. Importantly, dizziness as a symptom of an actual stroke may be misdiagnosed in the ED. Dizziness itself has numerous causes, and the very word "dizziness" means different things to different people, such as the sensation of passing out, lightheadedness, disequilibrium, gait instability, or weakness. However, in a strict sense, vertigo typically refers to the feeling of illusory movement of either the self or the environment, and is itself a category of dizziness. To the extent that a patient feels "dizzy," a degree of anxiety about falling may compound the initial dizziness. In this chapter, we use the generic term "dizziness" since we do not believe that the particular term used by a given patient is diagnostically meaningful.

Dizziness in the geriatric population can be associated with depression, falls, fatigue, and an overall higher incidence of serious CNS and cardiovascular causes [9–12]. Furthermore, dizziness is often caused by a variety of non-CNS or cardiovascular symptoms such as toxic-metabolic and infectious disorders. Additional issues are unique to older adults. For example, approximately 50% of patients older than 65 years take 5 or more medications, and 12% take 10 or more medications [13]. The inherent medication side effects, dose adjustments, drug–drug interactions, and delayed or impaired metabolism inherent to the geriatric population may all alter the pharmacokinetic properties of any of the medications and result in or compound and exaggerate an acute episode of dizziness [14]. Importantly, medications used to treat dizziness, such as meclizine, can paradoxically worsen dizziness in many instances and should be used selectively [15].

The evidence base for our understanding of the diagnosis and treatment of dizziness is weak, but it has increased substantially in the past several years. Even when a specific etiology cannot be found, some have hypothesized that dizziness in older adults is a distinct "geriatric syndrome" based on mild dysfunction of different age-related physiological changes [16] in cardiovascular and vestibular physiology, which can alter the presentation compared to younger patients. In addition, geriatric patients are more likely to have cardiovascular comorbidities, expanding the differential diagnosis and increasing the likelihood of serious vascular causes. Older adults are also more likely to be cognitively impaired, which can adversely affect their ability to provide a cogent history. For all these reasons, correct diagnosis is critically important but can be challenging. Moreover, even if the etiology of dizziness is benign, resultant falls, hip, and wrist fractures, and loss of independence have a greater impact in older adults.

Falls in older adults are common, and dizziness account for approximately one third of geriatric falls [17]. In the year 2000, there were over 10,000 fatal falls and 2.6 million nonfatal fall-related injuries in the United States in patients over 65 years of age [18]. The estimated direct cost of these ED visits alone was $4 billion [18]. Falls seem to be increasing in frequency, above and beyond what one would expect purely on demographic factors [19].

Dizziness and falls in older adults are important for three reasons. First, dizziness may be the cause of a patient's fall. Second, correctly diagnosing the cause of dizziness and treating the etiology is an important strategy in fall prevention. A large part of the morbidity due to dizziness in the geriatric patient has to do with repeated falls and resultant injuries. Finally, falls often have a significant impact upon dispositions, and subsequent loss of independence for an older patient may have huge psychosocial consequences. Even a relatively "minor" injury such as a distal radius fracture and its treatment can have a major impact on an older adult's independence, especially if it involves the dominant arm and the patient lives alone.

This chapter focuses on the most common and most serious etiologies of acute, episodic, and chronic entities causing dizziness in older adults and recent research published on specific testing for certain common conditions. As is usually the case, treatment flows from diagnosis, and given the long list of potential causes of dizziness, the list of potential treatments is equally long. We will only focus here on some of the treatments for a few selected vestibular and CNS causes.

Initial approach to the patient with dizziness and vertigo

The traditional diagnostic approach to dizziness is based upon the clinician starting by asking the question, "What do you mean dizzy?" This paradigm of "symptom quality" was first published in 1972 and is based on limited data from a small number of selected patients evaluated in a specialty clinic [20]. In the "symptom quality" paradigm, the patient's response to the question "What do you mean dizzy?" will place them into one of four categories – vertigo, presyncope, disequilibrium, or "other" nonspecific dizziness. The implication is that each category has etiologic significance. This approach concludes that vertiginous patients have vestibular causes, presyncopal patients have cardiovascular causes, disequilibrium patients have neurological causes, and nonspecific dizziness patients have psychiatric causes.

Despite the fact that this paradigm has been consistently used and taught across multiple specialties including emergency medicine, the evidence base for the "symptom quality" (dizziness "type") approach has serious limitations. The first has to do with the methodology of the original 1972 paper [20]. Recruited patients had to be fluent in English, healthy, and able to return on four separate half days for further testing in a specialty clinic. Of the 125 enrolled patients, 21 were rejected for inadequate data and another 9 for lack of a diagnosis. Thus, only 95 (76%) completed the study. A single author, who was a neurologist, assigned the diagnoses without independent verification, formal brain imaging, or any long-term follow-up. Since CT was not yet available, skull plain radiographs were the only "brain" imaging tests performed. Furthermore, some diagnoses known now

to be common causes of dizziness, such as vestibular migraine, had not yet been recognized as diagnostic entities. Nevertheless, when testing failed to identify a specific diagnosis, the type of dizziness was used to assign the final diagnosis (e.g., vertigo was assigned a peripheral vestibular cause if no other cause was found).

Although this paper was an important one at its time, its results have never been prospectively and properly validated. For the symptom quality paradigm, two conditions must first be true. First, patients must be able to reliably and consistently describe their dizziness type, and second, each type should be associated with a specific differential diagnosis. New research shows that neither condition is true [21].

In one study, patients were asked a series of questions designed at describing the dizziness type [22]. Within 10 minutes, they were asked the same questions, but given the answer choices in a different sequence. Half of the patients changed the category of dizziness that they had initially endorsed just a few minutes before, and most of the patients endorsed multiple dizziness symptom qualities. In addition to this, other data show that patients with cardiac causes of dizziness often use the word "vertigo" to describe what they are feeling [23]. In another study of older patients presenting to an ED with dizziness, the use of the word "vertigo" (as opposed to lightheadedness or dizziness) did not predict those who had a cerebrovascular cause [24]. The converse is also true. Patients with clear-cut vestibular disease often complain of vague lightheadedness or nonspecific "dizziness." Patients with benign paroxysmal positional vertigo (BPPV) with a positive Dix–Hallpike test were found to be referred by their primary care physicians to either an ear–nose–throat clinic or to a falls and syncope clinic depending on whether they used terms such as "dizzy" or "vertigo" to describe their symptoms. Although patients referred to the fall and syncope clinic were typically older, were taking more medications, and had more vascular comorbid conditions, they more often used terms other than "vertigo" to describe their symptoms [25]. All of this literature suggests that using the "symptom quality" paradigm for the diagnosis of undifferentiated dizzy patients has serious shortcomings. In the study showing that patients rapidly and frequently change their type of dizziness, their responses about

Table 17.1 ATTEST.

Associated symptoms	Associated signs/relevant history
Headache	New medication/dose
Neck pain	Neck pain
Ear pain or discharge	Recent ear surgery
Chest pain or palpitations	Antecedent illness
Dyspnea or other respiratory symptoms	Trauma
Abdominal pain	
Gastrointestinal blood or fluid loss	
Neurological symptoms including diplopia, dysphagia, dysarthria, other	
Timing	**Triggers**
Constant vs episodic	Positional vs paroxysmal
Frequent vs infrequent	
Waxing and waning vs intermittent	
Examination signs	
Abnormal vital signs (fever, tachy-/bradycardia, hyper-/hypotension, and tachy-/bradypnea)	
New murmur or gallop	
New rales or wheeze	
Gastrointestinal blood loss	
Any new abnormality in the basic neurological examination	
Testing	
Fingerstick glucose	
Pregnancy testing	
Urinalysis	
Electrocardiogram	

dizziness timing and triggers were far more reliable [22]. Thus, because the type of dizziness may not be etiologically useful, and because many of the major dizziness syndromes have reliable timing and triggers patterns, an alternative paradigm based on "timing and triggers" may be more useful to the clinician.

The "timing and triggers" paradigm can be summarized using the mnemonic of ATTEST, in which A stands for Associated symptoms and signs, TT for Timing and Triggers, ES for Examination Signs, and T for Testing (Table 17.1). Although the ATTEST approach has not been prospectively validated or systematically studied as a complete diagnostic paradigm, it seems to be more consistent with the current state of knowledge and may provide a more logical and algorithmic approach toward a dizzy patient.

First, one should inquire about **associated symptoms** that suggest a particular diagnosis or group of diagnoses. It is important to establish what symptoms accompany the dizziness since a large proportion of ED patients have various medical (and not vestibular or neurological) problems underlying their dizziness. For example, dizziness associated with chest pain, vomiting, and diarrhea, or fever and cough suggest other possible diagnoses. This step will often lead to a clear-cut limited differential diagnosis and workup for many patients, such as a chest X-ray study for a dizzy patient with fever, cough, and green sputum.

Next, ask questions designed to place the patient into one of four "timing and triggers" categories in which the history is used to define the onset, duration, constancy, and triggering or exacerbating features (Table 17.2). The categories include the following:

1 *Acute vestibular syndrome (AVS)*: acute onset of dizziness that persists for days to weeks.
2 *Spontaneous episodic vestibular syndrome (sEVS)*: acute onset of episodic dizziness lasting minutes to

Table 17.2 Common differential diagnoses presenting with dizziness.

Pathology	Associated Symptoms and Signs	Timing and Triggers	Exam Findings
Central causes			
Migrainous vertigo	Headache, phonophobia, photophobia	Gradual onset, spontaneous episodes which lasts hours, some times 1–2 days	May be normal, but quite variable
Posterior circulation stroke	Diplopia, dysphagia, dysarthria, ataxia (limb or truncal), weakness or numbness	Sudden onset, constant and lasts hours	Variable depending on location, must do full neurological exam
Cerebellar tumor or abscess	Same as for stroke	Gradual onset, long lasting	Variable
Peripheral causes			
BPPV	Nausea	Episodic, triggered by head movement, lasting <1 min	Absent focal neurological findings + Dix Hallpike test (posterior canal)
Meniere's (endolymphatic hydrops)	Tinnitus and sensorineural hearing loss or aural fullness	Spontaneous episodes each lasting hours	Conductive or sensorineural deafness, tinnitus
Vestibular neuritis/labyrinthitis	Disequilibrium (hearing loss/labyrinthitis)	Rapid onset, lasting days and preceded by viral syndrome. Head motion intolerance	Nystagmus usually unidirectional and contralateral and suppressed by visual fixation, head impulse test
Zoster (Ramsey Hunt Syndrome)	Hearing loss, tinnitus, ipsilateral facial paralysis, vesicles in ear	Same as vestibular neuritis	

Abbreviation: BPPV: benign paroxysmal positional vertigo.

hours and not triggered by head or body position changes.

3 *Triggered episodic vestibular syndrome (tEVS)*: brief episodes of dizziness, usually lasting less than 1 minute that have obligatory preceding triggers such as moving the head or assuming the upright position.

4 *Chronic vestibular syndrome (CVS)*: long-standing dizziness that lasts for weeks or longer, and that is always present.

Patients can generally describe these features of their histories more reliably than the "type" of dizziness [24]. In the authors' experience, the "timing and triggers" paradigm more often leads to making a specific diagnosis compared to the traditional "symptom quality" approach. The approach to patients with AVS and tEVS has been studied fairly extensively [26–29], but it is important to acknowledge that the "timing and triggers" or ATTEST approach has not been prospectively validated or systematically studied as a complete diagnostic paradigm. Each of these four categories suggests a particular differential diagnosis. Once the category is defined, physical examination findings and confirmatory tests are then used to further narrow the differential diagnosis and answer certain questions, including whether vital signs or the electrocardiogram is normal, whether the patient is mentating normally, whether there is nystagmus on primary gaze (staring straight ahead), whether there is a murmur or signs of heart failure, and whether there are signs of gastrointestinal bleeding. Some of the confirmatory tests include bedside oculomotor findings that help to distinguish central from peripheral vestibular disorders. Further confirmation with more sophisticated (nonbedside) tests is the final step. Many patients will not need these tests because the bedside examination findings and basic tests can establish some diagnoses (e.g., vestibular neuritis, BPPV, or a urinary tract infection).

Without some type of diagnostic strategy or algorithmic approach, diagnosis of the dizzy patient can be frustrating since numerous conditions and side effects from nearly every medication available can produce dizziness. As we have seen in the previous section, although the traditional "symptom quality" diagnostic paradigm suggests a limited differential diagnosis based upon the type of dizziness the patient endorses, the evidence base for this is very limited. Using the "timing and triggers" approach, the differential diagnosis is based on various temporal categories. Table 17.2 lists the more common and the more serious potential diagnoses and includes both vestibular, CNS, and other conditions.

Etiologies of vestibular syndromes

Acute vestibular syndrome (AVS)

AVS is characterized by the abrupt onset of dizziness and a feeling of imbalance, nystagmus, nausea, vomiting, head motion intolerance, or gait disturbance that last days to weeks [30, 31]. AVS can be due to central and peripheral vestibular causes as well as cardiovascular ones such as carotid and aortic stenosis or dissection, and transient low flow states including rotational vertebral artery syndrome, cardiac dysrhythmias, pulmonary embolism (PE), and acute coronary syndrome (ACS). As many as 25% of patients present with AVS harbor serious CNS pathology [32]. Dizziness as a manifestation of vertebrobasilar insufficiency can herald a subsequent basilar stroke and can even present in isolation as a transient ischemic attack (TIA) [32–35]. Less serious causes of AVS include vestibular neuritis, labyrinthitis, and multiple sclerosis.

The important differential diagnosis in AVS is stroke versus vestibular neuritis (also known as vestibular neuronitis) or labyrinthitis. Vestibular neuritis is inflammation of the vestibular portion of the eighth cranial nerve alone while labyrinthitis is inflammation of both cochlear and vestibular portions of the eighth cranial nerve. Although vestibular neuritis accounts for the majority of patients who present with AVS, cerebellar (or brainstem) stroke is another important possibility [36, 37]. Cerebellar strokes are important to detect early given the serious potential for deterioration from edema, mass effect, noncommunicating hydrocephalus, respiratory depression, and death.

Acute labyrinthitis and vestibular neuritis

The most common benign etiologies of AVS include vestibular neuritis or vestibular neuronitis (VN) and labyrinthitis. These conditions are presumed to be caused by viral or postviral nerve inflammation. The eighth cranial nerve has two components – the vestibular and the cochlear – both of which can be affected together or individually. Patients with acute sensorineural hearing loss have diminished hearing (and no dizziness) [49, 50]. Patients with vestibular neuritis have dizziness but no hearing loss [51, 52].

Patients also experiences nausea, vomiting, ataxia, and a falling tendency toward the affected side. Nystagmus is horizontal and unidirectional. Patients with labyrinthitis have both dizziness and hearing loss. Symptoms typically arise suddenly, increase over hours, and resolve over days. Because the organs of balance and hearing are colocated anatomically, coinvolvement of dizziness and hearing generally implicates a peripheral process, but as mentioned earlier, can also result from an AICA territory stroke. Patients with vestibular neuritis who present within 72 h of symptom onset benefit from "vestibular sedatives" including dimenhydrinate 100–300 mg, as well as a glucocorticoid (methylprednisolone 100 mg, tapered 20 mg every 4 days), unless there is a contraindication [53, 54]. Patients should be adequately hydrated given their tendency to become dehydrated from nausea and subsequent decreased oral intake. Finally, patients can be referred for vestibular physical therapy to promote reequilibration of peripheral vestibulopathy through central and vestibulospinal compensation exercises.

Classic teaching is that patients who have both dizziness and hearing loss always suffer from a peripheral problem. However, an exception to this rule is the AICA (anterior inferior cerebellar artery) syndrome. The labyrinth is supplied by the internal labyrinthine artery, which is a branch of the AICA. Thus, AVS in isolation from AICA syndrome or concomitant with an acute sensorineural hearing loss is actually the result of a stroke [38], although this mechanism is probably less common than benign peripheral causes. With AICA strokes, both balance and hearing are usually affected [36, 37, 39]. Isolated rotational vertigo only occurs rarely in patients with supratentorial stroke [40]. Other worrisome mimics of a peripheral vestibulopathy include metabolic derangements, drug intoxication or side effects, Wernicke encephalopathy, bacterial or viral meningoencephalitis, or environmental exposure (e.g., carbon monoxide, decompression sickness). In patients with AVS, factors that predict stroke include increasing age, vascular risk factors, coronary artery disease, abnormal tandem gait, and the physician's high concern for stroke [28, 41].

Spontaneous episodic vestibular syndrome (sEVS)

sEVS is characterized by recurrent episodes of dizziness that develop rapidly, and usually resolve over minutes to hours though they can sometimes last several days. By definition, triggers are absent in sEVS. Benign causes include vestibular migraine and Meniere's disease. The major serious cause is vertebrobasilar TIA. When present in patients with sEVS, associated brainstem symptoms that suggest a central cause include focal neurological motor and somatosensory deficits, visual disturbances, dysmetria or incoordination, confusion, dysarthria, or numbness. Episode duration and recurrences of TIAs and BPPV etiologies have significant overlap. Patients are asymptomatic between episodes.

Vestibular migraine

For patients who present with sEVS, vestibular migraine is the most common benign cause of dizziness. Migraine is extremely common in the general population, and in one series of dizzy patients older than 65 years, 13% were found to have vestibular migraine [42]. However, in older patients without a history of prior migraine, one should be hesitant to make this diagnosis since it becomes progressively less typical for geriatric patients to present with new-onset migraines.

While audiovisual, alimentary, environmental, sensory, or lifestyle triggers may occur, they are not obligatory, and they do not immediately precede dizziness as triggers do in patients with tEVS. Both central and peripheral features can occur with or without headache [43]. The evolution of a classic vestibular migraine is usually gradual and usually takes more than 30 minutes to reach peak intensity. Attack duration ranges from minutes to hours to days, but can last only seconds in 10% of patients. Head motion intolerance is common.

In patients with vestibular migraine, the suggested treatment is analogous to that of other migraines. However, to date there have been no large controlled trials proving the effectiveness of any particular medication in vestibular migraine.

Meniére's disease

Meniére's disease (MD) is another cause of sEVS and is associated with the triad of episodic vertigo lasting approximately 20 min, clinical and audiometric confirmation of hearing loss, and tinnitus or perception of aural fullness [44]. Symptoms last from minutes to hours [45]. Attacks are typically distinct and can occur as common as several times per week, or as seldom as once per year.

The mechanism involves impaired absorption of endolymphatic fluid, resulting in "endolymphatic hydrops" and vestibulocochlear dysfunction. The differential diagnosis includes central conditions including TIA, multiple sclerosis, vestibular schwannoma, and neurosyphilis, which can be investigated by MRI.

Treatment in the emergency setting is directed at ameliorating the acute symptoms by antihistamines, anticholinergics, and antiemetics. Patients should be referred to specialists to confirm the diagnosis and prevent further attacks.

Posterior circulation TIA

The classic teaching in posterior circulation TIA is that other brainstem symptoms, including dysarthria and diplopia, are nearly always associated with dizziness, at least in patients presenting with episodes occurring over more than 3 weeks [39]. Although this classic dogma, which dates back to an NIH consensus statement from 1975, states that isolated dizziness does not occur in TIA [46], more recent data demonstrate otherwise [47, 48]. Importantly, as with any TIA, there is increased risk for stroke in the following few days especially within the vertebrobasilar territory compared to the anterior circulation. Because these patients are often asymptomatic when in the ED, diagnosis is based purely on history and epidemiological context. Other possible causes of dangerous sEVS would be the same cardiovascular problems that cause AVS – dysrhythmias, PE, ACS, valvular heart disease, and other problems that might cause transient decreased flow.

Triggered episodic vestibular syndrome (tEVS)

tEVS is manifested by very brief episodes of dizziness, usually lasting less than 1 min, which are immediately preceded by some obligate trigger. The most common triggers are head movements, such as rolling in bed or looking up, and standing up from a sitting or supine position. Rare triggers include paroxysms of coughing, sneezing, and abrupt loud noises. The most common cause of tEVS is BPPV. Orthostatic hypotension is another common cause. While most

causes of orthostatic hypotension are benign, serious etiologies, such as blood loss or occult sepsis, can also occur.

Benign paroxysmal positional vertigo

BPPV is commonly caused by loose crystals (otoliths) that become displaced from the utricle and end up free-floating in one of three semicircular canals (canalithiasis). The posterior canal is most commonly involved though variants include otoliths in the other canals (most commonly the horizontal canal) or otoliths that are not free-floating, but are rather stuck to the cupula (cupulolithiasis). BPPV may be less well recognized in elderly patients [55].

The trigger for BPPV is usually positional or postural. The movement of otoliths in the semicircular canal leads to inappropriate stimulation of the receptor that leads to activation of the vestibular nerve and transmission to the vestibular nuclei in the pons. Cortical misinterpretation of these signals results in dizziness and vertigo. Patients typically report episodes lasting approximately 15–30 seconds that are triggered by head movement. Since many episodes occur at night while in bed, some patients have difficulty identifying the duration of the spells. This is one instance in which a history of symptoms that occur upon waking from sleep makes a benign diagnosis more likely.

BPPV patients may also complain of lightheadedness or dizziness that can easily be mistaken for orthostasis if symptoms occur on arising in the morning, as is often the case. The two can usually be distinguished, however, by inquiring whether the symptoms also occur on reclining or rolling over in bed, which should not occur in those with orthostatic hypotension. Patients with BPPV may feel an anticipation of dizziness and will sometimes report being constantly dizzy for days, but a careful history can tease out the true episodic nature of the dizziness. It also bears reemphasis that many patients with BPPV do not endorse true vertigo [25].

Untreated, BPPV can either resolve spontaneously, usually within weeks, or persist in roughly one third of cases [52]. The diagnosis is made via a characteristic history and a positive Dix–Hallpike test, which confirms the inappropriate presence of otoliths in the posterior semicircular canal (~85% of cases) [26, 56]. The treatment is a canalith repositioning maneuver, most commonly the Epley maneuver. In older adults, the neck should be assured to be sufficiently mobile before proceeding with the Epley maneuver. Recent studies demonstrated that canalith repositioning maneuvers, including the Epley maneuver, halted the symptoms of vertigo in 85% of patients with posterior canal BPPV after the first attempt [53, 54]. Postmaneuver therapies with vestibular suppressant medications, postural exercises, or postural restriction have been studied, albeit not in great detail. A recent double-blind, randomized, controlled clinical trial in a small number of patients with posterior canal BPPV compared the efficacy of Epley alone to combination medication therapy with the Epley maneuver. Addition of low-dose betahistine did not result in a statistically significant reduction in quality of life, as measured by four different vertigo assessment scales [57]. A number of similar but low-powered studies have also failed to show a significant difference when vestibular sedatives are added to the Epley maneuver at a mean follow-up of 4 weeks [58]. Although a vestibular sedative is commonly prescribed, the literature suggests that it plays a very limited role in symptom control and may actually impair vestibular compensation and cause excessive sedation, contributing to subsequent falls [53].

Some patients with a typical history of BPPV will have a negative Dix–Hallpike test and will not respond to an Epley maneuver. Some of these patients will have horizontal (lateral) canal BPPV, which can be diagnosed by the supine roll test. The horizontal semicircular canal variant can be treated with a Lempert barbeque-roll maneuver or Gufoni maneuver. These repositioning maneuvers are 60–72% effective [59]. Surgical treatment options are limited to intractable BPPV and include posterior canal or nerve ablation. Patients with atypical symptoms, such as sustained nystagmus, downbeat nystagmus, no latency, bilateral positive positional test, or lacking the fatigability of symptoms with repeated maneuvers or with visual fixation, should make the clinician concerned for a BPPV mimic, which can be due to various CNS lesions [60]. Even when canalith repositioning maneuvers improve or resolve older patients' symptoms, follow-up is important as some patients have persistent dizzy symptoms not directly related to BPPV [61].

Chronic vestibular syndrome (CVS)

CVS is marked by patients who feel dizzy for weeks to months or longer and who may exhibit a constant sensation of vague unsteadiness. Because all of the causes of dizziness referred to in the sections above are by definition short-lived, the conditions that cause CVS are different and are rarely caused by problems that require an emergency intervention. The most common causes are polysensory dizziness (sometimes called "presbylibrium" because it is much more frequent in older adults), degenerative neurologic disease, psychiatric syndromes, and drug-related symptoms.

Some patients with CVS, however, will have tumors, strokes, and other CNS lesions, usually in the posterior fossa [60, 62, 63]. Thus, gait/limb ataxia or instability, resting tremor, bradykinesias, long track signs, and distal weakness or sensory loss should be further investigated for an underlying central pathology.

An important cause of CVS in the older patient population is known as disuse disequilibrium, which is caused by a reduction in overall activity level due to other comorbid medical conditions, the fear of falling itself, and natural loss of muscle bulk and strength. Patients should be referred to their primary care providers and/or physical therapy, which can often ameliorate or abate symptoms and prevent future falls, with their attendant injuries that can severely impact an older adult's quality of life.

A recent retrospective study sought to determine the incidence of nonorganic vertigo in over 1500 patients presenting to a tertiary neuro-otology clinic [64]. Almost 20% of patients reported a prior episode of residual symptoms despite the absence of objective findings at the present neurovestibular examination. Moreover, almost 80% of patients presented with a concomitant psychiatric disorder. A recently established diagnosis known as migraine-anxiety-related dizziness (MARD) describes the combination of vestibular migraine along with anxiety.

With the exception of older adults who are at high fall risk (who may need acute case management or physical therapy interventions), and the rare patient with a posterior fossa tumor, abscess, or other significant lesion, patients with CVS can be discharged with outpatient follow-up as appropriate.

245

History and physical examination

The history is usually the most important part of any diagnostic evaluation since it helps the physician to develop a differential diagnosis, focus the physical examination, and direct any subsequent diagnostic testing. Thus, the clinician's focus will be different for a patient who presents with severe abrupt onset headache with dizziness compared to a dizzy patient who reports abdominal pain and diarrhea as associated symptoms, or if there are antecedent medication changes or head trauma suggestive of a drug side effect or posttraumatic BPPV, respectively. A history of head trauma can cause both central vertigo and peripheral vertigo. In the case of a cerebral concussion, for instance, accompanying symptoms can include a headache that worsens with stimulation, poor concentration, lightheadedness, and vertigo with positional features if a concomitant labyrinthine concussion is also present. We focus here on clues that may help pinpoint a diagnosis or at least help to narrow down a differential list of diagnoses.

Our approach is to use the ATTEST (Table 17.1) mnemonic to gather the important elements of the history and identify associated symptoms that may be clues as to the underlying etiology (Table 17.2). The clinician should also distinguish between "triggering" the dizziness and "exacerbating" the dizziness. "Triggered" dizziness suggests that something made a patient dizzy who started out not dizzy. An example is dizziness that is triggered by a Dix–Hallpike test. "Exacerbated" suggests that something increased a dizzy patient's preexisting symptoms. A hypovolemic patient, for example, may have worse dizziness upon changing position (standing up). Another example would be a patient with vestibular neuritis who feels dizzy at baseline while lying still in the stretcher, but on head motion, the dizziness increases. This is a very important distinction and highlights a common misconception about dizziness [65], which is that patients whose dizziness worsens with head motion have a peripheral vestibular cause of their dizziness. In reality, dizzy patients with a stroke, multiple sclerosis, or a cerebellar tumor will develop worsening dizziness with head movement.

Physical examination of the dizzy patient needs to be fairly comprehensive given the long list of possible causes, but it should always start with consideration of vital signs. Obviously, if the initial associated data suggests a particular problem or a type of problem, the examination should focus on that issue. For example, if a patient has dizziness with a new fever, then the source of the fever should be sought. If the fever is associated with cough, then a chest X-ray study is indicated. Dizziness and tachycardia should raise the suspicion of a gastrointestinal bleed or PE, or perhaps just dehydration from poor oral intake as a result of a vestibular disorder. Examination of the tympanic membrane may even show otitis media, a cholesteatoma, or vesicles in the external auditory canal from a Ramsay Hunt syndrome. Hearing should be tested as well as gait and other cerebellar tests, such as finger to nose testing, and their ability to sit up in the gurney. Having the patient try to sit up in the stretcher without holding on to the side rails (e.g., with arms crossed across the chest) will test for truncal ataxia. Comparison to baseline gait is crucial given older adults may already have preexisting gait abnormalities. Patients who normally use a cane or a walker should be tested using those devices to allow for a meaningful comparison to their baseline. A new gait abnormality, especially the inability to walk without falling, should suggest a central cause of dizziness or severe volume depletion.

Data suggest that in patients with AVS, a brief battery of three specific bedside oculomotor tests can identify posterior circulation stroke more accurately than MRI, at least in the first 48 h from symptom onset [27]. In patients presenting with an AVS, the presence of any of the worrisome findings is suggestive of stroke (or another central cause), whereas the absence of all the worrisome findings strongly suggests a peripheral problem. These three tests are the horizontal head impulse test (HIT) [56], testing for direction-changing gaze-evoked nystagmus, and alternate cover test for skew deviation [27]. They are collectively known as the HINTS tests (Head Impulse–Nystagmus–Test of skew).

See the reference section for links to video clips that demonstrate these bedside tests. An important caveat to this study is that it was done by trained neuro-otologists in patients with new onset vertigo. Although it has not been systematically studied, we believe that practicing emergency physicians can learn to perform and interpret these tests.

The HIT [56], otherwise known as head impulse test or head thrust test, was first described in 1988 [66]. The presence of a corrective saccade of the eyes back toward the examiner's nose after a rapid turn of the head to the side is a positive test and implicates a vestibular imbalance from a lesion located in the peripheral labyrinth. This maneuver tests the vestibulo-ocular reflex [66], a primitive reflex whose pathway runs through the rostral brainstem. Given the pathway does not loop through the cerebellum or caudal brainstem, it is typically absent (no corrective saccade) in patients with cerebellar or medullary strokes and present with strokes affecting the vestibular nerve root entry zone in the pons. Pooled results across four studies identified as part of a systematic review showed that a normal HIT was found in 85% of patients with stroke ($n = 152$) and only 5% of patients with a peripheral vestibular problem ($n = 65$) [28]. However, most patients with these brainstem strokes will have one of the other two eye findings (in the HINTS panel), which indicates the central nature of the lesion [27]. The HIT is a safe test although a single case of an induced transient complete heart block has been described [67]. There is one important issue with respect to the HIT that bears special emphasis, which is that it should only be performed in patients presenting with AVS. This is because it is the absent finding (no corrective saccade) that is worrisome for a stroke etiology. Thus, if one were to perform the HIT on normal individuals (or patients with pneumonia or fractured wrists), the result would be "negative," albeit in this case not worrisome for stroke. Therefore, if one were to do the HIT on a patient with unselected dizziness, it would also be falsely "normal" and incorrectly suggest a central cause.

The second component of HINTS is direction-changing nystagmus. Patients with both vestibular neuritis and cerebellar stroke may have nystagmus. Merely reporting the presence or absence of nystagmus is not particularly useful and certainly does not distinguish benign peripheral etiologies from serious central ones. It is the nature of the nystagmus that can help to differentiate the two groups. Patients with vestibular neuritis will have predominantly horizontal nystagmus, sometimes with a very slight torsional component [51, 53]. This will sometimes be present in primary (neutral) gaze and nearly always be present on gaze toward one side. When these patients look to the other side, they may still have nystagmus, but, if they do, the direction of the fast movement will be in the same direction as with the first side tested – that

is, it is unidirectional. The intensity of the nystagmus diminishes with fixation [53]. In patients with CNS causes of dizziness, however, nystagmus is usually still predominantly horizontal, but the direction of the fast component may "change direction." That is, when the patient looks to the left, the fast component beats to the left and when the patient looks to the right, the fast component beats to the right. Although only 20–50% of patients with central causes of AVS have direction-changing nystagmus, when present, it is very specific. Of note, some normal patients will have slight direction-changing nystagmus on extreme end gaze both right and left that resolves after a few beats and is symmetric; this physiologic nystagmus is not helpful diagnostically.

The third component of the composite HINTS is "the Test of Skew." Although not very sensitive, this finding is a very specific finding indicating a CNS lesion in dizzy patients [27, 28]. Skew deviation is tested by performing the "alternate cover" test. With the patient instructed to focus on a fixed point, each eye is alternately covered over and then uncovered sequentially. This forces the patient to take up visual fixation first with one eye and then the other, which allows the examiner to assess whether the eyes are vertically aligned. The examiner looks at the eyes to see if there is an upward or downward (hypertropia or hypotropia) correction as the eye is uncovered. This vertical misalignment is caused by any interruption in the otolith-ocular circuit [68]. Examiners should note that the presence of a horizontal misalignment (esophoria or exophoria) due to a residuum of childhood strabismus, eye muscle surgery, or prior oculomotor palsy does not convey the same meaning.

In conclusion, the HINTS test is 100% sensitive and 96% specific for the diagnosis of central causes of AVS in moderate- to high-risk patient population and appears to be more sensitive compared to MRI within the first 48 h of symptom onset [27, 69, 70]. Although stroke risk-stratification based on HINTS could be augmented by quantitative video-oculography, this composite test has positive and negative predictive values of stroke when performed by neurologists. Further studies should be directed at testing the performance of these tests by EPs.

On the other hand, in patients with sEVS, the physical examination is not generally useful if they are asymptomatic on presentation. In patients with the tEVS, the Dix–Hallpike test should be performed to test for the presence of otoliths in the posterior semicircular canal. This test should provoke positional vertigo and torsional nystagmus if the posterior semicircular canal is affected. The nystagmus and vertigo should extinguish in less than 45 seconds, and will recur in the opposite direction when the patient sits up. The intensity and duration of the dizziness and nystagmus will fatigue when the maneuver is repeated on the same side. If the Dix–Hallpike test is negative and the history is strongly suggestive of BPPV, then the horizontal canal should be tested by the supine roll test. Reliable video clips of both of these tests are readily found throughout the Internet. The Dix–Hallpike test should generally be positive on one side and negative on the other, and this is important because it tells you the starting position for the potentially curative Epley maneuver. As above, patients with any cause of persistent dizziness, including CNS ones, will feel worse on head movements so tests producing only additional symptoms or exacerbating preexisting horizontal nystagmus should not be interpreted as positive.

Diagnostic testing

While physical examination is very useful, in some patients, other diagnostic testing is necessary. CT imaging is the predominant form of imaging in the ED. It is very important to know the limitations of commonly used tests, especially head CT for posterior circulation stroke [71]. A recent study estimates the sensitivity of CT scan for acute posterior fossa stroke to be 42% [72], but studies with direct comparison to MRI scans suggest it could be as low as 16% in the first 24 h [73]. An MRI is clearly more sensitive for ischemic stroke than CT; however, it is less commonly available. Less commonly known is that the MRI is also imperfect and may miss up to 20% of posterior circulation strokes in the first 24–48 h after symptom onset [27, 28].

Unless a diagnosis is clear based on history and physical examination, and many times it will be (such as a patient with BPPV, vestibular neuritis, or hypovolemia), basic laboratory testing is also warranted. This is particularly true in older adults since the incidence of other diseases is increasingly common. Some older patients with a toxic-metabolic or infectious problem could present with an AVS, but the frequency with which this happens is probably low (<1%) [28], and many of these patients will likely be identified by attention to associated symptoms. Performing an electrocardiogram (ECG) may be useful in the geriatric patient with dizziness and no obvious cause by history or physical examination. Beyond these basic tests, imaging studies and other diagnostics should be targeted. If PE is the suspect diagnosis, a CT angiogram of the chest might be the best first test. If drug toxicity in a heart failure patient taking digoxin is considered, then a serum digoxin level might be an appropriate first test. Along the same vein, since medication side effects are an important cause of chronic dizziness, an outpatient trial of stopping a medication might be the appropriate "test," but, of course, this should be coordinated with the patient's primary care doctor.

Disposition

The disposition of an older adult with dizziness is a function of two issues – specific diagnosis and general environmental safety. Disposition is highly dependent on the underlying diagnosis. A patient with AVS due to an ischemic cerebellar stroke requires admission both to diagnose and treat the underlying vascular lesion and to observe for deterioration from posterior fossa edema. Another patient with the exact same presentation but due to vestibular neuritis can be sent home with oral steroids and short-term meclizine for symptomatic control. Although vascular risk factors may help stratify those at highest risk for TIA and stroke, care should be taken not to rely too heavily on age or related risks to exclude vascular disease – it is well documented that younger patients with vertebral artery dissection may present with dizziness or vertigo due to TIA or stroke [11] and are most likely to be misdiagnosed with dangerous consequences [66, 67].

The second issue is ensuring environmental safety. This is especially important in older dizzy patients. Dizzy patients may become dehydrated, which may worsen their symptoms whatever their initial cause. This can be compounded in older adults who have cardiovascular issues and are often taking multiple medications. Therefore, even benign appearing patients with AVS due to vestibular neuritis might require admission if they are dehydrated and still sufficiently symptomatic such that they cannot keep up with fluids. Most patients with BPPV can safely go home after canalith repositioning treatment.

However, an older BPPV patient who is somewhat dehydrated, volume sensitive, and who lives alone may require slow intravenous fluids as an inpatient prior to safe discharge. A home safety evaluation (either formally or by questioning the patient and their family about the home situation) prior to discharge is equally important. A patient who has a few steps to get to the bathroom and lives alone may also need a different disposition than another who normally has to climb a flight of stairs and lives with a healthy spouse.

Section IV: Decision-making

- Dizziness is a common presenting symptom in the ED and appears to be more endemic in the ever growing geriatric population
- Diagnosing dizzy older patients can be frustrating. However, when using a systematic, algorithmic method (such as the ATTEST method), the physician can often confidently make a specific diagnosis that leads to specific treatment
- An MRI is more sensitive than a CT scan for ischemic stroke and should be undertaken more frequently if readily available.
- Knowing the common peripheral vestibular causes of dizziness well and learning the beside oculomotor physical findings and HINTS while understanding the limitations of brain imaging will allow emergency physicians to make a specific diagnosis in the vast majority of elusive cases.

References

1 Baloh, R.W., Ying, S.H., and Jacobson, K.M. (2003) A longitudinal study of gait and balance dysfunction in normal older people. *Arch. Neurol.*, **60**, 835–839.

2 Ishiyama, G. (2009) Imbalance and vertigo: the aging human vestibular periphery. *Semin. Neurol.*, **29**, 491–499.

3 Kerber, K. (2010) Dizziness in older people, in *Vertigo and Imbalance: Clinical Neurophysiology of the Vestibular System* (eds S. Eggers and D. Zee), Elsevier, Philadelphia, PA, pp. 491–501.

4 Kerber, K.A., Ishiyama, G.P., and Baloh, R.W. (2006) A longitudinal study of oculomotor function in normal older people. *Neurobiol. Aging*, **27**, 1346–1353.

5 Neuhauser, H.K., Radtke, A., von Brevern, M. *et al.* (2008) Burden of dizziness and vertigo in the community. *Arch. Intern. Med.*, **168**, 2118–2124.

6 Colledge, N.R., Wilson, J.A., Macintyre, C.C., and MacLennan, W.J. (1994) The prevalence and characteristics of dizziness in an elderly community. *Age Ageing*, **23**, 117–120.

7 Lammers, W., Folmer, W., Van Lieshout, E.M. *et al.* (2011) Demographic analysis of emergency department patients at the Ruijin hospital, Shanghai. *Emerg. Med. Int.*, **2011**, 748274.

8 Newman-Toker, D.E., Hsieh, Y.H., Camargo, C.A. Jr. *et al.* (2008) Spectrum of dizziness visits to US emergency departments: cross-sectional analysis from a nationally representative sample. *Mayo. Clin. Proc.*, **83**, 765–775.

9 Royl, G., Ploner, C.J., and Leithner, C. (2011) Dizziness in the emergency room: diagnoses and misdiagnoses. *Eur. Neurol.*, **66**, 256–263.

10 Herr, R.D., Zun, L., and Mathews, J.J. (1989) A directed approach to the dizzy patient. *Ann. Emerg. Med.*, **18**, 664–672.

11 Cheung, C.S., Mak, P.S., Manley, K.V. *et al.* (2010) Predictors of important neurological causes of dizziness among patients presenting to the emergency department. *Emerg. Med. J.*, **27**, 517–521.

12 Yin, M., Ishikawa, K., Wong, W.H., and Shibata, Y. (2009) A clinical epidemiological study in 2169 patients with vertigo. *Auris Nasus Larynx*, **36**, 30–35.

13 Kaufman, D.W., Kelly, J.P., Rosenberg, L. *et al.* (2002) Recent patterns of medication use in the ambulatory adult population of the United States: the Slone survey. *J. Am. Med. Assoc.*, **287**, 337–344.

14 Shoair, O.A., Nyandege, A.N., and Slattum, P.W. (2011) Medication-related dizziness in the older adult. *Otolaryngol. Clin. North Am.*, **44**, 455–471, x.

15 Newman-Toker, D.E., Camargo, C.A. Jr., Hsieh, Y.H. *et al.* (2009) Disconnect between charted vestibular diagnoses and emergency department management decisions: a cross-sectional analysis from a nationally representative sample. *Acad. Emerg. Med.*, **16**, 970–977.

16 Tinetti, M.E., Williams, C.S., and Gill, T.M. (2000) Dizziness among older adults: a possible geriatric syndrome. *Ann. Intern. Med.*, **132**, 337–344.

17 Rubenstein, L.Z. (2006) Falls in older people: epidemiology, risk factors and strategies for prevention. *Age Ageing*, **35** (**Suppl. 2**), ii37–ii41.

18 Stevens, J.A., Corso, P.S., Finkelstein, E.A., and Miller, T.R. (2006) The costs of fatal and non-fatal falls among older adults. *Inj. Prev.*, **12**, 290–295.

19 Kannus, P., Parkkari, J., Koskinen, S. *et al.* (1999) Fall-induced injuries and deaths among older adults. *J. Am. Med. Assoc.*, **281**, 1895–1899.

20 Drachman, D.A. and Hart, C.W. (1972) An approach to the dizzy patient. *Neurology*, **22**, 323–334.

21 Edlow, J.A. (2013) Diagnosing dizziness: we are teaching the wrong paradigm!. *Acad. Emerg. Med.*, **20**, 1064–1066.

22 Newman-Toker, D.E., Cannon, L.M., Stofferahn, M.E. *et al.* (2007) Imprecision in patient reports of dizziness symptom quality: a cross-sectional study conducted in an acute care setting. *Mayo Clin. Proc.*, **82**, 1329–1340.

23 Newman-Toker, D.E., Dy, F.J., Stanton, V.A. *et al.* (2008) How often is dizziness from primary cardiovascular disease true vertigo? A systematic review. *J. Gen. Intern. Med.*, **23**, 2087–2094.

24 Kerber, K.A., Brown, D.L., Lisabeth, L.D. *et al.* (2006) Stroke among patients with dizziness, vertigo, and imbalance in the emergency department: a population-based study. *Stroke*, **37**, 2484–2487.

25 Lawson, J., Johnson, I., Bamiou, D.E., and Newton, J.L. (2005) Benign paroxysmal positional vertigo: clinical characteristics of dizzy patients referred to a Falls and Syncope Unit. *Q. J. Med.*, **98**, 357–364.

26 Fife, T.D., Iverson, D.J., Lempert, T. *et al.* (2008) Practice parameter: therapies for benign paroxysmal positional vertigo (an evidence-based review): report of the Quality Standards Subcommittee of the American Academy of Neurology. *Neurology*, **70**, 2067–2074.

27 Kattah, J.C., Talkad, A.V., Wang, D.Z. *et al.* (2009) HINTS to diagnose stroke in the acute vestibular syndrome: three-step bedside oculomotor examination more sensitive than early MRI diffusion-weighted imaging. *Stroke*, **40**, 3504–3510.

28 Tarnutzer, A.A., Berkowitz, A.L., Robinson, K.A. *et al.* (2011) Acute vestibular syndrome: does my patient have a stroke? A systematic and critical review of bedside diagnostic predictors. *Can. Med. Assoc. J.*, **84** (15), 1595–1604.

29 Kerber, K.A. and Fendrick, A.M. (2010) The evidence base for the evaluation and management of dizziness. *J. Eval. Clin. Pract.*, **16**, 186–191.

30 Hotson, J.R. and Baloh, R.W. (1998) Acute vestibular syndrome. *N. Engl. J. Med.*, **339**, 680–685.

31 Kim, H.A. and Lee, H. (2012) Recent advances in central acute vestibular syndrome of a vascular cause. *J. Neurol. Sci.*, **321**, 17–22.

32 Norrving, B., Magnusson, M., and Holtas, S. (1995) Isolated acute vertigo in the elderly; vestibular or vascular disease? *Acta Neurol. Scand.*, **91**, 43–48.

33 Karatas, M. (2011) Vascular vertigo: epidemiology and clinical syndromes. *Neurologist*, **17**, 1–10.

34 Kerber, K.A., Rasmussen, P.A., Masaryk, T.J., and Baloh, R.W. (2005) Recurrent vertigo attacks cured by stenting a basilar artery stenosis. *Neurology*, **65**, 962.

35 Moubayed, S.P. and Saliba, I. (2009) Vertebrobasilar insufficiency presenting as isolated positional vertigo or dizziness: a double-blind retrospective cohort study. *Laryngoscope*, **119**, 2071–2076.

36 Choi, K.D., Lee, H., and Kim, J.S. (2013) Vertigo in brainstem and cerebellar strokes. *Curr. Opin. Neurol.*, **26**, 90–95.

37 Lee, H., Sohn, S.I., Cho, Y.W. *et al.* (2006) Cerebellar infarction presenting isolated vertigo: frequency and vascular topographical patterns. *Neurology*, **67**, 1178–1183.

38 Lee, H., Kim, J.S., Chung, E.J. *et al.* (2009) Infarction in the territory of anterior inferior cerebellar artery: spectrum of audiovestibular loss. *Stroke*, **40**, 3745–3751.

39 Savitz, S.I. and Caplan, L.R. (2005) Vertebrobasilar disease. *N. Engl. J. Med.*, **352**, 2618–2626.

40 Brandt, T., Botzel, K., Yousry, T. *et al.* (1995) Rotational vertigo in embolic stroke of the vestibular and auditory cortices. *Neurology*, **45**, 42–44.

41 Chase, M., Goldstein, J.N., Selim, M.H. *et al.* (2014) A prospective pilot study of predictors of acute stroke in emergency department patients with dizziness. *Mayo Clin. Proc.*, **89** (2), 173–180.

42 Uneri, A. and Polat, S. (2008) Vertigo, dizziness and imbalance in the elderly. *J. Laryngol. Otol.*, **122**, 466–469.

43 Neuhauser, H. and Lempert, T. (2009) Vestibular migraine. *Neurol. Clin.*, **27**, 379–391.

44 Anonymous (1995) Committee on hearing and equilibrium guidelines for the diagnosis and evaluation of therapy in Meniere's disease. American Academy of Otolaryngology-Head and Neck Foundation, Inc. *Otolaryngol. Head Neck Surg.*, **113**, 181–185.

45 Sajjadi, H. and Paparella, M.M. (2008) Meniere's disease. *Lancet*, **372**, 406–414.

46 Anonymous (1975) A classification and outline of cerebrovascular diseases II. *Stroke*, **6**, 564–616.

47 Hoshino, T., Nagao, T., Mizuno, S. *et al.* (2013) Transient neurological attack before vertebrobasilar stroke. *J. Neurol. Sci.*, **325**, 39–42.

48 Paul, N.L., Simoni, M., and Rothwell, P.M. (2013) Transient isolated brainstem symptoms preceding posterior circulation stroke: a population-based study. *Lancet Neurol.*, **12**, 65–71.

49 Rauch, S.D. (2008) Clinical practice. Idiopathic sudden sensorineural hearing loss. *N. Engl. J. Med.*, **359**, 833–840.

50 Schreiber, B.E., Agrup, C., Haskard, D.O., and Luxon, L.M. (2010) Sudden sensorineural hearing loss. *Lancet*, **375**, 1203–1211.

51 Baloh, R.W. (2003) Clinical practice. Vestibular neuritis. *N. Engl. J. Med.*, **348**, 1027–1032.

52 Strupp, M. and Brandt, T. (2008) Diagnosis and treatment of vertigo and dizziness. *Dtsch. Arztebl. Int.*, **105**, 173–180.

53 Strupp, M. and Brandt, T. (2009) Vestibular neuritis. *Semin. Neurol.*, **29**, 509–519.

54 Strupp, M., Zingler, V.C., Arbusow, V. *et al.* (2004) Methylprednisolone, valacyclovir, or the combination for vestibular neuritis. *N. Engl. J. Med.*, **351**, 354–361.

55 Oghalai, J.S., Manolidis, S., Barth, J.L. *et al.* (2000) Unrecognized benign paroxysmal positional vertigo in elderly patients. *Otolaryngol. Head Neck Surg.*, **122**, 630–634.

56 Bhattacharyya, N., Baugh, R.F., Orvidas, L. *et al.* (2008) Clinical practice guideline: benign paroxysmal positional vertigo. *Otolaryngol. Head Neck Surg.*, **139**, S47–S81.

57 Guneri, E.A. and Kustutan, O. (2012) The effects of betahistine in addition to Epley maneuver in posterior canal benign paroxysmal positional vertigo. *Otolaryngol. Head Neck Surg.*, **146**, 104–108.

58 Sundararajan, I., Rangachari, V., Sumathi, V., and Kumar, K. (2011) Epley's manoeuvre versus Epley's manoeuvre plus labyrinthine sedative as management of benign paroxysmal positional vertigo: prospective, randomised study. *J. Laryngol. Otol.*, **125**, 572–575.

59 Kim, J.S., Oh, S.Y., Lee, S.H. *et al.* (2012) Randomized clinical trial for geotropic horizontal canal benign paroxysmal positional vertigo. *Neurology*, **79**, 700–707.

60 Dunniway, H.M. and Welling, D.B. (1998) Intracranial tumors mimicking benign paroxysmal positional vertigo. *Otolaryngol. Head Neck Surg.*, **118**, 429–436.

61 Gamiz, M.J. and Lopez-Escamez, J.A. (2004) Health-related quality of life in patients over sixty years old with benign paroxysmal positional vertigo. *Gerontology*, **50**, 82–86.

62 Carmona, S., Nicenboim, L., and Castagnino, D. (2005) Recurrent vertigo in extrinsic compression of the brain stem. *Ann. N. Y. Acad. Sci.*, **1039**, 513–516.

63 Johkura, K. (2007) Central paroxysmal positional vertigo: isolated dizziness caused by small cerebellar hemorrhage. *Stroke*, **38**, e26–e27; author reply e28.

64 Odman, M. and Maire, R. (2008) Chronic subjective dizziness. *Acta Otolaryngol.*, **128**, 1085–1088.

65 Stanton, V.A., Hsieh, Y.H., Camargo, C.A. Jr. *et al.* (2007) Overreliance on symptom quality in diagnosing dizziness: results of a multicenter survey of emergency physicians. *Mayo Clin. Proc.*, **82**, 1319–1328.

66 Halmagyi, G.M., Yavor, R.A., and McGarvie, L.A. (1997) Testing the vestibulo-ocular reflex. *Adv. Otorhinolaryngol.*, **53**, 132–154.

67 Ullman, E. and Edlow, J.A. (2010) Complete heart block complicating the head impulse test. *Arch. Neurol.*, **67**, 1272–1274.

68 Sharpe, J.A., Kumar, S., and Sundaram, A.N. (2011) Ocular torsion and vertical misalignment. *Curr. Opin. Neurol.*, **24**, 18–24.

69 Chen, L., Lee, W., Chambers, B.R., and Dewey, H.M. (2011) Diagnostic accuracy of acute vestibular syndrome at the bedside in a stroke unit. *J. Neurol.*, **258**, 855–861.

70 Newman-Toker, D.E., Kerber, K.A., Hsieh, Y.H. *et al.* (2013) HINTS outperforms ABCD2 to screen for stroke in acute continuous vertigo and dizziness. *Acad. Emerg. Med.*, **20**, 986–996.

71 Edlow, J. (2012) A physician's got to know his (test's) limitations. *J. Emerg. Med.*, **42**, 582–583.

72 Hwang, D.Y., Silva, G.S., Furie, K.L., and Greer, D.M. (2012) Comparative sensitivity of computed tomography vs magnetic resonance imaging for detecting acute posterior fossa infarct. *J. Emerg. Med.*, **42**, 559–565.

73 Chalela, J.A., Kidwell, C.S., Nentwich, L.M. *et al.* (2007) Magnetic resonance imaging and computed tomography in emergency assessment of patients with suspected acute stroke: a prospective comparison. *Lancet*, **369**, 293–298.

18 Weakness and functional decline

Colleen M McQuown

Department of Emergency Medicine, Summa Akron City Hospital, Northeast Ohio Medical University, Akron, OH, USA

Section I: Case presentation

A 90-year-old woman presents to the emergency department (ED) with a chief complaint of generalized weakness. The symptoms have been progressive over the prior 6 days, and today she required assistance to transfer from the chair. Her weakness is nonfocal. She denies chest pain, shortness of breath, dizziness, or lightheadedness. She is concerned because she had similar symptoms recently when she had a "heart attack."

Review of prior medical records confirms that she was admitted 3 weeks prior with a non-ST segment elevation myocardial infarction (NSTEMI) and mild congestive heart failure. Her chief complaint at that visit was generalized weakness with dyspnea on exertion. She chose not to undergo cardiac catheterization and was treated medically. She was started on an angiotensin-converting enzyme (ACE) inhibitor and hydrochlorothiazide (HCTZ) at that visit.

Her other past medical history is significant for hypertension, hypothyroidism, and a surgery for a prior hip fracture. She lives at home with a grandson who works second shift and ambulated independently until her last admission, when she began using a walker. She does not have home health services.

Physical examination reveals a thin woman, in no distress, with normal vital signs. The cardiopulmonary examination is normal, and there is no jugular venous distention or rales on examination. She has no lower extremity edema noted. The neurological examination revealed symmetric 5+ muscle strength in the upper and lower extremities, but with the up and go test, she needed assistance in transfer, and was unsteady with a slow gait using a walker.

Diagnostic studies revealed an unchanged electrocardiogram (EKG) and normal troponin-I; however, her sodium was 120, decreased from 135 at discharge 1 month ago.

Section II: Case discussion

Dr. Peter Rosen (PR): This is a fairly common complaint for the presentation of an acute myocardial infarction (MI) in the elderly. Here we have a patient with a recent NSTEMI, 3 weeks prior to this visit. I would have been personally guided toward the heart as a source of her problems.

Dr. Amal Mattu (AM): I would agree that acute MI should get the top of the differential list. The older the patient, the more atypical the presentations for acute MI become. It appears that elderly women over the age of 75 will often present with an abrupt onset of malaise as their "anginal equivalent." Acute coronary syndrome (ACS) being a killer, that is something that you need to consider early in a patient like this. Besides doing the history and physical examination, I would consider obtaining an early EKG, which would then direct where you are going to go with your evaluation.

PR: This is a 90-year-old woman. You don't get to be 90 without having a pretty good protoplasm. Do you think in the natural course of a disease, such as ischemic coronary disease, having an underlying

Geriatric Emergencies: A Discussion-Based Review, First Edition.
Edited by Amal Mattu, Shamai A. Grossman and Peter L. Rosen.
© 2016 John Wiley & Sons, Ltd. Published 2016 by John Wiley & Sons, Ltd.

ability to get to age 90, does that render you more able to tolerate it and ST segment elevation myocardial infarction (STEMI) compared to a 40 year old?

Dr. Don Melady (DM): That's a great point, and one that I make frequently. Old people tend to be very healthy. We tend to see them as sick all the time, given the large number of people that we see in the ED. However, your point is absolutely accurate. Only people who are vigorous and hardy get to be 90 years old. I noticed that this woman doesn't have a lot of comorbidities – hypothyroidism and a previous hip fracture is all about. So yes, I think that is much more likely that if she was going to do well if managed conservatively for this episode. There's an interesting component of the past history here. At the time of her previous MI, she "chose not to undergo cardiac catheterization." I would be very interested to know more about that discussion and the tone around it: did it include the perspective that the benefit might be considerably greater than the risk *for this particular patient*? My perspective is that just because she is 90, it doesn't make her any less likely to do well with cardiac catheterization, and actually the benefit in this woman would be much greater than in another frailer younger person. This is another example of "treat the patient, not the number," remembering that age is just a number! If she had had her arteries cleaned up 3 weeks ago, she might not be back in the ED now with more worries about having another heart attack.

Dr. Chris Carpenter (CC): David Alter published a very interesting analysis (American Journal of Medicine 2004; 116: 540–545) of the number needed to treat (NNT) and number needed to harm (NNH) for a geriatric ACS, using a data set of 71,000 patients, of whom 24,000 were over the age of 75. They adjusted the assumption of efficacy for acute revascularization of ACS in geriatrics patients down by 50%. In other words, the efficacy of reopening these vessels and keeping them open was assumed to be half what it was in younger patients and then they calculated the NNT for the 50 and older versus the 50 and younger age group. The NNT in the 50 and younger was 87 to prevent one death at 1 year. On the other hand, the NNT for over the age 75 was only 7. The point was that we need to take a closer look at NNT and NNH, which unfortunately is also lower in the older age population as we are having

these discussions with these patients in terms of their goals of care.

PR: Did they have any information whether this was the first episode or one on top of many others? I would think that in any age group, your ability to successfully open a vessel is going to be dependent on the number of previous stents placed and what is the pathology of the other vessels. This patient may have very well had single-vessel pathology.

CC: I agree and the Alter study did not provide these details.

PR: It says that at the time of her admission she was in mild failure, and, therefore, was started on a diuretic, HCTZ. Do you generally accompany a diuretic such as HCTZ with supplementary potassium, or do you not worry about that?

Dr. Robert Anderson (RA): With HCTZ, I usually worry about sodium levels. HCTZ and selective serotonin reuptake inhibitors (SSRIs) are two notorious drugs in the elderly but will cause hyponatremia within a couple weeks of treatment if you're not careful.

PR: What can you do to prevent this complication, and how would you quickly identify the cause as probably due to pharmacology rather than psychogenic polydipsia?

RA: Every presentation in the elderly is a medication effect until proven otherwise. Therefore, with any older patient, I assume there are going to be a lot of medications, that's where I go to first.

PR: Does her previous hypothyroidism have any effect on her in terms of what you're worried about?

Dr. Scott Wilber (SW): We can now get a thyroid-stimulating hormone (TSH) level a little quicker at our facility. I am concerned about hypothyroidism as a cause of her symptoms. I am not sure in her particular case there was anything to suggest that her hypothyroidism was not adequately treated in the past, or if she has been off of her medications. I certainly think about that in terms of her medications. Often with relatively vague symptoms, her hypothyroidism might not be adequately treated.

PR: I think a physical examination finding that we frequently forget about is the relaxation phase of the deep tendon reflex, which might give us a clue as to the efficacy of her treatment faster than a TSH level. We obtained a cardiogram that doesn't show any changes, but it doesn't necessarily mean that she's not having another acute NSTEMI. With a normal troponin, however, we can relax a little bit about cardiac causes. As we got that study back, we found her serum sodium to be markedly lowered. When you see such a low sodium level in an elderly patient, do you reach for an admission slip?

Dr. John Mark Hirshon (JMH): Yes, for many reasons. First of all, in just about anybody with such a low sodium level, I would reach her for an admission slip. Particularly in her, since she is weaker and her ability to function has decreased since her last admission. I want to try to understand what caused her hyponatremia. It could be that her medication is the likely source. But it might be something else. She could have pneumonia, or some other reason other than a syndrome of inappropriate antidiuretic hormone (SIADH) function. I would admit her, also because we need to correct her sodium, which cannot be fixed rapidly.

PR: You alluded to her therapy. Would you like to summarize how you would start on such a patient? I think we all agreed on admission. I have a saying that if something didn't develop quickly, it's something that is not going to be treated quickly. Metabolic changes frequently develop over time and are going to need time to get fixed.

RA: Even with sodium levels that aren't as impressive as 120, I feel strongly that there is no such thing as an asymptomatic hyponatremia in the elderly. With her history of falls and cognitive impairment, it is important to consider a sodium level of 130 as potentially contributory. How much workup is needed at that level in the ED is unclear especially if chronic. At a minimum, I would communicate the finding either directly or via your documentation with the primary care physician (PCP). I think with a sodium level of 120, the ED treatment of hyponatremia is relatively straightforward. If they are seizing, then you would start hypertonic saline. If they are dramatically volume depleted, the treatment IV is fluids. But for everyone else, you would fluid restrict and try to figure out why they are hyponatremic.

PR: The patient is not seizing from the history. Given her past history of cardiac failure, I would personally not race in giving her hypertonic saline, because normal saline is going to be relatively hypertonic for her. Nevertheless, if you want to start with therapy in the ED, you have to be cautious about how rapidly you want to give it.

This looks like a complication of medication rather than cardiac pathology. Would you consider reopening the question of cardiac catheterization after her metabolic derangements have been straightened out?

AM: I don't think I would necessarily do that in the ED. Once her metabolic problems are straightened out, I can revisit what her functional status is from a cardiac standpoint, and perhaps with a little bit more history, find out how she's been doing during the past few weeks since she had her NSTEMI. If she has been having functional problems that are attributable to worsened cardiac function since her NSTEMI, it might be worth reevaluating the issue of whether she needs a stent. If by history, you get the impression that she's been doing pretty well short of this new metabolic problem, then I don't know that I would rush to do a procedure. In previous discussions, we've talked about the studies that have looked at invasive versus noninvasive therapies for NSTEMIs. Many of those studies fail to show improvement with invasive therapies versus conservative therapies. Again, this is going to be completely based on her activities of daily living (ADLs), and how she's been doing at home as to whether she needs any further cardiac intervention of an urgent basis.

PR: They did a very nice assessment of her functional abilities, and it sounds like there has been a change that started probably with her MI 3 weeks ago. She has gotten progressively weaker, needing more assistance with moving about. Do you think this is probably the start of the steep portion of her decline curve, or do you expect her to turn around and perhaps get back to her baseline once her sodium has been corrected?

DM: I think folks interested in care of older people are natural optimists. I don't think this is necessarily the beginning of a rapid decline. I would even like to play the devil's advocate about whether she absolutely needs admission to the hospital. I think likely she would. But as the case suggests, her main problem is her functional decline not her sodium. Although the two are linked, I think the main thing we should be focusing on is her function. Depending on how optimistic you want to be – or possibly how cavalier – here is another approach: Almost certainly her weakness is because of her sodium. Almost certainly, her low sodium is because of the HCTZ she was started on, which, given she is not in failure, she doesn't need. So, what about saying, "well, if we stop her HCTZ, her sodium is going to improve. If her sodium improves, her function is going to improve." And then, "can we actually get her home in a safe way." She has lost one ADL in the last 6 days – ability to transfer – which means she can't be sent home safe – as is. But are we working in a setting where we could actually get her some supplementary support? Is there some community care agency that can provide it? My approach includes the knowledge that inpatient hospital admission wards are not the most senior-friendly places; unless there is going to be a clear benefit coming from that admission, we should really keep an open mind about alternatives to admission.

PR: I think that's a very strong point. I'm glad you made it. I personally, however, wouldn't have the courage to send someone out with a sodium level of 120, because, I don't think it's going to correct that quickly. I think that given that it's low enough she could get into trouble very fast, even though she's been declining into it slowly, I would personally be very nervous about sending her out as an outpatient until it was corrected.

DM: I would be nervous too, unless I can put enough in place that could counteract my nervousness. So, for example, if there was a good social support system in place: a visiting nurse, once a day or twice a day. In our place, it might be possible to get a visiting home physician the next day. If that were the case, your nervousness might be lower.

PR: Do you think we can stop in our workup? Or as we've discussed many times in the past, every time we think we have an answer in the elderly patient, we have nine other questions. Would you broaden your diagnostic workup in this patient?

CC: I probably would. I think of weakness, and I credit Rob Anderson in the chapter he wrote in the *North American Clinics of Geriatric Medicine*, "Assessment of Generalized Weakness," for this thought process. I think that weakness is a syndrome

rather than a specific diagnosis. A syndrome being a phenotypic manifestation of the interplay of multiple issues including the acute disease process, overlying comorbidities, physiologic reserve, and baseline conditioning as well as the patient's psychological state. All those things are what you see manifest in front of you as "weakness" in the chief complaint. Many things can go into that equation. Moreover, I don't think our initial encounter with the geriatric patient, 2–3 min of history and physical examination, reassessment, and when the laboratory tests and imaging studies return that we're necessarily going to pinpoint with real accuracy what the cause is. Therefore, I think that the general approach to the typical geriatric patient and with weakness in particular, reassessment, while in the ED, is probably merited, continuously reassessing your differential diagnosis.

PR: Along the lines of what Don was talking about, probably one of the worst places in the hospital for the geriatric patient is the intensive care unit (ICU). Would you think this patient needed the ICU, or would you feel comfortable keeping this patient on a medical ward?

JMH: I would prefer her to be on a medical ward. I would probably have to do a little bit of arguing to be able to get the folks upstairs to accept that. Part of that decision would be too, she would be in our ED for a number of hours, and I could watch and see how she would be doing from a clinical perspective, while correcting her sodium. So if I would be able to show that her sodium was improving, her clinical status was at least where she was when she came in perhaps a little bit better, then I could convince the residents upstairs to take her. My preference would be to not put this patient in the ICU. One option we haven't discussed in terms of between inpatient and outpatient would be an observation level. I don't think I would feel comfortable placing her with a sodium level of 120 in the ED observation unit. My preference would be to minimize her time in the hospital because I think it's not the healthiest place to be.

AM: I just want to add, I think the patient would be fine on a medical ward, provided that the house staff is absolutely diligent about not correcting that sodium too quickly. It's common teaching that you should not correct the sodium overzealously. Despite that, it happens too often when people write for some IV fluids, and fail to recheck the sodium as it corrects. During my second year out of residency, I admitted a hyponatremic patient, and he was corrected too quickly despite my conversation with the admitting team and he had a cardiac arrest the next morning. When I was in residency, I recall a pregnant patient who had hyponatremia that was corrected too quickly, who ended up quadriplegic. So, hyponatremia, although relatively common, can be relatively deadly from an iatrogenic standpoint. Whoever admits this patient needs to be really careful about correcting that sodium. This is definitely NOT the scenario where you write for some IV fluids, then run them throughout the night, get some morning laboratory tests, and forget about the patient until then, because that patient can have really serious problems if not carefully monitored.

PR: I think these patients are so brittle, that you have to work within your institution as to define what capacity they have while taking care of these on the floor. Historically, once we invented the ICUs, it became almost impossible to get any kind of decent nursing care on a regular floor. I think that's worse in some hospitals more than others. Moreover, since she's also got a cardiac problem that we need to be more concerned about, I think that in the average community hospital, she might not do so well on the floor and require at least a brief stay in the ICU until she can be stabilized. Do you have any thoughts on what they need to do to monitor her besides the frequent measuring of her serum sodium?

RA: I think because she is not volume depleted, her management would be fluid restriction, watch her neurologic status, and hold the HCTZ. Again, this would be another reason to admit her, to continue the workup, and to figure out what's going on with her. Maybe it's the sodium, maybe it's something else, or maybe it's hypothyroidism. Maybe you could start on one thing, give it the tincture of time and then expand your workup if you need to.

PR: I think that's a very strong point. I think the hardest thing you can do, as an emergency physician, is to not do anything. Sometimes, we do the wrong thing, but we're always willing to act and do something. Sometimes, not doing anything is much harder than doing the wrong thing.

RA: I just want to add; she is the exact kind of person who would run into trouble with rapid correction of her sodium. When you look at the folks that develop central pontine myelinolysis, it's the folks that develop hyponatremia over the period of several days to a week, not the marathon runners. It's people that develop it over 2 or more days. It's the older folks that you have to worry about that problem with. Younger folks that develop hyponatremia quickly are probably not going to develop CPM with rapid correction of the sodium.

SW: So in conclusion, this was an interesting case of a patient that presented twice with, in her mind, the exact same symptoms. Once from an MI, and the second time from hyponatremia, that was likely caused by a treatment that was started on the first visit. In her mind, the symptoms were indistinguishable. She was treated in the hospital as was suggested. This is not somebody who we can generally get to an alternative level of care very easily. She was treated in the hospital on a medical floor with holding of her HCTZ and fluid restriction and had a gradual return of her sodium back to normal, and was discharged home again with home health services for some physical therapy and nursing care. She was not catheterized on her second visit either. There is a group of 90 year olds, who have a very matter-of-fact attitude and don't want to have a lot of invasive procedures, and she was one of them. She said that she didn't want to have a heart catheterization and preferred medical management.

PR: Sometimes, I think we have to applaud the wisdom of people who are brave enough to refuse treatment that can make them worse as well as better. This was a very good outcome, and I have to compliment you for being able to perfect it so quickly. I think that as Don was saying, this was an elderly patient who will end up doing well for a much longer time, if we don't meddle too much.

Section III: Concepts

Background

ED visits and hospital admissions for older adults with weakness and functional decline are common and present diagnostic challenges. A clinician must decide whether an acute medical condition exists that causes the weakness or functional decline or whether the decline in function prompted the visit. A review of the National Ambulatory Medical Care Survey (NHAMCS) found that weakness and fatigue was the fifth most common ED chief complaint after trauma, dyspnea, chest pain, and abdominal pain [1]. A study done in the United Kingdom found 22% of patients aged 65 and older discharged from the hospital had a diagnostic code of an "ill-defined condition." [2]

Pathophysiology

Generalized weakness and functional decline are often associated with other geriatric syndromes such as delirium, falls, frailty, sarcopenia, and failure to thrive. There may be a shared pathophysiologic mechanism of multisystem dysregulation, inflammation, and atherosclerosis that contributes to the baseline functional impairment and impaired mobility seen in some older adults [3]. This may lead to the overlap of features seen with geriatric syndromes. One measure of function is gait speed, which declines with age and is an independent predictor of disability and healthcare utilization [4]. Maximal energy expenditure (VO_2 max) or the capacity to perform vigorous activity starts declining by about 10% per decade beginning at age 30 [4]. Eventually, daily tasks approach the VO_2 max and anaerobic metabolism is needed to meet energy demands and triggers feelings of fatigue. The theory is that this creates a cycle of fatigue leading to sedentary behavior, less endurance, and further decline in fitness leading to a decrease in VO_2 max [4]. Sarcopenia, which is the age-associated loss of skeletal muscle mass and function, contributes to frailty, functional decline, and generalized weakness. Sarcopenia is complex and involves multiple cell signaling pathways that contribute to the loss of skeletal muscle mass, slowing of contraction and relaxation phases, and a decrease in strength capacity [5]. The initial presentation of sarcopenia is a decline in function, strength, and self-reported mobility difficulty [6]. Sarcopenic patients are at increased risk for falls, functional decline, disability, and death [6–9]. Frailty and sarcopenia share common inflammatory pathways [9]. Frailty is also associated with falls, functional decline, and death [10]. In this chapter, we discuss generalized weakness as a chief complaint, functional decline, failure to thrive, and frailty. Falls and fear of falling are also associated with weakness,

functional decline, and frailty, which will be covered in further detail in Chapter 19.

Generalized weakness and nonspecific complaints

Older ED patients often present with nonspecific complaints. They may describe their symptoms as malaise, generalized weakness, falling, feeling ill, feeling tired, feeling "off," or feeling dizzy. Their caregiver, friend, family, or neighbor may bring them in or encourage them to call emergency medical services (EMSs) because they cannot care for themselves, but the patient may deny any symptoms. These vague, nonspecific complaints pose a diagnostic challenge. The clinician must proceed carefully to determine what workup must be done to rule out an emergent cause for the symptoms. The symptoms may be due to general aging progression, frailty, functional decline, sarcopenia, malnutrition, depression, loneliness, loss of social or caregiver support, financial difficulties, or a combination of these factors.

Older patients are more likely to have a chief complaint of generalized weakness and fatigue than young patients [1]. The Basel Nonspecific Complaints (BANC) study found that 20% of older ED patients had no specific complaint or complaints of generalized weakness, feeling exhausted, or recent falls [11]. The majority of the patients without a specific complaint were older, with a median age of 82 years; half of these patients had an acute medical problem [11]. A review of the NHAMCS study found that patients with weakness and fatigue had a larger total number of diagnostic tests and were more likely to have at least one procedure than patients without this presenting complaint [1]. They had longer ED lengths of stay and higher admission rates [1]. The study reviewed more than 181,000 visit observations and found that the top diagnoses in patients with weakness and fatigue were "other malaise and fatigue," pneumonia, urinary tract infection, syncope and collapse, congestive heart failure, volume depletion, fever, anemia, dehydration, and hemorrhage of the gastrointestinal tract [1]. A study of frail elderly whose chief complaint was "homecare impossible" had an acute medical condition 51% of the time, the most common being infection, cardiovascular, neurologic, delirium, and fracture [12]. In the BANC study, patients who were hemodynamically unstable in the ED were excluded from the study [11]. Despite excluding unstable patients, the mortality rate for patients with no specific complaint was 9% and the admission rate was 82% [11].

Given the seriousness and need for timely treatment for many of the diagnoses associated with generalized weakness, older patients who present with nonspecific complaints need a careful history, examination, and workup. Gait disturbance, a fall within 3 months, and lack of appetite were found in the BANC study to be predictors of a serious medical condition [11]. Although many of the diagnoses found in patients with generalized weakness as a chief complaint have a specific treatment, even those with the nonspecific final diagnosis of generalized weakness may need follow-up, admission, or referral for further services. A study to assess the rehabilitation potential of patients with "nondebility generalized weakness" (ICD-9 (international classification of disease) codes for muscle wasting and disuse atrophy, muscle weakness, and other malaise and fatigue/asthenia) found that they were more likely to respond to rehab and were more likely to be discharged home than the debility group (i.e., hip fracture) [13]. Their functional recovery was the same as patients in the debility diagnosis group [13]. Discovering a reason or developing a treatment plan for a generalized weakness is also important to prevent return to the ED. One study of patients aged 75 years and older found that generalized weakness had an OR (odds ratio) predictive of admission of 2.0 and an admit and return within 30 days OR of 1.57 [14]. A study of outcomes after admission of patients with ill-defined conditions in patients aged 65 years and older found that they were less likely to die in the 36 months of follow-up than patients with other admissions, but they were more likely than any other group to have readmissions for ill-defined conditions [2]. Their conclusion based on this study was that for this group of patients functional support needs may be more important than those of patients with other conditions [2].

Functional decline, cognitive decline, development of incontinence, or a history of falls may be found during history taking of patients with nonspecific complaints. Function can be assessed by a patient's ability to perform physical ADLs such as walking, dressing, transferring, bathing, grooming, continence, and eating and the ability to perform instrumental activities of daily living (IADLs) such as shopping, housework, transportation, meals, medicine, money, and communication [15]. A study of frail elderly with no specific complaint found that 90% had a problem with an instrumental activity of daily living and 61% had cognitive decline [12]. More than 50% had a problem with an ADL and 67% had a problem with falls [12]. Incontinence was also found in 48% of the frail patients without a specific complaint [12].

Adult failure to thrive, although it has many similar features to frailty, functional decline, and generalized weakness, actually has a unique ICD-9 code and diagnostic criteria. It is defined as weight loss greater than 5% of baseline, decreased appetite, poor nutrition, and inactivity [16]. It is associated with significant comorbidities and is found in 25–40% of nursing home patients and has an in-hospital mortality of about 16% [16]. Depression, malnutrition, impaired physical function, and cognitive impairment are all predictive of adverse events in patients with failure to thrive [16]. It is also associated with increased infection, hip fractures, and pressure sores. The workup for failure to thrive is similar to that of patients with frailty, functional decline, generalized weakness, or other nonspecific complaints and includes searching for a treatable condition and assessing for functional needs.

Frailty

Progressive generalized weakness that occurs over years and occasional prompts of an ED visit may be due to frailty. Frailty is a decline in function across multiple systems due to a heighted vulnerability to stressors. The Cardiovascular Health Study Collaborative Research Group defined frailty as three or more of the following: (1) unintentional weight loss in the previous year, (2) weakness (measured by grip strength), (3) exhaustion (self-report of poor endurance and energy), (4) slowness (defined as time to walk 15 ft), and (5) low physical activity (weighted score of kilocalories expended per week) [10]. Similarly, the Frailty Index defines frailty as three or more of the following: (1) unintentional weight loss (10 lbs or 5% of body weight), (2) exhaustion (in the last week at least 3–4 days), and (3) decline of physical activity (kilocalories per week expended, time to walk 15 ft or grip strength) [9]. This definition of frailty is similar to the diagnostic criteria for adult failure to thrive mentioned earlier, but with more specific measurements [16]. Other frailty identification tools include the Clinical Frailty Scale, Frailty Index-Comprehensive Geriatric Assessment, and Canadian Study of Health and Aging Frailty Index [9]. All of the frailty scale correlate with functional decline and increased risk of mortality and institutionalization.

The pathway to frailty is not well understood. Risk factors include chronic medical conditions, excessive drinking, smoking, depression, low physical activity, and both low and high body mass index (BMI = weight (kg)/(height (m))^2) [9]. Although these lifestyle choices and chronic medical conditions such as diabetes, arthritis, cardiovascular disease, pulmonary disease, obesity, and depression are associated with frailty, not all patients with these develop frailty [9, 10]. Frailty has been found to cause disability independent of clinical disease [10]. Frailty is associated with other geriatric syndromes such as falls, delirium, sarcopenia, and functional decline [9, 10, 17]. There is a shared pathophysiologic

process involving inflammation, undernutrition, and prothrombotic states [3, 6, 10, 17]. There is a pre-frail state that is clinically silent, where patients can recover completely from stressors [9, 18]. Once patients develop frailty, they have a slow and incomplete recovery from clinical and subclinical stressors. The frailty cycle consists of sarcopenia, lack of physical exercise, perception of increased exercise effort, downregulation of physiologic systems, inadequate nutrition, unhealthy environment, and decline in function, leading to more sarcopenia and restriction of physical activity [18] (Figure 18.1). With increased age and increased ratio of fat to lean mass there is an increase in the body's resting energy expenditure, or minimal amount of energy needed for independent living [4]. Undernutrition, sarcopenia, and obesity are precursors in the progression from pre-frail to frail [9]. When pre-frail patients perceive that it is increased work to physically exert themselves due to their sarcopenia and increased resting energy expenditure they might then enter the frailty cycle.

Frail patients are at increased risk for falls, delirium, functional decline, disability, nursing home placement, and death [9, 10, 17–20]. One study found that mortality was six times higher for frail patients versus nonfrail patients over a 3-year follow-up [10]. It is

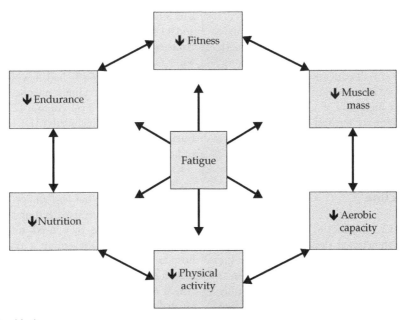

Figure 18.1 Cycle of frailty.

important for emergency physicians to understand the frailty syndrome and recommend further testing done as an outpatient or during admission. It may be that by identifying frail patients or pre-frail patients that are at risk for developing frailty, we can prevent functional decline associated with the downward spiral. Frailty first begins by affecting mobility [10]. Frail patients have a greater risk of falls and disability than prefrail or nonfrail patients [19]. A referral to a fall prevention clinic or a home fall assessment might prevent a pre-frail patient from falling, developing a fracture, and becoming a frail patient. Studies have found that exercise interventions decrease the risk of falls and increase balance and strength in frail older adults [18, 21]. Exercise interventions that combine strength, endurance, and balance training are the most effective [21]. Other home-based technologies such as a light path (device installed next to the patient's bed at home that turns on a light when the patient sets a foot on the ground) or tele-assistance (a medical alert bracelet that activates a transmitter that allows a provider to give assistance over an intercom in the house from a remote call center) may also reduce falls for frail older patients [22]. Nutritional interventions have showed mixed results with interventions based on caloric intake alone being found ineffective [18]. One study on protein supplementation found a reduction in the progression of functional decline [23].

It is important to recognize that frail patients may also have difficulty with IADLs or ADLs [18, 24]. This can affect discharge planning and follow-up. One study looked at frail patients who lived without needed help for an ADL disability [24]. The patients were found to have high rates of admission; however, when a multidisciplinary medical and social service program provided help to meet their ADL needs, their rates of admissions decreased significantly [24].

Functional decline

Patients with a chief complaint of generalized weakness may have a functional decline or a problem with an ADL that prompted them to seek care in the ED. An impaired functional status may be present in up to 50% of older ED patients [25]. A study of patients older than 65 years with an ED chief complaint of "home care impossible" found that

90% had a problem with an IADL and 53% had a problem with an ADL [12]. A study of ED patients 75 years and older with a subacute illness or injury at least 48 h old found functional decline was common and frequently contributed to their reason for a visit to the ED [15]. Functional decline was reported in 74% of the patients, 68% with an IADL, and 61% with an ADL [15]. Ninety-eight percent IADL decline involved shopping, transportation, meals, or housework. Eighty-eight percent of the ADL involved dressing, transferring, or walking [15]. Twenty-five percent of the patients said they could not take care of themselves if discharged home [15]. It is important to consider a patient's ADL and IADL functional decline when planning the patient's disposition or follow-up care from the ED regardless of his/her acute or subacute medical problem.

An illness or injury may prompt a decline in function after discharge from the hospital. A study of older patients discharged home after a fall reported that during home-based follow-up there was a functional decline in 35% [26]. Functional decline after a fall is associated with fractures, slower timed up and go (TUG) scores, and functional independence prior to the fall [26]. A study of older ED patients with blunt injuries who were discharged home from the ED found that 40% had a functional decline at 1-week follow-up [27]. At a 4-week follow-up, 35% had a functional decline, 15% had a repeat ED visit, and 11% needed to be admitted to the hospital [27]. Patients manifested their functional declines in other ways outside the ED. In the previous study, by the 4-week follow-up, 65% had new services initiated, mostly provided by family members and 56% had an unscheduled medical contact [27]. Predictors of functional decline included IADL dependence and fractures of the upper and lower extremities or trunk or head injuries [27].

Knowing which patients are at risk for a functional decline gives an ED physician an opportunity to intervene. Often one of the best things that a physician can do for older patients is getting them the support and follow-up care they need to prevent further injury and illness. Preventing a repeat visit to the hospital is important for patient care and also for the financial stability of the hospital as reimbursement is tied to readmission rates. There are several tools created for ED use to predict functional decline. One is the Identification of Seniors at Risk tool (ISAR) and another is Triage Risk Screening Tool (TRST) [25]. The ISAR is a self-completed six-item measure. It requires patient effort and asks patients to report premorbid function, acute change in function, recent hospitalization, impaired memory, impaired vision, and polypharmacy [25]. The TRST tool consists of six questions that a nurse completes at the time of triage. The questions are yes/no for the presence of cognitive impairment; difficulty walking, transferring, or recent falls; five or more medications; lives alone with no caregiver; ED use in the last 30 days; and nurse concern [25]. Patients who score positive on either screen need further attention.

Treatment and disposition

It is important to recognize when a patient with failure to thrive, functional decline, or frailty can no longer care for themselves at home. In the ED, the traditional option for these patients is to admit them to the hospital so that alternative arrangements may be made. These arrangements often included extended care in a skilled nursing home. To be eligible for Medicare's extended care benefit, a patient must have been inpatient in an acute care hospital for three consecutive calendar days (the three-midnight rule) [28]. Observation admissions do not count toward these nights, and the patient must have daily skilled services [28]. If the patient does not have to go directly to an extended care facility, he or she may still qualify if he or she has a return visit to the ED within 30 days of discharge. If a patient does not need to be admitted medically but still needs skilled nursing care, he or she may have to pay out of pocket for an admission to an extended care facility and arrange the admission on his or her own. Even if the patient is admitted to a skilled nursing facility as an extended Medicare benefit, it is important to realize that only the first 20 days are paid in full by Medicare, and the next 80 days require a daily co-pay depending on his or her supplemental insurance. After that the patient must pay for the nursing home out of pocket [28]. Medicare is looking closely at patients with short inpatient stays and may deny payment if they feel the patient should have been placed in observation rather than admission. Hospital case managers may help physicians decide whether a patient meets observation or inpatient admission criteria [29]. This

decision has financial consequences for the patient as well since Medicare part A does not cover observation, so the patient may have large out-of-pocket expenses [30, 31].

Some EDs, especially those described as "geriatric EDs," may provide referrals to visiting nurses, home physical therapy, home physician visits, help with housework or meals, and transportation aid. These services do not require an inpatient stay. A senior ED, made up of nurses, social workers, pharmacists, and physicians with extra training in geriatric emergency medicine may reduce the rate of admission [32]. A provider must understand the requirements for how to refer a patient to these home-based services and ideally care should be arranged prior to discharge. Typically, a patient must be homebound, defined by Medicare as follows: leaving the home is not recommended for the patient's condition, the patient requires aid to leave home (such as a walker), and leaving home is taxing to the patient [33]. Medicare does not cover housework or meals, but there may be resources through local affiliates with the Department of Health and Human Services Administration on Aging [34]. Home health must be ordered by a physician during a face-to-face visit, traditionally done during a follow-up appointment with the primary care doctor. This is counterproductive since the patient has difficulty leaving the house to go to the primary care doctor. ED physicians, assisted by a hospital coordinator, may be able to complete the face-to-face paperwork in the ED and speed up the process [35]. This is a change in the traditional role of an emergency physician but achieves the end goal of getting the right care to the patient.

Section IV: Decision-making

- Careful evaluation is required during the workup of older ED patients with generalized weakness or functional decline.
- Differential diagnoses include infection, metabolic derangements, and exacerbations of chronic conditions.
- Failure-to-address causes and consequences of functional decline may lead to further injury, illness, and decline.

- Referral for additional outpatient services may be warranted.
- A multidisciplinary approach in the ED may facilitate the workup and disposition.

References

1 Bhalla, M.C., Stiffler, K.A., Lowell, G.W., and Wilber, S. (2011) Weakness and Fatigue in older Emergency Department patients in the United States, 2003–2007. Abstracts of the SAEM (Society for Academic Emergency Medicine) Annual Meeting, Boston, MA, June 1–5, 2011. *Acad. Emerg. Med.*, **18** (**Suppl. 1**), S22.

2 Walsh, B., Addington-Hall, J., Roberts, H.C. *et al.* (2012) Outcomes after unplanned admission to hospital in older people: ill-defined conditions as potential indicators of the frailty trajectory. *J. Am. Geriatr. Soc.*, **60** (**11**), 2104–2109.

3 Inouye, S.K., Studenski, S., Tinetti, M.E., and Kuchel, G.A. (2007) Geriatric syndromes: clinical, research, and policy implications of a core geriatric concept. *J. Am. Geriatr. Soc.*, **55** (**5**), 780–791.

4 Schrack, J.A., Simonsick, E.M., and Ferrucci, L. (2010) The energetic pathway to mobility loss: an emerging new framework for longitudinal studies on aging. *J. Am. Geriatr. Soc.*, **58** (**Suppl. 2**), S329–S336.

5 Ryall, J.G., Schertzer, J.D., and Lynch, G.S. (2008) Cellular and molecular mechanisms underlying age-related skeletal muscle wasting and weakness. *Biogerontology*, **9** (**4**), 213–228.

6 Fielding, R.A., Vellas, B., Evans, W.J. *et al.* (2011) Sarcopenia: an undiagnosed condition in older adults. Current consensus definition: prevalence, etiology, and consequences. International working group on sarcopenia. *J. Am. Med. Dir. Assoc.*, **12** (**4**), 249–256.

7 Landi, F., Liperoti, R., Russo, A. *et al.* (2012) Sarcopenia as a risk factor for falls in elderly individuals: results from the ilSIRENTE study. *Clin. Nutr.*, **31** (**5**), 652–658.

8 Landi, F., Cruz-Jentoft, A.J., Liperoti, R. *et al.* (2013) Sarcopenia and mortality risk in frail older persons aged 80 years and older: results from ilSIRENTE study. *Age Ageing*, **42** (**2**), 203–209.

9 Kanapuru, B. and Ershler, W.B. (2009) Inflammation, coagulation, and the pathway to frailty. *Am. J. Med.*, **122** (**7**), 605–613.

10 Fried, L.P., Tangen, C.M., Walston, J. *et al.* (2001) Frailty in older adults: evidence for a phenotype. *J. Gerontol. A Biol. Sci. Med. Sci.*, **56** (**3**), M146–M156.

11 Nemec, M., Koller, M.T., Nickel, C.H. *et al.* (2010) Patients presenting to the emergency department with non-specific complaints: the Basel Non-specific Complaints (BANC) Study. *Acad. Emerg. Med.*, **17** (**3**), 284–292.

12 Rutschmann, O.T., Chevalley, T., Zumwald, C. *et al.* (2005) Pitfalls in the emergency department triage of frail elderly patients without specific complaints. *Swiss Med. Wkly.*, **135** (**9–10**), 145–150.

13 Haley, R., Sullivan, D.H., Granger, C.V., and Kortebein, P. (2011) Inpatient rehabilitation outcomes for older adults with nondebility generalized weakness. *Am. J. Phys. Med. Rehabil.*, **90** (**10**), 791–797.

14 LaMantia, M.A., Platts-Mills, T.F., Biese, K. *et al.* (2010) Predicting hospital admission and returns to the emergency department for elderly patients. *Acad. Emerg. Med.*, **17** (**3**), 252–259.

15 Wilber, S.T., Blanda, M., and Gerson, L.W. (2006) Does functional decline prompt emergency department visits and admission in older patients? *Acad. Emerg. Med.*, **13** (**6**), 680–682.

16 Robertson, R.G. and Montagnini, M. (2004) Geriatric failure to thrive. *Am. Fam. Physician*, **70** (**2**), 343–350.

17 Quinlan, N., Marcantonio, E.R., Inouye, S.K. *et al.* (2011) Vulnerability: the crossroads of frailty and delirium. *J. Am. Geriatr. Soc.*, **59** (**Suppl. 2**), S262–S268.

18 Lang, P.-O., Michel, J.-P., and Zekry, D. (2009) Frailty syndrome: a transitional state in a dynamic process. *Gerontology*, **55** (**5**), 539–549.

19 Tom, S.E., Adachi, J.D., Anderson, F.A. *et al.* (2013) Frailty and fracture, disability, and falls: a multiple country study from the global longitudinal study of osteoporosis in women. *J. Am. Geriatr. Soc.*, **61** (**3**), 327–334.

20 Fang, X., Shi, J., Song, X. *et al.* (2012) Frailty in relation to the risk of falls, fractures, and mortality in older Chinese adults: results from the Beijing Longitudinal Study of Aging. *J. Nutr. Health Aging*, **16** (**10**), 903–907.

21 Cadore, E.L., Rodríguez-Mañas, L., Sinclair, A., and Izquierdo, M. (2013) Effects of different exercise interventions on risk of falls, gait ability, and balance in physically frail older adults: a systematic review. *Rejuvenation Res.*, **16** (**2**), 105–114.

22 Tchalla, A.E., Lachal, F., Cardinaud, N. *et al.* (2012) Efficacy of simple home-based technologies combined with a monitoring assistive center in decreasing falls in a frail elderly population (results of the Esoppe study). *Arch. Gerontol. Geriatr.*, **55** (**3**), 683–689.

23 Kim, C.-O. and Lee, K.-R. (2013) Preventive effect of protein-energy supplementation on the functional decline of frail older adults with low socioeconomic status: a community-based randomized controlled study. *J. Gerontol. A Biol. Sci. Med. Sci.*, **68** (**3**), 309–316.

24 Sands, L.P., Wang, Y., McCabe, G.P. *et al.* (2006) Rates of acute care admissions for frail older people living with met versus unmet activity of daily living needs. *J. Am. Geriatr. Soc.*, **54** (**2**), 339–344.

25 Hustey, F.M., Mion, L.C., Connor, J.T. *et al.* (2007) A brief risk stratification tool to predict functional decline in older adults discharged from emergency departments. *J. Am. Geriatr. Soc.*, **55** (8), 1269–1274.

26 Russell, M.A., Hill, K.D., Blackberry, I. *et al.* (2006) Falls risk and functional decline in older fallers discharged directly from emergency departments. *J. Gerontol. A: Biol. Sci. Med. Sci.*, **61** (10), 1090–1095.

27 Wilber, S.T., Blanda, M., Gerson, L.W., and Allen, K.R. (2010) Short-term functional decline and service use in older emergency department patients with blunt injuries. *Acad. Emerg. Med.*, **17** (7), 679–686.

28 Birmingham, J. (2008) Understanding the Medicare "Extended Care Benefit" a.k.a. the 3-midnight rule. *Prof. Case Manag.*, **13** (1), 7–16; Quiz 17–18.

29 American College of Emergency Physicians. *Utilization Review FAQ* [Internet]. [cited 2014 Jan 16], http://www.acep.org/Clinical---Practice-Management/Utilization-Review-FAQ/ (accessed 4 September 2015).

30 Tergesen, A. (2013) Medicare's "Observation" Status Can Cost You Big - WSJ.com. The Wall Street Journal. [Internet]. [cited 2014 Jan 16], http://online.wsj.com/news/articles/SB100014240527023033769045791357 32284488114 (accessed 4 September 2015).

31 Anonymous. *Are You a Hospital Inpatient or Outpatient?* [Internet]. [cited 2014 Jan 16]. http://www.medicare.gov/Pubs/pdf/11435.pdf (accessed 4 September 2015).

32 Keyes, D.C., Singal, B., Kropf, C.W., and Fisk, A. (2014) Impact of a new senior emergency department on emergency department recidivism, rate of hospital admission, and hospital length of stay. *Ann. Emerg. Med.*, **63**, 517–524. [Internet]. [cited 2014 Jan 16], http://www.sciencedirect.com/science/article/pii/ S0196064413015527 (accessed 4 September 2015).

33 Visiting Nurse Associations of America (2013). *CMS Clarifies Definition of "Confined to the Home" (Homebound) for Medicare Purposes.* [Internet]. [cited 2014 Jan 16], http://vnaa.org/article_content.asp?article=406# .UtgoYPvPxpg (accessed 4 September 2015).

34 Eldercare Locator [Internet]. [cited 2014 Jan 16], http://eldercare.gov/Eldercare.NET/Public/Index.aspx (accessed 4 September 2015).

35 Anonymous. *Home-Health-Questions-Answers.pdf.* [Internet]. [cited 2014 Jan 16], http://www.cms.gov/Medicare/Medicare-Fee-for-Service-Payment/ HomeHealthPPS/Downloads/Home-Health-Questions-Answers.pdf (accessed 4 September 2015).

Emergency department evaluation of falls in the elderly

Tania D. Strout & Robert S. Anderson

Department of Emergency Medicine, Maine Medical Center, Tufts University School of Medicine, Portland, ME, USA

Section I: Case presentation

A 76-year-old woman presented to the emergency department (ED) after a fall. She was attending an event in the hospital when she fell on poorly lit stairs in an auditorium. She had been well recently without prior falls. As hospital staff and security wheel her into the ED, she expressed embarrassment and concern that she disrupted the event. She didn't remember hitting her head, she did not lose consciousness, and has isolated right ankle pain. Her glasses (bifocals) were broken during the fall.

Her medical history was notable for rheumatoid arthritis treated with chronic steroids. She had also been started on Coumadin for deep venous thrombosis (DVT) 2 weeks prior. She also took medicines for hypertension, hyperlipidemia, and diabetes. She had no surgical history and she is unclear what previous providers had told her about the reason for her DVT.

The vital signs were: temperature 37 °C, pulse 80 beats/min, respirations 15 breaths/min, blood pressure of 150/90 mmHg, pulse oximetry 98% on ambient air. There was no bony tenderness to her head or cervical spine. Her right ankle was swollen, deformed, and diffusely tender with range of motion limited by pain. Her dorsalis pedis pulse was easily palpated and she was able to wiggle her toes. Radiograph of the ankle revealed bimalleolar fracture with minimal displacement. Laboratory studies revealed an INR of 3.2.

Section II: Case discussion

PR: In reading the case one of the past medical facts was rheumatoid arthritis, do you have any note of which joints were affected in her?

RA: I don't know, which joints were affected in her.

PR: Ok, I think that becomes more interesting as we get into the issues of how to work this patient up. We essentially have an elderly woman who fell for the first time she believes, complaining of ankle pain. She doesn't give much of a history, but in the fall she also broke her glasses. Maura, would you like to begin for us how you would work her up? Any concerns you would have?

MK: I think part of it is trying to get as good of a fall history as possible. Was it simply dark in the hall with a trip hazard or was there an acute illness that made her less steady? A fall history, a recent medical history would be relevant. Thinking from the trauma perspective with falls you have to evaluate any preceding medical issues as well as do a trauma evaluation for injuries from the fall. The first question is do we need to do any imaging of her head? She says she doesn't remember hitting her head, but she doesn't explicitly say she didn't hit her head. She is on Coumadin and with her bifocals being broken during the fall, I would be more cautious and image her head. I would do a head computed tomography (CT) to rule out any intracranial bleeding. With regards to the neck I would be a little bit more conservative due to the rheumatoid arthritis and image her c-spine

Geriatric Emergencies: A Discussion-Based Review, First Edition.
Edited by Amal Mattu, Shamai A. Grossman and Peter L. Rosen.
© 2016 John Wiley & Sons, Ltd. Published 2016 by John Wiley & Sons, Ltd.

given potential for subluxation of c1-c2, though this may not necessarily be needed if you think the ankle isn't a distracting injury. Imaging the cervical spine whether or not she has any tenderness on her neck, though, this would be more controversial.

PR: I think those are really the most important issues for me. One of the things I think about in falls in the elderly, not so much if this is the first fall or an accidental fall, but if this is the presentation of a fall that the patient wasn't aware of. In other words, could the patient actually be having a subdural that is subacute and cause this fall. Anyone on Coumadin, I think this is a strong possibility and I go ahead and image the head. The neck, I hate to do X-rays of elderly people's necks, because they are almost always abnormal. While a CT may be helpful, we almost always need an MRI to truly work out the pathology in the neck. My original question to Rob was did she know she had severe arthritis in the neck, and if so I don't know if I would bother with a CT scan, I might go ahead and think about a MRI early on. One of the things about falls is we don't always know the reason why elderly people fall. One article about elderly hip fractures suggested that over half of falls in elderly woman were not due to the fall that produced the fracture, but the fracture that produced the fall. In other words, osteoporotic hip suddenly breaking on changes of position or changes in motion causing the patient falling. That being the case I don't worry too much about what caused the fall, but where the patient is hurting. That being said Rob do you have any thoughts about assessing the initial mechanism?

RA: I have been thinking a lot about falls in the elderly and have visited hundreds of elderly people in their homes after discharge from the ED for a fall related visit. I have read in the literature and observed in my practice, that history of fall is often poorly reported by the patient. I think much more important than the detail of a particular fall, is the tempo of the falls. Someone who has had a first fall or increased frequency of falls I think is more of a red flag. We should pay attention, has there been a change in medication, are they sick in some way, something is going on that we can change to improve their outcome. So tempo means something to me.

SG: We have reviewed a large case series in our institution of the elderly who fall, we have found the reason they fall is because something that is going on. It is an opportunity to do a workup that is different than if they just tripped. Why are they tripping today when they haven't tripped in the past 75 years? Or why have they tripped every day recently when they tripped once before in the past 75 years prior? The question becomes especially important if they don't have rheumatoid arthritis or aren't on Coumadin. Do they still need an aggressive workup with a head and neck CT? Do they also need their chemistries checked, a urinalysis checked, a hematocrit checked? I don't think we have a good answer to any of those questions. Our tendency at our institution is to be more conservative and so we tend to order these tests almost as a knee jerk reflex. We are concerned we are going to miss something and this is the only opportunity to catch something before the patient will deteriorate further after we discharge them.

RA: Those are great points. Ordering laboratory studies on a person with a new fall or increased frequency of falls might turn up surprising things. For example, I recently had a case of woman with significant hyponatremia attributable to recently started SSRI.

JH: I think you have to take into the account their frailty. One of the questions I have is: what kind of 76 year old this is, there is 76 and there is 76. There are some people at 76 who are still running and look great, and others who look frail and have real difficulty. Part of it is the clinical assessment, I am not sure we have a great tool for that. We as experienced clinicians use a gestalt. I think the points you raise are important: past medical history, recent event history, medications they are on are all things we take into account of whether you work them up.

PR: I think those are all reasons for being much more permissive in our workups then in a young patient who tripped over the cat who complains of a single limb pain that we can focus on that injury and be done with it. But here we have a patient who has lots of reasons to have a fall that they might not be aware of. We see a lot of type 2 diabetes, which doesn't often cause hypoglycemia on a regular basis, as compared to insulin dependent diabetics. While we might not check on a younger person, it would be reasonable to check a fingerstick on this person. Once we have started down the pathway of the workup, we seem to be embarrassed to do imaging studies that might be very useful.

265

I think we should be overly generous rather than to confine our efforts because these patients are so complex in terms of what hurts that they don't complain of.

JH: For me one of the issues in a person like this, elderly on Coumadin, altered mental status or not, I think you are obligated to get a head CT especially if it is unclear if she hit her head. She has age related atrophy so you have increased space for things to move in addition to Coumadin which increases the risk of bleeding. There is no question but to do the head CT.

PR: Do you think that chronic steroid consumption increases the risk of osteoporosis or the risk of fracture?

JH: Yes, I think that chronic steroids increases the frailty, and, particularly from a bone health perspective, it makes me more cautious of my workup and makes me more concerned. It would be helpful to know which steroid she has been on and for how long. X-rays might reveal her degree of osteopenia. I would be relatively compulsive in working this person up.

PR: Rob, you made a great point that a fall maybe a clue into a major change in status that the patient has in their daily lives. Particularly in patients who have a reason for chronic pain, we may not know that they have changed their pattern of motor movement and that the fall comes from a weakness due to inactivity. They may not be using a walker because no one thought to give them one and that they just sit in their chair and when they try to move they can't. So I think the overall assessment of general function is as critical as anything we do to find out what the acute injury is. Were there any other sources of discomfort for her other than the ankle?

RA: No

PR: And then we found a rather serious fracture.

RA: Yes, she actually had a bimalleolar ankle fracture. She had no other imaging and she did fine.

PR: Well once again, we have a fracture that in a younger patient would be easily be taken care of by casting and outpatient services. But now we need to discover just how much impairment this injury is going to produce in this woman's life. If she lives alone, she is not going to be able to do her daily activities, cook for herself, clean for herself, and take care of her personal hygiene needs. As we discussed in the person with the humerus fracture, in the elderly even a single limb immobility is enough to support an in increase in the services they need on a daily basis and even temporary placement in a nursing home.

RA: It is a very hard time to be an old person right now in light of increasingly stringent insurance rules. You mention a humerus fracture which is a great example. Currently an upper extremity fracture does not qualify as an inpatient diagnosis in a hospital by Medicare rules. So if you are 99 year old with a broken arm and get admitted to hospital because you are unable to go home safely, that admission will be observation status. This is important because observation admissions do not count toward overnight stays that qualify you for insurance-covered post-hospital rehabilitation. There are many rules and financial implications for the care of older patients that have now become our problem in the ED. It has been strange for me to have conversations with patients and families about insurance rules in the ED.

PR: It is very hard to find relatives who are willing to step in and give the kind of care that 50 years ago would be quite routine from any relative or most neighbors. So I think you are quite right it is a very difficult management issue for these kind of patients. Shamai, one of the hidden causes of fall is of course cardiac. How far you would you want to look for a dysrhythmia or some other cardiac cause for this patient's fall?

SG: The first issue is how reliable the patient is. If that patient can't give you a history you have to be far more concerned that this wasn't a fall at all, but an episode of syncope. For syncope, as we have discussed, there are risk factors for patients that predict an adverse outcome after syncope. Age isn't one of them. If you get to be old, and you haven't had any heart disease and you have a normal EKG, and you have a clear cause of what happened, and you didn't have a chest pain, shortness of breath or palpitations, then I can confidently send that patient home, and know at least at 30 days they are not going to have a bad outcome. Well if the patient can't tell me whether there was chest pain, palpitations, or shortness of breath, or they have a bunch of risk factors, then I need to worry and I need to start with EKG and possibly an admission for dysrhythmia monitoring.

PR: Rob, you have recorded her INR as 3.2 that seems a little high for a DVT therapy, was that normal for her, or was she supposed to be at that level?

RA: I think she was still figuring out her dosing at that time. It was a new medication for her.

PR: With an elevated INR and an acute fracture, we are faced with the issue of when you would reverse it. I suppose this is a place where 50 years ago we simply would have kept her in the hospital to make sure she didn't bleed too much into the fracture and to address her life problems. Today we do not have that luxury. Although I think elevated INR is an adequate reason for admitting a patient. One of the things that you suggested Rob is that we need to make sure that more falls aren't going to occur. Is there anything we can do to manage that in this patient, because most of the issues that are going to make her fall are going to be distorted now that she has an ankle fracture?

RA: Yes, so I can answer that by discussing my approach to falls. There is lots of literature about falls and it can be overwhelming. In an effort to simplify, I have broken it down into three causes for every fall in an older person. The first cause are changes related to aging for which one could teach an entire course of geriatric physiology. Maintaining upright posture is dependent on almost every organ system, some of which we can evaluate and treat to prevent future falls. This is why we order physical therapy in these folks because we can increase their balance and strength. This first reason probably explains the majority of the falls. The second reason older adults fall is related to medications and alcohol. Our job in the ED regarding this is consider this and look for changes in medications or addition of high risk medications like benzodiazepines, sedative-hypnotics, and anticholinergics. The third reason for falls is an acute illness that lead to the fall. This is the what we mean by atypical presentation of illness in the elderly. Examples that I've seen include cholecystitis presenting as a fall, delirium presenting as a fall, and even a case of rupturing aortic aneurysm presenting as a fall. So, for every fall I think about old age, I think about medications, and I think about acute illness.

PR: Maura, her blood pressure is a little elevated would that concern you in terms of the fall or in terms of managing it?

MK: To be honest, I don't get particularly concerned about 150/90 in a 76 year-old female. I think recent guidelines on blood pressure support 150/90 to be an acceptable blood pressure for this age. I would be more concerned about a systolic blood pressure of 120 in her, that would raise my concern for syncope or presyncope related fall. But at 150/90, I am not particularly concerned that has contributed to the fall. If I had the luxury of prior blood pressures to compare it to that would be great.

PR: I would be curious what her outpatient blood pressure goals were. Because of the history of hypertension I would worry about TIA as the cause of this fall. And again, that is why the history of this mechanism would be very important in terms of what we need to fear for in this patient's future. Jon, assuming that you were able to get this patient easily managed as an outpatient, and assuming she had some relatives to help her in her daily activities, what sort of concerns would you have about preventing further falls while she is incapacitated from her ankle cast?

JH: I worry that she is going to have a lot of difficulty if she can be ambulatory at all. If she is going to try to go home with her bimalleolar fracture and elevated INR, I would try to convince to keep her in for observation or possibly surgery depending on how bad the fracture is. If she did go home, I would try to get a PT consult in the ED and make sure that she has adequate resources including someone to help her with activities of daily living, a bedside commode and other things.

RA: Having physical therapy evaluate the patient in the ED would be ideal and should probably be the standard. If the evaluation reveals she needs acute rehabilitation or is unsafe to go home alone, our disposition options are more clear.

MK: While I agree with this fundamentally, I think this reflects more of our societal issues with Medicare when someone doesn't meet the criteria for a full admission and doesn't have supplemental insurance or cannot pay for rehab despite physical therapy recommending it. Hopefully we will have things changing particularly with the ACOs getting a waiver for the

2 day hospital stay. That has been a challenge at our institution.

PR: While I hope you are right Maura, I think it is going to go the opposite direction and we are going to see less and less resources for patients because they cost too much. Regardless, I think this woman meets criteria for admission even without a PT telling you she is immobile due to the Coumadin therapy, ankle fracture, and elevated INR. I think most institutions would admit her to medicine with an orthopedics consult even though she is primarily an orthopedics problem. I certainly would push for admission. I particularly have seen these ankles balloon up into huge hemarthrosis in the subsequent 48 hours, and I don't think that is something that is easily watched as an outpatient. Again, it would depend at what institution you are in as to how easy or how hard it would be. Probably she would be more readily admitted in rural America then urban America, but she still probably needs to come in. Rob, you made a great point about the fear of falling in the future also restricting this patient's activities, and I think that once a patient has sustained a fracture from falling that truly induces fear of mobility in them. I am not sure what we can do to truly reduce that aside from make sure they are not living alone and having others make sure that they can stay mobile. For people who are truly solitary, I think this is often the first step in the downward spiral of old age. Do you have any suggestions on that fear?

RA: I think we should be aware of the impact a fall can have of people and be supportive. Taking a minute to communicate with a patient and family will go a long way. Even something as simple as "Mrs. Jones, I'm sorry you had this fall and I know it may impact you at home. We are ordering physical therapy to help you recover and prevent future falls. Please connect back with your doctor for a full medication review and other resources for fall prevention."

PR: I remember reading a paper on falls that suggested patients who were able to cut their own toe nails had a lower incidence of falls then the patients who couldn't. As a result, I started asking that history, but I don't know what to do about it when they can't. It was a strange fact.

RA: I think this speaks to a person's functional capacity at home. It helps us understand how frail a person might be. One could ask about nail cutting or showering or other activities of daily living. They all give important information. A strong marker of frailty is an inability to get up from the floor even after a non traumatic fall. I take this for granted now and have a hard time envisioning a time in my life when I could not get up from the ground.

PR: Well, being an old man, I can tell you that it is not as rare as you think it is. A lot depends on your general muscular strength and the kind of resources you have in your house. But if you fall in the middle of the floor where you have no furniture to help brace you, you can in fact be trapped on the floor. If you don't have someone visiting you every day, you can be trapped for a couple of days. We see people like this all the time. The only thing I can relate it to is if you're a skier and then fall in powder, it can take you an hour to get up. That is what it is like to be old. It is a very difficult time of life when you start losing your function and you become afraid of even losing it more. I think that we are going to be see more and more patients like this, and as you all pointed out our difficulties in managing them are particularity concerned with financial resources. Maura, I hope you are right that we are going to see more resources, but I am skeptical. I think things that we were able to do easily with hospitalization and observation units are now not being done so easily, and I think that it is going to harm us even more in the future.

JH: I would echo what Maura says and for the first time in 10–15 years we are getting a dedicated social worker down in the ED. I think there is recognition that hospitalizations are a big cost driver and that reducing hospitalizations can be achieved through improved outpatient resources. I would be cautiously optimistic that in their effort to cut the cost of inpatient care they will improve the outpatient support.

PR: I hope you people are right. But I am skeptical.

SG: I think the pendulum is going to swing back to where it was 50 years ago where we rely on the family as the caregivers for the elderly and those who become incapacitated. This is what is done in healthcare systems where resources are far more limited. I think we are going to go there as well.

PR: Well I think it has some salutary benefits that it may restore some of the family functions that we have lost in our society, but having lost them I think they are going to be very hard to recover. Until then, we are going to be left with patients who we have limited resources to help medically and there are few social resources. But I hope that we get more social services and that families do take more care of each other.

RA: May I raise one more issue?

PR: Please do!

RA: One thing that should be mentioned in this chapter is falls as a trauma issue. When you look at geriatric trauma, falls is far and away the number one mechanism of injury. Falling is how older adults hurt themselves; they don't get shot, stabbed, or fall off motorcycles. They do suffer significant injuries none the less. We have to think about how we are going to deal with falls from a trauma standpoint in terms of resources and our surgical colleagues. This is a big challenge which we will discuss more in our trauma chapter, but I wanted to bring up here as well.

PR: Well that is a terrific point because we have created a special methodology for dealing with trauma. We might exclude the patients who more need it from receiving it because "the trauma isn't great enough." Unless they were lucky enough to fall off a flight of stairs or a mechanism of injury compatible with receiving the level of care they need. Well I hope that changes over time. Well we can discuss that more in the trauma chapter.

Section III: Concepts

Scope of the problem and the opportunities

Falling kills people, falling hurts people, and falling scares people. Falls are an extensive public health problem that will continue to vex primary care and emergency providers alike. Sorting out the etiology of a fall, in addition to addressing the traumatic injury from a fall, is a frequent, major challenge for a busy emergency provider. Acute management of traumatic injury is complicated by older age. The presence of an acute injury in an older adult may require a more extensive workup than that typical for younger patients. Additionally and importantly, a simple "mechanical" fall in an elderly patient, one not associated with an external force, is an opportunity to search for underlying cause that may prevent additional morbidity and fear.

Falls and their sequelae present serious threats to the health and well-being of older adults [1]. About one in three older adults, those 65 years of age or older, fall each year, with falls being the leading cause of injury-related death, nonfatal injury, and hospital admissions for traumatic injury in this group [2, 3]. In addition, in 2010, more than 1.6 million older adults were treated and released from United States EDs following an unintentional fall, with an additional 595,000 patients hospitalized after such falls [3]. In the year 2000, direct medical costs related to falls summed to more than $19 billion, $28.2 billion when translated to 2010 dollars [4, 5]. Falls have been noted to be one of the most expensive medical conditions among community-dwelling older adults, and the annual direct and indirect costs associated with fall-related injuries are expected to continue to rise dramatically as the population ages [6, 7].

Falls are the most common source of traumatic brain injuries in older adults and are also the cause of most fractures sustained by this population [8, 9]. The development of a fear of falling is also recognized as an important negative consequence of falls, frequently resulting in the deterioration of both physical and mental health [10]. Fear of falling has been associated with reduced physical activity, decreased performance of activities of daily living, lower perceived physical health status, decreased quality of life, and increased rates of institutionalization [11–17]. Fear of falling results in changes in physical activity that lead to muscle weakness and balance impairment, changes that ultimately result in a further increased risk of falling [18, 19]. In fact, when studied in the context of other chronic illness, fear of falling leads to more restricted activity days than any other condition [20].

Given the serious implications of falls and their sequelae, researchers have focused much attention on the development and evaluation of interventions aimed at reducing falls in older adults [21]. Several interventions have demonstrated some efficacy in the reduction of falls, including exercise interventions, home safety interventions, and multicomponent interventions [21, 22].

These considerations suggest that emergency personnel can contribute in important ways beyond acute trauma management, after the fall of an elderly person. Determination of the etiology of the fall is also critical for development of prevention strategies and alleviation of fear as a sequela. In this chapter, we describe strategies for the management of acute trauma sustained by older adults and present a simplified method to explain and evaluate all "mechanical" falls for elderly patients.

Acute trauma management

Common injury patterns

The patterns of injury observed in elderly patients following falls are different than those noted in their younger counterparts [23–25]. Common injuries sustained by elder patients during falls include soft tissue injuries and lacerations, fractures, thoracic injuries, intracranial injuries, and injuries to the spine. Hip fractures are exceedingly common in older adults who have fallen, accounting for 87% of fractures and 95% of hip fractures in this population [25–27]. In addition, fractures of the pelvis, wrist, humerus, forearm, and lower extremities are especially prevalent consequences of geriatric falls [27]. Pelvic fractures are important injuries for elderly patients, with mortality reportedly between 12% and 21% [28–30]. Fractures of the spine and spinal cord injury also occur frequently in geriatric fallers [23]. Long-standing rheumatoid arthritis can weaken the odontoid ligament leading to atlantoaxial instability with trauma. While injury between the occiput and second cervical vertebrae is more likely in elder patients experiencing a fall from a low height, fracture of the lower cervical vertebrae is more common in those falling from greater elevation. Older patients commonly sustain injuries to the cervical spine across multiple levels [31].

Rib fractures and thoracic injuries are often present in older adults who have fallen [25]. Early identification of rib fractures is critical to optimizing care for geriatric patients as morbidity and mortality are significantly increased for those with fractures [32, 33]. Bergeron and colleagues observed increasing mortality as the number of rib fractures increased in their population of elderly trauma victims. Mortality ranged from 4% for those with one to two fractures to 32% for those elders with six or more fractures [33]. Stawicki and colleagues note similar findings in elderly patients with rib fractures. In their sample, mortality varied from 12.3% for those with one to two fractures to 37.8% for those with seven or more fractures [32]. Important pulmonary complications associated with rib fracture include pneumonia, pleural effusion, and respiratory failure.

Intracranial injuries are frequently observed in elderly patients who have sustained a fall [24, 25]. Geriatric patients who have experienced only minor head injury have been noted to be at high risk for significant intracranial processes, even when no alternation in level of consciousness, fracture, or neurologic deficit is present upon examination [34, 35]. In addition, the use of anticoagulant or antiplatelet medications increases the risk of intracranial hemorrhage [36, 37]. While warfarin is a commonly appreciated high-risk medication, there is less familiarity with the newer anticoagulant agents, which also can cause great morbidity.

Workup following acute trauma

Given the morbidity and mortality associated with traumatic injury in older adults, the aggressive use of imaging in an elderly patient after a fall should be instinctive, particularly in the presence of new focal findings upon examination, alterations in mental status, or the use of medications affecting coagulation. This is especially true for suspected head and cervical spine injuries due to the importance of early diagnosis. In general, if imaging of the cervical spine is necessary, a computed tomography (CT) scan is the preferred method, although with the prior presence of arthritic changes such as osteoarthritic spurs, it may be necessary to obtain a magnetic resonance imaging (MRI) to assess the new pathology.

Radiographs and CT may be useful for elders with suspected bony deformities, fractures, or disordered gait. Considering the tremendous morbidity and mortality associated with rib fractures in the elderly, such injuries should be aggressively identified. They are often hard to find on plain films, and there is much superior visualization with ultrasound and CT scan imaging. Nevertheless, after a fall, if there is clinical tenderness over the rib cage, even before there is any proof of rib fracture, it is prudent to assume the presence of a fracture. The stability of the patient should trump diagnostic proof of the entity. Thus, it is wise to place a thoracostomy tube in any patient requiring intubation and ventilation even without imaging proof of the rib fracture. Detection of hip and pelvic fractures continues to follow the usual progression of plain films followed by advanced imaging with CT, MRI, or bone scan if there is continued pain. Ultrasonography can assist in the identification of traumatic intra-abdominal injuries sustained during falls.

Disposition

Triage to a trauma center should be strongly considered for the fallen elderly patient. Unfortunately, the undertriage of elders to trauma centers following traumatic injury is well documented in the literature [38–43]. Undertriage is of critical importance in this population because injured older adults, even those with seemingly minor injuries, are noted to experience much greater mortality than their younger counterparts [44–47]. Staudenmayer and colleagues recently reported, in a population-based analysis of 6015 older adults, that most of the patients who died following a traumatic injury had sustained minor injuries from low-impact energy mechanisms [43]. Greater than 80% of those who died in their sample were more than 75 years of age, had experienced a fall, were neurologically intact, were hemodynamically stable, and had Injury Severity Scores of less than 15. These findings are in keeping with other reports that elder patients frequently fail to meet the standard physiologic criteria for transfer to a trauma center, possibly due to the synergistic effects of decreased physiologic reserve, physiologic frailty, medication use, and comorbid conditions [42, 48–53].

Seniors managed by a multidisciplinary team fare better than those managed by a single discipline [54, 55]. Care teams with members from a variety of disciplines often recognize the serious impact that traumatic injuries can have on elderly patients, beyond the obvious disruptions in physical health.

Discharging an elderly patient to home following an injury sustained in a fall may require additional resources beyond those typically present in the ED. For example, a relatively trivial wrist fracture may have tremendous morbidity for a frail geriatric patient living alone. Teams that include care coordinators, discharge planners, occupational and physical therapists, nutritionists, and nurses are often in tune with the complexities patients and their families encounter when returning to the community setting.

Development of multifaceted discharge and follow-up plans can prevent unnecessary return ED and hospital visits while improving quality of life, comfort, and outcomes for patients [54, 55].

For patients who will be discharged to the community setting and are at risk for additional falls, clinical assessments of mobility, balance, and gait can be completed. Disposition home may involve changes to existing medications or discussion with the patient's prescribing physician.

A strategy for classifying the etiology of falls in older adults

Considering fall etiology in the emergency setting

Many elders evaluated in the ED following a fall have not clearly sustained serious traumatic injury, and often reasons for the fall are not obvious. For these patients, establishment of the key factors precipitating the fall is critical to ensuring that appropriate and effective treatments are initiated. Many frameworks for considering the reasons that ambulatory older adults fall have been proposed. Previous authors have described the factors precipitating falls in terms of intrinsic and extrinsic risk factors or modifiable and nonmodifiable risk factors [56–58]. However, the risk factor classification systems used by clinicians and researchers have not been consistent, limiting the ability to compare findings across studies and settings [58]. Furthermore, any geriatric patient in the ED after a fall is already *de facto* at high risk for falls.

For all these reasons, understanding and evaluating the complex interactions between intrinsic, extrinsic, modifiable, and nonmodifiable risk factors can be cumbersome and impractical for clinicians in the fast-paced emergency setting. Yet this analysis is essential for the well-being of the patient, and for systematic accumulation of data on this widespread problem. Therefore, we have developed an alternative evaluation strategy, focusing on three reasons underlying nearly every fall. Falls in older adults are typically caused by one of the following three factors, alone or in combination: age-related physiologic changes or disease, medications, and acute illnesses.

We will present in detail each of the three common causes of falls. This section will be followed by a brief illustrative case summary highlighting these three causes of geriatric falls.

Reason 1: Physiologic changes and disease related to aging

Functional decline during aging

Physiologic changes related to the aging process contribute to falls in older adults, and are probably the most common reason for the "mechanical" fall. The ability to maintain upright posture is key to avoiding falls, and depends upon input from the visual, proprioceptive, and vestibular systems. Declines in function are noted with aging in all three systems [59]. In addition, the muscle activation patterns of older adults are notably different than those of their younger counterparts [59, 60]. In older persons, the proximal muscles, such as the quadriceps, are activated prior to the more distal muscles, such as the tibialis anterior, representing a less-efficient and effective way to maintain postural stability. In addition, older adults experience greater cocontraction of antagonistic muscles, and the onset of muscle activation is delayed when compared to younger people. Changes in one's ability to regulate systemic blood pressure are also known to influence falls. Declines in baroreflex sensitivity to hypotensive stimuli, exhibited as failure to cardioaccelerate, increase the risk of a fall while typical stresses such as changing position may lead to hypotension more frequently in older patients [61]. Many elderly patients experience cerebral perfusion compromise due to the presence of vascular disease, so even small decreases in blood pressure may result in cerebral ischemia and falls. Older adults are more prone to dehydration, which may result in orthostatic hypotension and falls, due to a reduced total body water volume. Moreover, many elderly patients are taking beta-blocking medications, and often have exaggerated postural changes with orthostatic changes in position.

Chronic conditions associated with aging are often implicated in falls experienced by older adults. Neurologic disorders are associated with impaired strength, sensation, balance, gait, muscle tone, and coordination. Musculoskeletal diseases, such as arthritis, influence mobility, postural control, and the ability to safely ambulate. Dementia and other disorders of cognition may impair awareness, judgment, problem-solving ability, and gait [62]. Changes associated with Parkinson's disease, such as lower extremity rigidity, delayed initiation of movement, cognitive impairment, and medication effects can all contribute to falls [63]. The hypoglycemic episodes and neuropathy commonly associated with diabetes can play a role. Disorders of the urinary tract, including incontinence and nocturia have both been associated with falls by causing a distraction for those who may be challenged to maintain postural stability at baseline (Table 19.1).

Evaluation of aging-related functional decline as causative for falls

Many of the functional changes listed above will be discovered during routine ED workup. In addition, evaluations of gait and balance may be a helpful part of the physical examination for older adults who have fallen. In the emergency setting, where assessing gait and balance are not typically priorities and physical therapy evaluation is rarely available on a 24-hour

Table 19.1 Key emergency department assessments of alterations contributing to falls.

Organ/Organ System	Alteration	Example Assessments
Cardiac	Dysrhythmia	Auscultation and electrocardiogram
	Acute coronary syndrome	Electrocardiogram and laboratory testing
Circulation	Decreased cerebral perfusion	Low blood pressure, altered level of consciousness, lightheadedness, and carotid hypersensitivity
	Orthostatic hypotension	Positional change in blood pressure
Brain	Decreased attention	Executive function tasks: ability to perform dual tasks such as timed up and go with a cup of water
	Slowed motor processing	Movement speed: timed tapping and timed finger to nose test
	Impaired cognition	Three item recall, clock drawing test, and functional activities questionnaire

basis, simple and valid tools can be helpful to assess gait and balance, as described in Table 19.2. One example is the "Get Up and Go" test, described in Figure 19.1, which can be used to quickly and simply evaluate gait and strength [68, 64]. While this test is often timed, emergency clinicians typically need to identify major gait abnormalities contributing to falls and timing is not crucial to this purpose. Common gait disturbances that may contribute to falls in older adults are listed in Table 19.3.

Both balance and quadriceps strength are assessed with the "functional reach" test, a measure of the patient's neuromuscular base of support described in Figure 19.2 [61, 62, 65]. Simple measures of gait and mobility are provided in Table 19.2.

Reason 2: Acute illness

Acute illnesses contributing to falls

In older persons, falls are recognized as being a nonspecific presentation of an acute illness [63]. For example, cardiac dysrhythmias may cause an acute

reduction in cerebral blood flow, and a related loss of consciousness that results in a fall [63, 69, 70]. Acute infectious illnesses, often pneumonia or infections of the urinary tract, may contribute to falls by precipitating confusion and an impaired ability to maintain postural stability [71]. Acute exacerbations of chronic diseases, such as diabetes mellitus, congestive heart failure, and chronic obstructive pulmonary disease, may give rise to falls by impairing sensory, neurologic, or musculoskeletal functioning as well as by altering cerebral oxygenation or perfusion. Acute cerebrovascular events, including strokes and transient ischemic attacks, may cause weakness, vertigo, or loss of consciousness that can all lead to physical instability and falls.

Evaluation of acute illness as causative of falls

Considering the possibility that an acute illness has caused a fall in an older adult is an important first step. Diagnostic studies based on symptomatology observed during routine workup may be helpful. For

Table 19.2 Brief measures of balance and mobility.

Test	Population	Sample Assessments	Scoring
Timed up and go [64]	Ambulatory older adults with or without assistive devices	Patient rises from chair without use of arms, walks 10 feet, turns, and walks back to the chair	Time to complete task in seconds is measured; score is average of two test trials; <10 seconds is optimal, >30 seconds indicates that mobility may be impaired and physical therapy referral indicated
Functional reach [65]	Persons able to stand without support	While standing without shoes/socks, the patient reaches forward as far as possible without losing balance	Distance the patient is able to reach is measured; reaching less than 6 inches. is indicative of an impaired base of support
Berg balance scale [66]	Ambulatory older adults with or without assistive devices; those with limited endurance for walking-based tests	Standing with feet together, standing with eyes closed, tandem, and single-leg stance, functional reach, 360° turn, and transfer from sitting to standing; includes 14 tasks	Each task is scored 0–5; individual scores are sum yielding a total score of 0–56; scores 45 and below are indicative of increased fall risk
Short physical performance battery [67]	Ambulatory older adults	Includes a 4-meter walk; standing balance with feet together, in semitandem and tandem positions; five stands from a chair with arms across the chest	Times to task completion are converted to a 0–4 scale; scores on the three tasks are summed and ranged from 0 to 12, with 0 indicating the inability to perform any of the tasks

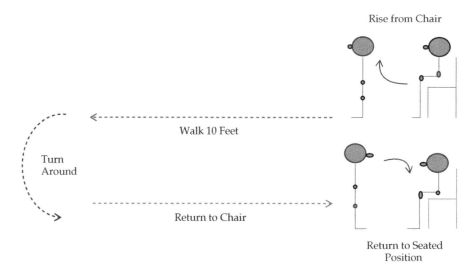

Figure 19.1 The timed "get up and go" test begins with the patient seated in a chair without arms. The patient is asked to (1) rise from the chair without using their arms, (2) walk 10 feet, (3) turn around, (4) walk back to the chair, and (5) return to the seated position. The clinician measures the length of time necessary to complete the task. Completion of the test in 30 seconds or more indicates impaired mobility. Observing the "get up" portion of the test allows the clinician to evaluate quadriceps strength, while the gait observation allows for the identification of hesitant starts, broad-based gait, a deviated path, failure of the patient's heels to clear the floor, and arm extension.

Table 19.3 Gait disturbances in ED fallers.

Gait Disturbance	Observed as	Cause
Myopathic gait	Presence of Trendelenburg sign – waddling gait, pelvis drops on contralateral side while walking	Weakened hip abductor muscles
Diplegic gait	Scissoring; legs or feet cross at midline	Parkinson's disease; tightness of hip adductor muscles
Lack of heel strike	Absence of heel strike when foot makes contact with the ground or initial heel strike followed by the foot "slapping" the ground; reduced toe clearance during swing phase	Weakness of ankle dorsiflexors, ankle plantarflexion contracture, peripheral neuropathy, severe L4 or L5 radiculopathies, and injury of the peroneal nerve due to trauma or compressive injury
Stance time asymmetry	Length of time in stance phase differs between legs	Sensory impairment, pain, weakness, flexion contracture of the knee or leg, and fear of falling
Trunk flexed gait	Pronounced lumbar flexion while walking, pronounced head protrusion, and thoracic kyphosis	Vertebral fractures, hip or knee contractures, weakened gluteal muscles or knee extensors, Parkinson's disease, and dementia
Wide-based gait	Increased step width, observable by watching patient's gait on a floor with 12-inch. tiles; gait is wide if the outside of the patient's feet do not stay within the tile	Sensory impairment, fear of falling, cerebellar disease, bilateral hip, or knee disease

A. Stand next to wall, extend arm to 90° with closed fist

B. Reach as far forward as possible without taking a step or losing balance

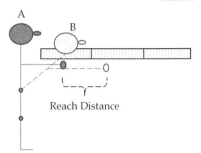

Reach Distance

Figure 19.2 Preparing the Functional Reach Test begins with the clinician attaching a yardstick to a wall at the patient's acromion level. The patient is asked to stand next to the wall and yardstick without touching them and is then asked to extend the arm closer to the wall to 90° of shoulder flexion with a closed fist, position A above. The location of the third metacarpal head on the yardstick is recorded as the starting position. The patient is asked to reach as far forward as possible without taking a step. The location of the third metacarpal is again recorded, position B above. The difference between the starting and ending positions is the reach distance. The inability to reach 6 inches. or more is indicative of an impaired base of support.

example, in the setting of cardiopulmonary symptoms, electrocardiography and chest radiography may be of benefit. Neurologic findings should prompt a search for brain ischemia. Infection should be considered, especially in view of the muted temperature and heart rate responses to infection observed in older patients. Infections in the elderly may go undetected as nearly half of older patients with confirmed bacterial infections do not display fever upon initial presentation [72].

Reason 3: Medications and substances

Medicines and substances contributing to falls
Medication use is a well-documented contributor to falls in older adults [62]. Many medications and classes of medications have been identified as increasing fall risk, including beta-blocking agents and other antihypertensives, benzodiazepines, antidepressants, antipsychotics, antiparkinsonian agents, narcotic analgesics, antihistamines, statins, diuretics, and glaucoma medications. Older patients are at risk, for example, for developing hyponatremia while on hydrochlorothiazide, or when commencing a SSRI.

Particular medication effects of concern are sedation, hypotension, myopathy, extrapyramidal effects, and pupillary constriction [73–75]. Recent changes in medication dosing, the use of multiple medications, particularly those that potentially influence the central nervous system have all been associated with falls and are particularly dangerous for older persons [76, 77]. Alcohol, even in small quantities, has been shown to be a substantial risk factor for falls in older patients, with both alcohol and prescription drug dependence occurring commonly in the elderly population [78–81].

Evaluation of medicines as causative for falls
This is the most challenging category for systematic workup as there are many possibilities (Table 19.4). Establishment of a definitive list may require a call to a primary care office, pharmacy, or long-term care facility. Identifying any new medications may provide clues. Routine laboratory testing is not recommended in this context, but may be reasonable as age and number of prescriptions rise. Medication-related electrolyte problems, renal insufficiency, and anemia can be detected. Especially, if the other two categories of causation are not likely, then detailed investigation of medicines and alcohol consumption could be worthwhile, indeed essential for further protective management of the patient. Many EDs are utilizing the services of a full-time pharmacist who can not only assist with drug dosages and mixing solutions, but also with information about complex and negative drug interactions.

Applying the "three causes for every fall" approach: The case of Mrs. Smith

Consider Mrs Smith, an 80-year-old woman, who fell at church.
Mrs Smith was an 80-year-old woman who presented to the ED after experiencing a fall at her church. She reports that she fell after tripping over a curb outside of the church, and when questioned, she denied striking her head. A deformity of Mrs. Smith's wrist was immediately apparent. While evaluating Mrs Smith, you consider the first of the "three causes for every fall," physiologic changes, and diseases related to the aging process.

Age-related physiologic changes in gait, balance, vision, proprioception, and many other body systems

Table 19.4 Medications contributing to falls in elders.

Medication Classes	Mechanism of Contributing to Falls
Benzodiazepines, narcotic analgesics, antidepressants, SSRIs, sedating antihistamines, antipsychotics, anticonvulsants, and ethanol	Sedation
Antihypertensives and beta-blockers, antiparkinsonian agents, antidepressants, antipsychotics, and antianginals	Orthostatic hypotension
Corticosteroids, high-dose statins, colchicine, interferon, and ethanol	Myopathy
Glaucoma medications, especially pilocarpine	Pupillary constriction (miosis)
Phenothiazines, SSRIs, metoclopramide, and antipsychotics	Extrapyramidal side effects

often contribute to falls in older adults. While Mrs. Smith may have been successfully navigating the same curb for decades, her status as an octogenarian most certainly places her at high risk for physiologic changes and age-related diseases that now challenge her ability to maintain postural stability and control. Considering this, her ED care might involve simple tests of balance and muscular strength such as the functional reach or "get up and go" tests described in this chapter. In addition to evaluating and treating Mrs Smith's wrist fracture, your follow-up plan may include arranging for an outpatient physical therapy evaluation.

Review of Mrs Smith's triage notes reveal that she has no history of previous falls and that a low-grade fever was documented at triage. On review of systems, Mrs Smith reports that she has had a cough for approximately 1 week.

Perhaps an underlying pneumonia has overtaxed her physiologic reserves, and has contributed to her fall. Mrs Smith's emergency care might now include acquisition of laboratory tests, a chest radiograph, and treatment of an underlying infectious process. Maintaining vigilance for the possibility of occult acute illness can dramatically change the ED course for elders who have fallen.

While reviewing Mrs Smith's medications, you noted that she was being treated with eight medications, prescribed by four different medical providers. Her medications include anxiolytics, antidepressants, and cardiac medications.

There should be little doubt that Mrs Smith's medications may have contributed to the fall through their effects on the central nervous and cardiovascular systems. In light of identifying medication use as a potential explanation for her fall, you consider obtaining orthostatic vital signs and a brief cognitive assessment as part of Mrs Smith's evaluation. In addition, you understand that communicating with Mrs Smith's primary care provider, either verbally or through the electronic medical record, will be an important part of ensuring that her medications do not contribute to future falls.

Section IV: Decision-making

- Falls in older adults are important, are associated with great morbidity and mortality, and often do not have an assignable external cause.
- After treatment of acute injuries, the ED clinical evaluation of the older adult who has fallen continues in order to discover reasons for the fall, which may need treatment or alleviation. This evaluation includes physical examination, the past medical history, medication history, brief cognitive examination, and laboratory and radiographic testing as indicated.
- In the setting of acute trauma in the elderly, early, and aggressive imaging is recommended.
- Under triage of the elderly to trauma centers is well documented, probably resulting in increased risk for older patients.
- Falls in older adults are almost always explained by one or more of the following factors:
  - Physiologic changes or diseases associated with the aging process
  - Acute illnesses
  - Medication use.
- Interdisciplinary teams are typically most successful at creating individualized interventions that can prevent future falls.

References

1 Van Nieuwehuizen, R.C., van Dijk, N., van Breda, F.G. et al. (2010) Assessing the prevalence of modifiable risk factors in older patients visiting an ED due to a fall using the CAREFALL triage instrument. *Am. J. Emerg. Med.*, **28**, 994–1001.

2 Hausdorff, J.M., Rios, D.A., and Edelber, H.K. (2001) Gait variability and fall risk in community-living older adults: a 1-year prospective study. *Arch. Phys. Med. Rehabil.*, **82** (8), 1050–1056.

3 Centers for Disease Control and Prevention, National Center for Injury Prevention and Control. (2013) *Web-based Injury Statistics Query and Reporting System (WISQARS)* [online] (accessed 31 December 2011) http://www.cdc.gov/injury/wisqars/pdf/ leading causes of non fatal injury 2013-a.pdf.

4 Stevens, J.A., Corso, P.S., Finkelstein, E.A. et al. (2006) The costs of fatal and nonfatal falls among older adults. *Inj. Prev.*, **12**, 290–295.

5 Centers for Disease Control and Prevention, National Center for Injury Prevention and Control. (2012) *Falls among Older Adults: An Overview* [online], http://www.cdc.gov/homeandrecreationalsafety/falls/adultfalls.html (accessed 12 December 2013).

6 Carroll, N.V., Slattum, P.W., and Cox, F.M. (2005) The cost of falls among the community-dwelling elderly. *J. Manag. Care Pharm.*, **11** (4), 307–316.

7 Englander, F., Hodson, T.J., and Terregrossa, R.A. (1996) Economic dimensions of slip and fall injuries. *J. Forensic Sci.*, **41** (5), 733–746.

8 Jager, T.E., Weiss, H.B., Coben, J.H. et al. (2002) Traumatic brain injuries evaluated in US emergency departments, 1992–1994. *Acad. Emerg. Med.*, **359**, 134–140.

9 Bell, A.J., Talbot-Stern, J.K., and Hennessy, A. (2000) Characteristics and outcomes of older patients presenting to the emergency department after a fall: a retrospective analysis. *Med. J. Aust.*, **173** (4), 176–177.

10 Jung, D. (2008) Fear of falling in older adults: comprehensive review. *Asian. Nurs. Res.*, **2** (4), 214–222.

11 Bruce, D.G., Devine, A., and Prince, R.L. (2002) Recreational physical activity levels in healthy older women: the importance of fear of falling. *J. Am. Geriatr. Soc.*, **50**, 84–89.

12 Delbaere, K., Crombez, G., Vanderstraeten, G. et al. (2004) Fear-related avoidance of activities, falls and physical frailty. A prospective community-based cohort study. *Age Ageing*, **33**, 368–373.

13 Fletcher, P.C. and Hirdes, J.P. (2004) Restriction in activity associated with fear of falling among community-based seniors using home care services. *Age Ageing*, **33**, 273–279.

14 Li, F., Fisher, J., Harmer, P. et al. (2003) Fear of falling in elderly persons: association with falls, functional ability, and quality of life. *J. Gerontol. B: Psychol. Sci. Soc. Sci.*, **58**, 283–290.

15 Cumming, R.G., Salkeld, G., Thomas, M. et al. (2000) Prospective study of the impact of fear of falling on activities of daily living, SF-36 Scores, and nursing home admission. *J. Gerontol. A Biol. Sci. Med. Sci.*, **55**, 299–305.

16 Martin, F.C., Hart, D., Spector, T. et al. (2005) Fear of falling limiting activity in young-old women is associated with reduced functional mobility rather than psychological factors. *Age Ageing*, **34**, 281–287.

17 Brouwer, B., Musselman, K., and Culham, E. (2004) Physical function and health status among seniors with and without a fear of falling. *Gerontology*, **50**, 135–141.

18 Friedman, S.M., Munoz, B., West, S.K. et al. (2002) Falls and fear of falling: which comes first? A longitudinal prediction model suggests strategies for primary and secondary prevention. *J. Am. Geriatr. Soc.*, **50**, 1329–1335.

19 Hill, K., Womer, M., Russell, M. et al. (2010) Fear of falling in older fallers presenting at emergency departments. *J. Adv. Nurs.*, **66** (8), 1769–1779.

20 Kosorok, M.R., Omenn, G.S., Diehr, P. et al. (1992) Restricted activity days among older adults. *Am. J. Public Health*, **82**, 1263–1267.

21 Carpenter, C.R. (2010) Preventing falls in community-dwelling older adults. *Ann. Emerg. Med.*, **55** (3), 296–298.

22 Gillespie, L.D., Robertson, M.C., Gillespie, W.J. et al. (2009) Interventions for preventing falls in older people living in the community. *Cochrane Database Syst. Rev.*, **2**: (Art. No.: CD007146). DOI: 10.1002/14651858.CD007143.pub3.

23 Aschkenasy, M.T. and Rothenhaus, T.C. (2006) Trauma and falls in the elderly. *Emerg. Med. Clin. North Am.*, **24**, 413–432.

24 Gowing, R. and Jain, M.K. (2007) Injury patterns and outcomes associated with elderly trauma victims in Kingston, Ontario. *Can. J. Surg.*, **50** (6), 437–444.

25 Ojo, P., O'Connor, J., Kim, D. et al. (2009) Patterns of injury in geriatric falls. *Conn. Med.*, **73** (3), 139–145.

26 Nordell, E., Jarnlo, G.B., Jetsen, C. et al. (2000) Accidental falls and related fractures in 65–74 year olds: a retrospective study of 332 patients. *Acta Orthop. Scand.*, **71**, 175–179.

27 King, M.B. (2009) Falls, in *Hazzard's Geriatric Medicine and Gerontology* (eds J. Halter, J. Ouslander, M. Tinetti et al.), McGraw-Hill (electronic version), http://www.r2library.com.library.mmc.org/resource/detail/0071488723/ch0054s1326 (accessed 26 August 2015).

28 Alost, T. and Waldrop, R.D. (1997) Profile of geriatric pelvic fractures presenting to the emergency department. *Am. J. Emerg. Med.*, **15** (6), 576–578.

29 Henry, S.M., Pollak, A.N., Jones, A.L. *et al.* (2002) Pelvic fracture in geriatric patients: a distinct clinical entity. *J. Trauma*, **53** (1), 15–20.

30 O'Brien, D.P., Luchette, F.A., Pereira, S.J. *et al.* (2002) Pelvic fracture in the elderly is associated with increased mortality. *Surgery*, **132** (4), 710–714.

31 Lomoschitz, F.M., Blackmore, C.C., Mirza, S.K. *et al.* (2002) Cervical spine injuries in patients 65 years old and older: epidemiology analysis regarding the effects of age and injury mechanism on distribution, type, and stability of injuries. *AJR Am. J. Roentgenol.*, **178**, 573–577.

32 Stawicki, S.P., Grossman, M.D., Hoey, B.A. *et al.* (2004) Rib fractures in the elderly: a marker of injury severity. *J. Am. Geriatr. Soc.*, **52**, 805–808.

33 Bergeron, E., Lavoie, A., Clas, D. *et al.* (2003) Elderly trauma patients with rib fractures are at greater risk of death and pneumonia. *J. Trauma*, **54** (3), 478–485.

34 Mack, L.R., Chan, S.B., Silva, J.C. *et al.* (2003) The use of head computed tomography in elderly patients sustaining minor head trauma. *J. Emerg. Med.*, **24**, 157–162.

35 Rathlev, N., Medzon, R., Lowery, D. *et al.* (2006) Intracranial pathology in the elderly with blunt head trauma. *Acad. Emerg. Med.*, **13**, 302–307.

36 Reynolds, F.D., Dietz, P.A., Higgins, D. *et al.* (2003) Time to deterioration of the elderly, anticoagulated, minor head injury patient who presents without evidence of neurologic abnormality. *J. Trauma*, **54**, 492–496.

37 Li, J., Brown, J., and Levine, M. (2001) Mild head injury, anticoagulants, and risk of intracranial injury. *Lancet*, **357**, 771–772.

38 Hsia, R.Y., Wang, E., Torres, H. *et al.* (2010) Disparities in trauma center access despite increasing utilization: data from California, 1999 to 2006. *J. Trauma*, **68**, 217–224.

39 Hsia, R.Y., Wang, E., Saynina, O. *et al.* (2011) Factors associated with trauma center use for elderly patients with trauma a statewide analysis, 1999–2008. *Arch. Surg.*, **146**, 585–592.

40 Vassar, M.J., Holcroft, J.J., Knudson, M.M. *et al.* (2003) Fractures in access to and assessment of trauma systems. *J. Am. Coll. Surg.*, **197**, 717–725.

41 Newgard, C.D., Zive, D., Holmes, J.F. *et al.* (2011) A multisite assessment of the American College of Surgeons Committee on Trauma field triage decision scheme for identifying seriously injured children and adults. *J. Am. Coll. Surg.*, **213**, 709–721.

42 Nakamura, Y., Daya, M., Bulger, E.M. *et al.* (2012) Evaluating age in the field triage of injured persons. *Ann. Emerg. Med.*, **60**, 335–345.

43 Staudenmayer, K.L., Hsia, R.Y., Mann, N.C. *et al.* (2013) Triage of elderly trauma patients: a population-based perspective. *J. Am. Coll. Surg.*, **217**, 569–576.

44 Shifflette, V.K., Lorenzo, M., Mangram, A.J. *et al.* (2010) Should age be a factor to change from a level II to a level I trauma activation? *J. Trauma*, **69**, 88–92.

45 Morris, J.A. Jr., MacKenzie, E.J., Damiano, A.M. *et al.* (1990) Mortality in trauma patients: the interaction between host factors and severity. *J. Trauma*, **30**, 1476–1482.

46 Rogers, A., Rogers, F., Bradburn, E. *et al.* (2010) Old and undertriaged: a lethal combination. *Am. Surg.*, **78** (6), 711–715.

47 Ferrera, P.C., Bartfield, J.M., and D'Andrea, C.C. (2000) Outcomes of admitted geriatric trauma victims. *Am. J. Emerg. Med.*, **18**, 575–580.

48 Demetriades, D., Sava, J., Alo, K. *et al.* (2001) Old age as a criterion for trauma team activation. *J. Trauma*, **51**, 754–757.

49 Phillips, S., Rond, P.C. III, Kelly, S.M. *et al.* (1996) The failure of triage criteria to identify geriatric patients with trauma; results from the Florida Trauma Triage Study. *J. Trauma*, **40**, 278–283.

50 Scalea, T.M., Simon, H.M., Duncan, A.O. *et al.* (1990) Geriatric blunt multiple trauma: improved survival with early invasive monitoring. *J. Trauma*, **30**, 129–136.

51 Demetriades, D., Karaiskakis, M., Velmahos, G. *et al.* (2002) Effect on outcome of early intensive management of geriatric trauma patients. *Br. J. Surg.*, **89**, 1319–1322.

52 Lehamann, R., Beekley, A., Casey, L. *et al.* (2009) The impact of advanced age on trauma triage decisions and outcomes: a statewide analysis. *Am. J. Surg.*, **197**, 571–575.

53 MacKenzie, E.J., Weir, S., Rivara, F.P. *et al.* (2010) The value of trauma center care. *J. Trauma*, **69**, 1–10.

54 Stenvall, M., Olofsson, B., Lundstrom, M. *et al.* (2007) A multidisciplinary, multifactorial intervention program reduces postoperative falls and injuries after femoral neck fracture. *Osteoporos. Int.*, **18**, 167–175.

55 Stenvall, M., Berggren, M., Lundstrom, M. *et al.* (2012) A multidisciplinary intervention program improved the outcome after hip fracture for people with dementia – subgroup analyses of a randomized controlled trial. *Arch. Gerontol. Geriatr.*, **54** (3), e284–e289.

56 Institute of Medicine, Division of Health Promotion and Disease Prevention (1992) Falls in older persons: risk factors and prevention, in *The Second Fifty Years: Promoting Health and Preventing Disability* (eds R.L. Berg and J.S. Cassells), National Academy Press, Washington, DC, pp. 263–290.

57 Kane, R., Ouslander, J., Abrass, I. *et al.* (2009) Falls, in *Essentials of Clinical Geriatrics*, 6th edn (eds R. Kane, J. Ouslander, I. Abrass, and B. Resnick), McGraw-Hill, Columbus, http://www.r2library.com/Resource/Title/ 0071498222 (accessed 26 August 2015).

58 American Geriatrics Society, British Geriatrics Society, and American Academy of Orthopaedic Surgeons Panel on Falls Prevention (2001) Guideline for the prevention of falls in older persons. *J. Am. Geriatr. Soc.*, **49**, 664–672.

59 Laughton, C.A., Slavin, M., Katdare, K. *et al.* (2003) Aging, muscle activity, and balance control: physiologic changes associated with balance impairment. *Gait Posture*, **18**, 101–108.

60 Collins, J.J., De Luca, C.J., Burrows, A. *et al.* (1995) Age-related changes in open-loop postural control mechanisms. *Exp. Brain Res.*, **104**, 480–492.

61 Schneider, D.C. and Mader, S.L. (2007) Falls, in *Primary Care Geriatrics: A Case Based Approach*, 5th edn (eds R.J. Ham, P.D. Sloane, G.A. Warshaw, and M.A. Bernard), Mosby, Philadelphia, PA, pp. 291–305.

62 Soriano, T.A., DeCherrie, L.V., and Thomas, D.C. (2007) Falls in the community-dwelling older adult: a review for primary-care providers. *Clin. Interv. Aging*, **2** (4), 545–553.

63 Fernandez, H.M. (2007) Instability and falls, in *Fundamentals of Geriatric Medicine: A Case-based Approach* (eds R.P. Soriano, H.M. Fernandez, C.K. Cassel, and R.M. Leipzig), Springer, New York, pp. 356–372.

64 Posiadlo, D. and Richardson, S. (1992) The timed "up and go" test: a test of basic functional mobility for frail elderly persons. *J. Am. Geriatr. Soc.*, **39**, 142–148.

65 Duncan, P.W., Weiner, D.K., Chandler, J. *et al.* (1990) Functional reach: a new clinical measure of balance. *J. Gerontol.*, **45** (6), M192–M197.

66 Berg, K.O., Wood-Dauphinne, S.L., Willliams, J.I. *et al.* (1992) Measuring balance in the elderly: validation of an instrument. *Can. J. Public Health Rev.*, **83** (**Suppl. 2**), S7–S11.

67 Guralnik, J.M., Simonsick, E.M., Ferrucci, L. *et al.* (1994) A short physical performance battery assessing lower extremity function: association with self-reported disability and prediction of mortality and nursing home admission. *J. Gerontol. Med. Sci.*, **49** (2), M85–M94.

68 Mathias, S., Nayak, U., and Issacs, B. (1986) Balance in elderly patients: the "get up and go" test. *Arch. Phys. Med. Rehabil.*, **67**, 387–389.

69 Shaw, F.E. and Kenny, R.A. (1997) The overlap between syncope and falls in the elderly. *Postgrad. Med. J.*, **73** (**864**), 635–639.

70 Lamarre-Cliché, M. (2007) Syncope in older adults. *Geriatr. Aging*, 10 (4), 236–240.

71 Tinetti, M.E. and Speechley, M. (1988) Risk factors for falls among elderly persons living in the community. *N. Engl. J. Med.*, **36**, 1701–1707.

72 Marco, C.A., Schoenfeld, C.N., Hansen, N.K. *et al* (1995) Fever in geriatric emergency patients: clinical features associated with serious illness. *Ann. Emerg. Med.*, **26**, 18.

73 MacDonald, J.B. (1985) The role of drugs in falls in the elderly. *Clin. Geriatr. Med.*, **1** (3), 621–636.

74 Ray, W.A., Thapa, P.B., and Gideon, P. (2000) Benzodiazepines and the risk of falls in nursing home residents. *J. Am. Geriatr. Soc.*, **48** (6), 682–685.

75 Sorock, G.S., Quigley, P.A., Rutledge, M.K. *et al.* (2009) Central nervous system medication changes and falls in nursing home residents. *Geriatr. Nurs.*, **30** (5), 334–340.

76 Weiner, D.K., Hanlon, J.T., and Studenski, S.A. (1998) Effects of central nervous system polypharmacy on falls liability in community-dwelling elderly. *Gerontology*, **44**, 217–221.

77 Perez-Ros, P., Martinez-Arnau, F., Navarro-Illana, E. *et al.* (2013) Relationship between the risk of falling and prescribed medication in community-dwelling elderly subjects. *Adv. Pharmacol. Pharm.*, **1** (**1**), 29–36.

78 Nelson, D.E., Sattin, R.W., Langlois, J.A. *et al.* (1992) Alcohol as a risk factor for fall injury events among elderly persons living in the community. *J. Am. Geriatr. Soc.*, **40**, 658–661.

79 Culberson, J.W. and Ziska, M. (2008) Prescription drug misuse/abuse in the elderly. *Geriatrics*, **63** (**9**), 22–31.

80 Onen, S.H., Onen, F., Mangeon, J.P. *et al.* (2005) Alcohol abuse and dependence in elderly emergency department patients. *Arch. Gerontol. Geriatr.*, **41** (2), 191–200.

81 Blazer, D.B. and Wu, L.T. (2009) The epidemiology of substance use and disorders among middle aged and elderly community adults: National Survey on Drug Use and Health. *Am. J. Geriatr. Psychiatry*, **17**, 237.

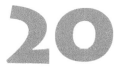

Trauma in the geriatric patient

Christopher R. Carpenter[1] & Peter L. Rosen[2]

[1]*Division of Emergency Medicine, Evidence Based Medicine, Washington University School of Medicine, St. Louis, MO, USA*
[2]*Division of Emergency Medicine, University of California, San Diego, CA, USA*

Section I: Case presentation

A 75-year-old man presented to the emergency department (ED) after a standing level fall. He arrived coherent and had been communicative several hours prior, but while awaiting evaluation in the waiting room, the triage nurse noted a rapid change in his mental status. He became agitated, nonverbal, and resisted care. The triage note listed a history of atrial fibrillation treated with warfarin for several years. In addition, his medications included treatment for hypertension and hyperlipidemia. Long-standing anxiety was also being managed with twice-daily benzodiazepine use for 30 years.

The vital signs were as follows: temperature of 37 °C, pulse of 70 beats/min, respirations of 25 breaths/min, blood pressure of 150/90 mmHg, and a pulse oximetry of 96% on 2 l of nasal cannula. His eyes were open, normal sized and reactive pupils were looking wildly around the room. He had a bruise on the left temple without any bony abnormality or crepitus palpated on his face or skull. The cardiopulmonary examination was normal and the abdomen soft.

Initial orders include a noncontrast head computed tomography (CT) scan, cervical spine X-ray studies, a complete blood count, and coagulation profile. While the patient was in the scanner, his family arrived and related that he fell while working in the garden earlier in the day resulting in a bruise to his head, a headache, and some confusion.

The CT scan revealed a subacute subdural hematoma. Shortly thereafter, he was flailing aimlessly, with all extremities. Rapid sequence intubation was performed without issue. A warfarin-induced intracranial hemorrhage protocol was initiated, but a repeat CT scan ordered several hours later by neurosurgery reveals a nonsurvivable extensive intracranial hemorrhage. In accord with the family, it was decided to discontinue mechanical ventilation, and the patient expired in the ED.

Section II: Case discussion

Dr Peter Rosen (PR): What do you consider to be the biggest issue in geriatric trauma?

Dr Chris Carpenter (CC): The biggest issue is that geriatric adults are not just older or middle-aged adults. They have unique physiology, psychosocial limitations, transfer limitations, and a unique response to therapy, not to mention they are treated with polypharmacy, and have often unrecognized underlying comorbidities such as dementia. All of these elements make the diagnostic evaluation for the emergency physician extremely difficult and we're very prone to getting fooled by a patient who looks well but quickly decompensates.

PR: There seems to be a predilection for underestimating the impact of trauma on the geriatric patient. I know Dr Carpenter has indicated that undertriage is a serious problem. I find that this starts in the field, and

Geriatric Emergencies: A Discussion-Based Review, First Edition.
Edited by Amal Mattu, Shamai A. Grossman and Peter L. Rosen.
© 2016 John Wiley & Sons, Ltd. Published 2016 by John Wiley & Sons, Ltd.

can remember several cases where a younger patient who was bleeding was sent by helicopter, but an older patient who wasn't bleeding, but who was absolutely much more seriously injured, was taken by ground transportation. Do you have any opinion about what we could do to overcome this reluctance to view the seriousness of the geriatric trauma patient?

Dr Rob Anderson (RA): I think there are two major components to this solution. Number one has to do with understanding and appreciating the mechanism of injury, especially ground-level falls as something that can cause major trauma in an older adult. We and our trauma colleagues are struggling with how to take care of or think about elderly fall patients. The Eastern Association for the Surgery of Trauma (EAST) management guidelines discuss this, and some of their editorials have said, we don't even know if a ground-level fall should count as a trauma activation or should involve the trauma service? Certainly, every elderly person who falls cannot have a trauma team activation, but we need to appreciate that these falls can lead to serious injuries in older adults. Older people don't hurt themselves by shooting each other or falling off motorcycles. They hurt themselves by falling. Second, we can think differently about our triage criteria. Undertriage is a well-documented problem. Fortunately, there has been some work done on this. There's a study from Ohio that Dr Carpenter alludes to later in this chapter that tries to identify what a geriatric trauma patient is, in terms of their physiology and mechanism. One key change might be appreciating that a blood pressure of 110 systolic could be an indication of acute or occult hypoperfusion and should lead to trauma team activation.

PR: I think that trauma center designation has, on the whole, been helpful. Nevertheless, it has produced some problems. The centers that are not designated trauma centers still receive some trauma, especially geriatric patients who are not perceived as trauma, and these nondesignated hospitals don't have reflexes for the management of trauma. Do you think we have created a problem that can only be solved by deliberately overtriaging to trauma centers? Or do we need to rediscover how to take care of trauma in nontrauma centers?

Dr Amal Mattu (AM): I think you make a great point. It has to do with what I would call the overregionalization of emergency medicine (EM). Emergency medicine is all about taking care of anyone who comes in; any age, with any complaint, and any time. A well-trained emergency physician should be able to figure out which patients have really severe problems, and which don't. But, in emergency medicine, generally speaking, things have become so regionalized with separate pediatric emergency medicine and separate trauma centers. People want to separate out cardiac arrest centers, STEMI (ST segment elevation myocardial infarction) centers, and so on. The result is that when a patient shows up in your ED, especially the geriatric trauma patient, and you're not a trauma center, there is a mindset that this must not be a major problem. It's analogous to the idea that when a patient with a serious problem shows up in fast track, the automatic assumption is that this patient must not have a serious problem because this is fast track. I think there is a problem with this overregionalization. I don't know that there is any way to turn that around. Perhaps we really need to focus on reeducating people about the undifferentiated patients. No matter what kind of ED you work in, you need to be ready for anything. Don't lower your guard because you're not a trauma center, you're not a cardiac arrest center, you're not a pediatric center, and so on.

CC: I don't disagree with any of that. I think that any emergency center needs to be able to deal with any emergency that comes through the door. As educators and clinicians, we need to remember that the trauma outcomes for geriatric patients and other patients is a longitudinal process, and is not just dependent on the care in the ED. It has to do with care from the trauma surgeons, the care the patient receives on the floor from trauma nurses, geriatric consultants, and the availability of specialists such as interventional radiologists, which is going to be hard for the small rural hospital to have access to.

PR: I think that's one of the upsides to trauma center designation. Clearly, it has made a positive impact on the management of major trauma. I believe we're seeing a marked decline in the untimely deaths we used to see because trauma patients weren't recognized and managed appropriately. Clearly, there are special considerations for the management of various classes of patients, including, why we're writing this book, the geriatric patient. I've been very impressed at how brittle the geriatric patient is. They look great 1 min and the next minute they are at death's door. Because of that, they probably deserve the trauma center more than many patients who get there. It's an almost unsolvable problem.

PR: One of the problems in this case is that in addition to a fall, the patient is anticoagulated. Could you comment on what that means for your workup for that patient? I'm not just talking about a CT scan. I would presume that anyone who has had a head injury and who is on an anticoagulant is going to get a head CT scan. Are there other aspects of management of these patients that need to be initiated early on?

CC: Modern anticoagulants, including antiplatelet therapies, throw another challenge at emergency physicians and surgical subspecialists. For example, clopidogrel, which is very common in our postcardiac patients, has a half-life of 5–7 days. Dabigatran has a half-life of 3 days, doesn't have a rapid reversal agent, and can only be removed by hemodialysis. Therapeutic warfarin increases mortality significantly in trauma patients. Nevertheless, we can reduce the mortality in geriatric patients to the level of nonanticoagulated, blunt head injury patients, which is about 10%, if we reverse that warfarin anticoagulation with vitamin K and fresh frozen plasma (FFP) within 2 h. Thus, we need to not only scan these patients aggressively and quickly identify any existing injuries, but we also need to reverse them quickly. What I would caution physicians is to not be reassured by a negative scan in these anticoagulated patients, because it has limited prognostic accuracy for a delayed bleed in the next 24–48 h.

PR: I think that's a critical point. We receive what we consider useful critical negative information, yet, it's only one point on the curve. We probably ought to be reversing these people earlier than we do. But then, of course, you're facing the issue of why they are anticoagulated in the first place and the concern that we could cause harm by reversing that anticoagulation.

PR: Here's a patient who is anticoagulated for atrial fibrillation. If we reverse him, what is the probability that he is going to flip an embolus?

SG: First, we're reversing him for the immediate future. We do know that your risk of throwing an embolus from atrial fibrillation doesn't kick in until you've had time for stasis of blood in the left atrium and an embolus to form. So if you're reversing him, you have at least 48 h before any risk. When we talk about risk for throwing an embolus in atrial fibrillation, we talk about a long-term risk, and not an immediate risk. If we say that the average person has a risk of 1 in 10,000 of having a stroke, we're talking about a long-term risk. It's certainly not happening contemporaneously. For atrial fibrillation, there's very little downside to immediate and full reversal. The issue is when we have a patient who has had a valve replacement and they really do need to be anticoagulated all the time, and their risk of clot or valve dysfunction is significantly greater. There is not good data on when we should reverse them. Here, we need to rely on good clinical judgment based on their injury and how dangerous it would be if we leave them anticoagulated. If we're talking about intracranial hemorrhage, I'm not sure we have any other choice but to reverse them. If we're talking about a negative head CT, I think no one would reverse their anticoagulation at the risk of clotting their mechanical valve.

PR: You mentioned clopidogrel (Plavix), which is a very commonly used drug in the geriatric population, what would you do to reverse it?

CC: The only reversal I know of is platelet transfusion.

PR: When would you consider doing that? Do you have to find a pathology or would you start transfusing platelets on anyone on Plavix who has a significant mechanism of injury?

CC: That's a good question that I have not seen addressed in the literature. However, it is striking that in traumatic head injuries in patients using anticoagulation or antiplatelet agents, the bleeding risk for antiplatelet agents is equal to or maybe even a little bit higher than patients on warfarin (Coumadin) in a couple of studies comparing the two. My personal practice, since I have not seen any data on proactive reversal in patients with head injury but no bleed, would be to start antiplatelet reversal in patients with intracranial bleed, but I would wait to see the bleed first.

PR: We say that any patient over a certain age probably should have a head CT even with the most minor mechanism of head injury. Do you agree with that? Or do you reverse that only for the anticoagulated? For example, an elderly patient bangs his head in the kitchen and may have a scalp laceration that will need a repair and has no other significant findings, but is over the age of 70. Would you do a head CT on that patient?

CC: Without reservation. I think the downsides of liberal CT use in these patients, the risk of radiation, and overdiagnosis, or finding something that you wouldn't have otherwise found that has no implications for the patient, is pretty small in this geriatric population. The benefits far outweigh the risks in this population.

PR: One of the issues in this case is the intracranial bleed. We know that in many older patients who survive intracranial bleeds we can never identify the mechanism that caused the bleed, and that rather than the fall causing the bleed, it may be the subdural that caused the fall. While I don't know of any good way of sorting that out, I think that we are somewhat cavalier about elderly patients and subdurals, based on whether our individual neurosurgeon is willing to operate for the relief of the subdural. Do you have any feelings about what size subdural needs to be admitted, or if all of these patients need to have a neurosurgical consultation?

RA: If I have a patient with a traumatic neurologic injury for which the only potential treatment other than some medications I can give in the ED is surgical, I'm going to request a neurosurgical consult on all these patients. I can't think of a scenario where I would not at least talk to them on the phone. Criteria for discharge would need to include no change in mental status, very small amount of blood, and assurance that serial neurological examinations can continue for the next few days.

PR: The reason I ask that question is that I think that it is the practice in virtually all tertiary centers, but remember that there are many EDs in this country that do not have access to a neurosurgeon. I know that when I was working Jackson Hole, the neurosurgeon that we would transfer to was about 90 mi. away and was often reluctant to see patients. We had a difficult time in having him accept patients in transfer, and he was quite convinced that as long as the subdural was

small that he didn't have to see the patient. I think this is a real issue in how to monitor these patients.

RA: I have recently started to use my phone to send photographs of injuries to my surgical consultants. Perhaps for a neurosurgeon, you can take a picture of the CT scan, keeping it HIPAA (Health Insurance Portability and Accountability Act) compliant with no patient identifiers, and send it to the surgeon. I have found that reaching out in this new way makes the consultant feel more involved and responsible.

AM: You can go one step further in the era of telemedicine and have the consultant evaluate the patient even if you're 100 mi. away in a snow storm. They can look at patients, talk to them, examine them, just as if they were there. There's no reason we can't take advantage of that technology in 2016 everywhere.

PR: We used to think there was a connection between the age of the subdural and its treatability at least neurosurgically, in that the acute subdural is rarely the cause of the patient's decline but more often due to the cerebral contusion and the trauma itself. The subacute subdural is more likely to be producing the increased pressure that needs relief, as well as the chronic subdural. We don't seem to make these distinctions quite as often any more. Do you think there is a change in physiology, or is it just old fashioned thinking based on the old CT scan findings?

SG: I am not aware of anyone who differentiates based only on the time frame of when the patient developed their subdural. One can envision a case where neurosurgery might defer intervention if the patient is 4 days out from their subdural and neurologically intact, and then 10 days out they develop a major deficit and need the OR. There's no one who could have predicted one way or the other what was going to happen with that subdural. I think generally the perception of our neurosurgeons today is that if it's a subdural that developed immediately, then we have to worry about it. If it's been there for awhile, then we probably don't. I don't think we have as strong of data here as we'd like to have.

AM: I will say that what I've seen more often in the last 10 years is that if someone comes in with a small subdural that is acute or subacute and their mental status is intact, I've seen neurosurgeons ask us to observe the patient and repeat the CT scan in 6–8 h. If there's no change in the patient's CT scan or clinical examination, then they will sign off on the case and have the patient follow up closely as an outpatient. I don't know if there is literature to back that up.

CC: I've seen that in St Louis as well, and I think it's rather cavalier practice. I've not seen literature to back it up.

SG: I haven't either. I found that in our institution, as emergency physicians we tend to be more conservative than our neurosurgeons. Our neurosurgeons will want to send them home after 6 h. We'll put them in observation for at least 24 h to watch them.

PR: Well, I think that there are different levels of anxiety in medicine, and I think that as emergency physicians we tend to be more anxious than our colleagues. Unfortunately, we are dependent on them for tertiary care.

PR: One of the issues in this case is that this patient is combative. Here, we have a man who has a known head injury, has a known complication of a head injury, and whose mental status is worsening. How would you suggest controlling that combativeness?

CC: There are recommendations for dealing with delirium in general which include limiting the use of pharmacologic agents, trying to use reasoning with the patient, correct lighting, trying to make sure the patient has familiar things around him. In the case of a head injury, I do not think I would follow the delirium recommendations, though. My concern would be making sure we have the best medical management as possible for a head injury with intracranial bleed, which means making sure we have his blood pressure appropriately controlled, not too high, not too low. We need to keep him as calm and comfortable as possible, and make sure he doesn't fall out of bed in his agitated state. My threshold for intubating and sedating this patient would be low. Of course, I would want to have a conversation with family about goals of care in any geriatric patient. One of our concerns in this case was that he ended up with a lot of tubes sticking out of every orifice, and died that way with his family around him, which perhaps wasn't the best way to go. For managing his agitation, I think sedation and early intubation would be my goal.

PR: I think that that's a difficult problem for us. I've had many neurosurgical consults say that you can't intubate and sedate him because we can't follow his mental status. I don't have an easy answer for that other than to say how much longer are you going to follow it before you decide to do something to treat it. I think sometimes we just have to accept the reality that we will take charge of intubating and sedating the patient, and not ask for permission to do it. I think it can be a difficult fight in some patients.

One of the issues in this case that you've alluded to is that he had a subsequent bleed even though he had been reversed, and it led to a downhill course and ultimate demise. Do you think there would have been a different outcome in this patient had he been initially triaged to a tertiary care center?

CC: That's a tough question. I think his best chance of neurologically intact survival would be for him to have been triaged to a trauma center where he would have access to definitive imaging and neurosurgical care. But the outcome of head-injured geriatrics patients is dismal. If you come in with a Glasgow Coma Scale (GCS) of less than 8, your overall mortality is 71%. Nobody over the age of 85 with that severity of a head injury survives either with or without surgery. He didn't have that severity when he presented, but I think his best chance of survival was a trauma center.

SG: I would agree but with the caveat that we are obligated to give the best possible care in the community as well. It doesn't excuse leaving a patient in the waiting room for 2 h after a head bleed. As an emergency physician, your training is to take care of a patient in any scenario, in any type of ED, anywhere you are. You must be vigilant to whatever comes into your waiting. I think that this patient's outcome may have been dramatically different even in the community setting had they been vigilant, and had there been appropriate treatment protocols for falls in the elderly.

PR: I sense that criticism of the care of this elderly patient in the nontrauma center. I am concerned that this was a patient who in the field was transported to a nontrauma center, and again I don't think that that was against anyone's protocol. I just think our protocols are wrong. I think it does make a big difference if we could somehow alter the consciousness of our prehospital as well as nontrauma center EDs as to the seriousness of elderly trauma patients.

PR: I wanted to change the discussion from head injury to the more general trauma status of patients. One of the common problems that I see is that we focus on individual organs. The elderly patient may have had a mild auto crash or minor auto versus pedestrian accident, and comes into the ED with an obvious hip fracture. How do we avoid focusing so much on the hip fracture that we miss that this patient is probably a major trauma patient, and needs a complete trauma workup rather than just a hip workup?

RA: I think this comes down to good trauma care regardless of the age group. In my mind, trauma care is designed to find blood or air somewhere in the body it shouldn't be or an acute neurologic injury, and having the right people around that can address the problems quickly. What is unique to geriatric trauma is that we are at risk of losing valuable time by inappropriate triage. Once any patient is in the resuscitation bay, I think we are primed to do a great job. The challenge is getting the appropriate older trauma patients to the bay in the first place. We can do this by recognizing the danger of ground-level falls, and by recognizing that a systolic blood pressure of 110 mmHg might be hypotension. So, for example, a person who comes in with a hip fracture, but with a pressure of 110 mmHg, should be triaged into the resuscitation room so we don't miss another injury. We know that if the patient is triaged to a resuscitation room, we get excited about them earlier, and they have a better chance at recovery.

PR: There's one other difference that I see a trauma center providing. I feel like trauma center workups tend to be more complete. They don't try to evaluate for the one injury they're looking at but they just put the patient through the complete workup. This is just as important in the young patient as the older patient because the younger patients can hide their injury too because they have such strong compensatory mechanisms. I think that what these patients all need is a complete and almost rote workup, where you put your brain in neutral and just coast, and get on with the business of evaluating the entire patient, not just the organ that appears to be most damaged.

PR: One of the frequent complications of even minor trauma is the exacerbation of concomitant diseases that the patient possesses. This is, of course, especially important in the geriatric patient. What

do you suggest about trying to prevent some of the cardiac complications that occur as the patients lose perfusion pressure?

SG: In my mind it revolves around the standard care that we try to give patients in emergency medicine, where we try and look at the entire patient from each perspective. We'll have a patient who presents for a single car motor vehicle crash, and while the trauma surgeon is concerned about the trauma event, we are equally concerned about what caused the event. Our differential might include a syncopal event, a myocardial infarction, a pulmonary embolus, or whatever it might be. I think that this is the way that we might avoid a pitfall of missing the different concomitant diseases in these patients; keeping our minds open but using our training as emergency physicians and realizing that we always need to look at the entire patient and the entire spectrum of disease and not be focused on one element of the acute process going on. If we steer ourselves in that direction, we will be less prone to missing the other processes going on.

RA: I think it comes down to trying to find markers of injury as well as markers of resuscitation. For example, following serum lactate or base deficit values. Unfortunately, we don't know the exact values we can use to help resuscitate these older adults in an effort to detect hypoperfusion to any organ whether it's the brain or anywhere else.

PR: I think that's part of the problem, we don't have any good markers. What we use is confusing such as the blood pressure cuff because the patient may be on antihypertensives, which further complicate the care. Moreover, what appears to be a normal pressure, as you've already indicated, may be an abnormal blood pressure. Probably, the most important consideration is to recognize how brittle the geriatric population is, and how much care they need in order to prevent that deterioration.

PR: What is the disposition practice of your institution? Do you admit these trauma patients to the trauma service, or are they more likely to be admitted to medicine if they are older with concomitant disease?

AM: Our trauma service is good about taking those patients on their service. I think part of that is the head of our trauma center has a particular area of expertise in geriatric trauma. He's a strong proponent of aggressive geriatric trauma care, and searching out signs of occult shock in the elderly patient. We're lucky that the leader of our trauma center is very on board with and in tune with the concerns that we've all been expressing pertaining to geriatric trauma. When I was in residency, granted this was a handful of years ago, probably before a lot of the research and teaching had gone out there, I think that we all probably missed cases, and the trauma service missed cases as well because we didn't know about all the issues that we're talking about. What we knew about trauma was based on what we all learned in advanced trauma life support (ATLS); and ATLS, at least back then, and probably even now, is based on studies in which elderly patients are thrown out of the studies. Consequently, a lot of those ATLS studies are largely irrelevant to geriatric patients.

A perfect example is this chart imprinted in my brain of the different classes of shock when they say this person has class one shock, this is their heart rate, class two shock, this is their heart rate, class three, class four, and so on. This is what their expected blood pressure is and mental status is and that's the material that everyone learns, including prehospital people. Yet, that is completely irrelevant to elderly patients who don't mount the tachycardia, plus they're on beta-blockers, plus they don't have hypotension until they're ready to crash, and we could go on forever. Although at our institution they're good about admitting these patients, I'm not sure if this teaching has been disseminated to institutions that are not particularly focused on geriatric care.

PR: No, unfortunately I think it is dependent on who is charge of the trauma service. I've been blessed through the years of having aggressive trauma surgeons who were willing to admit patients, but others are less fortunate.

PR: One of the issues that you addressed in one of my first questions to you were the sociologic consequences of trauma in elderly patients. Would you give a few examples of what we need consider for a trauma patient who has been evaluated and who has been deemed safe for discharge?

CC: There's ample literature now showing that even after mild blunt trauma in geriatric patients who we send home, or when they're not injured enough to need to come into the hospital or perhaps to even see trauma services, there is a significant number of them who have functional decline at 1–3 months. Functional decline means that where once they could make their own meals or get to the bathroom unassisted, now they require someone in the house to help them to do those things. We currently lack a good mechanism to identify which of those patients are the ones who are going to deteriorate, and that's a big problem. We can't arrange home services for every patient that we send home. However, we know that a large number of mild blunt trauma patients who are discharged home, perhaps one in three, will have functional deterioration at 3 months.

Another problem is that a significant percentage of them have underlying mental incapacity, mild cognitive impairment, or even frank dementia. Most of those patients pass through our EDs unrecognized with early stages of dementia that may not have been enough to impair their daily life before their injury. However, after their injury, these vulnerable patients may forget follow-up appointments or to take their medication. The only way that we can identify these patients is if we screen for cognitive impairment in these patients in the ED. This is currently not standard of care in the ED, because the instruments aren't easy to use, or are not part of our general medical education of the evaluation of the geriatric patient. Another issue to consider is that a lot of these patients have very limited transport ability at baseline. They don't drive, they don't have somebody to drive them to appointments, and they don't have someone to get them to the pharmacy. Anything that's going to impede their ability to walk to the bus stop, or use public transportation, or even to get to the phone at home to call a taxi, is going to impair their ability to recover from an injury.

PR: We've talked at some length in other cases about the impairment of the geriatric function from what would appear to be a minor injury. I think it is one of the areas where the tertiary care centers do a better job because they have more resources, not because they are any cleverer. They do have the social services, the physical therapy, and perhaps the experience of why it's required.

PR: Another issue that we've talked about in the past is specific protocols that we can implement for the care of geriatric trauma patients? I know that I have, personally, been somewhat opposed to this, but there are clearly so many areas in which you have to make a different decision. One thing that jumps into mind is rib fractures. I think in young adults, intercostal blocks work wonderfully, but in older patients I think two or more rib fractures is a very serious injury, and it needs a different disposition. Do you have any overall feelings about this?

CC: I do think that there are protocols that have been proposed that are worth looking at. Dr Anderson mentioned earlier the Ohio Geriatric Trauma Field Triage Criteria on the prehospital side, which is doing more to get patients that need tertiary trauma care to the tertiary trauma care center. Once they are in the ED, there are guidelines that have been proposed such as by the EAST committee for evidence-based care of geriatric trauma patients that have never been empirically tested. They are all consensus-based trauma surgeons' evaluation of the literature. Nevertheless, I think if I was in an ED that didn't have geriatric protocols, then I would see what the trauma surgeons are recommending as a general guideline for the care of these patients. We proposed in our Geriatric Emergency Department Guidelines work, orthopedic, geriatric, multidisciplinary team protocols to optimize care of patients that are in the ED until they leave the hospital, whether they are discharged home or admitted to the floor, and how best to get the care they need on the floor. For example, orthopedic surgeons managing hip fracture patients don't want to deal with the geriatric issues we just mentioned, the dementia and delirium, the functional limitations at baseline. Providing a geriatrician as a consultant to that service is definitely beneficial in getting that patient up and ambulatory and out of the hospital sooner. Not to say that they shouldn't be admitted to the surgical services – they should – but the geriatric consultants play a key role in getting them back to their baseline function.

PR: They're not going to be admitted to the surgical service in most institutions. I'm not talking about multiple trauma, I'm talking about the patient with a single orthopedic injury, at least at the institutions that I'm familiar with offhand, orthopedics is glad to consult the medical service, but they think all these patients should be admitted to the hospitalist. I think that is happening frequently, perhaps that's an area

where we need better education for patients and physicians.

RA: It's very helpful if these decisions are made in the light of day between the different departments, and it makes it easier for the providers in the ED. For example, in my hospital for every hip fracture, two pages go out automatically, one to orthopedics and the other to medicine and both teams come down to see the patient. This is the protocol, and there is no discussion, nobody is grumpy about it and it's very helpful.

SG: We have something similar, where the patient gets admitted to an interdisciplinary service that should involve geriatrics, trauma and orthopedics as well.

RA: It makes life so much easier for everybody up front, and is better for the patient down the road.

PR: That's a critical point. You can't resolve these issues over a single patient. It has to be done on a policy basis long before the patient comes to the ED. It's much easier to resolve when the policy is in place. You don't want to end up with a patient where everybody says, yes this is a sick patient but not on my service. I'm sure we have all dealt with that issue in the past. It's very difficult to resolve it without an advance policy.

PR: I once had a patient in Wyoming who presented this kind of difficult disposition problem. He was a house painter who fell off a scaffold. He presented to the ED as a multiple trauma. He had multiple fractures. He had a head injury. I said to myself, "why does a house painter who has been painting houses for 30 years fall off a scaffold?" Sure enough I did an electrocardiogram (EKG), and he was having an ST-elevation myocardial infarction (MI), and had a syncopal episode. Well, the orthopedics said, "we don't want to admit this patient because clearly his heart attack takes precedence." Neurosurgery said, "his head injury is minor and we certainly don't need to admit this patient." Cardiology said, "well, I can't take care of fractures and head injuries." There I had a patient who was sick enough to be on anyone's service, but no one would take him. This was in a rural hospital, where there was no trauma service, and I wonder if you could suggest what one is supposed to do in this situation.

SG: I think we're often stuck in many institutions admitting a patient that no service will take to the internal medicine service for better or worse, because the most difficult problem often involves the internal medicine parts of the patient's care, and they've become the so-called "dumping ground" for all patients that nobody wants. This is perhaps not ideal, but may be the only choice we have given the restraints of our healthcare system.

PR: I was very fortunate that evening that one of the very good internists in the hospital was listening to me make all these phone calls and said: "Admit the patient to me. I'll take care of him," and he did. I was very grateful because I simply had a patient for whom I could not do anymore, who was very complex. I think we do have an easier time at the tertiary care center in dealing with problems such as this because we have trauma services, and perhaps that's the reason that we've had such a benefit from the designation of trauma centers. But, there are many hospitals that don't have that luxury, but still have to resolve the issue of the complex emergency. This is one of the areas of trauma care, especially for the elderly, where we need to do a better job of developing in the future.

CC: Geriatric trauma patients, and the geriatric population as a whole, represent a canary in the coal mine for the healthcare system and trauma care. They are often fragile, potentially vulnerable, and it's not always easy for us to tell, looking at the patient and even with extensive testing, which ones are going to do well and which ones are not. We need to have strong ties with our medical and trauma services. Protocols and policies are going to go a long way in helping to care for these patients, regardless of whether they show up at the rural hospital or tertiary care center. The key is going to continue to perform research as to what constitutes effective care of this elder adult population in today's healthcare environment, from the prehospital setting until the day they return home back on their feet, recovered and hopefully back at baseline. I would encourage our educators, our clinicians, and our researchers to keep working to improve the care of these older adults because it is going to be a generational challenge for the world.

Section III: Concepts

Background

Epidemiology and trends

It is estimated that 90 million adults over age 65 will reside in the United States in 2050, which will represent over one fifth of the population [1, 2]. Geriatric adults presently represent 23% of trauma admissions, and traumatic injury is the fifth leading cause of death in this age group [3, 4]. In the 85 and older subset of geriatric adults, 1 in 5 is treated in an ED for injury every year in the United States [5]. Injury-related hospitalizations for geriatric adults continue to increase [6]. Standing level falls and motor vehicle accidents (MVAs) are the most common mechanisms of trauma [7, 8]. The challenges of an aging population are not isolated to the United States, and geriatric trauma is the most common presenting complaint for older adults worldwide [9, 10]. The EAST practice recently released updated management guidelines (Figure 20.1) [11]. One notable element of the EAST guidelines is the lack of strong recommendations, which highlights the critical need for ongoing research to identify which fall victims benefit from trauma services [12, 13].

Geriatric trauma patients are much harder to care for than younger populations [14]. They present to the ED with higher Injury Severity Scores, longer hospital and rehabilitation lengths of stay, and higher mortality than younger cohorts do [15]. When adjusted for Injury Severity Scores, geriatric trauma patients have a twofold increased mortality and significantly longer hospital length of stay (LOS) compared with younger populations [16]. Even minor trauma such as a ground-level fall can indicate a sentinel event for geriatric patients since up to 35% of older adults with minor blunt trauma who are discharged from the ED experience functional decline at 3 months [17–19]. Functional decline increases ED recidivism [20]. Unfortunately, no validated instruments exist to identify the subset that is most at risk for post-ED functional decline while they are still in the ED [21, 22].

Age-associated trauma mortality appears to increase beginning at age 70 [23]. In the "very old" (age > 80 years), management of trauma in nonaccredited centers increases hospital mortality in comparison to treatment in nontrauma centers [24]. Unfortunately, old age is an independent predictor of failure to provide advanced trauma care worldwide [25, 26]. Beginning at age 50, prehospital personnel undertriage trauma patients to designated trauma centers [6, 27]. The most common injuries in such undertriaged geriatric trauma patients are brain injuries and thoracic fractures [28]. Old age alone should be an important criterion to mobilize trauma resources [29]. Trauma team activation using age alone as a trigger with ED-based invasive hemodynamic and tissue perfusion monitoring, as

well as a low threshold for Intensive Care Unit (ICU) admission, decreases mortality from 53.8% to 34.2% [30].

Geriatric physiology and trauma

Older adults are vulnerable to serious injuries from blunt and penetrating trauma because the amount of energy required to produce injury decreases in the aging body [31]. Geriatric adults are more likely to have osteoporosis, fragile skin that is prone to

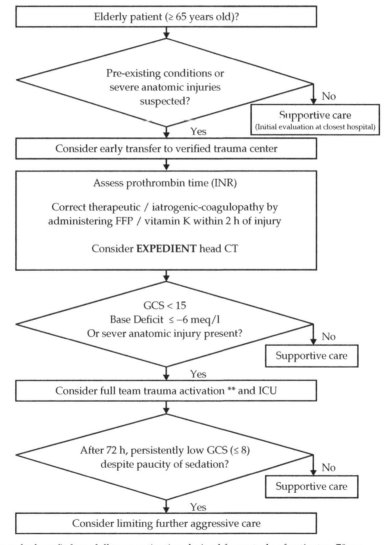

**Evidence for benefit from full team activation derived from study of patients > 70 y.o.

Figure 20.1 EAST guidelines for evidence-based care of the geriatric trauma victim.

tear, and diminished cardiac index and oxygen transport at baseline, limiting their functional reserve to respond to acute trauma [32, 33]. In addition to the age-related limitations in physiologic reserve that are produced by age, the geriatric patient often has concomitant disease that is poorly compensated, and severe organ dysfunction may be triggered by minor trauma. For example, they may be borderline anemic from many causes, which means that they cannot respond easily to even low-volume traumatic hemorrhage. Moreover, due to underlying poor respiratory function, what has been a barely compensated chronic lung disease may suddenly decompensate from a minor degree of thoracic blunt trauma, such as a single broken rib [34, 35]. Moreover, their volumes may already border on dehydration from chronic diuretic use to control blood pressure and heart failure. Furthermore, the barely compensated oxygen saturation will quickly turn to hypoxia with serious decompensation of cardiac and cerebral functions. Another source of decompensation is the medications the patient is taking, such as beta blockade, which prevents a response to volume loss [36].

Prehospital and ED management of geriatric trauma

Prehospital

Prehospital providers frequently transport geriatric trauma patients to hospitals lacking trauma accreditation. Emergency medical service (EMS) personnel identify three causal factors for undertriage to designated trauma centers: inadequate training, unfamiliarity with trauma protocols, and age bias [27].

Triage

Despite clinically significant injuries, critically ill geriatric patients frequently fail to exhibit hypotension, tachycardia, or pain [37, 38]. In patients over the age of 75, abnormal vital signs are only 73% sensitive and 50% specific (positive likelihood ratio 1.47, negative likelihood ratio 0.54) for predicting death or ICU admission [38]. Similarly, well-validated triage nurse instruments such as the Emergency Severity Index fail to identify over half of the geriatric patients who ultimately receive an immediate lifesaving intervention with sensitivity 42% and specificity 99% [39]. Adjusting the threshold of "normal" in existing screening instruments is one approach to improving prognostic accuracy. For example,

raising the GCS threshold for trauma activation from 13 to 14 improves sensitivity for clinically relevant injuries [40]. The state of Ohio recently proposed geriatric-specific criteria for prehospital personnel to use in triaging older trauma patients to the appropriate level of care [41]. (Box 20.1) Another modification to triage protocols could be initiating trauma protocols for any geriatric injury victim with a heart rate above 90 or systolic blood pressure below 110 mmHg since trauma-related mortality begins to increase at that threshold [42].

Box 20.1 Ohio geriatric trauma field triage criteria

If patients >70 years meet any of the following criteria following trauma, transport directly to a designated trauma center:
- GCS < 14 in the presence of known or suspected traumatic brain trauma
- Systolic blood pressure <100 mmHg
- Fall from any height with evidence of traumatic brain injury
- Multiple body system injuries
- Struck by a moving vehicle
- Presence of any proximal long bone fracture following motor vehicle trauma.

While an accurate prehospital or ED geriatric trauma triage instrument has yet to be developed, clinical research has identified risk factors that do increase mortality. Preexisting comorbidities such as hepatic disease, renal disease, and cancer increase trauma-related mortality [43]. Cardiac morbidity is associated with higher long-term mortality [44]. Similarly, pulmonary disease is associated with increased mortality [45].

Diagnostic and prognostic resources

Most laboratory tests are of low utility in the identification of specific injuries or their seriousness in geriatric trauma patients, but anticoagulation status should always be assessed [46]. Many older adults are prescribed anticoagulation therapy for atrial fibrillation and other indications because the risk-to-benefit trade-off favors stroke prevention [47]. Although warfarin use alone does not predict mortality, the duration and degree of anticoagulation do predict adverse outcomes in head injury patients [48–52]. There must be a low threshold for CT scanning in all geriatric patients, but particularly those who are on anticoagulants [11, 53, 54]. A history of a fall or the presence of neurological findings predicts an abnormal CT scan in confused geriatric patients with a traumatic head injury [55]. Unfortunately, a normal brain CT scan at the time of the initial ED evaluation does not eliminate the risk of a delayed intracranial hemorrhage in subsequent days. Head injury patients, and more importantly their caregivers, must be advised to carefully monitor the patient's mental status in the days following a traumatic head injury. While it has been thought prudent to arrange an observation admission and repeat CT scan for those on anticoagulation therapy, this strategy has not been adopted by US hospitals for a variety of reasons related to cost and crowding.

Vital signs are inaccurate to predict injury severity in geriatric patients. The product of age multiplied by shock index is a slightly more accurate predictor of mortality [56]. A base deficit of ≤−6 has been used as a laboratory marker of trauma-related mortality and anticipated prolonged ICU care [57]. While there is controversy over the value of central venous pressure monitoring, it is a particularly challenging modality of care in the elderly who can least afford an iatrogenic complication on top of their trauma [58]. More recently, venous lactate appears promising. As opposed to shock index and traditional vital signs, venous lactate is an independent predictor of geriatric trauma mortality when adjusted for age, GCS, and Injury Severity Score [37]. Using venous lactate-guided therapy to identify occult hypoperfusion with early trauma surgeon involvement is associated with improved survival [59]. Researchers are also developing nomograms to predict mortality-related complications such as wound infection, empyema, urinary tract infection, deep venous thrombosis, pressure ulcer, and pneumonia based on age, gender, and number of preexisting comorbidities [60, 61].

Therapeutics and role of trauma surgeon

Effective team-based care is essential for optimal geriatric trauma outcomes. Emergency medicine cannot and should not assume sole responsibility for these patients since the severity of their injury is often elusive and post-ED outcomes are often suboptimal even with ideal access to outpatient resources [22].

Similarly, Trauma Surgery cannot manage these complex patients alone. In the ED, models of an in-house geriatric trauma team have included physicians from emergency medicine, trauma services, and radiology with reliably rapid access to subspecialty services such as neurosurgery, orthopedics, and geriatrics [2]. The requirement to have these services available in-hospital, around the clock is one reason that a leveled trauma credentialing system exists and the reason why geriatric patients should routinely be triaged to credentialed trauma centers. Furthermore, the team-based approach to trauma care continues after admission as evidenced by the rapidly expanding number of orthogeriatric services [62].

Geriatric trauma protocols in the ED

Table 20.1 provides some overarching recommendations for geriatric trauma management within the context of current research evidence, while contemplating potential unintended consequences of these recommendations. It makes sense to mandate trauma center transport by local EMS systems for any patient above the age of 65, if there is a significant mechanism of injury. In addition, it is easy to underestimate the degree of trauma by history alone because of underlying dementia, inability to perceive or report pain, or because the wrong injury has the attention of the patient. For example, the patient might complain of wrist pain because of a fracture and never mention a head injury or abdominal discomfort. Therefore, all elderly patients who come to a trauma center should have a complete trauma evaluation, and not just focus upon a single organ. Specifically, all elderly patients with significant trauma merit chest and pelvis physical evaluation and imaging, as well as a head CT if this is a mechanism of multisystem trauma. While many decisions in EM are complex and difficult, any elderly patient on anticoagulation with head trauma must have a CT scan, and there may be a role for delayed observation in this population.

All elderly patients with three or more acute rib fractures warrant admission for pain management and respiratory therapy. Analgesia should include nerve blocks or epidural blocks. Furthermore, all patients should have an EKG and a chest X-ray study, with further imaging dependent upon the mechanism of injury. Carefully consider chest tubes in geriatric trauma patients who have blunt trauma to the chest with one or more rib fractures, if they must be

Table 20.1 Specific geriatric trauma management recommendations and level of evidence.

Management Recommendations	Examples	Level of Evidence[a]	Potential Problems or Disadvantages
All patients ≥65 with significant injury[b] mechanism should be initially evaluated at trauma center	EMS protocols to transport to closest Level I trauma center	C	Overtriage to Level I trauma centers, delays to care during transport, and underuse of safety net hospitals with consequent atrophy of trauma skills
	Accepting Level I trauma center systems to minimize transfer and treatment delays for geriatric trauma patients (remote access to outside hospital images so that consultants at bedside when patient arrives, air transport protocols)	E	
Triage protocols should be modified for geriatric trauma patients	Hypotension present below systolic blood pressure 110 mmHg	D	Overtriage of geriatric trauma patients resulting in delayed care to other ED populations
	Triage screening instruments such as the Emergency Severity Index should be used with caution	C	
Initial geriatric trauma victim evaluation (ATLS primary and secondary survey) in trauma center should aggressively and comprehensively seek trauma-related injury and resulting medical complications	Head-to-toe physical exam with clothing removed	C	Overutilization of diagnostic resources,[c] hypothermia, and patient discomfort
	Chest X-ray	C	
	ECG	E	
	Delirium	C	
Multiple rib fracture patients should be admitted for pain control and pulmonary care	Nerve blocks or epidural opioid analgesia should be provided	C	Oversedation and increased fall risk
	Anesthesiology consultants need to be available in the ED for early initiation of these interventions	E	
	Avoid NSAIDs	C	
	Incentive spirometry with respiratory therapy	C	
All geriatric patients with significant trauma will be assessed for abdominal injuries with bedside sonography to queue CT imaging prioritization or immediate CT	ED ultrasound (FAST, chest wall for pneumothorax) can prioritize timing of CT imaging but is insufficiently accurate to be definitive	C	IV-contrast renal injury or allergies and operative delays awaiting imaging
	Radiology will prioritize CT imaging and interpretation for geriatric trauma patients	E	

Table 20.1 (*continued*)

Management Recommendations	Examples	Level of Evidence[a]	Potential Problems or Disadvantages
Fractures will be routinely sought and obvious injuries managed aggressively before imaging	Splinting and analgesia for extremity fractures before imaging	E	Overutilization of diagnostic resources,[d] prolonged ED length of stay, and patient discomfort
	Pelvic X-ray for hip fractures in patients with significant injury mechanism	C	
Admission to a geriatric trauma service with multidisciplinary-derived and staffed care models is appropriate	Geriatric trauma services should include early and appropriate evaluation by geriatricians, physical therapy, pharmacy, and surgical subspecialists	B	Overcrowding of less critically injured trauma services limiting access to trauma beds for other populations, costs to healthcare payers, and increased ED length of stay for geriatric trauma patients awaiting trauma surgery evaluation/ admission orders
	Emergency medicine should provide input into early stage geriatric trauma management protocols, admission thresholds, and admitting services	E	

[a]Levels of evidence: A = systematic reviews of randomized controlled trials, B = multiple randomized controlled trials, C = multiple nonrandomized observational studies, D = single study (randomized or observational), and E = no published research evidence (anecdotal observation/opinion).
[b]Significant mechanism includes fatality in accident, >1 multitrauma patients from same accident, high-speed mechanism, open fractures, underlying comorbidity (ankylosing spondylitis, anticoagulation), or any alteration in vital signs.
[c]Overutilization is defined by diagnostic tests that are unlikely to improve patient-centric outcomes or that lead to overdiagnosis, overtreatment, and preventable harm.
[d]Overutilization is defined by diagnostic tests that are unlikely to improve patient-centric outcomes or that lead to overdiagnosis, overtreatment, and preventable harm.

ventilated either for management or as part of surgery for orthopedic injuries. Early analgesia before imaging is completed might include small repeated doses of an opioid intravenously. Nonsteroidal anti-inflammatory drugs (NSAIDs) should be avoided.

Geriatric trauma-related abdominal injuries cannot be underestimated, even if the patient's physical examination appears unremarkable [63]. Therefore, all patients should have an objective evaluation of the abdomen with ED clinician performed focused assessment with sonography for trauma (FAST) examination, if there is any delay in CT imaging or operative management. However, whether performed by ED staff, surgeons, or radiologists, the FAST examination is insufficient to definitively exclude life-threatening injury, so CT scans are necessary for all of these patients [64–67]. Early use of a nasogastric tube is useful in any patient with altered vital signs and blunt abdominal trauma. A rectal examination for blood and sphincter tone should be performed in all patients. A Foley catheter should be placed unless there is gross hematuria or blood at the meatus, in all patients with altered vital signs. A pelvis evaluation by physical compression should be performed in all patients, and supplemented by imaging with vital sign abnormalities.

Orthopedic injury management includes immediate splinting, with application of ice and administration of analgesia even before completion of imaging sstudies. Any geriatric patient triaged to a trauma center should be admitted to the trauma service rather than an individual subspecialty. For example, even patients with isolated head injury or orthopedic fractures should be admitted to the trauma service. However, geriatric trauma service and protocols/care pathways should evolve from multidisciplinary teams including geriatricians, surgical subspecialists, physical therapy, pharmacy, and emergency medicine.

Specific injuries

Head injuries
Although they rarely have neurosurgical intervention, hospitalization rates for older adults with head injuries are increasing [68, 69]. Traumatic brain injury (TBI) in geriatric patients leads to over 80,000 ED visits in the United States every year and 75% result in hospitalization [70]. Standing level falls and, to a much smaller degree, MVAs are the leading causes of head injuries in the elderly [69, 71, 72]. Antiplatelet agents such as clopidogrel increase long-term disability and mortality in head injury patients [73, 74]. Similarly, the length of time that patients are anticoagulated and the extent of anticoagulation increase head injury-related mortality [51, 52].

Overall, geriatric TBI patients have increased mortality and worse functional outcome than those with less severe head injuries [72, 75, 76]. Patients over the age of 75 are less likely to survive surgical intervention than younger populations following head injury [71]. In one review of geriatric TBI victims with initial GCS ≤ 8, the overall mortality was 70.8%, and no patients over the age of 85 survived with or without surgery [77]. The recovery potential of geriatric TBI patients has remained static for decades leading to statements that extensive research concerning factors impeding or improving reliable recovery in this population is a priority [72]. Given the dismal prognosis in this population, the EAST guidelines (Figure 20.1) recommend "discussions regarding the goals of care if no improvement in GCS is seen after the initial phase of care and after withdrawal of sedatives" after 72 h of aggressive trauma management [11].

Cervical spine injuries
Standing level falls are the most common injury mechanism preceding C-spine fractures, and c1 or

C2 fractures are more common in geriatric trauma patients than in younger patients [78]. Even minor degrees of trauma can cause fracture in a neck already damaged by osteoarthritis or other kinds of joint disease. Fortunately, many of these patients benefit significantly from operative stabilization of higher level C-spine fractures, so aggressive surgical management should be an option if it falls within the goals of care [79, 80]. Operative management of upper C-spine fractures leads to a 9.2% mortality rate and 12% of patients demonstrate nonunion [81].

The Canadian C-spine rule stratifies any blunt neck trauma patient over age 65 as high risk, but the NEXUS (National Emergency X-Radiography Utilization Study) criteria do not include age as a significant predictor [61, 82]. Nonetheless, clinicians often ignore the NEXUS criteria and image the C-spine and head in geriatric trauma patients [83, 84]. Geriatric-specific cervical spine decision aids have been derived retrospectively, but as yet are not used extensively [85]. What makes evaluation of the geriatric spine particularly difficult is the frequent presence of underlying arthritic changes, such as osteoarthritic spurs, making image interpretation confusing.

The optimal imaging modality is debatable and depends upon the objective. If the goal is to identify every possible C-spine injury than CT scan *and* magnetic resonance imaging (MRI) are ideal [86]. However, many injuries identified on CT scan that are missed by X-ray alone are clinically inconsequential, and require neither operative intervention nor spine immobilization that would not otherwise have been recommended. Compared with X-ray alone, CT scan undoubtedly identifies more injuries [87]. Clinicians need to balance the risk of finding trivial injuries against missing significant ones [88]. In addition, X-ray studies in geriatric patients are frequently suboptimal due to age-related degenerative changes, so imaging frequently proceeds to CT scan after X-rays are obtained, which delays the time to diagnosis. In the case of geriatric trauma patients, however, significant C-spine injuries are more likely, particularly C1 and C2 injuries, and the long-term risk of iatrogenic radiation-induced iatrogenic medical disease is far less likely. Therefore, CT is the cost-effective and preferred imaging strategy to evaluate for C-spine injuries for this population [87, 89]. MRI complements CT scan in the setting of a neurological deficit following neck trauma, or when attempting to clear the C-spine in patients who are obtunded or otherwise unobservable after a negative CT scan [86].

Rib fractures

Each year, 25% of trauma deaths result from chest trauma. Rib fractures are the most common injuries identified. Rib fracture–related mortality increases with age, and especially with an increased number of fractured ribs [90, 91]. Older adults with blunt chest trauma are more likely to suffer rib fractures than younger populations do [91]. Elderly patients with rib fracture are at increased risk for pneumonia and death [34, 35]. Vital capacity is one predictor of hospital length of stay, and could be used to determine disposition in these patients [92]. Rib fractures are a marker for significant solid organ injury, including spleen and liver [93]. Chest X-ray studies are a poor way to find broken ribs, and while CT scan and ultrasound imaging are more accurate, it may be most prudent to assume that a fracture is there in any elderly patient with blunt trauma to the chest, and localized tenderness over the lateral ribcage [34].

Elderly patients perceive pain poorly and often do underreport pain. Pain may be expressed with confusion rather than a direct complaint. The elderly patient often poorly tolerates analgesics as well. Medical-related risks include gastrointestinal bleeding after NSAID use and depressed respiratory drive or confusion after opiates. Therefore, it may be preferable to manage the pain of rib fractures with intercostal nerve blockade, or an epidural catheter if more than three ribs are fractured [94].

Pain is generally underdiagnosed and undertreated in older adults, a phenomenon called "oligoanalgesia." [95, 96] For example, older adult MVA victims are less likely to receive analgesia in the ED (35% vs 47%) or at home. (52% vs 65%) [15] Inadequate pain control exacerbates the complications of rib fractures, including respiratory failure and pneumonia. Nonpharmacologic interventions are also effective to prevent rib fracture complications. For example, hourly incentive spirometry is also important, and a decrease in performance may herald pulmonary deterioration [97].

The sociologic impacts of what are often deemed minor orthopedic injuries cannot be emphasized enough. A simple humeral fracture in elderly patients living alone may totally incapacitate those patients.

They can no longer cook, clean, or dress themselves. They may no longer be able to bathe if they have no shower but only a bathtub. They may not be able to rise from a chair or even the toilet. There is a paucity of short-term rehabilitation facilities that might be utilized to solve these problems, and sometimes a patient will require hospitalization for an injury that would otherwise be discharged to be followed as an outpatient because of sociologic necessities.

Hip fractures

Operative delays beyond 48 h increase mortality, but a geriatric fracture patient's surgical risk must be assessed carefully [98, 99]. Comanagement of hip fracture patients between trauma, orthopedics, geriatrics, and emergency medicine significantly reduces the length of hospital stay, surgical delays, complication rates, and mortality [100–102]. Figure 20.2 demonstrates one example of a comanagement model for ED hip fracture patients [103]. Hip fracture management should focus on functional recovery if the surgical risks and anticipated benefits coincide with the patient's goals of care [104].

One frequently challenging situation is the older adult patient with persistent pain or inability to bear weight despite unremarkable X-ray imaging [62]. Many fractures are hard to see even with multiple views on plain X-ray study. When an elderly patient has new pain and cannot ambulate, admission is mandatory, and the patient may ultimately require an MRI or bone scan to find the subtle fracture. Hip fractures that are not seen on the initial X-ray study occur in 2.9–4.4% of cases, and the sensitivity of two-view X-rays to detect these fractures is 90% [105–108]. A new inability to bear weight is 73% sensitive for occult hip fractures [109]. Other physical examination findings such as pain with straight leg raise (50% sensitive, 45% specific) or with passive internal rotation (61% sensitive, 59% specific) are less helpful [109]. In these situations, MRI is the most accurate imaging test with 100% sensitivity and 100% specificity in early trials [110]. Early use of an MRI during the ED evaluation is cost-effective and reduces the time to diagnosis by days [111, 112]. However, regardless of imaging findings, these nonambulatory patients need admission for pain control and physiotherapy even if no bony injury is identified [113].

A femoral nerve block is an effective pain management strategy for hip fracture patients, particularly in

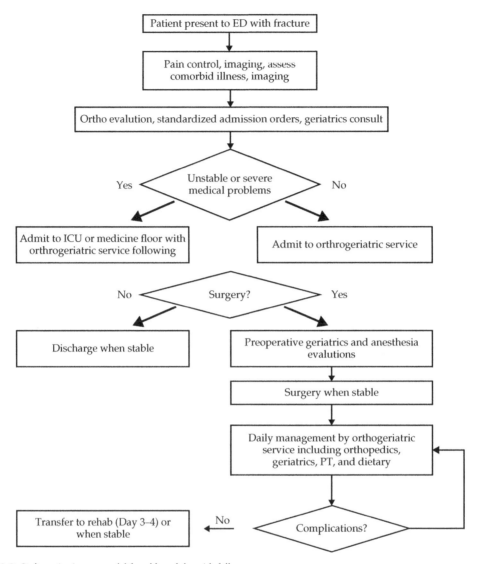

Figure 20.2 Orthogeriatric care model for older adults with falls.

those with hypotension or at risk for opioid-induced delirium [62, 114–119]. Ultrasound-guided femoral nerve block can decrease the time until effective analgesia is attained [120]. Another option is a nurse-led femoral nerve block service [121].

Special situations/considerations

Elder abuse and neglect
Up to 1.2 million older adults (4% of all senior citizens) suffer mistreatment in the United States with 450,000 new cases every year [122]. Elder abuse and neglect is a complex issue with multiple potential risk factors within the geriatric patient, perpetrator, relationship, and environment [123]. Most abuse does not occur in nursing homes, but in the home of community-dwelling older adults. Abuse is more likely in developed countries and in urban settings [124, 125]. Types of abuse include abandonment, psychological, financial, neglect, physical, sexual, or resident-to-resident aggression [122]. Physical abuse

is less common than psychological abuse and financial exploitation [124]. The elder abuse suspicion index is a six-question screen for this problem [126]. The American Medical Association has also developed a screening instrument [122, 127].

Driver safety

Large and increasing numbers of older adults, including those over age 85, are current drivers [128]. Although older adults are *less* likely to be the driver in MVAs, that is because they drive less frequently than younger populations. Most (78%) geriatric MVA victims are discharged home from the ED [15]. After assessing and treating MVA-related injuries, emergency providers have an obligation to assess the role of age and age-related comorbidities to prevent future MVA-related injuries to the patient and to society [129]. Multiple resources exist to guide clinicians, patients, and families to assess driving safety [130]. Office-based testing for driver safety is increasingly available, and cutoff norms are being established to increase the accuracy to predict future MVAs [131, 132]. If time, space, and personnel are available, ED-based driver safety testing is also feasible and accurate [133].

Fall risk

Fall-related injuries are common geriatric patient presenting complaint in EDs worldwide [134]. However, older adults in the ED usually do not have a fall risk assessment obtained as part of their ED evaluation [135]. About 10% of geriatric fall patients will fall again within 6 months after their ED evaluation [136]. One barrier to routine fall risk stratification in the ED is that instruments designed to do so lack validation in the emergency setting [137, 138]. Nonetheless, multiple fall risk factors exist and effective geriatric emergency medicine care includes an assessment of underlying fall risk [2, 138].

End-of-life issues

It is unrealistic to discuss geriatric trauma without discussing end-of-life issues. Few individuals would choose to die alone in a sterile hospital without family and friends. Every meaningful decision junction that involves invasive procedures, delayed testing, or operative management should include cognitively intact patients and their family [139]. The specific risks and benefits of surgery should be discussed and

quantified as much as possible to facilitate shared decision-making. Ethically, the cognitively impaired patient can share in decision-making via providing subject assent and designated decision-maker legal consent [140]. When aggressive care is contraindicated based upon goals of care and underlying comorbidities within the context of the injuries sustained, reliable ED palliative care is imperative [141].

Unanswered questions/future directions

The clinical science of efficient and effective geriatric trauma management continues to evolve. Several potentially high-yield questions exist that could quickly improve the management of these vulnerable trauma patients [13, 142]. In general, most evidence is retrospective and single center. High-quality diagnostic, prognostic, and therapeutic systematic reviews that follow published research guidelines and empirically assess the level of evidence of existing clinical research could provide an overall perspective of how certain clinicians are about what we currently claim as fact or consensus [143].

Specifically, the diagnostic accuracy of venous lactate and base deficit to identify high-risk geriatric trauma patients necessitating ICU admission should be prospectively assessed in ED settings [144]. Alternative noninvasive methods to assess fluid status should be evaluated by using accepted diagnostic research criteria [144–146]. In addition, prognostic instruments superior to existing instruments need to be developed to identify geriatric trauma patients that are most at risk for short-term functional decline [21, 22, 147]. Finally, efficient and acceptable (for EM and Trauma Surgery) diagnostic-therapy-disposition protocols for mild-to-moderate and severe blunt trauma, including standing level falls, need to be developed.

In summary, the management of the geriatric patient is difficult. The emergency physician must not only be alert for occult injury but also be a strong advocate for appropriate disposition. Elders who appear to have only minor injuries may also have multiple comorbidities, poor or no ability to be safely observed as outpatients, require time to develop the classical signs and symptoms of their trauma, and may require assistance in caring for themselves and hospitalization to relieve the pain of their injuries [22]. As with medical disease in geriatric patients, emergency physicians evaluating the older trauma victim should have a low threshold to order basic and advanced imaging, even while recognizing that imaging is imperfect and will miss some potentially life-threatening injuries.

Section IV: Decision-making

- Geriatric patients represent 23% of trauma admissions and standing level falls are the leading causes of older adult trauma mortality.
- Up to 35% of community-dwelling geriatric patients with minor blunt trauma discharged home from the ED experience functional decline at 3 months.
- Despite clinically significant injuries, critically ill geriatric patients often fail to exhibit hypotension, tachycardia, or pain.
- Clinicians should maintain a low threshold for CT scanning in all geriatric patients, particularly anti-coagulated individuals, but a normal brain CT scan at the time of the initial ED evaluation does not eliminate the risk of a delayed intracranial hemorrhage in subsequent days.
- Admit elderly patients with three or more acute rib fractures for pain management and respiratory therapy.
- Emergency providers must play a role in injury prevention via postaccident driver safety assessment and future fall management decisions prior to ED discharge.

References

1 Bonne, S. and Schuerer, D.J.E. (2013) Trauma in the older adult: epidemiology and evolving geriatric trauma principles. *Clin. Geriatr. Med.*, **29** (1), 137–150.

2 Carpenter, C.R., Bromley, M., Caterino, J.M. *et al.* (2014) Optimal older adult emergency care: introducing multidisciplinary geriatric emergency department guidelines from the American College of Emergency Physicians, American Geriatrics Society, Emergency Nurses Association, and Society for Academic Emergency Medicine. *Acad. Emerg. Med.*, **63** (5), e1–e3. doi: 10.1016/j.annemergmed.2014.03.002

3 Thompson, H.J., McCormick, W.C., and Kagan, S.H. (2006) Traumatic brain injury in older adults: epidemiology, outcomes, and future implications. *J. Am. Geriatr. Soc.*, **54** (10), 1590–1595.

4 Keller, J.M., Sciadini, M.F., Sinclair, E., and O'Toole, R.V. (2012) Geriatric trauma: demographics, injuries, and mortality. *J. Orthop. Trauma*, **26** (9), e161–e165.

5 Carter, M.W. and Gupta, S. (2008) Characteristics and outcomes of injury-related ED visits among older adults. *Am. J. Emerg. Med.*, **26** (3), 296–303.

6 Pracht, E.E., Langland-Orban, B., Tepas, J.J. *et al.* (2006) Analysis of trends in the Florida Trauma System (1991–2003): changes in mortality after establishment of new centers. *Surgery*, **140** (1), 34–43.

7 Yildiz, M., Bozdemir, M.N., Kilicaslan, I. *et al.* (2012) Elderly trauma: the two years experience of a university-affiliated emergency department. *Eur. Rev. Med. Pharmacol. Sci.*, **16** (**Suppl. 1**), 62–67.

8 Sharma, O.P., Oswanski, M.F., Sharma, V. *et al.* (2007) An appraisal of trauma in the elderly. *Am. Surg.*, **73** (4), 354–358.

9 Downing, A. and Wilson, R. (2005) Older people's use of Accident and Emergency services. *Age Ageing*, **34** (1), 24–30.

10 Salvi, F., Mattioli, A., Giannini, E. *et al.* (2013) Pattern of use and presenting complaints of older patients visiting an Emergency Department in Italy. *Aging Clin. Exp. Res.*, **25** (5), 583–590.

11 Calland, J.F., Ingraham, A.M., Martin, N. *et al.* (2012) Evaluation and management of geriatric trauma: an Eastern Association for the Surgery of Trauma practice management guideline. *J. Trauma Acute Care Surg.*, **73** (**5 Suppl. 4**), S345–S350.

12 Carpenter, C.R. and Gerson, L. (2008) Geriatric emergency medicine, in *A Supplement to New Frontiers in Geriatrics Research: An Agenda for Surgical and Related Medical Specialties*, 2nd edn (eds J. LoCicero, R.A. Rosenthal, M. Katic, and P. Pompei), The American Geriatrics Society, New York, pp. 45–71.

13 Carpenter, C.R., Shah, M.N., Hustey, F.M. *et al.* (2011) High yield research opportunities in geriatric emergency medicine research: prehospital care, delirium, adverse drug events, and falls. *J. Gerontol. A Biol. Sci. Med. Sci.*, **66** (7), 775–783.

14 McNamara, R.M., Rousseau, E., and Sanders, A.B. (1992) Geriatric emergency medicine: a survey of practicing emergency physicians. *Ann. Emerg. Med.*, **21** (7), 796–801.

15 Platts-Mills, T.F., Hunold, K.M., Esserman, D.A. *et al.* (2012) Motor vehicle collision-related emergency department visits by older adults in the United States. *Acad. Emerg. Med.*, **19** (7), 821–827.

16 Taylor, M.D., Tracy, J.K., Meyer, W. *et al.* (2002) Trauma in the elderly: intensive care unit resource use and outcome. *J. Trauma*, **53** (3), 407–414.

17 Shapiro, M.J., Partridge, R.A., Jenouri, I. *et al.* (2001) Functional decline in independent elders after minor traumatic injury. *Acad. Emerg. Med.*, **8** (1), 78–81.

18 Wilber, S.T., Blanda, M., Gerson, L.W., and Allen, K.R. (2010) Short-term functional decline and service use in older emergency department patients with blunt injuries. *Acad. Emerg. Med.*, **17** (7), 679–686.

19 Sirois, M.J., Emond, M., Ouellet, M.C. *et al.* (2013) Cumulative incidence of functional decline following minor injuries in previously independent older Canadian emergency department patients. *J. Am. Geriatr. Soc.*, **61** (10), 1661–1668.

20 Wilber, S.T., Blanda, M.P., and Gerson, L.W. (2006) Does functional decline prompt emergency department visits and admission in older patients? *Acad. Emerg. Med.*, **13** (6), 680–682.

21 Bissett, M., Cusick, A., and Lannin, N.A. (2013) Functional assessments utilised in emergency departments: a systematic review. *Age Ageing*, **42** (2), 163–172.

22 Carpenter, C.R. (2013) Deteriorating functional status in older adults after emergency department evaluation of minor trauma-opportunities and pragmatic challenges. *J. Am. Geriatr. Soc.*, **61** (10), 1806–1807.

23 Caterino, J.M., Valasek, T., and Werman, H.A. (2010) Identification of an age cutoff for increased mortality in patients with elderly trauma. *Am. J. Emerg. Med.*, **28** (2), 151–158.

24 Meldon, S.W., Reilly, M., Drew, B.L. *et al.* (2002) Trauma in the very elderly: a community-based study of outcomes at trauma and nontrauma centers. *J. Trauma*, **52** (1), 79–84.

25 Grant, P.T., Henry, J.M., and McNaughton, G.W. (2000) The management of elderly blunt trauma victims in Scotland: evidence of ageism? *Injury*, **31** (7), 519–528.

26 Lane, P., Sorondo, B., and Kelly, J.J. (2003) Geriatric trauma patients – are they receiving trauma center care? *Acad. Emerg. Med.*, **10** (10), 244–250.

27 Chang, D.C., Bass, R.R., Cornwell, E.E., and Mackenzie, E.J. (2008) Undertriage of elderly trauma patients to state-designated trauma centers. *Arch. Surg.*, **143** (8), 776–781.

28 Scheetz, L.J. (2012) Comparison of type and severity of major injuries among undertriaged and correctly triaged older patients. *J. Emerg. Med.*, **43** (6), 1020–1028.

29 Demetriades, D., Sava, J., Alo, K. *et al.* (2001) Old age as a criterion for trauma team activation. *J. Trauma*, **51**, 754–757.

30 Demetriades, D., Karaiskakis, M., Velmahos, G.C. *et al.* (2002) Effect on outcome of early intensive management of geriatric trauma patients. *Br. J. Surg.*, **89**, 1319–1322.

31 Morris, A., Welsh, R., Frampton, R. *et al.* (2003) Vehicle crashworthiness and the older motorist. *Ageing Soc.*, **23**, 395–409.

32 Epstein, C.D., Peerless, J., Martin, J., and Malangoni, M. (2002) Oxygen transport and organ dysfunction in the older trauma patient. *Heart Lung*, **31** (5), 315–326.

33 Belzberg, H., Wo, C.C.J., Demetriades, D., and Shoemaker, W.C. (2007) Effects of age and obesity on hemodynamics, tissue oxygenation, and outcome after trauma. *J. Trauma*, **62** (5), 1192–1200.

34 Bulger, E.M., Arneson, M.A., Mock, C.N., and Jurkovich, G.J. (2000) Rib fractures in the elderly. *J. Trauma*, **48** (6), 1040–1046.

35 Bergeron, E., Lavoie, A., Clas, D. *et al.* (2003) Elderly trauma patients with rib fractures are at greater risk of death and pneumonia. *J. Trauma*, **54** (3), 478–485.

36 Havens, J.M., Carter, C., Gu, X., and Rogers, S.O. (2013) Preinjury beta blocker usage does not affect the heart rate response to initial trauma resuscitation. *Int. J. Surg.*, **10** (9), 518–521.

37 Salottolo, K.M., Mains, C.W., Offner, P.J. *et al.* (2013) A retrospective analysis of geriatric trauma patients: venous lactate is a better predictor of mortality than traditional vital signs. *Scand. J. Trauma Resusc. Emerg. Med.*, **21**, 7.

38 LaMantia, M.A., Stewart, P.W., Platts-Mills, T.F. *et al.* (2013) Predictive value of initial triage vital signs for critically ill older adults. *West. J. Emerg. Med.*, **14** (5), 453–460.

39 Platts-Mills, T.F., Travers, D., Biese, K. *et al.* (2010) Accuracy of the Emergency Severity Index triage instrument for identifying elder emergency department patients receiving an immediate life-saving intervention. *Acad. Emerg. Med.*, **17** (3), 238–243.

40 Caterino, J.M., Raubenolt, A., and Cudnik, M.T. (2011) Modification of Glasgow Coma Scale criteria for injured elders. *Acad. Emerg. Med.*, **18** (10), 1014–1021.

41 Werman, H.A., Erskine, T., Caterino, J.M. *et al.* (2011) Development of statewide geriatric patients trauma triage criteria. *Prehosp. Disaster Med.*, **26** (3), 170–179.

42 Heffernan, D.S., Thakkar, R.K., Monaghan, S.F. *et al.* (2010) Normal presenting vital signs are unreliable in geriatric blunt trauma victims. *J. Trauma*, **69** (4), 813–820.

43 Grossman, M.D., Miller, D., Scaff, D.W., and Arcona, S. (2002) When is an elder old? Effect of pre-existing conditions on mortality in geriatric trauma. *J. Trauma*, **52** (2), 242–246.

44 Gallagher, S.F., Williams, B., Gomez, C. *et al.* (2003) The role of cardiac morbidity in short- and long-term mortality in injured older patients who survive initial resuscitation. *Am. J. Surg.*, **185** (2), 131–134.

45 Yilmaz, S., Karcioglu, O., and Sener, S. (2006) The impact of associated diseases on the etiology, course

and mortality in geriatric trauma patients. *Eur. J. Emerg. Med.*, **13** (5), 295–298.

46 Williams, T.M., Sadjadi, J., Harken, A.H., and Victorino, G.P. (2008) The necessity to assess anticoagulation status in elderly injured patients. *J. Trauma*, **65** (4), 772–777.

47 Gage, B.F., Birman-Deych, E., Kerzner, R. *et al.* (2005) Incidence of intracranial hemorrhage in patients with atrial fibrillation who are prone to fall. *Am. J. Med.*, **118** (6), 612–617.

48 Kennedy, D.M., Cipolle, M.D., Pasquale, M.D., and Wasser, T. (2000) Impact of preinjury warfarin use in elderly trauma patients. *J. Trauma*, **48** (3), 451–453.

49 Kirsch, M.J., Vrabec, G.A., Marley, R.A. *et al.* (2004) Preinjury warfarin and geriatric orthopedic trauma patients: a case-matched study. *J. Trauma*, **57** (6), 1230–1233.

50 Cohen, D.B., Rinker, C., and Wilberger, J.E. (2006) Traumatic brain injury in anticoagulated patients. *J. Trauma*, **60** (3), 553–557.

51 Pieracci, F.M., Eachempati, S.R., Shou, J. *et al.* (2007) Degree of anticoagulation, but not warfarin use itself, predicts adverse outcomes after traumatic brain injury in elderly trauma patients. *J. Trauma*, **63** (3), 525–530.

52 Pieracci, F.M., Eachempati, S.R., Shou, J. *et al.* (2007) Use of long-term anticoagulation is associated with traumatic intracranial hemorrhage and subsequent mortality in elderly patients hospitalized after falls: analysis of the New York State Administrative Database. *J. Trauma*, **63** (3), 519–524.

53 Mack, L.R., Chan, S.B., Silva, J.C., and Hogan, T.M. (2003) The use of head computed tomography in elderly patients sustaining minor head trauma. *J. Emerg. Med.*, **24** (2), 157–162.

54 Riccardi, A., Frumento, F., Guiddo, G. *et al.* (2013) Minor head injury in the elderly at very low risk: a retrospective study of 6 years in an Emergency Department (ED). *Am. J. Emerg. Med.*, **31** (1), 37–41.

55 Hardy, J.E. and Brennan, N. (2008) Computerized tomography of the brain for elderly patients presenting to the emergency department with acute confusion. *Emerg. Med. Australas.*, **20** (5), 420–424.

56 Zarzaur, B.L., Croce, M.A., Magnotti, L.J., and Fabian, T.C. (2010) Identifying life-threatening shock in the older injured patient: an analysis of the National Trauma Data Bank. *J. Trauma*, **68** (5), 1134–1138.

57 Davis, J.W. and Kaups, K.L. (1998) Base deficit in the elderly: a marker of severe injury and death. *J. Trauma*, **45** (5), 873–877.

58 Stewart, R.M., Park, P.K., Hunt, J.P. *et al.* (2009) Less is more: improved outcomes in surgical patients with conservative fluid administration and central venous catheter monitoring. *J. Am. Coll. Surg.*, **208** (5), 725–737.

59 Bar-Or, D., Salottolo, K.M., Orlando, A. *et al.* (2013) Association between a geriatric trauma resuscitation protocol using venous lactate measurements and early trauma surgeon involvement and mortality risk. *J. Am. Geriatr. Soc.*, **61** (8), 1358–1364.

60 Min, L., Burruss, S., Morley, E. *et al.* (2013) A simple clinical risk nomogram to predict mortality-associated geriatric complications in severely injured geriatric patients. *J. Trauma Acute Care Surg.*, **74** (4), 1125–1132.

61 Pines, J.M., Carpenter, C.R., Raja, A., and Schuur, J. (2013) *Evidence-Based Emergency Care: Diagnostic Testing and Clinical Decision Rules*, 2nd edn, Wiley-Blackwell Publishing, Oxford.

62 Carpenter, C.R. and Stern, M.E. (2010) Emergency orthogeriatrics: concepts and therapeutic alternatives. *Emerg. Med. Clin. North Am.*, **28** (4), 927–949.

63 Nishijima, D.K., Simel, D.L., Wisner, D.H., and Holmes, J.F. (2012) Does this adult patient have a blunt intra-abdominal injury? *J. Am. Med. Assoc.*, **307** (14), 1517–1527.

64 Moylan, M., Newgard, C.D., Ma, O.J. *et al.* (2007) Association between a positive ED FAST examination and therapeutic laparotomy in normotensive blunt trauma patients. *J. Emerg. Med.*, **33** (3), 265–271.

65 Lee, B.C., Ormsby, E.L., McGahan, J.P. *et al.* (2007) The utility of sonography for the triage of blunt abdominal trauma patients to exploratory laparotomy. *AJR Am. J. Roentgenol.*, **188** (2), 415–421.

66 Natarajan, B., Gupta, P.K., Cemaj, S. *et al.* (2010) FAST scan: is it worth doing in hemodynamically stable blunt trauma patients? *Surgery*, **148** (4), 695–700.

67 Carpenter, C.R. (2012) *The Prognostic Accuracy of FAST Exam in Hemodynamically Stable Blunt Trauma*, Washington University Emergency Medicine Journal Club, http://emed.wustl.edu/education/Emergency MedicineJournalClub/Archive/July2012.aspx (accessed 29 January 2014).

68 Lawes, D. (2002) A retrospective review of emergency admission for head injury in the over 75s. *Injury*, **33** (4), 349–351.

69 Jamieson, L.M. and Robrets-Thomson, K.F. (2008) Hospitalized head injuries among older people in Australia, 1998/1999 to 2004/2005. *Inj. Prev.*, **13** (4), 243–247.

70 Papa, L., Mendes, M.E., and Braga, C.F. (2012) Mild traumatic brain injury among the geriatric population. *Curr. Transl. Geriatr. Exp. Gerontol. Rep.*, **1** (3), 135–142.

71 Bouras, T., Stranjalis, G., Korfias, S. *et al.* (2007) Head injury mortality in a geriatric population: differentiating an "edge" age group with better potential for benefit than older poor-prognosis patients. *J. Neurotrauma*, **24** (8), 1355–1361.

72 Mohindra, S., Mukherjee, K.K., Gupta, R., and Chhabra, R. (2008) Continuation of poor surgical outcome after elderly brain injury. *Surg. Neurol.*, **69** (5), 474–479.

73 Ohm, C., Mina, A., Howells, G. *et al.* (2005) Effects of antiplatelet agents on outcomes for elderly patients with traumatic intracranial hemorrhage. *J. Trauma*, **58** (3), 518–522.

74 Wong, D.K., Lurie, F., and Wong, L.L. (2008) The effects of clopidogrel on elderly traumatic brain injured patients. *J. Trauma*, **65** (6), 1303–1308.

75 Susman, M., DiRusso, S.M., Sullivan, T. *et al.* (2002) Traumatic brain injury in the elderly: increased mortality and worse functional outcome at discharge despite lower injury severity. *J. Trauma*, **53** (2), 219–224.

76 LeBlanc, J., De Guise, E., Gosselin, N., and Feyz, M. (2006) Comparison of functional outcome following acute care in young, middle-aged and elderly patients with traumatic brain injury. *Brain Inj.*, **20** (8), 779–790.

77 Mitra, B., Cameron, P.A., Gabbe, B.J. *et al.* (2008) Management and hospital outcome of the severely head injured elderly patient. *ANZ J. Surg.*, **78** (7), 588–592.

78 Wang, H., Coppola, M., Robinson, R.D. *et al.* (2013) Geriatric trauma patients with cervical spine fractures due to ground level fall: five years experience in a level one trauma center. *J. Clin. Med. Res.*, **5** (2), 75–83.

79 Huybregts, J.G., Jacobs, W.C., and Vleggeert-Lankamp, C.L. (2013) The optimal treatment of type II and III odontoid fractures in the elderly: a systematic review. *Eur. Spine J.*, **22** (1), 1–13.

80 Vaccaro, A.R., Kepler, C.K., Kopjar, B. *et al.* (2013) Functional and quality-of-life outcomes in geriatric patients with type-II dens fracture. *J. Bone Joint Surg. Am.*, **95** (8), 729–735.

81 Jubert, P., Lonjon, G., de Loubresse, C.G., and Bone and Joint Trauma Study Group GETRAUM (2013) Complications of upper cervical spine trauma in elderly subjects. A systematic review of the literature. *Orthop. Traumatol. Surg. Res.*, **99** (6 Suppl), S301–S312. doi: 10.1016/j.otsr.2013.07.007. Epub 2013 Aug 22.

82 Stiell, I.G., Clement, C.M., McKnight, R.D. *et al.* (2003) The Canadian C-spine rule versus the NEXUS low-risk criteria in patients with trauma. *N. Engl. J. Med.*, **349** (26), 2510–2518.

83 Barry, T.B. and McNamara, R.M. (2005) Clinical decision rules and cervical spine injury in an elderly patient: a word of caution. *J. Emerg. Med.*, **29** (4), 433–436.

84 Morrison, J. and Jeanmonod, R. (2014) Imaging in the NEXUS-negative patient: when we break the rule. *Am. J. Emerg. Med.*, **32** (1), 67–70.

85 Bub, L.D., Blackmore, C.C., Mann, F.A., and Lomoschitz, F.M. (2005) Cervical spine fractures in patients 65 years and older: a clinical prediction rule for blunt trauma. *Radiology*, **234** (1), 143–149.

86 Schoenfeld, A.J., Bono, C.M., McGuire, K.J. *et al.* (2010) Computed tomography alone versus computed tomography and magnetic resonance imaging in the identification of occult injuries to the cervical spine: a meta-analysis. *J. Trauma*, **68** (1), 109–114.

87 Holmes, J.F. and Akkinepalli, R. (2005) Computed tomography versus plain radiography to screen for cervical spine injury: a meta-analysis. *J. Trauma*, **58** (5), 902–905.

88 Hoffman, J.R. and Cooper, R.J. (2012) Overdiagnosis of disease: a modern epidemic. *Arch. Intern. Med.*, **172** (15), 1123–1124.

89 Grogan, E.L., Morris, J.A., Dittus, R.S. *et al.* (2005) Cervical spine evaluation in urban trauma centers: lowering institutional costs and complications through helical CT scan. *J. Am. Coll. Surg.*, **200** (2), 160–165.

90 Ziegler, D.W. and Agarwal, N.N. (1994) The morbidity and mortality of rib fractures. *J. Trauma*, **37** (6), 975–979.

91 Sharma, O.P., Oswanski, M.F., Jolly, S. *et al.* (2008) Perils of rib fractures. *Am. Surg.*, **74** (4), 310–314.

92 Bakhos, C., O'Connor, J., Kyriakides, T. *et al.* (2006) Vital capacity as a predictor of outcome in elderly patients with rib fractures. *J. Trauma*, **61** (1), 131–134.

93 Lee, R.B., Bass, S.M., Morris, J.A., and Mackenzie, E.J. (1990) Three or more rib fractures as an indicator for transfer to a Level I trauma center: a population-based study. *J. Trauma*, **30** (6), 689–694.

94 Wardhan, R. (2013) Assessment and management of rib fracture pain in geriatric population: an ode to old age. *Curr. Opin. Anaesthesiol.*, **26** (5), 626–631.

95 Hwang, U., Richardson, L.D., Harris, B., and Morrison, R.S. (2010) The quality of emergency department pain care for older adult patients. *J. Am. Geriatr. Soc.*, **58** (11), 2122–2128.

96 Hwang, U. and Platts-Mills, T.F. (2013) Acute pain management in older adults in the emergency department. *Clin. Geriatr. Med.*, **29** (1), 151–164.

97 Wuermser, L.A., Achenbach, S.J., Amin, S. *et al.* (2011) What accounts for rib fractures in older adults? *J. Osteoporos.*, **2011**, 457591.

98 Radcliff, T.A., Henderson, W.G., Stoner, T.J. *et al.* (2008) Patient risk factors, operative care, and outcomes among older community-dwelling male veterans with hip fracture. *J. Bone Joint Surg. Am.*, **90A** (1), 34–42.

99 Egol, K.A. and Strauss, E.J. (2009) Perioperative considerations in geriatric patients with hip fracture: what is the evidence? *J. Orthop. Trauma*, **23** (6), 386–394.

100 Friedman, S.M., Mendelson, D.A., Kates, S.L., and McCann, R.M. (2008) Geriatric co-management of proximal femur fractures: total quality management

and protocol-driven care result in better outcomes for a frail patient population. *J. Am. Geriatr. Soc.*, **56** (7), 1349–1356.

101 Biber, R., Singler, K., Curschmann-Horter, M. *et al.* (2013) Implementation of a co-managed Geriatric Fracture Center reduces hospital stay and time-to-operation in elderly femoral neck fracture patients. *Arch. Orthop. Trauma Surg.*, **133** (11), 1527–1531.

102 Grigoryan, K.V., Javedan, H., and Rudolph, J.L. (2014) Ortho-geriatric care models and outcomes in hip fracture patients: a systematic review and meta-analysis. *J. Orthop. Trauma*, **28** (3), e49–e55.

103 De Jonge, K.E., Christmas, C., Andersen, R. *et al.* (2001) Hip fracture service -- an interdisciplinary model of care. *J. Am. Geriatr. Soc.*, **49** (12), 1737–1738.

104 Buecking, B., Struewer, J., Waldermann, A. *et al.* (2014) What determines health-related quality of life in hip fracture patients at the end of acute care?--a prospective observational study. *Osteoporos. Int.*, **25** (2), 475–484.

105 Pandey, R., McNally, E., Ali, A., and Bulstrode, C. (1998) The role of MRI in the diagnosis of occult hip fractures. *Injury*, **29** (1), 61–63.

106 Lee, Y.P., Griffith, J.F., Antonio, G.E. *et al.* (2004) Early magnetic resonance imaging of radiographically occult osteoporotic fractures of the femoral neck. *Hong Kong Med. J.*, **10** (4), 271–275.

107 Dominguez, S., Liu, P., Roberts, C. *et al.* (2005) Prevalence of traumatic hip and pelvic fractures in patients with suspected hip fracture and negative initial standard radiographs--a study of emergency department patients. *Acad. Emerg. Med.*, **12** (4), 366–369.

108 Cannon, J., Silverstri, S., and Munro, M. (2009) Imaging choices in occult hip fracture. *J. Emerg. Med.*, **37** (2), 144–152.

109 Hossain, M., Barwick, C., Sinha, A.K., and Andrew, J.G. (2007) Is magnetic resonance imaging (MRI) necessary to exclude occult hip fracture? *Injury*, **38** (10), 1204–1208.

110 Verbeeten, K.M., Hermann, K.L., Hasselqvist, M. *et al.* (2005) The advantages of MRI in the detection of occult hip fractures. *Eur. Radiol.*, **15** (1), 165–169.

111 Rubin, S.J., Marquardt, J.D., Gottlieb, R.H. *et al.* (1998) Magnetic resonance imaging: a cost-effective alternative to bone scintigraphy in the evaluation of patients with suspected hip fractures. *Skeletal Radiol.*, **27** (4), 199–204.

112 Lubovsky, O., Liebergall, M., Mattan, Y. *et al.* (2005) Early diagnosis of occult hip fractures MRI versus CT scan. *Injury*, **36** (6), 788–792.

113 Smith, J.E., Jenkin, A., and Hennessy, C. (2009) A retrospective chart review of elderly patients who cannot weight bear following a hip injury but whose initial x rays are normal. *Emerg. Med. J.*, **26** (1), 50–51.

114 McGlone, R., Sadhra, K., Hamer, D.W., and Pritty, P.E. (1987) Femoral nerve block in the initial management of femoral shaft fractures. *Arch. Emerg. Med.*, **4** (3), 163–168.

115 Finlayson, B.J. and Underhill, T.J. (1988) Femoral nerve block for analgesia in fractures of the femoral neck. *Arch. Emerg. Med.*, **5** (3), 173–176.

116 Haddad, F.S. and Williams, R.L. (1995) Femoral nerve block in extracapsular femoral neck fractures. *J. Bone Joint Surg. Br.*, **77** (6), 922–923.

117 Parker, M.J., Griffiths, R., and Appadu, B. (2002) Nerve blocks (subcostal, lateral cutaneous, femoral, triple psoas) for hip fractures. *Cochrane Database Syst. Rev.*, (1Art. No.: CD001159). doi: 10.1002/14651858.CD001159

118 Fletcher, A.K., Rigby, A.S., and Heyes, F.L.P. (2003) Three-in-one femoral nerve block as analgesia for fractured neck of femur in the emergency department: a randomized, controlled trial. *Ann. Emerg. Med.*, **41** (2), 227–233.

119 Mutty, C.E., Jensen, E.J., Manka, M.A. *et al.* (2007) Femoral nerve block for diaphyseal and distal femoral fractures in the emergency department. *J. Bone Joint Surg. Am.*, **89** (12), 2599–2603.

120 Reid, N., Stella, J., Ryan, M., and Ragg, M. (2009) Use of ultrasound to facilitate accurate femoral nerve block in the emergency department. *Emerg. Med. Australas.*, **21** (2), 124–130.

121 Layzell, M. (2007) Pain management: setting up a nurse-led femoral nerve block service. *Br. J. Nurs.*, **16** (12), 702–705.

122 Bond, M.C. and Butler, K.H. (2013) Elder abuse and neglect: definitions, epidemiology, and approaches to emergency department screening. *Clin. Geriatr. Med.*, **29** (1), 257–273.

123 Johannesen, M. and LoGiudice, D. (2013) Elder abuse: a systematic review of risk factors in community-dwelling elders. *Age Ageing*, **42** (3), 292–298.

124 Sooryanarayana, R., Choo, W.Y., and Hairi, N.N. (2013) A review on the prevalence and measurement of elder abuse in the community. *Trauma Violence Abuse*, **14** (4), 316–325.

125 Eulitt, P.J., Tomberg, R.J., Cunningham, T.D. *et al.* (2014) Screening elders in the emergency department at risk for mistreatment: a pilot study. *J. Elder Abuse Negl.*, **26** (4), 424–435.

126 Yafee, M.J., Wolfson, C., Lithwick, M., and Weiss, D. (2008) Development and validation of a tool to improve physician identification of elder abuse: the Elder Abuse Suspicion Index (EASI). *J. Elder Abuse Negl.*, **20** (3), 276–300.

127 Geroff, A.J. and Olshaker, J.S. (2006) Elder abuse. *Emerg. Med. Clin. North Am.*, **24** (2), 491–505.

128 Betz, M.E. and Lowenstein, S.R. (2010) Driving patterns of older adults: results from the Second Injury Control and Risk Survey. *J. Am. Geriatr. Soc.*, **58** (10), 1931–1935.

129 Carr, D.B. (2004) Commentary: the role of the emergency physician in older driver safety. *Ann. Emerg. Med.*, **43** (6), 747–748.

130 Carr, D.B. and Ott, B.R. (2010) The older adult driver with cognitive impairment: "It's a very frustrating life". *J. Am. Med. Assoc.*, **303** (16), 1632–1641.

131 Molnar, F.J., Patel, A., Marshall, S.C. *et al.* (2006) Clinical utility of office-based cognitive predictors of fitness to drive in persons with dementia: a systematic review. *J. Am. Geriatr. Soc.*, **54** (12), 1809–1824.

132 Ott, B.R., Davis, J.D., Papandonatos, G.D. *et al.* (2013) Assessment of driving-related skills prediction of unsafe driving in older adults in the office setting. *J. Am. Geriatr. Soc.*, **61** (7), 1164–1169.

133 Molnar, F.J., Marshall, S.C., Man-Son-Hing, M. *et al.* (2007) Acceptability and concurrent validity of measures to predict older driver involvement in motor vehicle crashes: an Emergency Department pilot case-control study. *Accid. Anal. Prev.*, **39** (5), 1056–1063.

134 Schrijver, E.J.M., Toppinga, Q., de Vries, O.J. *et al.* (2013) An observational cohort study on geriatric patient profile in an emergency department in the Netherlands. *Neth. J. Med.*, **71** (6), 324–330.

135 Carpenter, C.R., Griffey, R.T., Stark, S. *et al.* (2011) Physician and nurse acceptance of geriatric technicians to screen for geriatric syndromes in the emergency department. *West. J. Emerg. Med.*, **12** (4), 489–495.

136 Carpenter, C.R., Scheatzle, M.D., D'Antonio, J.A. *et al.* (2009) Identification of fall risk factors in older adult emergency department patients. *Acad. Emerg. Med.*, **16** (3), 211–219.

137 Carpenter, C.R. (2009) Evidence based emergency medicine/rational clinical examination abstract: will my patient fall? *Ann. Emerg. Med.*, **53** (3), 398–400.

138 Carpenter, C.R., Stern, M., and Sanders, A.B. (2009) Caring for the elderly, in *Evidence-Based Emergency Medicine* (eds B.H. Rowe, E.S. Lang, M.D. Brown *et al.*), Wiley-Blackwell, Chichester, pp. 260–270.

139 Chang, T.T. and Schecter, W.P. (2007) Injury in the elderly and end-of-life decisions. *Surg. Clin. North Am.*, **87** (1), 229–245.

140 Buckles, V.D., Powlishta, K.K., Palmer, J.J. *et al.* (2003) Understanding of informed consent by demented individuals. *Neurology*, **61** (12), 1662–1666.

141 Rosenberg, M., Lamba, S., and Misra, S. (2013) Palliative medicine and geriatric emergency care: challenges, opportunities, and basic principles. *Clin. Geriatr. Med.*, **29** (1), 1–29.

142 Carpenter, C.R., Heard, K., Wilber, S.T. *et al.* (2011) Research priorities for high-quality geriatric emergency care: medication management, screening, and prevention and functional assessment. *Acad. Emerg. Med.*, **18** (6), 644–654.

143 Moher, D., Liberati, A., Tetzlaff, J., and Altman, D.G. (2009) Preferred reporting items for systematic reviews and meta-analyses: the PRISMA statement. *Ann. Intern. Med.*, **151** (4), 264–269.

144 Bossuyt, P.M., Reitsma, J.B., Bruns, D.E. *et al.* (2003) The STARD statement for reporting studies of diagnostic accuracy: explanation and elaboration. *Ann. Intern. Med.*, **138** (1), W1–W12.

145 Marik, P.E., Baram, M., and Vahid, B. (2008) Does central venous pressure predict fluid responsiveness? A systematic review of the literature and the tale of seven mares. *Chest*, **134** (1), 172–178.

146 Marik, P.E., Cavallazzi, R., Vasu, T., and Hirani, A. (2009) Dynamic changes in arterial waveform derived variables and fluid responsiveness in mechanically ventilated patients: a systematic review of the literature. *Crit. Care Med.*, **37** (9), 2642–2647.

147 Cousins, G., Bennett, Z., Dillon, G. *et al.* (2013) Adverse outcomes in older adults attending emergency department: systematic review and meta-analysis of the Triage Risk Stratification Tool. *Eur. J. Emerg. Med.*, **20** (4), 230–239.

21 Surgical considerations in the elderly

Charles W. O'Connell, Davut Savaser & Colleen Campbell
Department of Emergency Medicine, University of California San Diego Health System,
San Diego, CA, USA

Section I: Case presentation

A 76-year-old woman presented to the emergency department (ED) with nausea and vomiting and "indigestion" for the past 2 days. The patient has a history of hypertension, hypothyroidism, and hyperlipidemia, and had been recently diagnosed with a deep vein thrombosis (DVT) in her left leg just 3 months ago after sustaining a fall while walking her dog. She remarked that she had vomited three times and that the vomit had no bile; however, the most recent episode had some "blood streaks," but not more than a tablespoon in quantity. She described the "indigestion" as cramping in her abdomen that started right after dinner two nights prior and had become progressively dull in nature. She stated that her entire abdomen "just aches" and attributed this to her vomiting. In addition to being on warfarin therapy for her DVT, she had also been on both a beta-blocker and diuretic for her hypertension, thyroid hormone replacement therapy, and a baby aspirin. The vital signs were normal with a blood pressure of 118/76 mmHg, pulse of 76 bpm, respiratory rate of 18 breaths/min, oral temperature of 37.4°C (99.3°F), and pulse oximetry of 97% on room air (RA). The physical examination was normal except for hyperactive bowel sounds, a mildly distended abdomen, and diffuse tenderness without rebound or guarding.

The 12-lead electrocardiogram (EKG) was noted to have left ventricular hypertrophy and some nonspecific ST-T segment abnormalities. The cardiac markers were normal. She had an upright plain abdominal film as well as single anteroposterior (AP) view chest X-ray studies performed, which revealed no free air under the diaphragm and a nonobstructive, nonspecific bowel gas pattern in her abdomen. The laboratory results were significant for a complete blood cell count (CBC) with an elevated white blood cell (WBC) count to 12,300 cells/mm³ and a thrombocytosis to 530,000 cells/mm³, and an international normalized ratio (INR) of 2.3, a normal basic metabolic panel except for mild hypochloremia to 92 mEq/l (normal range 95–105 mEq/l) and hyperglycemia to 128 mg/dl (normal range 70–130 mg/dl) with a normal anion gap. A prompt computed tomography (CT) scan of the abdomen and pelvis with IV contrast revealed an acute appendicitis with perforation and abscess formation with the abscess measuring 3 × 3 × 4 cm, and no free air in the abdomen.

Case outcome

The patient was made nil per os (NPO), administered IV piperacillin-tazobactam, and admitted to the surgical service, with internal medicine and interventional radiology (IR) services in consultation. The patient's INR was promptly reversed with blood products, vitamin K and factor supplements, intravenously, back to a level of 1.4. A percutaneous IR-guided drain was placed intra-abdominally to drain the

Geriatric Emergencies: A Discussion-Based Review, First Edition.
Edited by Amal Mattu, Shamai A. Grossman and Peter L. Rosen.
© 2016 John Wiley & Sons, Ltd. Published 2016 by John Wiley & Sons, Ltd.

abscess, and an IVC-filter was placed as well, given an in-hospital ultrasound revealed persistence of her left lower leg DVT. On hospital Day 3, the patient was taken to the operating room and an appendectomy with drainage and washout of the abdominal abscess was performed. The patient did well postoperatively and was discharged on hospital Day 6 to her home with follow-up in surgery clinic 1 week later. She was restarted on therapeutic dosing of heparin at the 1 week follow-up visit and placed back on her warfarin therapy.

Section II: Case discussion

Dr Peter Rosen (PR): In summary, this is an elderly woman who presented with abdominal pain and nausea and vomiting. Being a geriatric patient, there are all sorts of concomitant diseases and distractors from her principal problem. What makes you think of a surgical disease in a patient with an acute onset of disease?

Dr Vaishl Tolia (VT): Especially in our geriatric population, the initial presentation and any change with the chronic underlying disease process with new onset of symptoms and even an acute onset of vague symptoms could be concerning for a possible surgical process. We know that elderly patients are more likely to present with generalized discomfort because their symptoms are of longer duration, and they may not present early in their disease course. Their delay in presentation can lead to an evolving surgical process. That is the first thing we need to tease out in any geriatric patient especially with any abdominal or acute onset of symptoms. The other concern we need to think about is polypharmacy. Most of our patients in this age group are on a long list of medications, and oftentimes the medications themselves can be responsible for sudden onset of symptoms, particularly with any dose change or if they are unable to take their medications for whatever reason.

PR: Another point to remember is that abdominal disease can present as almost anything and is most likely to require surgical therapy in the elderly patient. No matter how diffuse and how unlocalized it appears to be, it's always prudent to consider the possibility that the patient early on is going to require a surgical consult. This is a patient in whom it would be very easy to get led away from her major surgical problem by potential complications of her therapy. Specifically, she is on warfarin. We know that patients who are on warfarin for a significant length of time are more likely to have complications from warfarin. What do you do to quickly assess this as the potential cause of the entire disease state?

Dr Chris Carpenter (CC): It's very important in geriatric patients to recognize the medications that they are on, which in itself is a real challenge given they often don't come to us with a written list of what their medications are. Getting an accurate list of medications is the first step. Next, one must ascertain whether their medications, warfarin in particular, is the cause or related to their problem. I usually look for other signs of iatrogenic coagulopathy in these patients, and ask for easy bruising, bleeding in other sites such as their nose or their urine. For gastrointestinal (GI) complaints, when I'm trying to distinguish medications from other causes of GI illness, abdominal pain, vomiting, diarrhea, and constipation, I always have my residents spend an extra minute with the patient to make sure that they obtain a complete GI history including any recent travel history, sick contacts at home or at work, duration of illness, and what kind of foods did the patient ingest the last couple meals before the symptoms started, and ensure that this gets documented in the medical record. I think a careful history helps distinguish between medication-related problems from other causes of abdominal pain.

PR: Do you think that this a patient in whom an early rectal examination is important?

Dr Shamai Grossman (SG): I think that rectal examination could be very useful, especially if the patient is on warfarin, and we are concerned that this may be a GI bleed. The issue is what happens if it's positive? If you found melenic stools, I think that would be useful. If you found some blood tinged stool, I think it would be less useful.

PR: I think that it does depend upon the amount of blood in the stool. Melena is helpful, and a large quantity of blood is helpful. Blood tinged stool isn't helpful, whether the patient is on warfarin or not. We have a patient who would appear to have an active surgical disease from the presentation. What is your custom with nasogastric (NG) intubation of such patients?

Dr Don Melady (DM): I think it's unlikely that I would put an NG tube into this woman. I can't see what value it would have. She has vomited. She is not actively vomiting. It doesn't appear that the symptoms are mostly obstructive. There's an important principle of geriatric management here, specifically, that it is good practice in older patients to decrease tethers, restraints, and irritants. So I wouldn't put a catheter in until there was a good reason for it. An NG tube decreases her mobility, adds another irritant, and makes the possibility of developing delirium even greater. Not much benefit and probably quite a lot of risk from that intervention.

PR: I think that's probably a standard attitude toward using an NG tube. I would like to suggest a counter. First of all, we don't know that she isn't bleeding actively into her stomach, and the fastest way to determine that is to place an NG tube. Second, she is described as having a distended abdomen with diffuse tenderness. I don't think that you can say at this point that she is not obstructed. The fact that she is vomiting doesn't mean that she is not obstructed. It just means that there is something going on that's causing her to vomit. If she is obstructed, then an NG tube is not only therapeutic but it may also be diagnostic, because it would allow your imaging studies to provide evidence for obstruction. Thirdly, if she has something other than a bowel obstruction, like a bowel perforation, such as an early mesenteric thrombosis, then you do need to decompress her. Even though I agree with you totally, about the increased risk of confusion, I think the part of surgical disease that is most often omitted today is decompression of the abdomen. Wanganstein showed probably close to 75 years ago now, how much better patients with obstruction do when decompressed with an NG tube, while sorting out whether or not they need surgery. While I would be quick to remove the NG tube, once I've evaluated the cause of the surgical abdomen, I would be quicker to place it until I've discovered what in fact was the pathology that we were aiming for.

How early do you tend to involve surgical consultation in these geriatric patients? Do you complete your workup, with imaging studies and laboratory studies? Or do you tend to involve them early on before you've commenced most of your workup?

VT: In someone that I'm fairly convinced has surgical disease or that has a surgical abdomen, I would definitely try to get them involved early. Oftentimes, culturally, especially at academic medical centers, it's challenging to do that especially when you have a junior surgical resident evaluating the patient. But that's probably the main reason why I like to get them involved early. Consultation tends to require multiple phone calls, a junior talking to a senior, then talking to an attending, all of which can take some time. Informing them of what my initial concern is early and letting them know that this is my workup that I've planned tends to work pretty well.

PR: I think those are really important points. The surgical house staff like the complete package, but they don't understand the process of surgical decision-making and the earlier you can get a surgical senior to see the patient, the earlier the surgical decision-making can occur. The first question for the surgeon is not "what is the pathology," but "does this patient need an operation?" The more senior the surgeons, the more likely they are to be asking and answering that question, without an enormous body of information.

We've discussed many times in the past, the need for a broad-based evaluation of these patients. This particular patient is no exception. It isn't surprising that a CT scan of the abdomen was ordered on the patient. There is no way to evaluate what's going on with this patient without such a study. I can't say that the result of this scan is particularly surprising. If you go back and look at the history, it's not a bad history for appendicitis: pain starting somewhere and then moving somewhere else, with pain worsening and the patient getting sicker over time. I think she actually perforated fairly early, but we don't really know how long her disease has been going on. The history of perforation with appendicitis is more common in the elderly. Thirty percent seem to be perforated before they ever see a physician, and this would appear to be another such case. Do you have any particular studies that you think are critical in the evaluation of such patients before you obtain your images?

CC: No, I agree completely with what you just said. The emergency physicians and our surgical colleagues need to have a very low threshold to get a CT scan, and not delude themselves that the laboratory studies or the plain films are going to make a diagnosis, because they're not. There is very good data, individual trials and meta-analysis data looking into abdominal X-ray studies and CT scan for abdominal obstruction, if that's the reason why you're ordering the studies. The plain abdominal X-ray study changes nothing. The positive likelihood ratio across multiple studies is 1. Your negative likelihood ratio, however, hovers around 0.5, which is not diagnostically helpful. If you think your patient has a surgical abdomen and your surgical consultants need CT scan verification of that to take them to the operating room, get the CT scan early and don't hesitate. There is not really a downside; the same is true for laboratory studies, the WBC count is one test that irritates me in that surgical consultants and some of my emergency medicine colleagues think it's going to tell them something. There is no good data that WBC count is going to be helpful for the diagnosis of appendicitis in the elderly. Twenty percent of these patients are going to have a WBC count below 10. That's not a study you should wait for.

SG: I might add that in this patient they did do an upright chest X-ray, which I think has some utility in this patient population because were they to have seen free air, I think that may have pushed the surgeon to have taken the patient to the operating room sooner rather than later. Although, again the case is somewhat more confusing because the patient is anticoagulated.

PR: I'm puzzled at the need to reverse the anticoagulation. For years, we've been doing surgery for hip replacement and hysterectomy by deliberately anticoagulating people probably to within the range that this patient was in to prevent postoperative embolus. Yet, here we took the time to delay treating this patient surgically to reverse the anticoagulation. Is this a peculiarity of this surgical service, or is that a change in attitude toward operating on anticoagulating patients?

VT: The key in this case besides the medical, surgical, and emergency medicine services is that we've added a fourth element, and that's IR. IR in our institution generally will not perform any sort of procedures on a patient with an INR above 1.5. I think that is why they waited until the INR was 1.4. They do that even when inpatients get paracentesis, which we know are safe regardless of the INR, because often cirrhotics have INRs in the high 1 or 2 s. They will not do procedures until that INR is lowered to 1.5.

PR: I guess that's dependent on the tertiary care consultant. But it is an interesting conflict in philosophies.

As one would have confidently predicted, the EKG was abnormal. What abnormalities would stop you from operating on such patient?

SG: I would think, none unless you actually saw an acute ST-elevated myocardial infarction (MI) on your EKG, in a patient without known cardiac history. If there was a cardiac history, it might make sense to start the patient on a beta-blocker perioperatively. I imagine also dysrhythmias, although that could also be controlled, if it's a bradydysrhythmias, with a pacemaker perioperatively. Given this patient's pathology, I don't think that from a cardiac perspective, I would see any other good reason to hold her back from going to the Operating Room (OR).

PR: This is a patient who is on her way to some kind of surgical therapy, and clearly the reason for doing an interventional rather than open laparotomy was the abscess formation. What is your practice for starting antibiotics for these patients? Do you wait for your surgical consult, or do you just routinely start them as you are starting your patient evaluation?

DM: It's hard to say what "routine practice" would be in this rather atypical and usually unpredictable situation. My sense is that surgeons, at least junior surgical residents, like to get antibiotics started earlier. After the diagnosis of an abscess has been made and the expectation is that there is now going to be an open procedure, it sounds reasonable to start antibiotics. Another consideration is how sick this woman is, since we are all in agreement that sometimes older people are much sicker than they appear to the untrained eye. Could this woman be septic already? She's someone whose vital signs are going to be difficult to interpret. She is not tachycardiac – only 76 – but she is beta blocked. She is not hypotensive by standard definition – 118/76 – but given she is usually hypertensive, maybe her blood pressure represents relative hypotension. She is not febrile, but older patients often do not mount a fever with infection. She does not meet systemic inflammatory response syndrome (SIRS) criteria – but she could still be septic. Starting antibiotics early may well be a good idea.

PR: The point about how sick is she is really an important one. It is really hard to measure this in these patients because our usual external parameters are not helpful. Yet, this is a patient who sounds sick from the description. Did she have the appearance of illness, or did she just look like a frail old lady?

VT: On initial evaluation, she did not look that ill. They were more concerned by her history of vomiting and abdominal discomfort. She was a fairly stoic lady. After reassessing her several times, they realized that there was more than meets the eye because she was being very stoic.

DM: I guess that's one of the reasons I'm hesitant to get early surgical intervention. Somehow I feel that this woman is in better hands with me until it's absolutely clear that she has a surgical presentation and that her only management options are surgical. The senior-friendly emergency physician is aware of a lot of the variable parameters of looking after old people. For one thing, from the history, it sounds like this woman is not a frail older person. She had her hip fracture a few weeks ago while walking her dog. So it sounds like she is a fairly robust person. I'm factoring that into my assessment when I'm looking at her now. Does she look like the robust person who is now looking very ill or a robust person who still looks pretty good? I don't want to disparage anyone, but I think that a lot of these subtleties are lost on surgical residents or surgeons in general. A good emergency physician is more likely to keep a broad differential and an open mind about complex older patients.

PR: It's hard to not disagree with that. On the one hand, I believe the emergency physician is more used to finding a wide variety of diseases other than surgery. On the other hand, as an ex-surgeon, there is value in getting patients to surgery sooner rather than later. This is particularly true with GI bleeds, where years ago we showed that the longer you delay surgical intervention in the bleed, the greater the mortality. The same thing is true for peritonitis. The longer the patient has peritonitis before the repair, the greater the mortality and it's almost linear. Once again, we're walking a calculus problem of involving a team who may be too precipitous in focusing on a single disease as opposed to taking away the chance of survival in someone who has a time-dependent critical disease. I think you have to use some judgment

again as to when you involve your surgical service. Dr Carpenter, in your institution if your patient were to be managed by IR, even though she has a surgical disease, would she be admitted to surgery or to medical intensive care?

CC: At Washington University, this patient would go to surgery with the anticipation that they would be going for operative intervention in the next few days.

SG: In Boston, if they were very clear the patient would ultimately end up in the operating room, it's more likely the patient would go to surgery intensive care. Where it isn't clear then, our surgeons like to wash their hands in these cases and say, "'we'll consult," and the patient would get admitted to the medical intensive care unit (ICU) for better or worse.

PR: I think this can be a terrific problem around the country because the decision to operate is not well made by the people who don't do the surgery. I think where there is the potential need for an open operation, the patient belongs on a surgical service. Nevertheless, that's become less of a custom throughout the country as Dr Grossman just indicated. I think you're going to have to go with what is the practice of your institution. I personally believe that this is surgical problem and a surgical disease, even if there is a delayed surgical repair. It sounds like ultimately she got her appendectomy and did quite well with the delayed drainage of the abscess and subsequent surgery.
Do you have any summary thoughts for us?

VT: I would add to one of the comments that was made about the CT scan in particular. This patient did receive IV contrast, which is important. I think oral and IV contrast are often overused particularly in general for the diagnosis of acute appendicitis. I think in the hands of trained radiologists who feel confident especially in elderly patients in whom you may have acute kidney injury and chronic underlying kidney disease, that usually for cases such as this, contrast may be unnecessary, particularly for acute appendicitis and even bowel obstruction. I think that in general, early surgical consultation, for us is important and something that the emergency house staff don't do as frequently just because they may get rebuffed from the surgical house staff. As a trauma center with a surgeon in house 24 h a day, I think that it's useful to get your surgical colleagues involved at an appropriate time. This patient not only got surgical consultation but also internal medicine, which in a complex patient, with multiple medical problems, on Coumadin and on a lot of other medications, is very appropriate. Dealing with IR can oftentimes can be challenging especially when a patient like this is not going to go to the operating room immediately. So coordinating that is part of the role in emergency medicine as well as keeping that broad differential while we get our surgical colleagues involved.

PR: There is going to be some institutional variation, depending on how your colleagues work together. I think it is rare to have formal internal medicine consults on ED patients. I think this is the place that even if the patient would be admitted to the surgical ICU, an internist would be well involved in the care of the patient. In Boston, that might be the hospitalist.

Section III: Concepts

Background

Geriatric patients require special consideration due to age-related changes associated with the process of senescence. The impact of the geriatric population on US emergency medicine departments will continue to grow for the foreseeable future. Between 2012 and 2050, the United States will experience a considerable growth of its older population, projected to almost double from 43.1 million in 2012 to 83.7 million in 2050 [1]. Thirteen percent of the US population is aged 65 or older, but they account for nearly 20% of all ED encounters. Both of these proportions are predicted to continue to rise [1, 2]. Elderly visits to the ED are increasing more rapidly than in any other age group [2]. This increasing influx will prove a challenge to EDs and hospitals. Visits by the elderly population are generally associated with higher acuity. They are also associated with increased utilization of laboratory testing, radiology imaging acquisition, extended stays, and higher admission rates [3]. As the population ages, there will be a resultant total increase in surgical necessity among geriatric aged patients.

Elderly patients are more likely to have serious medical illness when seen in the ED than nonelderly patients, 32% and 19%, respectively [4]. Many of these serious illnesses will be of surgical nature in etiology. Marco *et al.* report a 22.1% requirement for surgical intervention in elderly patients presenting to the ED with abdominal pain [5]. It has been projected that the need for surgery in this age population may exceed the rate of physician growth [6]. It has also been reported that many emergency physicians have not been trained in geriatric-specific approaches, and many feel less comfortable in dealing with older patients [7]. It is imperative that EDs, surgical services, and healthcare organizations are equipped to handle this impending wave of geriatric patients. This chapter strives to highlight pertinent evaluative strategies to ensure optimal care to geriatric surgical patients encountered in the ED.

Elderly physiology

It is the physiological age, not simply the chronological age of a patient that primarily dictates the response to surgical pathology and resultant biological stress. Physiological studies of aging have shown that basal function of organ systems is relatively uncompromised by the aging process per se [6]. However, functional reserve certainly diminishes with aging, which leads to a reduction in the ability to compensate for physiological stress due to illness and surgery. Various medical comorbidities in addition to the aging process can alter core function and the ability to adapt to stressors. An understanding of the physiology of aging will provide a keener scope for evaluation and management of these patients.

Cardiac complications are the leading cause of perioperative morbidity and death in surgical patients of all age groups, particularly in the elderly. Atherosclerosis and systolic arterial hypertension increase with age, and are associated with an increased incidence of ventricular hypertrophy. Hypertrophied myocardium increases wall stress, myocardial oxygen demand, and susceptibility to ischemia. Ventricular hypertrophy also leads to diastolic dysfunction, impairing the ability to adjust stroke volume and impeding passive refill. In addition, there is thought to be age-related impairment to catecholamine response [8]. The intrinsic resting contractility and cardiac output are generally unaltered with age [6]. However, when faced with physiological stress, the elderly cardiovascular system less effectively buffers changes in circulatory volume. Consequently, the elderly are more susceptible to hypotension and ischemia due to inadequate cardiac output.

Changes in pulmonary function parallel cardiac changes. Diminished elasticity and structural thoracic changes cause decreased forced expiratory volume and vital capacity. Alveolar dead space increases, which impairs oxygen diffusion capacity [9]. These changes ultimately result in decreased maximum minute ventilation and increased work of breathing to meet oxygen demands. Older patients have decreased response to hypoxia and hypercapnia, causing increased propensity for respiratory failure during high demand states [9]. Weakened respiratory muscles and decreased ciliary function impair cough and airway clearance [10, 11]. Compromised pulmonary function increases susceptibility to and severity of hypoxia, atelectasis, and pneumonia in the postoperative period.

The function of the renal system declines with age as well. There is an average 30–50% loss of renal parenchyma between the ages of 20 and 90 years [12]. This corresponds to a progressive decrease in glomerular capillary surface and glomerular filtration rate (GFR). Reduction of basal blood flow causes the kidneys in the elderly to be more susceptible to injury in low perfusion states, including hypotension, hemorrhage, hypovolemia, and low cardiac output [13]. Chronic kidney disease is a common comorbidity in the elderly secondary to long-standing conditions such as hypertension and diabetes. The incidence of recognized chronic kidney disease in those aged 65 years or older more than doubled from 1.8% to 4.3% from 2000 to 2008 [14]. Decreased renal clearance should also be a consideration during drug administration, especially for analgesic and anesthetic choices.

A subtle but steady decline occurs in both the central and peripheral nervous systems during the aging process. Aside from the well-known age-related cerebral atrophy, over time there is a reduction in the complexity of neuronal connections, decreased synthesis of neurotransmitters, and increase in enzymes responsible for postsynaptic degradation [15]. Skeletal musculature innervations decrease, translating into a loss of motor units and decrease in strength and fine motor control [16]. This cumulative degradation of the neuronal network contributes to the elderly propensity for falls, potential for drug toxicity, and medically induced delirium. Sympathetic and parasympathetic neurons are also lost over time and associated with impaired cardiovascular reflexes [17].

Diagnosis

As always, the task of the emergency physician is to determine the cause and the extent of present illness. Those with advanced age are more likely to have comorbid conditions, chronic disease, impaired nutrition, cognitive decline, dementia, and social isolation. These factors compound to make the surgical evaluation and management exceedingly more complex. These confounding age-related factors can influence history acquisition, physical presentation of illness, and diagnostic interpretation. Chronologic age is not the main determinant in the complexity and management strategies of these cases. It is a composite of the physiological and pathologic states of the individual that should be used as the yardstick to measure age [18]. Chronological age should not be an independent contraindication to surgery; management should be tailored to the patient's symptoms, overall health and functional status.

A multifaceted approach in acquiring a clear, comprehensive history is optimal in the evaluation of elderly patients. This includes primary history from patients, communication with family members, Emergency Medical Services (EMS) documentation, and prior health records. This provides necessary information to determine comorbidities and other surgical risk factors. If multiple complaints are present, they should be addressed in order of priority and "red flag" issues should be promptly identified. Evaluation of complaints in elderly patients requires more time and care than similar complaints among younger adult populations [19]. Optimizing communication with the elderly is ideal to ensure the most accurate and complete record. Encouraging the use of devices such as dentures, eyeglasses, and hearing aids can mitigate communicative breakdown. Also, adequate lighting and minimization of surrounding visual and auditory distraction will improve exchange of information.

The review of systems is often helpful to ascertain details that the patient may have neglected to report. Elderly patients may fail to report symptoms that they attribute to normal aging such as constipation, incontinence, falls, and dizziness. A review of systems should also be supplemented with a brief functional assessment and identification of new difficulties in activities of daily living along with a change in chronic symptoms. A comprehensive social history including living situation, access to transportation, and availability of caretakers is essential to the eventual proper disposition of elderly patients. The assembly of a complete medication list of both active medications and recent changes can be invaluable. The elderly are the largest users of prescription drugs. Many of these medications have effects that may alter presentation or pose a potential interaction with planned interventions.

Initial, expedient review and consideration of the patient's vital signs identifies fever, hemodynamic instability, hypoxia, and respiratory distress. Review of vital signs yields both diagnostic information and signals necessary for immediate intervention to stabilize. Fever, the cardinal sign of infection, may be absent or blunted in 20–30% of the time in the elderly [20]. The exact physiological mechanism for the blunted temperature response in the elderly has not been completely elucidated. Fever is more likely associated with a serious viral or bacterial infection compared to younger patients [20]. Infection frequently accompanies many surgical processes. Early and accurate detection of infection is important in all populations, especially among the elderly who are known to have increased morbidity and mortality rates from common infections [21]. The acquisition of the temperature value may be affected by patients who are altered, uncooperative, demented, or with neurobehavioral disorders. Tongue tremors, mouth breathing, ingestion of hot or cold fluids, and variations in the rate and depth of respiratory patterns can affect the measurement of oral temperatures. The recorded temperature can be affected by the mode of acquisition. A study of 73 geriatric patients shows oral and axillary temperatures are 0.66°C and 0.88°C lower than rectal, respectively [22]. Rectal temperature as shown by Darowski *et al.* has a greater sensitivity, 88%, for detection of fever in geriatric patients with definite infections compared to sublingual (66%) and axillary (32%) [23].

A thorough but focused physical examination is essential. It remains an important element of the geriatric examination. However, the physical examination of the elderly population can be fraught with diagnostic uncertainty. Much of the literature and conventional diagnostic criteria upon which we rely are based on studies of younger individuals. This convention may be a source of serious error in geriatric emergency medicine. We know key findings, such as fever, hypotension, abnormal bowel sounds, and physical findings suggestive of peritonitis are associated with significant morbidity and mortality [5]. However, the absence of these findings does not preclude significant surgical disease, especially in the elderly [5]. The most common causes of peritonitis in the elderly are mesenteric infarction, malignancy, intestinal obstruction, perforated peptic ulcer, cholecystitis, and diverticulitis [5, 24]. A retrospective analysis of geriatric patients shows that abdominal pain is identified in only 55% of surgery or autopsy proven cases of peritonitis [24]. However, there is typically some indication, for there were no cases of absolutely silent peritonitis based on symptoms and the physical examination. In addition, there is no difference in the identification of peritonitis in those given analgesics [24]. Findings of nausea, vomiting, constipation, fever, tachycardia, hypotension, abdominal tenderness, peritoneal inflammation, and malaise should all raise concern for a surgical etiology of disease.

A disease-specific approach may not work as well in the geriatric population. They frequently have atypical presentations, alterations in mental status, or masking coexisting conditions that preclude this manner of evaluation. A patient-centered approach, taking into account comprehensive health and functional status, may prove to be more fruitful diagnostically. In addition to making the correct surgical diagnosis, it is crucial to identify existing comorbid disease such as pneumonia, congestive heart failure, coronary ischemia, and urinary tract infection. Given these challenges, the provisional diagnosis is often less accurate in elderly patients [25]. Not surprisingly, diagnostic inaccuracy has shown to adversely affect outcomes. Morbidity is increased when there is discrepancy between the provisional diagnosis and the final discharge diagnosis. The morbidity is nearly three times higher in elderly (45%) than nonelderly (16%) when this occurs [26]. For this reason, it is extremely important to expand the early differential diagnosis and maintain an early and high concern for surgically relevant disease within the geriatric population.

Laboratory diagnostics

Laboratory diagnostics serve as useful adjuncts to a thorough history and physical examination. Laboratory evaluations can help to evaluate for common medical causes of abdominal pain such as coronary ischemia, pancreatitis, hepatitis, and urinary tract infections. Laboratory screening will have a higher diagnostic yield in the elderly due to higher prevalence of disease and a frequent absence of clinical symptoms. A urinalysis is especially useful because elderly patients will frequently manifest more generally with symptoms of altered mental status, fatigue, weakness, or loss of appetite. Useful blood tests may include complete blood count, coagulation studies, electrolytes, liver panel, coagulation, lactate and albumin in ill-appearing elderly patients. The utility of a WBC count is often unhelpful as fever and elevated WBC are absent in 30% of surgical geriatric emergencies. The independent utility of WBC count in differentiating between surgical and nonsurgical conditions is also limited [27]. There has not been a correlation with an abnormal creatinine, cell blood count, coagulation profile, or electrolyte abnormality as a predictor of surgical risk. The level of lactate elevation has been correlated with mortality in elderly patients and can also be used as a guide to resuscitation.

Preoperative screening should be guided by the type of surgery and underlying comorbidities [28]. A urinalysis can be used to screen for asymptomatic urinary tract infections, often seen in elderly patients [29]. The detection of significant metabolic abnormalities in terms of electrolyte balance, glucose, and renal dysfunction may be helpful for preoperative optimization [28]. A blood gas may elucidate the presence of carbon dioxide retention in the setting of pulmonary dysfunction.

Radiographic diagnostics

Imaging studies are frequently necessary in the evaluation of the elderly, because geriatric patients have a significantly higher proportion of urgent surgical diagnoses than nongeriatric populations [4, 30]. The choice of imaging studies will vary based on the presenting symptoms and suspected underlying pathology. Each diagnostic test has its own merits and limitations.

The CT scan has become a mainstay diagnostic tool. One study shows that abdominal CT scan modifies the suspected diagnosis in nearly 50% of cases. This same study shows that a CT scan modifies the decision for admission in 26% of cases, need for surgery in 12%, and antibiotic treatment in 21% of cases [31]. It offers many advantages over traditional two-dimensional radiography. The superimposition of structures outside the area of interest is eliminated with CT imaging. The invasive catheter and specialization required for angiography have been largely obviated by the advent of CT angiograms.

There is associated ionizing radiation with acquisition of CT images. Age is thought to play a significant role in the lifetime risk of developing cancer associated with CT scan radiation. For instance, a 40 year old is estimated to have half the risk compared to a 20 year old. The geriatric population is thought to have substantially less risk given the exposure is much later in life [32]. A more pertinent risk in the elderly is complications associated with the use of intravenous contrast. Minor complications such as nausea, vomiting, itching, and rash are not uncommon. Anaphylaxis was seen with a higher incidence with the use of older radiocontrast agents, but the introduction of less osmotically active agents has significantly lowered the rate of this occurrence. Age is a main risk factor for contrast-induced nephropathy. Risk factors implicated in the development of this complication include underlying renal impairment, diabetes, chronic heart failure, and reduced intravascular volume, all of which are seen with a higher frequency in the elderly [33, 34]. Optimizing intravascular volume before intravenous contrast load is a putative goal to improve outcomes [35]. It is also advisable to avoid contrast administration in those with moderate-to-severe kidney impairment. Although it may affect the diagnostic yield, noncontrast CT scans and ultrasound may be the most appropriate tests for patients at high risk for renal complication.

Ultrasound has emerged as a useful diagnostic utility for specific indications. It is portable, acquired in real time, and uses sound waves instead of ionizing radiations. Its role has been well established with the Focused Assessment with Sonography for Trauma (FAST) examination in the trauma setting for the identification of free fluid within the intra-abdominal and pericardial spaces. It has also widely become the imaging modality of choice for evaluation of cholecystitis and DVT and has shown useful sensitivity for screening of abdominal aortic aneurysm, pneumothorax, pleural effusion, small bowel obstruction, and subcutaneous abscess. Its bedside application has become instrumental in rapid assessment of hypotensive patients to ascertain the presence of free fluid in the abdomen or lung, intravascular filling within the inferior vena cava and relative contractility of the heart, to help guide resuscitation. Its safety, ease of use, and rapid image acquisition have allowed emergency physicians to employ it as an ultrasonic stethoscope in every evolving field of medicine. Its universal application is limited due to challenges in quality imaging acquisition due to bone, bowel gas, external interferences such as bandages, splints and casts, and excessive soft tissue and adipose.

Chest radiography is certainly indicated for unexplained respiratory symptoms and distress, concern for pneumonia, trauma, or other underlying symptomatic pulmonary processes. However, empiric preoperative chest radiography has little clinically significant yield. In a large meta-analysis, it is found to change management in only 0.1% of cases [36].

Management of surgical issues

In addition to accurate diagnosis, timely stabilization and treatment are essential. Thoughtful age-specific considerations should be applied to the management of geriatric patients. For example, the expected tachycardiac response for a given presentation may be absent due to the blunted cardiovascular response of the elderly and the frequent use of heart rate–slowing medications. Normal vital signs can lead to a false sense of security and lead to inadequate resuscitation. Complications of surgical disease such as respiratory failure, sepsis, and hypoperfusion all require urgent management, but may all have less apparent presentations. Even despite increased mortality rates of elderly surgical patients compared to younger populations, aggressive management has demonstrated favorable long-term outcomes among acute geriatric surgical populations [37, 38].

Maintenance of a patent airway is a primary concern in critically ill patients. The anatomic variation in the elderly including poor dentition, presence of dentures, and both cervical and temporomandibular arthritis often contribute to more difficult intubations. In concert with airway management, impairment of the pulmonary function should be rapidly addressed. Weakened respiratory muscles and degenerative changes of the spine and chest wall result in diminished effective ventilation. This risk of compromised respiration is compounded by blunted response to hypoxia, hypercarbia, and acidosis. These factors contribute to delay the onset of clinical distress and its detection. Failure to recognize indications for early intubation is a serious mistake, especially within geriatric patients associated with major trauma and critical illness with a higher risk of mortality.

It is crucial to optimize hemodynamics and perfusion to tissues. Both medical and traumatic surgical patients often present in a relative state of hypovolemia. Elderly patients often have a chronic decrease in total body water due to increased free water clearance and decreased thirst and urinary concentrating ability [39]. This relative state of dehydration is also exacerbated by frequent use of diuretics. This predisposition provides susceptibility for fluid disorders and can presage a state of profound hypovolemia. The elderly may have a blunted chronotropic and cardiovascular response to hypovolemia, especially if they are taking heart rate–controlling medications such as beta-blockers. Another consideration is that chronic hypertension, a common entity in elderly patients, may obscure relative hypotension in those presenting with blood pressures within normal appearing parameters. A "normal" heart rate and blood pressure do not always imply normal cardiac output. Vigilant hemodynamic monitoring should be provided in potentially ill patients to optimize management of fluid status. Consider judicious volume replacement in this population given the high prevalence of elderly patients with heart failure, renal impairment, and limited pulmonary reserve to avoid complications of fluid overload.

Rapid neurologic evaluation to assess for intracranial and spinal cord injury is an important initial consideration in regard to surgical patients in the trauma setting. Clinical symptoms from compressive effects of intracranial bleeds may be delayed to due to brain atrophy in the elderly. It is a grave error to assume alterations in mental status are due solely to underlying dementia or senility.

Pain management

Pain is typically associated with most surgical emergencies. Coexisting conditions such as aphasia or advanced dementia, particularly common in the elderly, may limit expression or communication of the presence pain or its severity. There is a frequent failure to recognize new acute pain due to chronic underlying painful conditions. Pain in these geriatric populations may manifest as failure to move in bed or ambulate, anorexia, or depressive affect.

The first axiom in providing analgesia is thoughtful assessment of the patient and the comorbidities. Pain is often undertreated in the elderly populations. Generally, the goal should be to adequately treat the pain with the least amount of medication necessary in an effort to mitigate adverse effects. Ideally, this can be accomplished with analgesic options and other adjuncts that minimize systemic effects.

Opiates and opioids are a mainstay of analgesia, but central nervous system depression can be seen with their use. Specifically, respiratory depression and apnea are risks that should be taken into account. Opiate use also confers a risk of constipation, and, therefore, should be coupled with a bowel regimen of stool softeners and laxatives. Multimodal approaches may help to optimize pain control and decrease side effects as well. Acetaminophen and nonsteroidal anti-inflammatory drugs (NSAIDs) may be appropriate initial agents, alternatives, or adjuncts. NSAIDs can be associated with renal impairment, platelet inhibition, and irritation to gastric mucosa. This may limit their use in many elderly patients especially with chronic use. Local anesthetics, nerve blocks, and topical ice packs may be advantageous alternatives and supplements.

The route of analgesia administration should also be taken into account as well. Oftentimes the intravenous route is preferred due to ease and comfort with existing IV access or need for repeated doses. It is also preferred when the patient has poor oral tolerance of medications or malabsorptive issues. Intramuscular and subcutaneous injections can be very painful in cachectic, frail elderly patients [40]. Oral and rectal medications may not be absorbed well in those patients with nausea, vomiting and dehydration or with inherent malabsorption. Sublingual, intranasal, and buccal routes are all alternative considerations if applicable to the specific treatment option.

Pharmacology

Elderly patients are the largest users of prescription drugs. Obtaining the most comprehensive list available of the patient's medications is a vital part of the assessment of elderly patients. Medications may have both expected and unexpected effects, which can be exacerbated by the interactions between other medications, vitamins, and supplements. The physiological changes of the elderly influence the efficacy, distribution, and metabolism of pharmaceuticals. The body composition changes with age. The elderly typically have decreases in lean body mass and total body water and increased adipose, which affects the distribution of medications. Also, decreased protein binding and increased free fraction of drugs can potentially increase pharmacological effect [40]. Diminished cardiac output and lessened renal and hepatic clearance can all influence the effects of drug concentration.

There are certain medications that have both broad use and significant consequences. Beta-blockers, certain calcium channel blocking medications, and other rate-slowing medications can blunt cardiovascular response masking the tachycardia expected with hypovolemia, fever, and other physiological stressors. As a result, seemingly normal vital signs can lull a physician into a false sense of confidence. There is a lack of conclusive evidence regarding the cost-benefit of beta-blockers in the perioperative setting in regard to mortality benefit [41, 42]. A large meta-analysis of perioperative beta-blocker use has shown there is small decrease in nonfatal MIs, but conversely a small increase in nonfatal but debilitating strokes and bradycardia with hypotension [42]. The general consensus is that a thoughtful evaluation of the risk of surgery and comorbidities should take place before administration.

Many geriatric patients are pharmaceutically anticoagulated for a host of medical indications such as management of DVT and embolism, mechanical heart valves, and stroke risk reduction for atrial fibrillation.

There is no clear consensus for the management of anticoagulated patients in the preoperative setting. It is best to consider a patient-centered approach based on risk stratification profile taking into account the patient and procedural risk factors for thrombosis and bleeding. The risk profile among reversal for anticoagulation varies widely according to the indication for its use. The reversal of anticoagulation with a prosthetic mechanical valve carries a much greater consequence than those who are anticoagulated for stroke risk reduction. Many different products are used for the purpose of anticoagulation, each with unique mechanism of action and ability and ease of reversal. Warfarin, which interferes with vitamin K recycling and production of clotting factors, has been a mainstay for generations. Many other products such as fractionated heparins and the newer oral anticoagulants such as thrombin inhibitor, dabigatran, and factor Xa inhibitors, rivaroxaban, edoxaban and apixaban have become more frequently used. The new oral agents carry the advantage of less drug–drug and food–drug interactions and do not require laboratory monitoring compared to warfarin. That being said, current common laboratory diagnostics lack the ability to distinguish those who are effectively anticoagulated as the INR is used with warfarin. Moreover, there are no drug-specific reversal agents, and the cost of the drug is very high at present.

In the case of emergency surgery or life-threatening hemorrhage, anticoagulation should typically be fully reversed when possible. The product of choice is generally prothrombin complex concentrate (PCC) where available [43]. PCC has the advantage over fresh frozen plasma (FFP) in regard to more rapid infusion due to lack of a need for a thawing period and less volume per dose, and contains more predictable factor concentrations [43]. When PCC is not available, FFP should be used, with consideration given to volume constraints in patients susceptible to fluid overload. There is a paucity of evidence to dictate the manner of anticoagulation reversal with newer oral anticoagulants. The general consensus suggests the use of PCC is a reasonable approach, and that FFP would likely be of low yield [43]. The half-life and duration of effect are much shorter in these agents than with warfarin. Of note, dabigatran has significantly more renal clearance than either apixaban or rivaroxaban [42]. Patients who develop renal insufficiency while taking dabigatran are at increased risk for supratherapeutic effects. Hemodialysis has been suggested as a possible method of reducing dabigatran concentration and its anticoagulative effects. New reversal agents for these new oral anticoagulants are in production and will potentially be a more sufficient means of reversal.

Preoperative clearance

There is no clear consensus for single standard presurgical assessment for elderly patients in the emergency setting [44]. Geriatric assessment tools developed for elective and outpatient surgeries often do not apply to surgical cases seen within the ED. Classically, whenever a surgical procedural intervention is used within the ED, the American Society of Anesthesiologists (ASA) physical status classification system is employed to assess surgical risk. This system is based on the fitness of individuals preoperatively on a graded scale I–VI based on the degree and threat of systemic disease (Table 21.1). The physical classification is followed by an "E" when the surgery is defined as emergency in nature. The ASA scale does have loosely

Table 21.1 ASA classification.

ASA Classification	Definition
ASA I	Normal healthy patients
ASA II	Patients with mild systemic disease (e.g., hypertension and well controlled)
ASA III	Patients with severe systemic disease that is limiting but not incapacitating (e.g., complicated diabetes)
ASA IV	Patients with incapacitating disease that is a constant threat to life (symptomatic coronary artery disease, hepatic, or renal failure)
ASA V	Moribund patients with dismal prognosis (e.g., cardiogenic shock)
ASA VI	A declared brain-dead patient whose organs are being removed for donor purposes
E	Patients requiring emergency surgery

defined definitions, which can cause confusion when assigning the grading scale designation. Increased ASA classification has shown to increase the odds of mortality in surgical patients of geriatric age, in addition to impairment of activities of daily living and emergency operation (E). Conversely, a low ASA classification (grades 1 and 2) does predict a low overall mortality odds ratio across all age groups [45].

Pulmonary function tests and cardiac stress tests are helpful if available, but are infrequently present upon arrival, and are impractical to obtain in the ED and may be independent of emergency surgical disposition. Geriatric electrocardiograms (ECG) will often show abnormalities, but have shown limited value in predicting postoperative complications in patients undergoing noncardiac surgery [46]. There is no consensus on need for 12-lead ECG, but it is warranted in older patients, if for no other reason, then to establish a preoperative baseline [47]. Abnormalities are common in preoperative geriatric ECG, but have limited value in predicting postoperative complications in patients undergoing noncardiac surgery [46]. Chest radiographs should be obtained if clinical presentation suggests respiratory pathology or if prior patient history warrants imaging.

Elective versus emergent surgery

Emergency physicians are often faced with diagnosis and management of surgically correctable disease processes. However, it is not the role of the emergency physician to provide definitive surgical treatment. Many conditions such as symptomatic hernias and gallstones are frequent, reoccurring diagnoses made within the ED. These may not require immediate surgical need, but negatively impact quality of life. Such etiologies are often amenable to elective procedures providing cure, but the elderly may not be deemed surgical candidates due to advanced age and comorbidities. It should be emphasized that these procedures done electively have much improved and safer outcomes in the medically optimized elderly patient as opposed to those necessitated by surgical emergencies [45]. Conversely, elderly patients may be able to tolerate the surgical procedure but not the complications that may ensue. Elective surgeries are not without risk. Infection, wound complications,

bleeding, damage to surrounding structures, cardiac events, and venous thrombus are some of the realized risks with any surgical procedure and the postoperative period.

Emergency surgery, defined as nonelective surgery that is performed with the aim to prevent morbid or fatal health consequence of a surgically treatable condition, poses considerable risk to the elderly population [35]. It is quite clear that geriatric patients have a higher incidence of morbidity and mortality associated with emergency surgery than younger patients [48]. Recent literature has shown that elective surgical outcomes between young and old do not represent the disparity often believed; elective surgical outcomes are quite similar among different age groups [48, 49]. Even at the extreme of ages, this phenomenon can be seen. A study of individuals 90+ years of age undergoing elective operations reports a 5-year survival not significantly different than age-matched populations [49].

It can be very difficult to determine the risk–benefit ratio in relation to the elderly and surgical procedures. Every surgery does indeed pose risk, which may deter elective procedures in the elderly. Unfortunately, the delay of elective surgery may also necessitate emergency surgical management at a later time that carries a much higher risk for complications and mortality. In addition, the lengthy wait or deference of needed surgery experienced by many geriatric patients represents a burden in terms of chronic, unrelieved symptoms and poor health-related quality of life [50]. When assessing outcomes and risks, the overall quality of life should be considered in addition to mortality concerns. Prognostication of factors regarding return to function, activities of daily life, and placement in nursing care facility are all assessed in the preoperative evaluation of the elderly. Given the relative low risk of morbidity and mortality of elective surgery, in a subset of symptomatic elective surgical cases, it may fall within the purview of the emergency physician to be an advocate for more expedient surgical correction.

Postoperative complications are more prominent in elderly patients. Early complications are associated with long-term morbidity and mortality [51]. The most common postoperative complications for elderly postsurgical patients include respiratory, wound, and cardiac-related complications that, in one study, occur in 39.5%, 16.3%, and 12.4% of all elderly postsurgical patients, respectively [52]. Both MI and pneumonia may tend to present as vague abdominal complaints and may be the only presenting symptom in this population [31, 53]. Postoperative delirium is another complication that can occur in 15% to >50% in varying populations [54]. Postoperative delirium will often lead to delays in discharge, increased morbidity due to prolonged exposure to the hospital environment, and a higher probability of discharge to a higher level of care [55]. The exact cause of such delirium is not completely understood, but it is hypothesized that the etiology may be an imbalance between the central nervous system cholinergic and dopaminergic signaling. The elderly may be more susceptible to an excess of dopaminergic signaling and cholinergic signaling suppression. This can be altered further with the addition or withdrawal of medications that alter these neurochemical-signaling pathways.

In addition to delirium, another postoperative complication is infection. Elderly patients will often have increased susceptibility to infections from depressed immune system function, and may not be accurately or timely diagnosed with sepsis due to atypical presentations. Focal signs or symptoms may be lacking in this population. Instead, patients may present with isolated fever or nonspecific anorexia, weakness, fatigue, and functional decline as the only evidence of infection. The most frequent sites of infection include the urinary tract, lungs, and the surgical site. Urinary tract infections often arise from a prolonged course of bladder catheterization in more than one quarter of hospitalized patients having bladder catheters inserted at some point in time during hospitalization. Bladder catheterization is more frequent in elderly populations due to a myriad of reasons including immobility, prior incontinence, prostate difficulties, impaired mobility, and neurogenic bladder. Elderly urinary tract infections may lack the classic associated lower urinary tract symptoms, and only present as simple confusion or altered mental status, or be completely asymptomatic [56]. Nosocomial pneumonia is another common complication. Iatrogenic interventions such as orotracheal intubation, NG tubes, aspiration, and chest and lung surgeries place elderly patients at increased risk for this type of infection [57]. Surgical site infections (SSIs), a significant postoperative complication, will account for ~38% of nosocomial infections in the elderly population [58]. Certain factors such as maintenance of normothermia and euglycemia both

perioperatively and during the surgical procedure, avoidance of shaving of the surgical site until just prior to the procedure, and appropriate antibiotic selection all lead to improved outcomes for elderly patients undergoing surgical procedures, and reduce the risk of SSI by ~27% [59, 60]. In addition to postoperative complications, elderly patients often experience longer hospitalizations, more frequent readmissions, and increased medical costs secondary to these infections [59]. Geriatric patients with a higher number of comorbidities are at a higher risk for complications, which should be taken into account when assessing risk for postoperative complications [61]. Also, patients and families optimally will have the opportunity to make an informed decision regarding the risks and benefits of the procedure.

End-of-life issues

Advanced directives

Medicine in the United States operates on the principle of a patient's right to autonomy and self-determination. The individual's decision-making takes precedence over the physician's judgment. However, it is the physician's role to advocate and navigate a clinical course to optimize medical care within the patient's beliefs and desires. This is often blurred with the use of life-sustaining treatments because patients are frequently unable to participate in medical decision-making. Advance directives and living wills allow competent individuals to extend their right to self-determination to future situations where physical incapacitation would limit this ability. These documents often address predetermined life-support and resuscitative measures. Often, a surrogate for medical decision-making responsibilities is designated in these documents as well. However, the effectiveness of such documents is limited by inattention to these predesignated decisions, or by shift of priority to considerations other than the patient's autonomy [62]. Whenever possible, query into the presence of advanced directives and living wills should be made to respect the rights and wishes of patients.

Palliative care

Palliation may seem contradictory to the curative surgical philosophy, but may be in the patient's best interest in terms of mitigating suffering and quality of life. The American Medical Association provides ethical standards that state, "physicians have an obligation to relieve pain and to promote the dignity and autonomy of dying patients in their care. This includes providing effective palliative treatment even though it may foreseeably hasten death". [63] It can be a difficult decision to make, but may be appropriate when the disease is incurable, injury irreparable or death is inevitable despite further aggressive care. The key to harmonious palliation is an alleviation of symptoms with minimization of risk laden or futile intervention. One of the most important aspects to successful implementation of palliative care is respect of patient and family autonomy with open, honest communication about prognosis, even if difficult to predict. The risks should be discussed in an effort to optimize quality of life and mitigate undue suffering.

Palliative surgery is targeted at alleviation of patient's symptoms through surgical intervention to improve quality of life and minimize suffering. There is no demonstrated improved outcome of palliative surgery in younger populations compared to disease-matched older populations. Once again, chronological age should not be the main determinant in designation of surgical candidates. An individually tailored, comprehensive approach should be employed to assure decisions are allowed to maximize quality of life. The focus should hearken on maximum benefit with least invasive means.

Section IV: Decision-making

- Careful consideration is needed regarding physiologic age of geriatric patients, not just the chronological age when making surgical assessment.
- A patient-centered approach as opposed to disease-oriented evaluative process will prove to be more beneficial in the elderly.
- Physical examination features such as fever, tachycardia, and peritoneal findings may be blunted in the elderly.
- Polypharmacy and medications, such as beta-blockers and anticoagulants, can complicate the diagnosis and management of surgical etiologies.
- More liberal use of diagnostic imaging is required given higher rates of incidence and atypical presentation.

- Despite an inherent higher mortality rate when faced with surgical pathology, geriatric patients benefit from early accurate diagnosis and aggressive medical and surgical care.
- Emergency surgery carries a much higher risk than elective surgeries in the elderly.
- Autonomy and respect to end-of-life issues should be maintained as much as possible in the care of the advanced age population.

References

1 Ortman, J., Velkoff, V.A., and Hogan, H. (2014) *An Aging Nation: The Older Population in the United States.* US Bureau of Statistics, Issued May 2014, http://www .census.gov/content/dam/Census/library/publications /2014/demo/p25-1140.pdf (accessed 26 August 2015).

2 Roberts, D.C., McKay, M.P., and Shaffer, A. (2008) Increasing rates of emergency department visits for elderly patients in the United States, 1993 to 2003. *Ann. Emerg. Med.*, **51** (6), 769–774.

3 Singal, B.M., Hedges, J.R., Rousseau, E.W. *et al.* (1992) Geriatric patient emergency visits part I: comparison of visits by geriatric and younger patients. *Ann. Emerg. Med.*, **21** (7), 802–807.

4 Ettinger, W.H., Casan, J.A., Coon, P.J. *et al.* (1987) Patterns of use of the emergency department by elderly patients. *J. Gerontol.*, **42** (6), 638–642.

5 Marco, C.A., Schoenfeld, C.N., Keyl, P.M., and Menkes, E.D. (1998) Abdominal pain in geriatric emergency patients: variables associated with adverse outcomes. *Acad. Emerg. Med.*, **5** (12), 1163–1168.

6 Cook, D.J. and Rooke, G.A. (2003) Priorities in perioperative geriatrics. *Anesth. Analg.*, **96** (6), 1823–1836.

7 Grief, C.L. (2003) Patterns of ED use and perceptions of the elderly regarding their emergency care: a synthesis of recent research. *J. Emerg. Nurs.*, **29** (2), 122–126.

8 Pfeifer, M.A., Weinberg, C.R., Cook, D. *et al.* (1983) Differential changes of autonomic nervous system function with age in man. *Am. J. Med.*, **75** (2), 249–258.

9 Sharma, G. and Goodwin, J. (2006) Effect of aging on respiratory system physiology and immunology. *Clin. Interv. Aging*, **1** (3), 253–260.

10 Kronenberg, R.S. and Drage, C.W. (1973) Attenuation of the ventilatory and heart rate responses to hypoxia and hypercapnia with aging in normal men. *J. Clin. Invest.*, **52** (8), 1812–1819.

11 Zaugg, M. and Lucchinetti, E. (2000) Respiratory function in the elderly. *Anesthesiol. Clin. North Am.*, **18** (1), 47–58.

12 Aymanns, C., Keller, F., Maus, S. *et al.* (2010) Review on pharmacokinetics and pharmocodynamics and the aging kidney. *Clin. J. Am. Soc. Nephrol.*, **5**, 314–327.

13 Epstein, M. (1996) Aging and the kidney. *J. Am. Soc. Nephrol.*, **7** (8), 1106–1022.

14 U.S. Department of Health and Human Services National Institutes of Health NIH Publication No. 12–3895 June 2012

15 Creasey, H. and Rapoport, S.I. (1985) The aging human brain. *Ann. Neurol.*, **17** (1), 2–10.

16 Muravchik, S. (1997) Peripheral and autonomic nervous system, in *Geroanesthesia: Principles for Management of the Elderly Patient* (ed L. Craven), Mosby, St Louis, MO, pp. 114–148.

17 Phillips, P.A., Hodsman, G.P., and Johnston, C.I. (1991) Neuroendocrine mechanisms and cardiovascular homeostasis in the elderly. *Cardiovasc. Drugs Ther.*, **4** (6), 1209–1213.

18 Dudgeon, H.R. (1950) Geriatric surgery. *Am. J. Surg.*, **79** (3), 417–419.

19 Sanders, A.B. (1992) Care of the elderly in emergency departments: conclusions and recommendations. *Ann. Emerg. Med.*, **21** (7), 830–834.

20 Keating, M.J. III, Klimek, J.J., Levine, D.S., and Kierman, F.J. (1984) Effect of aging on the clinical significance of fever in ambulatory adult patients. *J. Am. Geriat. Soc.*, **32**, 282–287.

21 Yoshikawa, T.T. (1997) Perspective: aging and infectious diseases: past, present, and future. *J. Infect. Dis.*, **176**, 1053–1057.

22 Downton, J.H., Andrews, K., and Puxty, J.A.H. (1987) Silent pyrexia in the elderly. *Age Ageing*, **16**, 41–44.

23 Darowski, A., Najim, Z., Weinberg, J.R., and Guz, A. (1991) The febrile response to mild infections in elderly hospital inpatients. *Age Ageing*, **20**, 193–198.

24 Wroblewski, M. and Mikulowski, P. (1991) Peritonitis in geriatric inpatients. *Age Ageing*, **20** (2), 90–94.

25 De Dombel, F.T. (1994) Acute abdominal pain in the elderly. *J. Clin. Gastroenterol.*, **19** (4), 331–335.

26 Kizer, K.W. and Vassar, M.J. (1998) Emergency department diagnosis of abdominal disorders in the elderly. *Am. J. Emerg. Med.*, **16** (4), 357–362.

27 Cardall, T., Glasser, J., and Guss, D.A. (2004) Clinical value of the total white blood cell count and temperature in the evaluation of patients with suspected appendicitis. *Acad. Emerg. Med.*, **11** (10), 1021–1027.

28 Dzankic, S., Pastor, D., Gonzalez, C., and Leung, J.M. (2001) The prevalence and predictive value of abnormal preoperative laboratory tests in elderly surgical patients. *Anesth. Analg.*, **93** (2), 301–308.

29 Sewell, J.M., Spooner, L.L., Dixon, A.K., and Rubenstein, D. (1981) Screening investigations in the elderly. *Age Aging*, **10**, 165–168.

30 Samaras, N., Chevalley, T., Samaras, D., and Gold, G. (2010) Older patients in the emergency department: a review. *Ann. Emerg. Med.*, **56** (3), 261–269.

31 Esses, D., Birnbaum, A., Bijur, P. *et al.* (2004) Ability of CT to alter decision making in elderly patients with acute abdominal pain. *Am. J. Emerg. Med.*, **22** (4), 270–272.

32 Furlow, B. (2010) Radiation dose in computed tomography. *Am. Soc. Radiol. Technol.*, **81** (5), 437–450.

33 Gussenhoven, M.J., Ravensbergen, J., van Bockel, J.H. *et al.* (1991) Renal dysfunction after angiography; a risk factor analysis in patients with peripheral vascular disease. *J. Cardiovasc. Surg.*, **32**, 81–86.

34 Kini, A.S., Mitre, C.A., Kim, M. *et al.* (2002) A protocol for prevention of radiographic contrast nephropathy during percutaneous coronary intervention: effect of selective dopamine receptor agonist fenoldopam. *Catheter. Cardiovasc. Interv.*, **55** (2), 169–173.

35 Akinbami, F., Askari, R., Steinberg, J. *et al.* (2011) Factors affecting morbidity in emergency general surgery. *Am. J. Surg.*, **201**, 456–462.

36 Archer, C., Levy, A.R., and McGregor, M. (1993) Value of routine preoperative chest X-rays: a meta-analysis. *Can. J. Anaesth.*, **40** (11), 1022–1027.

37 Battistella, F.D., Din, A.M., and Perez, L. (1998) Trauma patients 75 years and older: long-term follow-up results justify aggressive management. *J. Trauma*, **44** (4), 618–624.

38 Perdue, P.W., Watts, D.D., Kaufmann, C.R., and Trask, A.L. (1998) Differences in mortality between elderly and younger adult trauma patients: geriatric status increases risk of delayed death. *J. Trauma*, **45** (4), 805–810.

39 Lucky, A.E. and Parsa, C.J. (2003) Fluid and electrolytes in the aged. *Arch. Surg.*, **13**, 1055–1060.

40 Lamy, P.P. and Wiser, T.H. (1990) Geriatric anesthesia, in *Pharmacotherapeutic Considerations in the Elderly Surgical Patient* (ed M.R. Katlic), Urban & Schwarzenberg Inc, Baltimore, MD, pp. 209–239.

41 Lindenauer, P.K., Pekow, P., Wang, K. *et al.* (2005) Perioperative beta-blocker therapy and mortality after major noncardiac surgery. *N. Engl. J. Med.*, **353** (4), 349–361.

42 Bangalore, S., Wetterslev, J., Pranesh, S. *et al.* (2008) Perioperative β blockers in patients having non-cardiac surgery: a meta-analysis. *Lancet*, **372** (9654), 1962–1976.

43 Thachil, J., Gatt, A., and Martlew, V. (2008) Management of surgical patients receiving anticoagulation and antiplatelet agents. *Br. J. Surg.*, **95** (12), 1437–1448.

44 Cheema, F.N., Abraham, N.S., Berger, D.H. *et al.* (2011) Novel approaches to perioperative assessment and intervention may improve long-term outcomes after colorectal cancer resection in older adults. *Ann. Surg.*, **253**, 867–872.

45 Turrentine, F.E., Wang, H., Simpson, V.B., and Jones, R.S. (2006) Surgical risk factors, morbidity, and mortality in elderly patients. *J. Am. Coll. Surg.*, **203** (6), 865–877.

46 Liu, L.L., Dzankic, S., and Leung, J.M. (2002) Preoperative electrocardiogram abnormalities do not predict postoperative cardiac complications in geriatric surgical patients. *J. Am. Geriatr. Soc.*, **50** (7), 1186–1191.

47 Goldberger, A.L. and O'Konski, M. (1986) Diagnostic decision utility of the routine electrocardiogram before surgery and on general hospital admission critical review and new guidelines. *Ann. Intern. Med.*, **105** (4), 552–557.

48 Arenal, J.J. and Bengoechea-Beeby, M. (2003) Mortality associated with emergency abdominal surgery in the elderly. *Can. J. Surg.*, **46** (2), 111–116.

49 Warner, M.A., Hosking, M.P., Lobdell, C.M. *et al.* (1988) Surgical procedures among those greater than or equal to 90 years of age. A population-based study in Olmstead, Minnesota, 1975–1985. *Ann. Surg.*, **207** (4), 380–386.

50 Derrett, S., Paul, C., and Morris, J. (1999) Waiting for elective surgery: effects on health-related quality of life. *Int. J. Qual. Health Care*, **11** (1), 47–57.

51 Story, D.A. (2008) Postoperative complications in elderly patients and their significance for long-term prognosis. *Curr. Opin. Anaesthesiol.*, **21** (3), 375–379.

52 Seymour, D.G. and Pringle, R. (1983) Post-operative complications in the elderly surgical patient. *Gerontology*, **29** (4), 262–270.

53 Hustey, F.M., Meldon, S.W., Banet, G.A. *et al.* (2005) The use of abdominal computed tomography in older ED patients with acute abdominal pain. *Am. J. Emerg. Med.*, **23** (3), 259–265.

54 Agnosti, J.V. and Inouye, S.K. (2003) Delirium, in *Principles of Geriatric Medicine and Gerontology*, 5th edn (eds W.R. Hazzard, J.P. Blass, J.P. Halter *et al.*), McGraw-Hill, New York.

55 Robinson, T.N., Raeburn, C.D., Tran, Z.V. *et al.* (2009) Postoperative delirium in the elderly. Risk factors and outcomes. *Ann. Surg.*, **249**, 173–178.

56 Beliveau, M.M. and Multach, M. (2003) Perioperative care for the elderly patient. *Med. Clin. North Am.*, **87**, 273–289.

57 Feldman, C. (2001) Pneumonia in the elderly. *Med. Clin. North Am.*, **85**, 1441–1459.

58 Neumayer, L., Hosowana, P., Itani, K. *et al.* (2007) Multivariable predictors of postoperative surgical site infection in general and vascular surgery: results from the patient safety in surgery study. *J. Am. Coll. Surg.*, **204** (6), 1178–1187.

59 Barie, P.S. and Eachempati, S.R. (2005) Surgical site infections. *Surg. Clin. North. Am.*, **85** (6), 1115–1135.

60 Dellinger, E.P., Hausmann, S.M., Bratzler, D.W. *et al.* (2005) Hospitals collaborate to decrease surgical site infections. *Am. J. Surg.*, **190** (1), 9–15.

61 Roche, J.J., Wenn, R.T., Sahota, O., and Moran, C.G. (2005) Effect of comorbidities and postoperative complications on mortality after hip fracture in elderly people: prospective observational cohort study. *Br. Med. J.*, **331** (7529), 1374.

62 Danis, M., Southerland, L.I., Garrett, J.M., and Smith, J.L. (1991) A prospective study of advance directives for life-sustaining care. *N. Engl. J. Med.*, **324** (13), 882–888.

63 American Medical Association (1994) *Ethical Standards E-2.20* [Internet]. [Place unknown] Issued December 1984. Updated June 1994. http://www.ama-assn.org/ama/pub/physician-resources/medical-ethics/code-medical-ethics/opinion220.page (accessed 26 August 2015).

22 Oncologic emergencies

Gabriel Wardi, Alexander Bromfield & Leslie C. Oyama
Department of Emergency Medicine, UCSD Medical Center, San Diego, CA, USA

Section I: Case presentation

A 76-year-old man presented to the emergency department (ED) with a chief complaint of productive cough that had worsened in the prior few days. He described minimal wheezing, and stated he had dull right-sided chest pain that worsened with deep inspiration. He also mentioned that during the preceding month, he had noticed worsening fatigue, generalized weakness, and occasional fevers that often occurred at night. He denied any nausea, vomiting, diaphoresis, back pain, focal neurological changes, and had no blood in his urine or stools. His pain did not radiate to either arm, and he denied any associated dyspnea on exertion or leg swelling.

The past medical history was significant for well-controlled hypertension, a remote history of myocardial infarction, and no report of pulmonary disease. He took hydrochlorothiazide, metoprolol, atorvastatin, and a baby aspirin. He occasionally drank alcohol, but denied a prior smoking history.

Initial vitals were as follows: temperature 37.5 °C, heart rate 106 beats/min, blood pressure 135/78 mmHg, respiratory rate 16 breaths/min, and oxygen saturation 95% on room air. The patient was placed on 2 l of oxygen. On evaluation, the patient was in no apparent distress, speaking in full sentences. He exhibited slight pallor, had numerous 1–2 soft, mobile, nontender cervical lymph nodes. The cardiopulmonary examination was significant for right-sided rales with scant expiratory wheezes. He had mild splenomegaly but no abdominal tenderness or hepatomegaly. He had no evidence of jugular venous distention, peripheral edema, leg asymmetry, rashes, or petechiae. The remainder of the physical examination was unremarkable.

An electrocardiogram (EKG) was performed, which revealed a sinus tachycardia 110 beats/min and was otherwise unremarkable. Laboratory analysis was remarkable for a leukocytosis of 71,000 with a lymphocytic predominance, hemoglobin 10.2, and 122,000 platelets. The metabolic panel revealed a potassium of 3.2 meq/dl and was otherwise unremarkable. Serial troponins were negative. A chest X-ray study showed a possible early right-sided lobar pneumonia.

The patient was admitted to the general medicine service, and antibiotics to treat the community-acquired pneumonia were started. The pneumonia quickly resolved. The oncology service was consulted given the severely elevated white count and concern for a hematologic malignancy. Bone marrow biopsy and flow cytometry were consistent with chronic lymphocytic leukemia (CLL). Therapeutic options were discussed with the patient, who was initially reluctant to start any chemotherapeutics, but eventually agreed to undergo therapy.

Section II: Case discussion

Dr Peter Rosen (PR): This is a patient who appears to have a respiratory problem who enters your ED. We've discussed repeatedly how elderly patients need a broad workup no matter how focal their appearance is in terms of their disease process, and this would simply fall into the same category. In

Geriatric Emergencies: A Discussion-Based Review, First Edition.
Edited by Amal Mattu, Shamai A. Grossman and Peter L. Rosen.

this case, after this the patient's workup, he would appear to have pneumonia. Yet, I think the definition of community-acquired pneumonia may be hard to follow, and I wonder if it needs to be modified for patients who are otherwise healthy as opposed to patients who might have an underlying problem such as AIDS or some other immunosuppression. Could you enlighten us on that issue?

Dr Vaishal Tolia (VT): I think that we do have to be cognizant of our geriatric population, and consider some of the underlying pathogens that could be at play given not only the medical history, but oftentimes the multiple comorbidities, medications, living situations, and exposures that they could have as well as their vulnerability to certain pathogens. So, before even obtaining the blood work and going down the pathway that this case does, I think we need to consider that not only should we cover typical and some atypical organisms, but in this population we should at least initially consider, because of their exposures, a broader antibiotic coverage. This is especially true if we are able to obtain blood cultures, which is a controversial topic in and of itself, especially for someone not going to the intensive care unit (ICU), but also sputum culture, as well as any tissue that could help us with making a diagnosis, and eventually narrowing antibiotic therapy. Although broad-spectrum antibiotics are a good choice in the ED particularly in patients such as this who may have other serious comorbidities or other reasons for having a more resistant organism, but antibiotics themselves can also be problematic in causing side effects, such as *Clostridium difficile* infections. Most hospitals, including ours in San Diego, have antibiotic protocols for community-acquired pneumonia, healthcare-associated pneumonia, and then those patients who have pneumonia with underlying lung disease who may be at a higher risk for an organism such as pseudomonas. Unfortunately, we don't have guidelines specific to geriatrics or a list that includes elderly patients that may be immunocompromised.

PR: Dr Melady, I was wondering if there is a difference between Canada and the United States, in how much workup is expected from the ED. It used to be true that we identified a sick patient, admitted him, and then the workup was performed in the hospital,

but over the past 50 years, I would say it has become more and more difficult to get a workup in the hospital, and more and more of our hospitals are expecting a complete workup in the ED. Now that's for a specific emergent disease, but I also was wondering about the concomitant diseases that might be present that again in the past would have been worked up electively. How is that managed in Canada?

Dr Don Melady (DM): I don't want to be the spokesperson for all 35 million of us, but I think in general it's probably pretty much the same and quite similar to what you're describing. When I started my career 25 years ago, the decision was "is this person coming in or not?" If they're coming in, the rest was done in hospital. Today, that's not the case. Certainly, with the subpopulation we're interested in, older people, I think that's a good development. If we really expand what we're doing in the ED, we can often avoid completely the need for admission to the hospital. With reference to this case in particular, I was a bit surprised when the punch line was he was admitted to the general medicine service. I'm not sure that is what would have happened at our institution, or at least what I would have done. I can't see much in this case that required this seemingly pretty healthy, fit person, with not a lot of comorbidities except the new pneumonia that would require him to be in hospital. So, I would be interested in knowing how practice varies on that front. I think quite possibly this person would have gone home from our ED on oral antibiotics, avoiding all the hazards of hospitalization, and had prompt referral to our own hospital's hematology service. His workup for the leukocytosis would have happened as an outpatient. I think he would probably do better at home than stuck in a hospital for the next 4 or 5 days.

PR: Dr Tolia, was the reason for admission for a potential oncological emergency, or was it simply because he was a geriatric patient who looked sicker than the report would have suggested?

VT: The initial concern from the treating physician in this case was that he did look a little more ill in his appearance on ED presentation. Apparently, this man was pretty functional and very active, but had a fairly precipitous decline over several days. They didn't think it was just simply explainable by the pneumonia, and then they saw the leukocytosis and had a conversation with the on-call heme/onc fellow who recommended the admission to expedite the workup. Nevertheless, I think Dr Melady's point is well taken. Avoiding an admission is something we have control over, something we should consider when possible when we can expedite the outpatient follow-up and workup for a patient. In this case, however, I think it was both the concern of his rapid decline and the oncology fellow's insistence that he comes in to get some more tests done that produced the admission.

PR: I don't think anyone can argue against that kind of prudence, but to change the facts slightly, if this patient didn't look as ill and hadn't had a rapid decline but basically appeared to be an elderly man with an acute but not terribly systemically disturbing pneumonia, how would you feel about putting him in the observation unit, giving him a dose or two of IV antibiotics, see how he responds in terms of his appearance over the next day, and then discharging him to arrange a follow-up for the possible oncological problem as an outpatient?

Dr Shamai Grossman (SG): I think that would be reasonable. I think more and more, we're using the observation unit for this very purpose, where we have a borderline patient who looks relatively well, but may have more associated comorbidities that make us hesitant to send him home. Moreover, we're actually getting pushed by administration to use the observation unit in this manner for this. We're not getting reimbursed for many of these admissions. In addition, if you take away some of those comorbidities: for example, you take away the weakness and fevers and general decline, the most likely diagnosis in this patient is early CLL, and there is really no treatment. In any event, we have a patient with a chronic disease and concomitant pneumonia, and at many institutions, he might get sent home, but putting him in the observation unit would be a very reasonable option.

PR: One of the problems that I see happening in modern emergency medicine is that we have one set of medical recommendations that are based on cost, hospital admission requirements, or bed capacity, and another set that are based on what happens if we make an error when we send someone out. Does your hospital feel pressure to admit someone with what looks like a minor acute medical emergency with an underlying oncologic disease that has yet to be defined simply because you don't want to risk losing him to follow-up?

Dr Amal Mattu (AM): I wish I had a simple answer for that. It's a question that I think we face every single day in the ED. Moreover, there is a problem of follow-up in our inner-city tertiary care type of EDs in the United States. Almost daily, we face pressures from our financial compliance advisors who are constantly looking at the charts to figure out whether that person's admission is going to be reimbursed or not. Now they're looking at ED charts to figure out before the patient gets admitted, whether the patient is going to qualify for admission, and if the patient doesn't, they're very insistent that such a patient not be admitted. Nevertheless, we oftentimes feel very nervous about sending out a patient who has multiple comorbidities or an underlying condition for which we're not sure they're going to get a prompt follow-up. This case would be a great example. This is a 70-some-year-old man who right off the bat we're feeling a bit uncomfortable about, and even if he can get good follow-up, we're very uncomfortable about sending him out, yet there may be guidelines saying that he doesn't justify an emergency admission. Compounding that, primary care physicians and office-based physicians are also overcrowded and have very limited resources as well. Thus, when we send somebody out to follow up with the primary care doctor, we often get a call back from them saying "what exactly did you expect us to do? We can't do extensive oncologic workups here in the office either." It is a very difficult situation, and I think the saving grace in many cases has been the observation unit that is somewhat more reimbursable for the hospital and enables us to feel a bit more comfortable that the patient will probably get better follow-up care because the patient will have the time for this to be arranged from the observation unit.

PR: Is there a similar magnitude of medical malpractice push and paranoia in Canada? I was quite impressed the last time I was in Italy where I found a burgeoning malpractice burden that previously they hadn't had to face, and I'm hearing the very same kind of magical words "we have to do this or else we're going to get sued" and the same kind of illogical medical testing that we've been living with in the United States.

DM: Mercifully that contagion is not as widespread in Canada. Rates of litigation are significantly lower than in the United States. We all know that the daily, hourly consideration that "I have to do something so it will look good if anything bad happens and will prevent me from getting sued" is bad for patient care.

DM: One of the reasons for our lack of litigation is that there is a single provider of malpractice insurance in Canada, which is owner-operated. That is, all physicians in Canada are the shareholders in the Canadian Medical Protective Association, and that is effectively the only insurance in Canada. That is relevant in shaping the whole malpractice scene and culture as well as the insurance industry. Or maybe Canadians are just easygoing, more congenial people, and we just don't sue each other as much!

PR: I believe that may be a difference in human beings, but I suspect the lawyers haven't found the economic pot of gold. When they do, people will be people, and start looking for money from litigation.

AM: I wonder whether what we do is maybe less based on worry of lawyers, although we tend to blame the lawyers for all the extra laboratory testing and imaging studies that we order, but perhaps the excessive ordering of everything is very largely based on this culture we have in medicine whereby we're taught from the day we start medical school that a good physician is complete and thorough, and never misses anything. No one ever compliments you for doing a cost-effective workup or efficient workup, but you'll always be criticized if you didn't order the serum "porcelain level, and, God forbid, the patient comes back with porcelinemia."

PR: I think another part of excessive testing stems from a human psychology that is efficiency driven. We noticed in Denver that our house officers ordered every laboratory test that was available. Therefore, we were able to reduce the cost of laboratory testing by making fewer tests available. We didn't take them off of the menu completely in that you couldn't get a "serum porcelain" if you really needed one, but it wasn't on the original list that you could order from. In order to get it, you had to consult the pathologist and the attending emergency physician (EP). That one

change reduced our laboratory testing by about 30%. California doesn't seem to be much different than any other state in terms of worrying about malpractice even though there has been a tort reform for many decades, and I would guess that the general attitude toward medical malpractice is pretty similar throughout the United States. The one exception might be right now in Texas, where they seemed to have produced a tort reform that has really lowered the number of malpractice cases enormously, but in talking with doctors who practice there, it hasn't changed their medical practice that much. Perhaps it is a more basic issue of how we're taught to think about medicine rather than the explanation we constantly give that we're trying to avoid being sued. Concerning this case, I'm not sure that we have a setup to do good oncologic emergency care in the ED whether or not it's a geriatric patient. Do you have any recommendations for how we can change our practice to make it a little safer? I know there was at one time in San Diego where we said: cancer patient and fever equals admit, and that was the end of our thinking process. Yet then the oncologists were unhappy with "unnecessary admissions."

VT: In our institution, things have definitely evolved now that one of our two hospitals is connected to a regional cancer center. What has evolved, and is still is evolving, is increased communication, not only in real time but also ahead of time as to how to manage these patients. Not only do we have regular oncology patients, but we have a lot of bone marrow patients as well as those with all sorts of acute febrile illness with ongoing chemotherapy. The default management of anyone who has cancer and some sort of systemic illness was to admit these people. More recently, even febrile neutropenic patients without an obvious source in an otherwise stable patient are beginning to be managed as outpatients. More and more of oncology patients have greater potential for outpatient management. They have access to nurse practitioners and case managers as well as being at the cancer center, there's a large staff who are dedicated to their care. I think that having a system in place where patients such as this don't necessarily have to be admitted, and they can get antinausea medication, IV fluids, via an infusion center, because most of these patients will have indwelling ports, is ideal and is a better alternative than just being in an inpatient bed for a prolonged period of time. I'm curious about some of the patients with complex disease and comorbidities, who often don't fit the typical inclusion criteria for an observation unit but may become observation candidates with good communication with the oncology service. I'm just curious too if some of you folks who would put this patient in observation in your facility, do you get that sort of degree of responsive communication? For those of you who are using observation units for patients like this, do you find your oncology service supportive?

SG: When we first opened our observation unit, we were very dogmatic. We had very strict criteria about who we could put into the unit, but as you acclimate your physicians and nursing staff to observation care, you find that rigidity is no longer necessary. Nevertheless, you have to have clear-cut outcomes. You need to identify clear goals for the observation stay, and you need to have a patient who you think is going to get discharged quickly from the hospital, within 24 h, as this is the primary motivator for putting the patient in the observation unit. We found that once you have set goals in place, and you have a staff that is used to taking care of observation patients, you can be more malleable. We found that our consultants actually like seeing patients in the observation unit, like the way they get expedited care, and are quite comfortable with the process. If we need to have oncology, come see the patient in the observation unit, they can and they will, and that's true for any other subspecialty service.

VT: I think that's interesting and a model we may need to move toward because I think that it's prudent to not immediately discharge this kind of patient, although many of our patients that we see with cancer, have fever, weakness, vomiting, dehydration, and so on, yet even though we're admitting them to the hospital, most of them are being discharged within 24–36 h. Perhaps they would benefit from that sort of extended ED observation care even though our traditional teaching has taught us to admit folks such as this, to do broad workups.

PR: Do you use observation units in Canada?

DM: I cannot speak for all of Canada, but I have no such experience in any of the three large hospitals where I've worked. We don't have one and the tone of this discussion doesn't sound very familiar to me. I think for the most part our decision hinges on: can we do enough in the ED to turn this person around, or do they need admission to the hospital?

PR: Other countries are moving in this direction, too. In Italy, they've developed what we would call a step-down unit, but what I would call a step-up unit. They take patients who are under the control of the ED and admit them to an emergency unit unless they need intubation, in which case they would be admitted to an ICU bed. They've been able to manage a fair number of cases that otherwise in our country would have been directly admitted to the hospital or to an ICU. There are political and financial reasons for this in addition to medical reasons, but it seems to work quite well. The one unintended consequence I have observed is that they frequently don't intubate patients whom we would, so that they don't lose control of the patient to the ICU. I don't think that's always prudent, but that's probably my biased viewpoint because we have so many more ICU beds than they do, and are much more accustomed to using them.

DM: Once we have already decided on an admission, I would bring up a couple of topics that are specific to older people. The most important is a discussion of goals of care and advanced care planning even in the ED. While we've established that this man seems like a basically healthy, functioning person, we've already established that he is over the age of 70 and is coming into the hospital with a significant problem, probably has cancer, and seems to require admission. I think that it's never too early, including in the ED, to start talking about advanced care planning. I don't mean in simplistic terms, like "do you want to be intubated and have chest compressions, or not?" But to actually start a conversation about: "Where do you think things going? What do you see ahead of you? If you were to get even sicker than you already are, what would you want to be done? If you weren't able to speak for yourself, what direction have you given to your substitute decision-makers?"

SG: Our problem here is number one there's increasing pressure, looking at the criteria for reimbursement, to shorten the length of stay for patients in the ED. That's actually what's prompting this push toward more observation unit care, and finishing up workups outside of the ED. I think rushing a patient through a discussion about whether or not they want to be resuscitated or what are their goals of care in the ED isn't always a great idea. In fact, often I think it may be detrimental to have a patient make a sudden decision.

PR: I was going to raise this question but more on the lines of the frustration we feel in the ED of oncology patients who either have not had advanced directives, or any advice about the direction of their cancer. They come in with the expectation of cure when otherwise they're on a downward spiral, and I think that I agree with Dr Grossman, that the place to start the discussion is not the ED, but I don't think there's anything wrong with trying to communicate with patients to find out what are their expectations. I certainly don't think there's anything wrong with getting all the oncologists and saying, "how about commencing this discussion?"

DM: I think an important distinction that you made is that advanced care planning is a *process* not an *event*. It seems to me that it's never the wrong time or too early or too late to start the process. There may not be one single, unique answer, but it is always a good idea to start people thinking about the process of making their own decisions about where their care is going. I tell my colleagues and residents that we can't be critical of other people, of other physicians, for not initiating goals of care or advanced care planning discussion if we're not willing to do it ourselves! We complain, "the oncologists didn't talk about it the last time they were in clinic," "the family doctor didn't bring it up," or "the hospitalist should have done it." But we in the ED are equally at fault ("I was too busy on that shift") if we're not going to participate in that conversation either. Patients consistently say that there is no opportunity to talk about the "bigger issues" associated with their health and illness: they're literally dying to talk about these issues, and we are not providing them with the opportunity. You *et al.* (in CMAJ April 1, 2014 186:425–432) discuss strategies and explore scripts that can be used even in EDs to initiate a goals of care discussion.

SG: I don't disagree. In fact, I think we often need to have a more fundamental conversation. We have found enumerable patients who have newly discovered malignancies who aren't even informed

of the possibility of having malignancies in the ED, and that's something that has to do with a mindset of decisions, a mindset of surgeons, and even emergency medicine practitioners who become very reluctant to have any kind of conversation whatsoever with the patient about prognosis or diagnosis. Some of that has to do with a lack of knowledge of the disease, and some of that has to do with a simple avoidance of responsibility. I do agree that at least fundamentally there needs to be some conversation with the patient about what's going on with him, and then that conversation might lead to where their goals of care may be. Nevertheless, I don't think the ED is the appropriate venue to start having prolonged conversations and certainly for decision-making processes or in determining what their goals of care are.

PR: I have been reluctant to even tell patients that they have cancer, even if looks probable, before there is a chance to work the disease up, and prove its presence. You have to go case by case, and there's nothing wrong with perhaps hinting there's a serious problem here, but I find that there are a number of patients I've seen who I've thought had cancer in fact had something else. I would hate to have labeled them in the ED without any available evidence, so I think you have to be careful about initiating that kind of conversation. Do you have any closing thoughts for us on this case?

VT: I think the practice of emergency medicine is really changing, and in many cases we're expected to do a lot more in the ED. Sometimes, for good reasons, it is prudent to avoid an admission to the hospital. Discussing goals of care is a controversial subject, and one that is continuing to evolve. I think communication, not only with the family but also with our subspecialists and outpatient primary care physicians, is paramount for the best care for our patients, particularly because we only see them for a short period of time and reveal a lot of significant findings in that short time.

Section III: Concepts

Background

As the general population ages and cancer treatments continue to evolve, individuals are living longer with malignancy [1]. Given this, it follows that more and more patients with a diagnosis of malignancy will seek treatment in the ED. These patients present unique pathology and challenges for the EP. The term "oncologic emergencies" is often used to describe a unique set of malignancy-related syndromes requiring a prompt evaluation and care. These conditions are often categorized into four main sections: (1) those secondary to hematologic disease, (2) those secondary to biochemical derangement, (3) local tumor effects, and (4) those related to therapy.

Oncologic emergencies and geriatrics

The field of oncology is unique in that, with the average age of first diagnosis for all cancer at age 66, nearly 53% of newly diagnosed malignancies occur after age 65, making it a uniquely geriatric-focused specialty [2]. The majority of therapy in oncologic emergencies remains the same across all ages; however, several special considerations must be made in the geriatric population. Older patients have a higher likelihood of comorbid disease, have less physiologic reserve, and are more sensitive to pharmacologic agents. For example, throughout the following chapter, many of the treatments discussed will involve the administration of intravenous fluids. Geriatric patients are more sensitive to intravenous fluids, especially those with renal insufficiency, congestive heart failure (CHF), liver disease, and other volume-sensitive conditions [3–5]. Therapy must be tailored and modified to accommodate a frailer patient.

Another important consideration, especially when dealing with malignancy and the elderly, is the patient's goals of care [6, 7]. Seventy-five percent of patients aged 65 and older will visit the ED within the last 6 months of life [8]. Advanced directives and community awareness of them are increasing. Evidence suggests that advance care planning increases quality of life, and the provider should make every attempt to identify the patients' wishes prior to initiating aggressive therapy [9]. This conversation can often start in the ED.

Specific oncologic emergencies

Neutropenic fever

The definition of fever is a single oral temperature >38.3 °C (101.0°F) or >38.0 °C (100.4°F) for more than 1 h [10]. Neutropenia guidelines vary from institution to institution, but severe neutropenia that conveys risk of clinically important infection is usually defined as an absolute neutrophil count (ANC) <500 cells/µl or an ANC that is expected to fall below 500 cells/µl in the next 48 h (recent chemotherapy with evidence of downward trend) [11]. The ANC may be calculated by multiplying the total white blood cell count (WBC) by the percentage of polymorphonuclear cells (PMNs) and bands.

Neutropenia may occur at any time during cancer treatment. It is common for a nadir in ANC to occur 5–10 days from the start of systemic chemotherapy [10]. Ten percent to 50% of patients with solid tumors and >80% of patients with hematologic malignancies will develop fever during or after the first cycle of chemotherapy [12]. Fever in the neutropenic cancer patient has a variety of causes with only 50% attributable to infection and bacteremia present in ~20% of those cases [11].

The first step in evaluation of febrile neutropenia is risk stratification. Careful physical examination is crucial. Importantly, immunocompromised patients' reduced ability to mount an inflammatory response may limit localizing signs and symptoms. Fever may be the only finding [13]. However, attention should be given to areas of pain, mucosal disruption, frontal and maxillary sinuses, and indwelling catheter sites. Patients with signs of sepsis or septic shock should be treated according to early goal-directed therapy. Stable patients require extensive workup, antibiotics, and likely admission. Initial workup includes a complete blood count with differential, complete metabolic panel, and at least two sets of blood cultures (with one set collected from an existing central venous catheter, preferably from each lumen of a multilumen catheter if present). Urinalysis and culture along with a chest radiograph are also recommended [11, 14].

Treatment is similar to treating serious bacterial infections in immunocompetent individuals. Sepsis should be addressed accordingly with isotonic fluid administration, antibiotics, vasopressor support, intubation, and early goal-directed therapy. The early administration of antimicrobials is essential with studies showing a correlation between early administration and improved patient outcomes. In febrile cancer patients with neutropenia, empiric dosing of antibiotics should precede advanced workup or culture results [11, 15, 16]. The choice of antibiotics is frequently changing as organism complexity and resistance patterns evolve. Current guidelines by the Infectious Disease Society of America (IDSA) recommend high-risk patients receive monotherapy with an antipseudomonal beta-lactam agent (i.e., cefepime, piperacillin–tazobactam) or carbapenem (meropenem or imipenem–cilastatin). Vancomycin is not routinely recommended but should be added if clinical appearance exhibits skin/soft tissue infections, pneumonia, indwelling devices, or prior gram-positive infection. Penicillin allergic patients often tolerate cephalosporins; however, alternative therapy includes ciprofloxacin plus clindamycin or aztreonam plus vancomycin. Antifungal and antiviral medication is not routinely recommended and is often administered based on clinical course and culture results as an inpatient [11]. On rare occasions, certain patients who are expected to have brief neutropenic periods (less than or equal to 7 days), have few or no medical comorbidities, and are not on prophylactic antibiotics may be candidates for outpatient oral antibiotic therapy [11]. The decision to treat as an outpatient is not ordinary and should be made in consultation with the patients' oncologist.

IDSA guidelines for empiric antibiotics – Neutropenic Fever

Drug Class	Example	Modifications
Antipseudomonal, beta-lactam, or carbapenem	Cefepime, piperacillin–tazobactam, meropenem, imipenem–cilastatin	Soft tissue infection, prior gram-positive infection, pneumonia, or clinical concern for MRSA then add vancomycin, clindamycin
Penicillin allergic	Ciprofloxacin + clindamycin or aztreonam + vancomycin	Many penicillin allergic patients can tolerate cephalosporin therapy
Fluoroquinolone + clindamycin or aztreonam + vancomycin		

MRSA; methicillin-resistant *Staphylococcus aureus*.

Biochemical emergencies

Tumor lysis syndrome

Tumor lysis syndrome (TLS) occurs as a result of spontaneous or therapy-induced cell death causing a massive influx of electrolytes and nucleic acids into the circulation. TLS classically occurs more frequently in rapidly proliferative hematologic malignancies such as acute lymphoblastic leukemia (ALL), acute myelogenous leukemia (AML), and Burkitt's lymphoma [17]. However, TLS is well documented in a variety of hematologic and solid tumors [18]. The time of onset is also highly variable: occurring spontaneously prior to therapy, shortly after initiation of therapy (chemotherapy, radiation, ablation, and surgery), or with delays of up to several weeks in solid malignancies [14, 18, 19].

The Cairo–Bishop classification is a well-accepted set of criteria that diagnoses TLS based on laboratory and clinical grounds [20]. For the EP, diagnosis is a combination of history, laboratory abnormalities (hyperkalemia, hyperuricemia, hyperphosphatemia, and hypocalcemia), and renal, cardiac, or central nervous system (CNS) dysfunction. Acute renal failure is the most common cause of morbidity and usually results from uric acid and calcium phosphate precipitation in the renal tubules. Aggressive fluid hydration with isotonic normal saline to maximize glomerular filtration rate (GFR), renal blood flow, and ion exchange remains the mainstay of therapy [18]. Suggested regimens include initiating two to four times daily maintenance fluid (3 l/m (2)/day) to maintain urine output $\geq$100 ml/m (2)/h [20]. Adding a loop diuretic such as furosemide (2–4 mg/kg) is not routinely recommended, but may be considered in patients with oliguria/anuria [20].

Cardiac rhythm disturbances are mainly secondary to hyperkalemia. Treatment for this condition is the same as with other causes of hyperkalemia; IV calcium (1000 mg IV calcium gluconate), insulin (0.1 U/kg IV) and dextrose (25% 2 ml/kg), sodium bicarbonate (1–2 meq/kg), and beta2-agonists to shift potassium intracellular, followed by removal through binding resins like sodium polystyrene sulfate or dialysis [21].

Hypocalcemia, hyperphosphatemia, and hyperuricemia are other metabolic derangements that may require urgent treatment beyond hydration.

Hypocalcemia may cause tetany and seizures; treatment consists of IV calcium (bolus of 1000 mg or slow administration of 50–100 mg/kg IV calcium gluconate) with the caveat that it may worsen calcium–phosphate precipitation [21]. Hyperphosphatemia very rarely requires emergency intervention and is usually treated with phosphate restriction and use of phosphate binders such as aluminum hydroxide. Hyperuricemia is usually not addressed beyond fluid hydration in the emergency setting secondary to the toxic effects of uric acid lowering medications. Allopurinol is almost exclusively used as prophylaxis rather than treatment; rasburicase is a recombinant urate oxidase that shows potential, but as of 2008, it was not approved in the geriatric population. Hemodialysis corrects all abnormalities in TLS and is still required in up to 5% of patients with TLS [22]. Geriatric patients with preexisting renal dysfunction or fluid-restrictive disorders, such as CHF or liver failure, or those with severe metabolic derangements and advanced clinical presentations should be considered for dialysis early, with nephrology consultation and involvement often while the patient is still in the ED. All patients with TLS should be admitted to the hospital, most to an ICU setting given the potential for life-threatening cardiac dysrhythmias.

Summary of metabolic imbalance and treatment in TLS.

Metabolic Abnormality	Treatment
Hyperkalemia	IV hydration. Calcium gluconate 1000 mg IV, insulin (0.1 U/kg IV) with dextrose (25% solution 2 ml/kg), NaHCO$_3$ (1–2 meq/kg), PO/PR binding resin or dialysis
Hypocalcemia	IV calcium gluconate 1 g bolus or 50–100 mg/kg slow infusion
Hyperphosphatemia	IV hydration, phosphate restriction, and binders Rarely requires immediate treatment beyond fluid
Hyperuricemia	IV hydration with normal saline

Hypercalcemia

Hypercalcemia will be experienced by up to one third of cancer patients at some point. Along the same lines, those patients presenting with hypercalcemia, malignancy is the most common underlying cause [23]. It is frequently an ominous sign with 30-day mortality approaching 50%. In spite of this, correction of hypocalcemia has palliative benefit, and therapy is recommended [24]. Malignancy affects calcium homeostasis in four primary ways. Solid malignancies are prone to produce parathyroid hormone–related protein, binding parathyroid receptors and thereby stimulating release of calcium from bone and increasing renal reabsorption of calcium [25]. Malignancies predisposed to bony metastasis such as primary lung, breast, and multiple myeloma produce increasing calcium levels through stimulation of osteoclast activity and direct bone destruction [26, 27]. Lastly, lymphomas such as Hodgkin's disease are known to produce analogues of vitamin D, which increase intestinal absorption of calcium [28]. Rarely, tumors can primarily produce parathyroid hormone [29].

Regardless of the cause, hypercalcemia produces similar symptoms, the severity of which is proportional to the rate of increase in serum levels. A slow increase in serum calcium may produce minimal and vague symptoms (i.e., lethargy and weakness), whereas abrupt change will have a more dramatic effect [17]. In general, a patient will show some signs at levels above 14 mg/dl [30]. In diagnosis, the old adage "stones, groans, bones, and psychiatric overtones" refers to renal calculi, abdominal pain, diffuse bone pain, and altered mental status. At higher serum levels, hypercalcemia can present with dysrhythmia [31]. Reports vary, but the leading physical sign and symptom is generally related to CNS dysfunction, and given that elderly patients increased susceptibility to delirium, this is likely the most common complaint seen in geriatric hypercalcemia [24].

As with TLS, the initial priority in the ED is normalization of intravascular volume with IV normal saline or equivalent crystalloid administration. Hypercalcemia produces an osmotic diuresis, and patients are often significantly volume depleted. IV fluid promotes calciuresis in working kidneys and dilutes existing blood calcium. In those who are expected to tolerate IV fluid well, an initial rate of 200–300 ml/h that is then adjusted to maintain the urine output at 100–150 ml/h is recommended [21].

After euvolemia is achieved, a point of contention remains regarding the use of loop diuretics such as furosemide. While theoretically enhancing calciuresis, studies suggest that it provides little benefit over normal saline alone and is not universally recommended [32]. Adjunctive therapies consist of glucocorticoids, bisphosphonates, and calcitonin. Glucocorticoids work by a direct lympholytic effect in hematogenous malignancies, inhibiting cytokine and prostaglandin stimulation of osteoclasts, and direct suppression of macrophage-mediated calcitriol release [14]. Bisphosphonates are a powerful class of drugs that block bone resorption by osteoclasts. They have an extensive side effect profile and do not acutely lower calcium levels. They are an essential component of therapy but often may be delayed until the patient is admitted [33, 34]. Calcitonin acts more rapidly to reduce serum calcium levels, but its predilection to tachyphylaxis and rebound hypercalcemia is well documented [35]. As such, it should not be used as monotherapy. Gallium, mithramycin, and phosphates are no longer routinely used in clinical practice secondary to toxicity. As with TLS, those that are unable to tolerate IV hydration in sufficient enough quantity secondary to CHF or other fluid-sensitive diseases should be considered for urgent dialysis [36, 37].

Summary of emergency treatment of malignancy-related hypercalcemia.

Treatment	Comments
IV hydration	Mainstay therapy. Normal saline 200–300 ml/h then titrated to urine output of 100–150 ml/h
Glucocorticoids	Considered in hematogenous malignancies
Loop diuretics	Controversial. An agent such as furosemide (0.5–2 mg/kg) may be tried, but not universally recommended
Bisphosphonates	Not recommended in the emergency setting. Does not acutely lower calcium levels
Calcitrol	Not recommended in emergency setting because of tachyphylaxis and rebound hypercalcemia
Dialysis	Considered in patients who cannot tolerate aggressive fluid hydration or when advanced renal failure prevents diuresis

Hyponatremia

Hyponatremia will affect a large number of patients with malignancy with an incidence of around 30% when hyponatremia is defined as a serum sodium less than 135 meq/l [38]. Malignancy can affect serum sodium by the syndrome of inappropriate antidiuretic hormone (SIADH) as a side effect from medical therapy, and by exacerbating underlying conditions such as liver failure and CHF. One should be aware of the more common etiologies of hyponatremia, and these should be first on the differential. Malignancy-related hyponatremia from SIADH results in retention of free water by the kidneys and less than maximally dilute urine. Antidiuretic hormone (ADH) may be directly secreted by the tumor, but malignancy also indirectly stimulates ADH release, and many medications either stimulate release or potentiate its effect [39–41]. The diagnosis of SIADH requires meeting certain criteria [42], and maintaining increased suspicion in those with lung (especially small cell), pleural, and brain malignancies [43]. The physical examination usually reveals a euvolemic-appearing patient [39, 44], and the serum potassium and bicarbonate levels are usually within the normal range [45].

While the exact etiology is important to determine, the EP should be focused on the treatment of life-threatening severe hyponatremia. Signs and symptoms of hyponatremia include anorexia, nausea, malaise, headache, confusion, obtundation, seizures, and eventually coma. The severity of symptomatic presentation is proportional to the rate of sodium level decline [39, 46]. Those patients with levels above 125 meq/l are generally asymptomatic, and free water restriction (500–100 ml/day) is the mainstay of therapy, whereas those who present with a level less than 105 meq/l invariably have symptoms. Those patients with minimal or no symptoms may require the addition of loop diuretics to increase sodium levels, whereas those patients who present with seizures, altered mental status, or coma will require hypertonic saline [14, 17]. Three percent hypertonic saline (510 meq/l) is the preferred treatment for severe symptoms. Great care must be taken with the rate of infusion to avoid osmotic demyelination syndrome (central pontine myelinolysis) [47–49], a devastating neurologic complication of rapid overcorrection. Infusion rates are based on animal models and clinical expertise. An infusion rate of 25–100 ml/h resulting in a serum increase of 0.5–1.0 meq/l/h, not exceeding 12 meq/l in the first 24 h and 18 meq/l in 48 h is considered safe [50, 51]. Although generally not used by EPs, demeclocycline, in doses of 600–1200 mg/day or intravenous conivaptan (20 mg over 30 min followed by 20 mg over 24 h) will produce a diabetes insipidus effect and blocking of ADH receptors, respectively, causing dilute urine and sodium retention [14]. Severe hyponatremia with symptoms should always be treated promptly, but evidence also suggests correcting chronic asymptomatic hyponatremia in cancer patients improves outcomes [52, 53].

Overview of emergency treatment of hyponatremia.

Presentation	Treatment	Comments
Asymptomatic and sodium >125 meq/l	Fluid restriction 0.5–1 l per day	–
Asymptomatic and sodium <125 meq/l	Fluid restriction and consider small and slow NS infusion	The goal is to prevent further decrease in serum sodium levels, not immediate correction
CNS symptoms such as altered mental status, seizure, and coma	Hypertonic saline 25–100 ml/h or small boluses of 50–100 cc	Titrate to symptoms. Frequent sodium checks. Do not exceed 12 meq over 24 h

Adrenal failure

Adrenal failure in malignancy is usually secondary to invasion of adrenal tissues or adrenal suppression following chronic glucocorticoid therapy. The diagnosis should be suspected in those patients presenting with vasomotor collapse without a clear source or those patients with an alternative cause refractory to standard therapy. These patients may present with the clinical picture of an acute abdomen. Other clues include a metabolic profile consistent with steroid deficiency (hyponatremia, hyperkalemia, and hypoglycemia). A random serum cortisol may aid in diagnosis; however, this test is often not rapidly available.

If considering this diagnosis, stress dose steroids should be empirically given as the benefits generally outweigh the risks of therapy. In a patient without a previous diagnosis of adrenal insufficiency, dexamethasone (4 mg IV bolus) is preferred because it is not detected on serum cortisol assays [54].

Local tumor effects

Airway obstruction

Acute airway compromise from malignancy is a true emergency. In the majority of cases, obstruction is a slow process from the tumor growth near or in the airway [55]. Acute exacerbations may arise from inflammation related to treatment (radiation therapy, laser therapy, and biopsy/excision), superimposed infection, hemorrhage, or loss of muscular tone. A reasonable first step in evaluating a stable patient is defining the area of obstruction. Generally, obstructions involve the upper airway (opening of the mouth and nares to the vocal cords) or the central airway (below the vocal cords to the carina). One may further differentiate the tumor based on whether or not it involves the lumen of the airway. Careful history taking and external physical examination will help to differentiate and allow a more focused therapy [56].

Evaluation involves a combination of plain radiographs, CT, and endoscopy. During attempts to secure the airway, great caution must be taken in cases of malignant obstruction because direct laryngoscopy may precipitate bleeding and swelling of friable tissue and result in worsening airway compromise. This is especially true of endoluminal tumors. Along the same lines, paralyzing a patient with rapid sequence intubation (RSI) before direct visualization may result in an inability to secure an airway that was initially at least partially patent. Therefore, while it would be preferable to avoid it, a surgical airway may be the only route to maintain ventilation and oxygenation.

Definitive therapy is preferably with stenting by bronchoscopy in a controlled environment [56, 57]. Emergent stabilization begins initially with optimizing the airway. Positioning, supplemental humidified oxygen, suction, and nasopharyngeal adjuncts will help relieve symptoms and improve oxygenation [56]. Complete obstruction requiring mechanical intervention is rarely present. If necessary, direct passage of an endotracheal tube might best be done without RSI [58]. Awake fiber-optic intubation with a 5-0 or 6-0 reinforced essential thrombocytosis (ET) tube is the preferred method. The final step when other measures fail is to perform a surgical airway. Depending on the level of obstruction, a tracheostomy may be necessary because a cricothyrotomy would be above the level of the obstructing tumor. While expected to be technically more difficult secondary to increased vasculature or cutting into a tumor itself, these are lifesaving interventions in most cases and will bridge the patient to more definitive therapy.

Bone disease and pathologic fractures

Malignancy affects bone health through a variety of pathways. The aforementioned effects of calcium resorption on bone through parathyroid hormone–related protein, infection, primary bone tumor destruction, and metastatic lesions all impact bone health. The most common tumors causing an impact on bone in the elderly population are multiple myeloma and hematogenous spread of solid malignancies (higher incidence in breast, lung, prostate, and skin) to areas of high flow such as the long bones, pelvis, and very often the spine [59]. A majority of patients will have a known malignancy; however, occasionally pathologic fractures may be the initial finding. The diagnosis is made through a combination of radiographic imaging and the clinical presentation. A history of low-impact fractures, advanced age, a history of bone pain preceding the fracture, and clinical signs of malignancy (i.e., weight loss, weakness, and laboratory abnormalities) should all suggest a pathologic fracture. Plain radiographs are usually sufficient although a CT scan, with IV contrast if possible, may help in finding subtle fractures and extravasation into soft tissue. Magnetic resonance imaging (MRI) and positron emission tomography (PET) scans are often unnecessary in the acute setting as most of these patients will require admission, and these studies may be obtained as inpatients. Radiographs usually display loss of distinct cortical margins, a focal increase (osteoblastic) or decrease (osteoclastic) in bone density and a localized periosteal reaction [59, 60].

The main function of the EP is proper analgesia and salvage of function. Reduction and stabilization of fractures with neurovascular compromise or significantly displaced fracture sites should be performed. Spinal fractures require careful neurologic examination and spinal precautions to avoid exacerbating the injury. Metastatic malignancy of the bone is notoriously painful, and most patients end up on high doses of long-acting opioids; thus, proper dosing of analgesia should be individualized. After initial stabilization, treatment often includes palliative radiotherapy or operative repair [59]. Many elderly patients, or those with advanced malignancy, are poor surgical candidates, and management may focus on palliation. Unfortunately, pathologic fractures have a strong correlation with poor outcomes and often mark significant clinical decline in elderly patients [61].

Spinal cord disease

Three percent to six percent of all cancer patients will develop spinal cord compression. Early detection is essential to preserving function. Most individuals with malignant spinal cord compression will have pain often described as unrelenting, progressive, deep, worse in a supine position, and different than his/her usual back pain [62–64]. Metastases have a predilection for the thoracic spine (up to 60%), and new back pain in this region should trigger a search for metastasis [63]. Arguably, all elderly patients with new back pain, and certainly all those with known malignancy, should undergo imaging.

A careful neurologic examination should be performed to assess for signs of neurologic compromise. Lower extremity weakness, decreased sensation, and bowel or bladder dysfunction are all signs of spinal cord compromise. Examination of elderly patients may be difficult as coexisting neuropathy, diffuse weakness, and incontinence associated with age can mask acute change. One should attempt to determine the patient's baseline examination and function with assistance from the patient, old notes, and family members. Plain radiographs may help to identify metastatic changes of the vertebrae but lack sensitivity and specificity to diagnose spinal cord pathology. The imaging modality of choice for spinal cord disease is MRI [63]. In cases where MRI is unavailable or contraindicated (i.e., noncompatible pacemaker and prior orthopedic hardware), a CT scan with or without myelography is an alternative [65].

Initial treatment consists of adequate analgesia, initiation of spinal precautions, and prompt specialty consultation (i.e., radiation oncology and spinal surgery). The administration of IV corticosteroids continues to be a mainstay of therapy, but there is insufficient evidence as to the appropriate dose. An initial dose of dexamethasone 10 mg IV followed by 4–6 mg IV every 4 h is often used [14].

Definitive treatment for these cases is highly variable, and early consultation with spinal surgery, radiation oncology, and medical oncology is recommended [63]. Radiotherapy is often essential, making acute compromise of the spinal cord secondary to malignancy one of the rare indications for emergent radiotherapy [63, 66]. Combining radiotherapy with surgery has shown improved outcomes in select patients [66].

Pericardial effusion and tamponade

In patients with malignancy, fluid accumulation in the pericardium results from metastases, direct tumor invasion, or treatment [67]. The degree of physiologic distress is proportional to the rate of pericardial fluid accumulation. Patients with slow fluid accumulation may be asymptomatic despite a large pericardial volume (with case reports of up to 2 l), whereas rapid accumulation of even 100 ml may lead to tamponade and cardiovascular collapse [68, 69].

Beck's triad of distended neck veins, muffled precordium, and hypotension is rarely seen in malignancy (most likely secondary to slow fluid accumulation). More frequently, patients will present with shortness of breath, dyspnea, and chest pain. The physical examination may reveal distant heart sounds, distended neck veins, narrow pulse pressure, and pulsus paradoxus. EKG findings include diffuse low voltage, electrical alternans (often from large fluid collections), and nonspecific ST-T wave changes [17, 68]. Echocardiography is fast, is inexpensive, and has good sensitivity and specificity for pericardial fluid collections. In the current age of rapid bedside ultrasound (US), any patient with known malignancy who presents acutely short of breath should be evaluated using ultrasound when available [70].

Treatment for pericardial effusion depends on the patient's clinical status. There is little advantage of performing emergent pericardial drainage if the patient has minor symptoms and is stable [71, 72]. Besides the risk of procedure, removal of large volumes of fluid can produce a paradoxical hemodynamic instability [73]. However, those with signs of tamponade and cardiovascular collapse (hypotension, altered mental status, and shock) require emergent pericardiocentesis. In these cases, multiple studies have shown the superiority of using ultrasound guidance, and ultrasound should be used as time and equipment permits [70, 74, 75]. A catheter is often left in place to permit drainage as a bridge to definitive therapy.

Superior vena cava syndrome

A superior vena cava syndrome (SVCS) results from any process that obstructs venous return in the superior vena cava (SVC). The etiology of SVCS has shifted over time from predominantly untreated infection to the present era when malignancy is the primary cause. However, there is an increasing incidence of vascular thrombosis secondary to indwelling catheters and pacemakers [76, 77]. Early on in malignancy-related SVCS, symptoms are subtle with dyspnea, cough, and subtle face and upper extremity swelling. Dyspnea is reported as the most common initial finding. The classic presentation of facial swelling, head fullness, cough, arm swelling, chest pain, dysphagia, and headache is usually later in the disease progression [78–80]. The time course of symptoms and patient history may aid in differentiating the cause of SVCS. A rapid onset with or without an indwelling catheter suggests thrombosis, whereas a gradual onset suggests malignancy. Regardless of the cause, the majority of patients do not require immediate therapy in the ED [81, 82]. The one exception is if the patient presents with signs of elevated intracranial pressure.

The diagnosis is confirmed on imaging. The majority of patients will have an abnormal chest X-ray study, but the CT scan allows for accurate visualization of malignant masses and thromboembolism [83]. MRI offers several potential advantages, including increased soft tissue visualization, and since most stenting procedures are done with iodinated contrast, a double contrast load may be avoided. Venography is the most conclusive diagnostic tool to assess the exact location of SVC stenosis but is often obtained after a CT scan or an MRI [84].

Immediate management of SVCS is based largely on alleviating venous congestion. Although definitive data is lacking, head elevation and supplemental oxygen likely aid in relieving symptoms. Glucocorticoid therapy is reasonable in cases of known steroid responsive tumors such as lymphoma or thymoma.

Diuretics provide a theoretical benefit; however, definitive evidence is lacking. One study shows no significant difference between diuretics, steroids, or combination therapy [81]. Definitive treatment has long been a combination of chemotherapy, radiation, and intravascular stenting. Radiation therapy is widely advocated in the treatment of SVCS with a large proportion of patients experiencing relief. Over the past few years, intravascular stenting has become the first-line treatment of SVCS from benign causes, and the literature suggests it can be extrapolated to malignancy. In patients with CNS symptoms, vascular stenting may be more readily available and provides a more rapid resolution of symptoms than radiation does. Often, all three therapies will be used in conjunction [85–87]. Regardless of the cause, a diagnosis of malignancy-related SVCS is a poor prognostic factor, with most patients dying within 1 year and median survival of 5 months [17].

Hematologic emergencies

Background

Hematologic emergencies can be easily overlooked, especially in the elderly. Geriatric patients often have comorbidities that can make diagnosis more difficult, and oftentimes, more severe in the setting of decreased physiologic reserve. The hematologic system undergoes numerous changes that may affect almost every organ system in these patients. The elderly have a decreased ability to produce new blood cells. Fortunately, this is not readily apparent unless a significant stress that exceeds the body's ability to create more blood cells is present. Significant decreases in blood counts should not be attributed to aging, but are known to be associated with chronic disease and inflammation. Studies of bone marrow indicate that approximately one third of marrow cellularity is lost during an adult's life [88]. However, a compensatory proliferative effect has also been noted, which allows for normal levels of peripheral blood cells, in the absence of chronic disease or inflammation [89].

Leukocytosis and fever

Leukocytosis can be a sign of underlying infection. The etiology of leukocytosis in the elderly is varied, and inflammation, tissue necrosis, myeloproliferative disorders (MPDs), malignancy, thyroid abnormalities, and certain medications, including epinephrine and steroids, are known to cause significant leukocytosis. Studies have shown that there is no significant change in the absolute number of leukocytes in the elderly [88]. However, these cells are often less likely to become mobilized during significant physiologic stress in the geriatric age group. Furthermore, levels of neutrophil enzymes released during degranulation are reduced. Defects in the ability of the leukocyte to migrate have also been noted in elderly patients [90]. Although it is uncertain why this occurs, it has been suggested that an age-related decrease in chemotactic peptide receptor expression occurs. Although the mechanism of why leukocytes are less active remains a source of clinical and basic science research, it is clear that in the elderly, the absence of a leukocytosis should not allay any concerns for a potential infectious process.

The presence of a fever is a much more specific indicator of infection in the elderly. While the presence of an elevated temperature in younger patients can be associated with trivial bacterial or viral causes, elderly patients, especially those older than 80 years, are much more likely to have a serious cause of their fever [91, 92]. Interestingly, even in the presence of serious infection, 20–30% of geriatric patients will not manifest a fever [93]. The lack of fever is thought to be multifactorial, including a decreased baseline temperature in the elderly, diminished thermoregulatory responses, and decreased production and response to endogenous pyrogens (interleukin-1, interleukin-6, and tumor necrosis factor). An increase in baseline temperature of 1.3 °C has been shown to be suggestive of infection. Rectal temperature is the most sensitive method of temperature measurement in the elderly [94]. A study performed in elderly patients with "definite" infections finds that an elevated temperature greater than 38 °C is found in 86% of patients rectally, compared to 66% via the oral route and 32% by axillary measurement [94].

Anemia

Anemia is the most common hematological disorder encountered in the elderly. It is defined as an absolute reduction in the number of effective red blood cells, typically below 13 g/dl in men and 12 g/dl in women although some variations of this exist. It should be remembered that this is usually not a primary disease, but rather a sign of underlying pathology. In the general adult population, the lowest prevalence of anemia is 1.5% among men from 17 to 49 years old, and highest in men over 85 years old at 26% [95]. The most recent National Health and Nutrition Examination Survey finds that 10.6% of community-dwelling persons older than 65 have anemia [96]. The prevalence of anemia is even higher in elderly nursing home residents and has been reported in up to 53% [97]. Even a mild anemia is associated with a decreased quality of life, cognitive decline, impaired strength and mobility, worsening of comorbidities, and even an increase in mortality.

As with the general population, it is helpful to categorize elderly patients with either an acute or chronic anemia. An acute anemia is frequently seen in the presence of bleeding, and can require transfusion or emergent surgical correction of the underlying cause. Less common causes include autoimmune hemolytic anemia, oxidative stress with severe glucose-6-phosphate dehydrogenase (G6PD) deficiency, cold agglutinin hemolysis, and certain toxins such as brown recluse spider bites. Autoimmune hemolytic anemia is associated both with malignancies (CLL, CML (chronic myelogenous leukemia)) and numerous medications (ethacrynic acid, oral hypoglycemic agents, etc.) that are not rare in the elderly. Aplastic anemia may also cause an abrupt drop in hemoglobin in the elderly population, and causative agents include chloramphenicol, phenylbutazone, anticonvulsants, sulfonamides, and gold [98]. Typical laboratory tests that aid in the diagnosis of an uncertain acute anemia of uncertain etiology are found in Table 22.1.

Geriatric patients with an acute drop in their hemoglobin often present with weakness, altered mental status, a sharp drop in their blood pressure, and, less frequently, angina or high-output heart failure. The presence of pallor in the nail beds, conjunctiva, or the palmar creases suggests hemoglobin less than 8 mg/dl. Tachycardia may not be present, either from medications that suppress the autonomic nervous system, or from blunted physiologic responses. The initial presentation of anemia can be due to end-organ dysfunction from the underlying anemia in these scenarios.

Elderly patients with a chronic anemia typically present with nonspecific complaints, including fatigue, decreased exercise tolerance, and positional dizziness. As opposed to younger patients, who usually have a cause that is easily identified, elderly patients have numerous etiologies of their anemia. The typical classification of microcytic, normocytic, and macrocytic anemia are useful in determining the type of anemia, but is oftentimes complicated as geriatric patients may have multiple etiologies of their anemia. Diagnostic tests to determine the type of chronic anemia can be found in Table 22.2.

These patients have a degree of chronic inflammation, renal insufficiency, and nutritional deficiencies confounding the exact etiologies. Interestingly, even with the correction of the suspected factors that lead to anemia, a sizable percentage of these patients remain anemic, leading to the creation of the term "anemia of senescence" to describe anemia of uncertain etiology in the elderly [99]. Characteristics of this condition can be seen in Table 22.3. It should be emphasized that this is a diagnosis of exclusion and will often not be diagnosed in the ED.

Iron-deficiency anemia in the elderly is concerning not only for the drop in hemoglobin but also for the possibility of gastrointestinal (GI) malignancy. Studies have shown that of geriatric patients with iron-deficiency anemia, 10–15% have an underlying GI cancer [100, 101]. The proportion of patients

Table 22.1 Diagnostic tests for an acute anemia of uncertain cause.

Complete blood count including red blood cell indices
Peripheral blood smear
Direct and indirect Coombs' test
Lactate dehydrogenase
Bilirubin levels, specifically indirect level
Haptoglobin levels
Reticulocyte count, both percentage and index
Coagulation studies

Table 22.2 Suggested laboratory analysis for an uncertain chronic anemia.

Complete blood count, including RBC indices
Peripheral smear
Iron studies
B12 and folate levels
TSH
Haptoglobin levels

Table 22.3 Characteristics of the "anemia of senescence" seen in the geriatric population.

Hemoglobin	10.5–12 g/dl
MCV	80–95 fl
Reticulocyte index	Low
TIBC	Normal
Serum iron	Mildly low to normal
% iron saturation	Mildly low to normal

with macrocytic anemia from folic acid deficiency decreased sharply following a legislative policy change in the folic acid fortification act in 1998, from 16% to 0.5% of the general population [102]. B12 deficiency remains a problem in geriatric patients, and the macrocytic indices can be decreased to lower values due to other coexistent etiologies of anemia. Interestingly, B12 anemia in the elderly is generally due to cobalamin malabsorption, rather than pernicious anemia or dietary insufficiency.

von Willebrand's Disease

von Willebrand's disease (vWD) is the most common inherited bleeding disorder with an estimated prevalence of 1% in the general population; however, the prevalence of those with symptomatic bleeding is 30–100 cases per million [103]. von Willebrand's factor functions to bind platelets to the injured endothelium and also between adjacent platelets; its quantitative or qualitative absence manifests as an increased bleeding time. The majority of cases are due to a quantitative defect in von Willebrand's factor, a smaller subset due to decreased function of normal levels, and the most uncommon type a decrease in both quantitative and qualitative function of von Willebrand's factor. For those with concerning bleeding, desmopressin is recommended as it induces the release of platelets and factor VIII into the plasma; fresh frozen plasma (FFP) can also be given for more serious bleeding. Most elderly patients with vWD are aware of their diagnosis, and management is no different than the rest of the population. There is an acquired form of vWD that is more prevalent in the elderly and is associated with lymphoproliferative diseases, autoimmune conditions, cancer, and aortic stenosis [104]. This condition remains very rare, and the management typically involves correcting the underlying cause. In emergent situations, desmopressin, FFP, and intravenous immunoglobulin (IVIG) can be given [104].

Primary and secondary immune thrombocytopenia

Primary immune thrombocytopenia (ITP) is an autoimmune bleeding disorder in which IgG auto-antibodies are directed against antigens on the surface of platelets, leading to their eventual destruction. Its true incidence is unknown; however, it has been reported to be between 6 and 10 per 100,000 in the United States, with lower rates in Northern Europe, and with a female predominance [105]. Once thought to be a disease of the young, epidemiologic data now suggests that the prevalence of ITP increases with age [106, 107]. Secondary ITP is caused by numerous conditions, most commonly antiphospholipid syndrome, systemic lupus erythematosus, hepatitis C, HIV, and CLL. There is an association between chronic ITP and either current or past infection with *Helicobacter pylori* [108]. There is mixed data on the benefit of eradication of *H. pylori* in these patients, and thus treatment for eradication of *H. pylori* is typically not recommended in the ED [109].

Elderly patients with ITP typically present to the ED with bleeding, especially in the oral mucosa or along their viscera, complaining of blood either in their urine or stool. Alternatively, a low platelet level can be an incidental finding during laboratory analysis for an unrelated complaint. The diagnosis should be clinical. However, there is an assay to evaluate for the presence of antibodies on platelets, but it is associated with false positives.

For patients presenting with new-onset ITP and a platelet level less than 30,000, current guidelines suggest therapy. Management of the initial episode of ITP requires the administration of high-dose oral steroids, although this may need to be appropriately lowered in elderly patients. Other treatment strategies include intravenous immune globulin, rituximab, danazol, and thrombopoietin receptor antagonists, but these should be instituted in conjunction with hematologist consultation. Patients with persistent platelet counts less than 30,000 after a few months of therapy with steroids often undergo splenectomy. This is especially important to note in the elderly, as it predisposes these patients to serious bacterial infections. Elderly patients who present with ITP and have an intracranial bleed, internal bleeding, or require emergency surgery need aggressive management, which includes high-dose methylprednisolone, intravenous immune globulin, and an immediate infusion of platelets [110].

Drug-induced thrombocytopenia

Numerous medications can cause thrombocytopenia, especially those commonly prescribed to the elderly. Upward of 300 drugs have been confirmed to cause secondary thrombocytopenia. Some of these include very common medications used in the geriatric population such as acetaminophen, aspirin, cimetidine, hydrochlorothiazide, penicillin, quinine, trimethoprim/sulfamethoxazole, and vancomycin [111]. Thrombocytopenia typically develops 1–2 weeks following the initiation of a new drug or suddenly after a dose of a medication a patient has taken intermittently. Drug-induced thrombocytopenia is often misdiagnosed as ITP. Many serious complications have resulted from this condition, including intracranial hemorrhage, despite the common usage of many of these medications and seemingly innocuous profile.

Heparin-induced thrombocytopenia

Heparin-induced thrombocytopenia (HIT) deserves a special mention in geriatrics and is classified as either nonimmune or immune-mediated [112]. The far more benign and common type is nonimmune, in which patients have a slight decrease in platelets without clinical consequence. Immune-mediated HIT is caused by antibodies directed against complexes on platelet factor 4, and heparin can result in dangerously low platelet levels as well as thrombosis in both venous and arterial systems. Many patients who are hospitalized are started on heparin or its adjuncts for deep vein thrombosis prophylaxis. EPs will often see recently discharged patients who received heparin during their hospitalization. Since HIT usually develops 5–10 days following the initiation of therapy, EPs must remain vigilant for this condition as it can occur even after heparin has been discontinued. HIT is known to occur more commonly in patients following orthopedic procedures or those involved in traumatic injuries [113]. If the patient is still on heparin and develops HIT, it should be discontinued immediately. In addition, the initiation of either a direct thrombin inhibitor (lepirudin, argatroban, or bivalirudin) or antifactor Xa therapy (danaparoid) should be instituted [112].

Senile purpura

The most common cause of purpura in the elderly is termed senile purpura. It typically occurs on the extensor surfaces of the forearms and hands. It is thought to develop due to the loss of subcutaneous fat and deterioration in connective tissues that make small vessels much more prone to shear. This can be seen in healthy geriatric patients without any underlying hematological abnormalities.

Thrombocytopenic thrombotic purpura

The classic pentad in thrombocytopenic thrombotic purpura (TTP) of fever, microangiopathic hemolytic anemia, thrombocytopenia, neurologic abnormalities, and renal failure were first described in 1965 [114]. Fortunately, this condition is rare, with an estimated prevalence of 4–11 cases per million people in the United States [115]. The underlying cause of this condition is a deficiency of ADAMTS 13, a metalloprotease that cleaves von Willebrand factor into smaller multimers. In its reduction or absence, von Willebrand factor creates large mesh networks that shear red blood cells as they pass, leading to the formation of schistocytes and a destructive anemia. Platelets become sequestered in this mesh with resultant microthrombi that tend to accumulate in CNS and renal microvasculature.

Elderly patients, like the majority of those with TTP, generally present with rather nonspecific complaints of abdominal pain, nausea, vomiting, and generalized weakness. CNS effects, most commonly seizures or fluctuating focal neurological signs, are present in the course of ~50% of patients [116]. Fevers are typically of low grade or absent in the elderly, and a temperature greater than 102°F with chills should prompt the search for an infectious agent [117]. Laboratory analysis is central to the diagnosis, and geriatric patients with TTP should have an acute anemia with thrombocytopenia in the absence of leukopenia. Lactate dehydrogenase and reticulocytes are generally elevated. Schistocytes are suggestive of a microangiopathic anemia but not always present. Approximately one third of patients will have an elevation of their baseline creatinine, and renal failure is infrequent. Clopidogrel and ticlopidine are both associated with TTP [118].

The management of TTP requires plasma-exchange therapy; prior to this, the mortality of TTP approached 90% [119]. The function of plasma exchange is to remove the auto-antibodies directed against ADAMTS 13 and replace ADAMTS 13. If this cannot be initiated, FFP should be initiated until exchange transfusion can be given. Adjunctive therapy should include steroids, although the optimal amount has yet been determined. High-dose methylprednisolone (1 mg/kg/day) has been recently studied, and may have higher survival rates than that of standard therapy, although this difference was not statistically significant [120]. Other adjunctive therapies such as rituximab and cyclosporine should be initiated only following a discussion with a hematologist. Platelet transfusions should be avoided, except in the setting of life-threatening bleeding or intracranial bleeding [119].

Disseminated intravascular coagulation

Disseminated intravascular coagulation (DIC) is one of the more common acquired coagulopathies in the elderly. It represents uncontrolled coagulation and suppression of fibrinolysis leading to significant bleeding, consumption of platelets, and coagulation factors with small vessel obstruction and tissue ischemia from fibrin deposition. This condition can develop either from serious surgical or medical pathology in patients of any age; in the elderly, it is most commonly seen as a result from cancers, serious infections, burns, and trauma. The management of this in elderly patients is no different from other patients. In the ED, recognition and treatment of the underlying condition should be initiated, and identification and treatment of the underlying cause should be started. Therapy is typically tailored to each patient depending on the relative degree of coagulation and fibrinolytic activity. Those with significant bleeding typically receive replacement of the deficient blood products; however, it remains controversial if heparin is beneficial in those with significant thrombosis and fibrin deposition [121].

Hemophilia

The prevalence of geriatric hemophiliacs has increased in the past few decades. These patients are typically born with deficiencies in either factor VIII or IV, although a small proportion develop an acquired hemophilia. Severe hemophiliacs have less than 1% factor activity, moderate hemophiliacs have 1–5% factor activity, and mild hemophiliacs have greater than 5% factor activity (with normal activity ranging from 50% to 150%). Rarely women who possess the trait (symptomatic carriers) may exhibit symptoms of mild hemophiliacs as they possess a lower level of factor activity.

In the early 20th century, the median life expectancy of a hemophiliac was 11 years [122]. With advances in plasma-derived factor concentrate, effective screening for HIV, hepatitis C, and the presence of specialized hemophilia treatment centers, these patients continue to live longer. Currently in the United States, 2% of hemophiliacs are older than 65 years and in Italy, 8% are older than 65 and the number of geriatric hemophiliacs continues to increase [122, 123]. Complicating the care of these patients are significant comorbidities. Prior to safe transfusion techniques, the majority of hemophiliacs acquired HIV or viral hepatitis. Between 85% and 93% of hemophiliacs born before 1975 have hepatitis C and 27–51% have hepatitis B [124]. In the 1990s, the life expectancy of hemophiliacs dropped from 68 years old to 49, largely due to HIV infection [125]. Many of the guidelines on the management of geriatric hemophiliacs are based on very few studies or observations. With regard to the care of the bleeding or injured hemophiliac, the EP should identify the type of hemophilia, the degree of hemophilia, and discuss the case with a hematologist.

Bleeding in the elderly hemophiliac is one of the more common complications seen in this patient population. The amount of factor replacement is based upon the degree of bleeding and the type of hemophilia, with one unit of factor representing the amount of factor activity in $1 mm^3$ of fresh plasma. Generally, the infusion of 1 U of factor per kilogram will increase factor VIII by 2% and factor IX by 1%, with a half-life of 18–24 h. Table 22.4 shows guidelines for the management of bleeding for hemophilia A; those with hemophilia have very similar guidelines. Any significant hemorrhage requires immediate infusion to raise factor levels to 80–100%.

Intracranial hemorrhage is one of the three leading causes of death in geriatric hemophiliacs, along with complications from HIV and hepatitis [126]. The majority of these bleeds are atraumatic and carry

Table 22.4 Guidelines for the management of bleeding for hemophilia A.

Cause of Bleed	Initial Amount of Factor Required	Comments
Joint	40–60% factor activity	1–2 days, longer if treatment is inadequate
Muscle –except iliopsoas	40–60% factor activity	2–3 days, longer if treatment is inadequate
Iliopsoas bleed	80–100% factor activity	1–2 days, then goal 30–60% factor activity for 1–3 days
CNS bleed	80–100% factor activity	1–7 days, then goal 50% for days 8–14
Throat and neck	80–100% factor activity	1–7 days, then goal 30% for days 8–14
Gastrointestinal	80–100% factor activity	1–6 days, then goal 30% for days 7–14
Renal	50% factor activity	3–5 days
Deep laceration	50% factor activity	5–7 days
Abrasion	None needed	–

Adapted from "Guidelines for the Management of Hemophilia from the World Federation of Hemophilia, 2005."

a very high mortality rate, ~30% in patients older than 50. Any elderly hemophiliac with a headache, a change in the neurological examination, or an unexplained change in level of consciousness should have an immediate noncontrast computed tomography scan of the head. Those with a traumatic head injury should have factor therapy initiated as soon as possible, ideally before imaging. Treatment for an intracranial bleed requires immediate infusion of factor to a level of 100% activity.

Hemophilia appears to have a protective component against cardiovascular disease. This is felt to be due to decreased thrombus formation, although it remains uncertain if there is an effect against atherosclerosis [127]. In the rare event that a hemophiliac experiences an acute myocardial infarction, thrombolytics are contraindicated; however, patients have been given aspirin and unfractionated heparin without significant bleeding [128]. This is best done in conjunction with both cardiology and hematology services. No formal guidelines exist on the management of an acute myocardial infarction in a hemophiliac patient.

Acquired hemophilia is a very rare condition caused by the development of auto-antibodies against factor VIII, which results in neutralization or rapid clearance of this factor. The incidence of this condition is between 1.3 and 1.5 people per million per year and has a bimodal distribution, although the elderly are most likely to develop this [129]. The majority of cases appear to be idiopathic, although numerous conditions, such as malignancy and autoimmune diseases are associated with this condition. The bleeding pattern is different than in congenital hemophiliacs,

and typically occurs in muscles, GI, genitourinary, and soft tissues, while sparing the joints. High rates of mortality, up to 44% have been reported, with most deaths in the first few weeks of diagnosis [129]. This diagnosis should be considered in patients with an unexplained activated partial thromboplastin time (aPTT) and an acute onset of bleeding without prior history. Management of acquired hemophilia involves reversal of the bleeding and supportive management of the associated conditions in the ED. These patients are typically started on immunosuppressive therapy during hospitalization [127].

Myelodysplastic syndromes (MDS)

Myelodysplastic syndrome (MDS) is a category of hematological malignancies characterized by improper hematopoiesis and early apoptosis in myeloid precursor cells with a resultant deficiency in these cell lines. At diagnosis, ~80% will have a macrocytic anemia, 30–40% will have thrombocytopenia, and 40% will have neutropenia [130]. The World Health Organization classification scheme of the different types of MDS is shown in Table 22.5 [131].

Geriatric patients may present with complications from MDS, such as ease of bleeding or infection, or as an incidental laboratory abnormality. These patients are also at risk for conversion to AML. It is most typically encountered in the elderly, with over 80% of cases diagnosed in patients older than 60 years of age, with a median age of 76 [132]. There are ~60,000 persons in the United States with this condition, and 10,000 new diagnoses each year [132]. A recent study found that one in six elderly patients with

Table 22.5 World Health Organization classification of types of myelodysplastic syndromes.

Name of MDS	Characteristics
Refractory cytopenia with unilineage dysplasia	Isolated low levels of myeloid cell types, either refractory anemia, refractory thrombocytopenia, or refractory neutropenia 20% of patients with MDS have this Rarely progresses to AML, good prognosis
Refractory cytopenia with ring sideroblasts	Similar to refractory cytopenia with unilineage dysplasia but also has 15% of erythrocyte precursors with high iron content (sideroblasts) 3–10% of patients with MDS have this Rarely progresses to AML, good prognosis
Refractory cytopenia with multilineage	At least two types of myeloid cells are low 40% of patients with MDS have this 10% progress to AML, high mortality
Refractory anemia with excess blasts-1	One of more myeloid cells are low in the blood and abnormal in the marrow, blasts are increased in the marrow, but <10% 40% of patients with MDS have this 25% progress to AML, high mortality
Refractory anemia with excess blasts-2	One of more myeloid cells are low in the blood and abnormal in the marrow, blasts are increased in the marrow, ranging from 10% to 20% Rare Up to 50% progress to AML
MDS associated with isolated del(5q)	Only abnormality in marrow is missing segment of chromosome 5, typically have low hemoglobin, normal leukocytes, and elevated platelets <5% of patients with MDS have this Favorable prognosis
MDS, unclassified	Does not fit into above classifications Uncommon Variable prognosis, progression to AML

an unexplained macrocytic anemia had MDS.[133] It typically arises from de novo mutations, or can be acquired from radiation, chemotherapy, or environmental exposure to numerous agents, including benzene [95]. The diagnosis should be entertained in elderly patients with an unexplained new-onset cytopenia or pancytopenia. Follow-up is essential, and unfortunately, this syndrome may take years for proper diagnosis, which typically includes a bone marrow biopsy that shows more than 10% dysplasia. Some patients may require routine transfusions to help support failing marrow and may need chelation therapy to prevent iron overload. Mortality and morbidity is generally associated with progression to AML or as a result of infections and bleeding from the respective cytopenias. Prognosis is difficult, but longitudinal studies suggest that patients with de novo mutations, women, and those with single-cell cytopenias do better. Furthermore, the life expectancy of those diagnosed at age 70 is unchanged compared to the general population [134].

Myeloproliferative disorders (MPD), polycythemia, thrombocytosis

The MPDs are a group of conditions defined by an abnormally elevated production and hypercellularity of a type of myeloid cell line (red blood cells, platelets, and granulocytes) or increased bone marrow fibrosis in the absence of a secondary cause and absence of dysplasia. They are considered neoplasms by the World Health Organization. The MPDs are more commonly diagnosed in the elderly; recent data shows that persons older than 80 have a prevalence of 13.25 per 100,000, whereas in those less than 40, it is 0.27

Table 22.6 Common causes of thrombocytosis.

Reactive Thrombocytosis
  Trauma, blood loss
  Iron deficiency
  Infection or inflammation
  Asplenia
  Medications (epinephrine, vincristine)
Malignancy
  Myeloid (including essential thrombocytopenia,
    polycythemia vera, chronic myeloid leukemia, and
    primary myelofibrosis)
  Nonmyeloid malignancies
Familial, congenital thrombocytosis

per 100,000 [135]. Classically, the four MPDs are polycythemia vera (PV), ET, primary myelofibrosis (PMF), and CML although more recently some very rare conditions have been added. The Philadelphia chromosome, a translocation between chromosomes 9 and 22, defines CML. This mutation results in increased cellular signaling and control pathways that cause uncontrolled cellular proliferation. PV, ET, and PMF lack the Philadelphia chromosome, but typically possess a Janus kinase 2 (Jak-2) mutation that is felt to be responsible for abnormal cellular growth [136]. These are characterized by an increased thrombotic risk, increased hemorrhagic risk, and a risk of transformation to acute leukemia [137].

Patients with thrombocytosis are often asymptomatic; however, a minority present with complaints related to thrombosis. The causes of thrombocytosis are numerous and are found in Table 22.6. The most common etiologies of thrombocytosis in the elderly are related to iron deficiency, chronic inflammatory processes, and nonmyeloid cancers. Patients with solid malignancies, particularly lung cancer, and those with inflammatory bowel disease occasionally have platelet levels greater than 1,000,000 per mm^3.

Primary causes of thrombocytosis are uncommon and make up ~10% of cases. Of these, CML and ET are the most common etiologies and should be diagnoses of exclusion in the ED. Geriatric patients with platelets persistently greater than 450,000 cells per mm^3 and the absence of an obvious cause should have appropriate follow-up as the risk for an underlying malignancy is high. Those with a primary etiology have abnormal functioning platelets and are thus at

risk of numerous complications, including thrombotic or bleeding events. Low-dose aspirin is typically started in those at risk for thrombotic complications.

Erythrocytosis and polycythemia are terms often used interchangeably, although erythrocytosis refers to an increase in the volume of hematocrit and polycythemia includes the elevation of other myeloid cell lines. Erythrocytosis is not diagnosed until hematocrit levels are above 16 mg/dl, and above this point, the risk of thrombosis from increased viscosity increases exponentially [138]. Patients with severely elevated hemoglobin levels may present with flushing, tinnitus, headache dizziness, and severe itching, or more serious complications such as stroke, myocardial infarction, or venous thrombosis. Burning sensations are not uncommon as transient occlusions in the microvasculature occur. Spurious polycythemia occurs when plasma volume is decreased and commonly seen in dehydrated elderly patients. True elevations in hemoglobin are typically caused by one of three mechanisms in elderly patients, as seen in Table 22.7.

Conditions such as chronic obstructive pulmonary disease (COPD) or smoking are responsible for the majority of cases of polycythemia. PV is typically found in middle-aged or geriatric patients and ~30% present with symptomatic complaints of thrombosis including stroke, myocardial infarction, and deep vein thrombosis. Characteristics and diagnostic criteria of PV are shown in Table 22.8. It is the only MPD with erythrocytosis and can be quickly differentiated from secondary causes as erythropoietin (EPO) levels will be low.

Table 22.7 Causes of erythrocytosis.

Primary Erythrocytosis
  Polycythemia vera
EPO-mediated erythrocytosis
  Central hypoxia (chronic lung disease, carbon monoxide
    poisoning, smoker's erythrocytosis, and right-to-left
    cardiopulmonary shunts)
  Renal hypoxia (end-stage renal disease, renal artery
    stenosis, and polycystic kidney disease)
  Tumor/pathologic production (renal cell carcinoma,
    pheochromocytoma, and hepatocellular carcinoma)
Medications associated with EPO
  Androgen preparations
  Exogenous EPO in postrenal transplant patients

Adapted from "Guidelines for the diagnosis, investigation, and management of polycythemia/erythrocytosis" [139].

Table 22.8 Characteristics and diagnostic criteria of polycythemia vera.

Characteristics of Polycythemia Vera
  Hematologic abnormalities (erythrocytosis, thrombocytosis, and granulocytosis)
  Thrombosis (intra-abdominal venous, intracranial vessels, coronary arteries, and pulmonary vasculature)
  Splenomegaly
WHO Diagnostic Criteria (either both major criteria OR one major and two minor criteria)
  Major

1. Hemoglobin >18.5 g/dl in men, >16.5 g/dl in women
2. Presence of JAK2(V617F) other functionally similar mutation

  Minor

1. Biopsy showing hypercellularity with trilineage myeloproliferation
2. Serum EPO levels below the normal values
3. In vitro formation of endogenous erythyroid colony

Patients with PV typically receive phlebotomy to lower their hematocrit to below 45%, are started on a low-dose aspirin, and may take varying types of cytoreductive therapy depending on their age [139]. Asymptomatic geriatric patients who lack PV but have hematocrit greater than 60% are at risk of thrombosis and cautious phlebotomy should be considered in these patients.

Hematologic malignancies

Patients with hematologic malignancies typically present to the ED in three ways: the initial diagnosis, an unrelated complaint, or as a direct complication of the cancer. Given the increased prevalence of these in the elderly, the EP should be aware of both the underlying malignancies and possible complications. TLS, complications related to infection, and induction of therapy were discussed earlier in this chapter.

CLL is a B-cell lymphoma that is predominately seen in the elderly. It constitutes 30% of all hematologic malignancies, making it the most common leukemia [140]. There are almost no cases in patients younger than 30 years and 10% of cases occur in those younger than age 55 [141]. Typical complaints in undiagnosed patients are nonspecific and include fatigue, weight loss, and malaise. The physical examination findings typically include painless, nontender lymphadenopathy, and hepatosplenomegaly. Bruising may be present from thrombocytopenia, either from bone marrow failure or secondary autoimmune hemolytic anemia. The diagnosis should be suspected in elderly patients who have a marked leukocytosis and a predominance of lymphocytes. Numerous chemotherapeutic agents can cause significant morbidity to these patients, and they are at very high risk for TLS and neutropenic fever following induction therapy. These patients are also at a higher risk for infection from encapsulated organisms as they develop hypogammaglobulinemia. Bruising typically develops due to thrombocytopenia. In contrast to the traditional teaching that these patients typically do not die from CLL, geriatric patients have poor 10-year survival rates once the diagnosis is made [142]. However, there has been a generalized increase in survival in these patients in the past 30 years; it has been felt that this is due to improved chemotherapy regimens and a most noticeable improvement in healthy patients younger than 70 years [143].

AML is another hematogenous malignancy that is predominately seen in geriatric patients. More than two thirds of patients diagnosed with AML are older than 60 and the incidence of new diagnosis is nearly 10 times greater in those older than age 65 [144]. As with many of these malignancies, geriatric patients with AML present with initial complaints of weakness, fatigue, and weight loss. Their physical examination is notable for the absence of lymphadenopathy and slight, if any, splenomegaly. Ten percent of patients will have a new rash, whereas others have petechiae. There may be a significant leukocytosis, leukopenia, or decreased levels of red blood cells or platelets and the presence of circulating leukemic blasts. Diagnosis requires a bone marrow biopsy. These patients are also at much high risk for intracranial hemorrhage than both the general population and those with other malignancies of the blood. A recent study finds the incidence of intracerebral hemorrhage (ICH) in these patients to be 6.1% versus 1.1% in patients with other hematologic malignancies [145]. These devastating bleeds have a high mortality and thought to be due to an underlying hyperleukocytosis, sepsis, DIC, or platelet dysfunction. In particular, the acute promyelocytic subtype of AML is particularly notorious for coagulation dysfunction, with very high mortality from an ICH [146]. The majority of these intracranial bleeds are intraparenchymal, with a smaller subset of subdural hematomas [145].

CML, also referred to as chronic granulocytic anemia, is a myeloproliferative malignancy defined by the uncontrolled growth of mature granulocytes with normal differentiation. It is caused by an abnormal fusion of chromosomes 9 and 22, which is referred to as the Philadelphia chromosome. The median age at diagnosis is between 60 and 65 years of age and is one of the more common hematologic malignancies seen in the elderly [147]. It typically has a triphasic course: a chronic phase, an accelerated phase, and a blast crisis phase that resembles an acute leukemia. Around 85% of these patients are diagnosed in the chronic phase and generally are found on routine laboratory analysis, in which a leukocytosis typically above 100,000, or platelets elevated to 600,000–700,000 are present [148]. Patients typically report fatigue, weight loss, abdominal fullness, excessive sweating, or spontaneous bleeding. Patients may present with left upper quadrant pain, which typically occurs due to splenomegaly or splenic infarction. A blast crisis is the final stage of CML and represents the progression from a relatively benign chronic phase into a terminal stage, which resembles an acute leukemia, which is not responsive to chemotherapy [149]. The diagnosis depends on the number of blasts seen on a peripheral blood smear or marrow analysis; a blast count greater than 20% is generally considered diagnostic along with the evidence of clonal evolution [149]. The most worrisome complications occur from either infection or leukostasis at this stage.

Hyperleukocytosis and leukostasis are uncommon complications of hematologic malignancies. Hyperleukocytosis refers to an abnormally elevated amount of WBCs, generally above 100,000 cells per milliliter and is a poor prognostic marker [150]. Leukostasis, also referred to as symptomatic hyperleukocytosis, is a medical emergency in which WBCs inhibit perfusion in the microvasculature, generally in the lungs or in the CNS [150]. It is hypothesized to occur due to either secondary to increased blood viscosity in the microvasculature, or local hypoxemia due to the exceedingly high metabolic rate of the blast cells and resultant release of cytokines [151]. In the geriatric population, it is seen in those with AML or CML in blast crisis and is associated with a high mortality

Table 22.9 Signs and symptoms of leukostasis.

Central Nervous System
  Tinnitus, stupor, ataxia, coma, dizziness, and confusion
  Focal neurological changes, retinal hemorrhages
Pulmonary system
  Dyspnea, tachypnea, rales, and hypoxemia
Priapism (rare)
Renal vein thrombosis (rare)
Acute leg ischemia (rare)

rate. Signs and symptoms of leukostasis can be seen in Table 22.9.

There should be a very low threshold for imaging of the head and chest as the microvasculature in these regions is commonly occluded. Arterial pO2 can be falsely depressed as a high number of white cells utilize a significant portion of oxygen in the drawn sample and is referred to as "leukocyte larceny." [152] Other common abnormalities include a spuriously elevated platelet count, and elevated potassium due to release from blasts. Approximately 15–40% of patients develop DIC, and a smaller percentage develop spontaneous TLS [153]. Management of patients with leukostasis involves cytoreduction, induction chemotherapy, and leukapheresis; these patients need their care managed in consultation with an oncologist and transfusionist, as this is a rare and challenging condition to diagnosis and manage [153]. In situations in which a clear diagnosis of leukostasis is made and leukapheresis is not available, phlebotomy with concurrent blood and plasma transfusion may be used as a brief temporizing measure [150].

Section IV: Decision-making

- Neutropenic fever patients are at high risk of infection, and antibiotics should be given empirically if a source is not identified.
- Emergent conditions such as TLS and a variety of metabolic derangements deserve close attention, rapid evaluation and treatment, and consultation where appropriate.
- Subtle and vague complaints that are new in the geriatric patient should be taken seriously, such as new-onset bone pain, as this can be an early manifestation of malignancy.
- Fever is less commonly seen with infection in the elderly.

References

1 Buchanan, N.D., King, J.B., Rodriguez, J.L. *et al.* (2013) Changes among US Cancer Survivors: comparing demographic, diagnostic, and health care findings from the 1992 and 2010 National Health Interview Surveys. *ISRN Oncol.*, **2013**, 238017. doi: 10.1155/2013/238017

2 Surveillance, Epidemiology, and End Results Program (2013) Previous Version – SEER Cancer Statistics Review, 1975–2010, http://seer.cancer.gov/csr/1975_2010/sections.html (accessed 23 August 2013).

3 Halter, J., Ouslander, J., Tinetti, M. *et al.* (2009) *Hazzard's Geriatric Medicine and Gerontology*, 6th edn, McGraw-Hill.

4 Tsiompanou, E., Lucas, C., and Stroud, M. (2013) Overfeeding and overhydration in elderly medical patients: lessons from the Liverpool Care Pathway. *Clin. Med.*, **13** (3), 248–251. doi: 10.7861/clinmedicine.13-3-248

5 Allison, S.P. and Lobo, D.N. (2004) Fluid and electrolytes in the elderly. *Curr. Opin. Clin. Nutr. Metab. Care*, **7** (1), 27–33, http://www.ncbi.nlm.nih.gov/pubmed/15090900 (accessed 23 August 2013).

6 Torke, A.M., Moloney, R., Siegler, M. *et al.* (2010) Physicians' views on the importance of patient preferences in surrogate decision-making. *J. Am. Geriatr. Soc.*, **58** (3), 533–538. doi: 10.1111/j.1532-5415.2010.02720.x

7 Rosenberg, M., Lamba, S., and Misra, S. (2013) Palliative medicine and geriatric emergency care: challenges, opportunities, and basic principles. *Clin. Geriatr. Med.*, **29** (1), 1–29. doi: 10.1016/j.cger.2012.09.006

8 Smith, A.K., McCarthy, E., Weber, E. *et al.* (2012) Half of older Americans seen in emergency department in last month of life; most admitted to hospital, and many die there. *Health Aff. (Millwood)*, **31** (6), 1277–1285. doi: 10.1377/hlthaff.2011.0922

9 Bischoff, K.E., Sudore, R., Miao, Y. *et al.* (2013) Advance care planning and the quality of end-of-life care in older adults. *J. Am. Geriatr. Soc.*, **61** (2), 209–214. doi: 10.1111/jgs.12105

10 Hughes, W.T., Armstrong, D., Bodey, G.P. *et al.* (2002) 2002 guidelines for the use of antimicrobial agents in neutropenic patients with cancer. *Clin. Infect. Dis.*, **34** (6), 730–751. doi: 10.1086/339215

11 Freifeld, A.G., Bow, E.J., Sepkowitz, K.A. *et al.* (2011) Clinical practice guideline for the use of antimicrobial agents in neutropenic patients with cancer: 2010 update by the infectious diseases society of America. *Clin. Infect. Dis.*, **52** (4), e56–e93. doi: 10.1093/cid/cir073

12 Klastersky, J. (2004) Management of fever in neutropenic patients with different risks of complications. *Clin. Infect. Dis.*, **39** (Suppl. 1), S32–S37. doi: 10.1086/383050

13 Sickles, E.A., Greene, W.H., and Wiernik, P.H. (1975) Clinical presentation of infection in granulocytopenic patients. *Arch. Intern. Med.*, **135** (5), 715–719, http://www.ncbi.nlm.nih.gov/pubmed/1052668 (accessed 22 August 2013).

14 Lewis, M.A., Hendrickson, A.W., and Moynihan, T.J. (2011) Oncologic emergencies: pathophysiology, presentation, diagnosis, and treatment. *CA Cancer J. Clin.* doi: 10.3322/caac.20124

15 Link, H., Böhme, A., Cornely, O.A. *et al.* (2003) Antimicrobial therapy of unexplained fever in neutropenic patients-guidelines of the Infectious Diseases Working Party (AGIHO) of the German Society of Hematology and Oncology (DGHO), Study Group Interventional Therapy of Unexplained Fever, Arbeitsgemein. *Ann. Hematol.*, **82** (Suppl. 2), S105–S117. doi: 10.1007/s00277-003-0764-4

16 Dellinger, R.P., Levy, M.M., Carlet, J.M. *et al.* (2008) Surviving Sepsis Campaign: international guidelines for management of severe sepsis and septic shock: 2008. *Crit. Care Med.*, **36** (1), 296–327. doi: 10.1097/01.CCM.0000298158.12101.41

17 Behl, D., Hendrickson, A.W., and Moynihan, T.J. (2010) Oncologic emergencies. *Crit. Care Clin.*, **26** (1), 181–205. doi: 10.1016/j.ccc.2009.09.004

18 Coiffier, B., Altman, A., Pui, C.-H. *et al.* (2008) Guidelines for the management of pediatric and adult tumor lysis syndrome: an evidence-based review. *J. Clin. Oncol.*, **26** (16), 2767–2778. doi: 10.1200/JCO.2007.15.0177

19 Gemici, C. (2006) Tumour lysis syndrome in solid tumours. *Clin. Oncol. (R. Coll. Radiol.)*, **18** (10), 773–780, http://www.ncbi.nlm.nih.gov/pubmed/17168213 (accessed 24 August 2013).

20 Cairo, M.S. and Bishop, M. (2004) Tumour lysis syndrome: new therapeutic strategies and classification. *Br. J. Haematol.*, **127** (1), 3–11. doi: 10.1111/j.1365-2141.2004.05094.x

21 Kelen, G. and Hsu, E. (2011) Fluids and electrolytes, in *Tintinalli's Emergency Medicine: A Comprehensive Study Guide*, 7th edn (eds R. Cydulka and G. Meckler), McGraw-Hill, New York.

22 Jeha, S., Kantarjian, H., Irwin, D. *et al.* (2005) Efficacy and safety of rasburicase, a recombinant urate oxidase (Elitek), in the management of malignancy-associated hyperuricemia in pediatric and adult patients: final results of a multicenter compassionate use trial. *Leukemia*, **19** (1), 34–38. doi: 10.1038/sj.leu.2403566

23 Huncharek, M. (1993) Incidence of hypercalcemia in patients with malignancy referred to a comprehensive cancer center. *Cancer*, **72** (3), 956–957, http://www

.ncbi.nlm.nih.gov/pubmed/8334649 (accessed 23 August 2013).

24 Ralston, S.H., Gallacher, S.J., Patel, U. *et al.* (1990) Cancer-associated hypercalcemia: morbidity and mortality. Clinical experience in 126 treated patients. *Ann. Intern. Med.*, **112** (7), 499–504, http://www.ncbi.nlm.nih.gov/pubmed/2138442 (accessed 23 August 2013).

25 Stewart, A.F. (2005) Clinical practice. Hypercalcemia associated with cancer. *N. Engl. J. Med.*, **352** (4), 373–379. doi: 10.1056/NEJMcp042806

26 Deftos, L.J. (2002) Hypercalcemia in malignant and inflammatory diseases. *Endocrinol. Metab. Clin. North Am.*, **31** (1), 141–158, http://www.ncbi.nlm.nih.gov/pubmed/12055985 (accessed 23 August 2013).

27 Roodman, G.D. (1997) Mechanisms of bone lesions in multiple myeloma and lymphoma. *Cancer*, **80** (**Suppl. 8**), 1557–1563, http://www.ncbi.nlm.nih.gov/pubmed/9362422 (accessed 23 August 2013).

28 Seymour, J.F. and Gagel, R.F. (1993) Calcitriol: the major humoral mediator of hypercalcemia in Hodgkin's disease and non-Hodgkin's lymphomas. *Blood*, **82** (5), 1383–1394, http://www.ncbi.nlm.nih.gov/pubmed/8364192 (accessed 23 August 2013).

29 Chen, L., Dinh, T.A., and Haque, A. (2005) Small cell carcinoma of the ovary with hypercalcemia and ectopic parathyroid hormone production. *Arch. Pathol. Lab. Med.*, **129** (4), 531–533. doi: 10.1043/1543-2165 (2005)129<531:SCCOTO>2.0.CO;2

30 Bajorunas, D.R. (1990) Clinical manifestations of cancer-related hypercalcemia. *Semin. Oncol.*, **17** (**2 Suppl. 5**), 16–25, http://www.ncbi.nlm.nih.gov/pubmed/2185549 (accessed 24 August 2013).

31 Mahon, S.M. (1989) Signs and symptoms associated with malignancy-induced hypercalcemia. *Cancer Nurs.*, **12** (3), 153–160, http://www.ncbi.nlm.nih.gov/pubmed/2743297 (accessed 24 August 2013).

32 Fallah-Rad, N. and Morton, A.R. (2013) Managing hypercalcaemia and hypocalcaemia in cancer patients. *Curr. Opin. Support. Palliat. Care*, **7** (3), 265–271. doi: 10.1097/SPC.0b013e3283640f5f

33 Gucalp, R., Theriault, R., Gill, I. *et al.* (1994) Treatment of cancer-associated hypercalcemia. Double-blind comparison of rapid and slow intravenous infusion regimens of pamidronate disodium and saline alone. *Arch. Intern. Med.*, **154** (17), 1935–1944, http://www.ncbi.nlm.nih.gov/pubmed/8074597 (accessed 23 August 2013).

34 Hurtado, J. and Esbrit, P. (2002) Treatment of malignant hypercalcaemia. *Expert Opin. Pharmacother.*, **3** (5), 521–527. doi: 10.1517/14656566.3.5.521

35 Davidson, T.G. (2001) Conventional treatment of hypercalcemia of malignancy. *Am. J. Health Syst. Pharm.*, **58** (**Suppl. 3**), S8–S15, http://www.ncbi.nlm.nih.gov/pubmed/11757206 (accessed 23 August 2013).

36 Koo, W.S., Jeon, D.S., Ahn, S.J. *et al.* (1996) Calcium-free hemodialysis for the management of hypercalcemia. *Nephron*, **72** (3), 424–428, http://www.ncbi.nlm.nih.gov/pubmed/8852491 (accessed 23 August 2013).

37 Pelosof, L.C. and Gerber, D.E. (2010) Paraneoplastic syndromes: an approach to diagnosis and treatment. *Mayo Clin. Proc.*, **85** (9), 838–854. doi: 10.4065/mcp.2010.0099

38 Lassen, U., Osterlind, K., Hansen, M. *et al.* (1995) Long-term survival in small-cell lung cancer: posttreatment characteristics in patients surviving 5 to 18+ years--an analysis of 1,714 consecutive patients. *J. Clin. Oncol.*, **13** (5), 1215–1220, http://www.ncbi.nlm.nih.gov/pubmed/7738624 (accessed 24 August 2013).

39 Castillo, J.J., Vincent, M., and Justice, E. (2012) Diagnosis and management of hyponatremia in cancer patients. *Oncologist*, **17** (6), 756–765. doi: 10.1634/theoncologist.2011-0400

40 Salido, M., Macarron, P., Hernández-García, C. *et al.* (2003) Water intoxication induced by low-dose cyclophosphamide in two patients with systemic lupus erythematosus. *Lupus*, **12** (8), 636–639, http://www.ncbi.nlm.nih.gov/pubmed/12945725 (accessed 23 August 2013).

41 Tsujita, Y., Iwao, N., Makino, S., and Ohsawa, N. (1998) Syndrome of inappropriate secretion of antidiuretic hormone and neurotoxicity induced by vincristine and alkylating agents during chemotherapy for malignant lymphoma of thyroid gland. *Gan To Kagaku Ryoho*, **25** (5), 757–760, http://www.ncbi.nlm.nih.gov/pubmed/9571977 (accessed 23 August 2013).

42 Ellison, D.H. and Berl, T. (2007) Clinical practice. The syndrome of inappropriate antidiuresis. *N. Engl. J. Med.*, **356** (20), 2064–2072. doi: 10.1056/NEJMcp066837

43 Raftopoulos, H. (2007) Diagnosis and management of hyponatremia in cancer patients. *Support. Care Cancer*, **15** (12), 1341–1347. doi: 10.1007/s00520-007-0309-9

44 Onitilo, A.A., Kio, E., and Doi, S.A.R. (2007) Tumor-related hyponatremia. *Clin. Med. Res.*, **5** (4), 228–237. doi: 10.3121/cmr.2007.762

45 Graber, M. and Corish, D. (1991) The electrolytes in hyponatremia. *Am. J. Kidney Dis.*, **18** (5), 527–545, http://www.ncbi.nlm.nih.gov/pubmed/1835285 (accessed 24 August 2013).

46 Adrogué, H.J. and Madias, N.E. (2000) Hyponatremia. *N. Engl. J. Med.*, **342** (21), 1581–1589. doi: 10.1056/NEJM200005253422107

47 Laureno, R. and Karp, B.I. (1997) Myelinolysis after correction of hyponatremia. *Ann. Intern. Med.*, **126** (1), 57–62, http://www.ncbi.nlm.nih.gov/pubmed/ 8992924 (accessed 12 August 2013).

48 Brito, A.R., Vasconcelos, M.M., Cruz Júnior, L.C. *et al.* (2006) Central pontine and extrapontine myelinolysis: report of a case with a tragic outcome. *J. Pediatr. (Rio J)*, **82** (2), 157–160. doi: 10.2223/JPED.1463

49 Lin, C.-M. and Po, H.L. (2008) Extrapontine myelinolysis after correction of hyponatremia presenting as generalized tonic seizures. *Am. J. Emerg. Med.*, **26** (5), 632.e5–632.e6. doi: 10.1016/j.ajem.2007.10.007

50 Soupart, A. and Decaux, G. (1996) Therapeutic recommendations for management of severe hyponatremia: current concepts on pathogenesis and prevention of neurologic complications. *Clin. Nephrol.*, **46** (3), 149–169, http://www.ncbi.nlm.nih.gov/pubmed /8879850 (accessed 23 August 2013).

51 Verbalis, J.G., Goldsmith, S.R., Greenberg, A. *et al.* (2007) Hyponatremia treatment guidelines 2007: expert panel recommendations. *Am. J. Med.*, **120** (**11 Suppl. 1**), S1–S21. doi: 10.1016/j.amjmed.2007 .09.001

52 Ayus, J.C. and Arieff, A.I. (1999) Chronic hyponatremic encephalopathy in postmenopausal women: association of therapies with morbidity and mortality. *J. Am. Med. Assoc.*, **281** (24), 2299–2304, http:// www.ncbi.nlm.nih.gov/pubmed/10386554 (accessed 23 August 2013).

53 Adrogué, H.J. (2005) Consequences of inadequate management of hyponatremia. *Am. J. Nephrol.*, **25** (3), 240–249. doi: 10.1159/000086019

54 Taylor, R.L. (2004) Quantitative, highly sensitive liquid chromatography-tandem mass spectrometry method for detection of synthetic corticosteroids. *Clin. Chem.*, **50** (12), 2345–2352. doi: 10.1373/clinchem .2004.033605

55 Wood, D.E., Liu, Y.-H., Vallières, E. *et al.* (2003) Airway stenting for malignant and benign tracheobronchial stenosis. *Ann. Thorac. Surg.*, **76** (1), 167–172; discussion 173–174, http://www.ncbi.nlm .nih.gov/pubmed/12842534 (accessed 2 January 2014).

56 Chen, K., Varon, J., and Wenker, O.C. (1998) Malignant airway obstruction: recognition and management. *J. Emerg. Med.*, **16** (1), 83–92, http:// www.ncbi.nlm.nih.gov/pubmed/9472765 (accessed 2 January 2014).

57 Mathisen, D.J. and Grillo, H.C. (1989) Endoscopic relief of malignant airway obstruction. *Ann. Thorac. Surg.*, **48** (4), 469–473; discussion 473–475, http:// www.ncbi.nlm.nih.gov/pubmed/2478088 (accessed 2 January 2014).

58 Theodore, P.R. (2009) Emergent management of malignancy-related acute airway obstruction. *Emerg. Med. Clin. North Am.*, **27** (2), 231–241. doi: 10.1016/j.emc.2009.01.009

59 Torbert, J.T. and Lackman, R.D. (2011) in *Fractures in the Elderly* (eds R.J. Pignolo, M.A. Keenan, and N.M. Hebela), Humana Press, pp. 43–54. doi: 10.1007/978-1-60327-467-8

60 Blackburn, P. (2011) Emergency complications of malignancy, in *Tintinalli's Emergency Medicine: A Comprehensive Study Guide*, 7th edn (eds R. Cydulka and G. Meckler), McGraw-Hill, New York.

61 Saad, F., Lipton, A., Cook, R. *et al.* (2007) Pathologic fractures correlate with reduced survival in patients with malignant bone disease. *Cancer*, **110** (8), 1860–1867. doi: 10.1002/cncr.22991

62 Halfdanarson, T.R., Hogan, W.J., and Moynihan, T.J. (2006) Oncologic emergencies: diagnosis and treatment. *Mayo Clin. Proc.*, **81** (6), 835–848. doi: 10.4065/81.6.835

63 Cole, J.S. and Patchell, R.A. (2008) Metastatic epidural spinal cord compression. *Lancet Neurol.*, **7** (5), 459–466. doi: 10.1016/S1474-4422(08)70089-9

64 Prasad, D. and Schiff, D. (2005) Malignant spinal-cord compression. *Lancet Oncol.*, **6** (1), 15–24. doi: 10.1016/S1470-2045(04)01709-7

65 Kwok, Y., Tibbs, P.A., and Patchell, R.A. (2006) Clinical approach to metastatic epidural spinal cord compression. *Hematol. Oncol. Clin. North Am.*, **20** (6), 1297–1305. doi: 10.1016/j.hoc.2006.09.008

66 Patchell, R.A., Tibbs, P.A., Regine, W.F. *et al.* (2005) Direct decompressive surgical resection in the treatment of spinal cord compression caused by metastatic cancer: a randomised trial. *Lancet*, **366** (9486), 643–648. doi: 10.1016/S0140-6736(05)66954-1

67 DeCamp, M.M., Mentzer, S.J., Swanson, S.J., and Sugarbaker, D.J. (1997) Malignant effusive disease of the pleura and pericardium. *Chest*, **112** (**Suppl. 4**), 291S–295S, http://www.ncbi.nlm.nih.gov/pubmed/ 9337306 (accessed 3 January 2014).

68 Spodick, D.H. (2003) Acute cardiac tamponade. *N. Engl. J. Med.*, **349** (7), 684–690. doi: 10.1056/NEJMra022643

69 Reddy, P.S., Curtiss, E.I., O'Toole, J.D., and Shaver, J.A. (1978) Cardiac tamponade: hemodynamic observations in man. *Circulation*, **58** (2), 265–272, http:// www.ncbi.nlm.nih.gov/pubmed/668074 (accessed 3 January 2014).

70 Tsang, T.S., Freeman, W.K., Sinak, L.J., and Seward, J.B. (1998) Echocardiographically guided pericardiocentesis: evolution and state-of-the-art technique. *Mayo Clin. Proc.*, **73** (7), 647–652. doi: 10.1016 /S0025-6196(11)64888-X

71 Tsang, T.S. and Seward, J.B. (1999) Management of pericardial effusion: safety over novelty. *Am. J. Cardiol.*, **83** (**4**), 640, http://www.ncbi.nlm.nih.gov/pubmed/10073886 (accessed 3 January 2014).

72 Mercé, J., Sagristà-Sauleda, J., Permanyer-Miralda, G., and Soler-Soler, J. (1998) Should pericardial drainage be performed routinely in patients who have a large pericardial effusion without tamponade? *Am. J. Med.*, **105** (**2**), 106–109, http://www.ncbi.nlm.nih.gov/pubmed/9727816 (accessed 3 January 2014).

73 Wagner, P.L., McAleer, E., Stillwell, E. *et al.* (2011) Pericardial effusions in the cancer population: prognostic factors after pericardial window and the impact of paradoxical hemodynamic instability. *J. Thorac. Cardiovasc. Surg.*, **141** (**1**), 34–38. doi: 10.1016/j.jtcvs.2010.09.015

74 L'italien, A.J. (2013) Critical cardiovascular skills and procedures in the emergency department. *Emerg. Med. Clin. North Am.*, **31** (**1**), 151–206. doi: 10.1016/j.emc.2012.09.011

75 Tsang, T.S.M., Enriquez-Sarano, M., Freeman, W.K. *et al.* (2002) Consecutive 1127 therapeutic echocardiographically guided pericardiocenteses: clinical profile, practice patterns, and outcomes spanning 21 years. *Mayo Clin. Proc.*, **77** (**5**), 429–436. doi: 10.4065/77.5.429

76 Otten, T.R., Stein, P.D., Patel, K.C. *et al.* (2003) Thromboembolic disease involving the superior vena cava and brachiocephalic veins. *Chest*, **123** (**3**), 809–812, http://www.ncbi.nlm.nih.gov/pubmed/12628882 (accessed 3 January 2014).

77 Bertrand, M., Presant, C.A., Klein, L., and Scott, E. (1984) Iatrogenic superior vena cava syndrome. A new entity. *Cancer*, **54** (**2**), 376–378, http://www.ncbi.nlm.nih.gov/pubmed/6722752 (accessed 3 January 2014).

78 Rice, T.W., Rodriguez, R.M., and Light, R.W. (2006) The superior vena cava syndrome: clinical characteristics and evolving etiology. *Medicine (Baltimore)*, **85** (**1**), 37–42. doi: 10.1097/01.md.0000198474.99876.f0

79 Bell, D.R., Woods, R.L., and Levi, J.A. (1986) Superior vena caval obstruction: a 10-year experience. *Med. J. Aust.*, **145** (**11–12**), 566–568, http://www.ncbi.nlm.nih.gov/pubmed/3796366 (accessed 3 January 2014).

80 Bagheri, R., Rahim, M., Rezaeetalab, F. *et al.* (2009) Malignant superior vena cava syndrome: is this a medical emergency? *Ann. Thorac. Cardiovasc. Surg.*, **15** (**2**), 89–92, http://www.ncbi.nlm.nih.gov/pubmed/19471221 (accessed 3 January 2014).

81 Schraufnagel, D.E., Hill, R., Leech, J.A., and Pare, J.A. (1981) Superior vena caval obstruction. Is it a medical emergency? *Am. J. Med.*, **70** (**6**), 1169–1174, http://www.ncbi.nlm.nih.gov/pubmed/7234887 (accessed 3 January 2014).

82 Cohen, R., Mena, D., Carbajal-Mendoza, R. *et al.* (2008) Superior vena cava syndrome: a medical emergency? *Int. J. Angiol.*, **17** (**1**), 43–46, http://www.pubmedcentral.nih.gov/articlerender.fcgi?artid=2728369&tool=pmcentrez&rendertype=abstract (accessed 3 January 2014).

83 Parish, J.M., Marschke, R.F., Dines, D.E., and Lee, R.E. (1981) Etiologic considerations in superior vena cava syndrome. *Mayo Clin. Proc.*, **56** (**7**), 407–413, http://www.ncbi.nlm.nih.gov/pubmed/7253702 (accessed 3 January 2014).

84 Ganeshan, A., Hon, L.Q., Warakaulle, D.R. *et al.* (2009) Superior vena caval stenting for SVC obstruction: current status. *Eur. J. Radiol.*, **71** (**2**), 343–349. doi: 10.1016/j.ejrad.2008.04.014

85 Cheng, S. (2009) Superior vena cava syndrome: a contemporary review of a historic disease. *Cardiol. Rev.*, **17** (**1**), 16–23. doi: 10.1097/CRD.0b013e318188033c

86 Rizvi, A.Z., Kalra, M., Bjarnason, H. *et al.* (2008) Benign superior vena cava syndrome: stenting is now the first line of treatment. *J. Vasc. Surg.*, **47** (**2**), 372–380. doi: 10.1016/j.jvs.2007.09.071

87 Rowell, N.P. and Gleeson, F.V. (2002) Steroids, radiotherapy, chemotherapy and stents for superior vena caval obstruction in carcinoma of the bronchus: a systematic review. *Clin. Oncol. (R. Coll. Radiol.)*, **14** (**5**), 338–351, http://www.ncbi.nlm.nih.gov/pubmed/12555872 (accessed 4 January 2014).

88 Lipschitz, D.A., Udupa, K.B., Milton, K.Y. *et al.* (1984) Effect of age on hematopoiesis in man. *Blood*, **63**, 502–509.

89 Resnitzky, P., Segal, M., Barak, Y. *et al.* (1987) Granulopoiesis in aged people: inverse correlation between bone marrow cellularity and myeloid progenitor cell numbers. *Gerontology*, **33**, 109–114.

90 MacGregor, R.R. and Shalit, M. (1990) Neutrophil function in healthy elderly subjects. *J. Gerontol.*, **45**, 55–60.

91 Darowski, A., Najim, Z., Weinberg, J.R. *et al.* (1991) The febrile response to mild infections in elderly hospital inpatients. *Age Ageing*, **20**, 193–198.

92 Wasserman, M., Levinstein, M., Keller, E. *et al.* (1989) Utility of fever, white bloodcell, and differential count in predicting bacterial infections in the elderly. *J. Am. Geriatr. Soc.*, **37**, 537–543.

93 Norman, D.C., Grahn, D., and Yoshikawa, T.T. (1985) Fever and aging. *J. Am. Geriatr. Soc.*, **33**, 859–863.

94 Schoeinfeld, C.N., Hansen, K.N., Hexter, D.A. *et al.* (1995) Fever in geriatric emergency patients: clinical features associated with serious illness. *Ann. Emerg. Med.*, **26**, 18–24.

95 Guralnik, J.M., Eisenstaedt, R.S., Ferrucci, L. *et al.* (2004) Prevalence of anemia in persons 65 years and

older in the United States: evidence for a high rate of unexplained anemia. *Blood*, **104** (8), 2263–2268.

96 Astor, B.C., Muntner, P., Levin, A. *et al.* (2002) Association of kidney function with anemia: the Third National Health and Nutrition Examination Survey (1988–1994). *Arch. Intern. Med.*, **162** (12), 1401–1408.

97 Robinson, B., Artz, A.S., Culleton, B. *et al.* (2007) Prevalence of anemia in the nursing home: contribution of chronic kidney disease. *J. Am. Geriatr. Soc.*, **55** (10), 1566–1570.

98 Silver, B.J. and Zuckerman, K.S. (1980) Aplastic anemia: recent advances in pathogenesis and treatment. *Med. Clin. North Am.*, **64**, 607.

99 Lipschitz, D.A., Mitchell, C.O., and Thompson, C. (1981) The anemia of senescence. *Am. J. Hematol.*, **11**, 47–54.

100 Retzlaff, J.A., Hagedorn, A.B., and Bartholomew, L.G. (1961) Abdominal exploration for gastrointestinal bleeding of obscure origin. *J. Am. Med. Assoc.*, **177**, 104–107.

101 Coban, E., Timuragaoglu, A., and Meric, M. (2003) Iron deficiency anemia in the elderly: prevalence and endoscopic evaluation of the gastrointestinal tract in outpatients. *Acta Haematol.*, **110** (1), 25–28.

102 Pfeiffer, C.M., Caudill, S.P., Gunter, E.W. *et al* (2005) Biochemical indicators of B vitamin status in the US population after folic acid fortification: results from the National Health and Nutrition Examination Survey 1999–2000. *Am. J. Clin. Nutr.*, **82** (2), 442–450.

103 Wood, A.J. (2004) Treatment of von Willebrand's disease. *N. Engl. J. Med.*, **351**, 683–694.

104 Federici, A.B., Rand, J.H., Bucciarelli, P. *et al.* (2000) Acquired von Willebrand syndrome: data from an international registry. *Thromb. Haemost.*, **84**, 345–349.

105 Michel, M. (2009) Immune thrombocytopenic purpura: epidemiology and implications for patients. *Eur. J. Haematol.*, **82** (s71), 3–7.

106 Neylon, A.J., Saunders, P.W.G., Howard, M.R. *et al.* (2003) Clinically significant newly presenting autoimmune thrombocytopenic purpura in adults: a prospective study of a population-based cohort of 245 patients. *Br. J. Haematol.*, **122**, 966–974.

107 Frederiksen, H. and Schmidt, K. (1999) The incidence of idiopathic thrombocytopenic purpura in adults increases with age. *Blood*, **94**, 909–913.

108 Stasi, R., Sarpatwari, A., Segal, J.B. *et al.* (2009) Effects of eradication of *Helicobacter pylori* infection in patients with immune thrombocytopenic purpura: a systematic review. *Blood*, **113** (6), 1231–1240.

109 Franchini, M., Crurciani, M., Mengoli, C. *et al.* (2007) Effect of *Helicobacter pylori* eradication on platelet count in idiopathic thrombocytopenic purpura: a systemic review and meta-analysis. *J. Antimicrob. Chemother.*, **60** (2), 237–246.

110 Neunert, C., Lim, W., Crowther, M. *et al.* (2011) The American Society of Hematology 2011 evidence-based practice guideline for immune thrombocytopenia. *Blood*, **117** (16), 4190–4207.

111 George, J.N. and Aster, R.H. (2009) Drug-induced thrombocytopenia: pathogenesis, evaluation, and management. *Hematol. Am. Soc. Hematol. Educ. Program*, **1**, 153–158.

112 Arepally, G.M. and Ortel, T.L. (2006) Heparin-induced thrombocytopenia. *N. Engl. J. Med.*, **355** (8), 809–817.

113 Greinacher, A., Farner, B., Kroll, H. *et al.* (2005) Clinical features of heparin-induced thrombocytopenia including risk factors for thrombosis. *Thromb. Haemost.*, **94**, 132–135.

114 Amorosi, E.L. and Ultmann, J.E. (1966) Thrombotic thrombocytopenic purpura: report of 16 cases and review of the literature. *Medicine*, **45**, 139–159.

115 Terrell, D.R., Williams, L.A., Vesely, S.K. *et al.* (2005) The incidence of thrombotic thrombocytopenic purpura-hemolytic uremic syndrome: all patients, idiopathic patients, and patients with severe ADAMTS-13 deficiency. *J. Thromb. Haemost.*, **3**, 1432–1436.

116 Vesely, S.K., George, J.N., Lammle, B. *et al.* (2003) ADAMTS13 activity in thrombotic thrombocytopenic purpura-hemolytic uremic syndrome: relation to presenting features and clinical outcomes in a prospective cohort of 142 patients. *Blood*, **102**, 60–68.

117 George, J.N. (2006) Thrombotic thrombocytopenic purpura. *N. Engl. J. Med.*, **354**, 1927–1935.

118 Rock, G.A., Shumak, K.H., Buskard, N.A. *et al.* (1991) Comparison of plasma exchange with plasma infusion in the treatment of thrombotic thrombocytopenic purpura. Canadian Apheresis Study Group. *N. Engl. J. Med.*, **325**, 393–397.

119 Balduini, C.L., Gugliotta, L., Luppi, M. *et al.* (2010) High versus standard dose methylprednisolone in the acute phase of idiopathic thrombotic thrombocytopenic purpura: a randomized study. *Ann. Hematol.*, **89**, 591–596.

120 Kessler, C.S., Bilal, A.K., and Lai-Miller, K. (2012) Thrombotic thrombocytopenic purpura: a hematologic emergency. *J. Emerg. Med.*, **43** (3), 538–544.

121 Levi, M., Toh, C.H., Thachil, J. *et al.* (2009) Guidelines for the diagnosis and management of disseminated intravascular coagulation. *Br. J. Haematol.*, **145** (1), 24–33.

122 Philipp, C. (2010) The aging patient with hemophilia: complications, comorbidities, and management issues. *Hematol. Am. Soc. Hematol. Educ. Program*, **2010**, 191–196.

123 Tagliaferri, A., Rivolta, G.F., Iorio, A. *et al.* (2010) Mortality and causes of death in Italian persons with haemophilia, 1990–2007. *Haemophilia*, **16** (3), 437–446.

124 Soucie, J.M., Richardson, L.C., Evatt, B.L. *et al.* (2001) Risk factors for infection with HBV and HCV in a large cohort of hemophiliac males. *Transfusion*, **41**, 338–343.

125 Chorba, T.L., Holman, R.C., Clarke, M.J., and Evatt, B.L. (2001) Effects of HIV infection on age and cause of death for persons with hemophilia A in the United States. *Am. J. Hematol.*, **66**, 229–240.

126 Reitter, S., Waldhoer, T., Vutuc, C. *et al.* (2009) Survival in a cohort of patients with haemophilia at the haemophilia care center in Vienna, Austria, from 1993 to 2006. *Haemophilia*, **15**, 888–893.

127 Schutgens, R.E., Tuinenburg, A., Roosendaal, G. *et al.* (2009) Treatment of ischaemic heart disease in haemophilia patients: an institutional guideline. *Haemophilia*, **15**, 952–958.

128 Collins, P.W., Hirsch, S., Baglin, T.P. *et al.* (2007) Acquired hemophilia A in the United Kingdom: a 2-year national surveillance study by the United Kingdom Haemophilia Centre Doctors' Organisation. *Blood*, **109** (5), 1870–1877.

129 Delgado, J., Jimenez-Yuste, V., Hernandez-Navarro, F., and Villar, A. (2003) Acquired haemophilia: review and meta-analysis focused on therapy and prognostic factors. *Br. J. Haematol.*, **121** (1), 21–35.

130 Huth-Kuhne, A., Baudo, F., Collins, P. *et al.* (2009) International recommendations on the diagnosis and treatment of patients with acquired hemophilia A. *Haematologica*, **94** (4), 566–575.

131 Steensma, D.P. and Bennett, J.M. (2006) The myelodysplastic syndromes: diagnosis and treatment. *Mayo Clin. Proc.*, **81**, 104–130.

132 Steensma, D.P. (2009) The changing classification of myelodysplastic syndromes: what's in a name? *Hematol. Am. Soc. Hematol. Educ. Program*, **81**, 645–655.

133 Ma, X. (2012) Epidemiology of myelodysplastic syndromes. *Am. J. Med.*, **125** (7), S2–S5.

134 Hofmann, W.K. and Koeffler, H.P. (2005) Myelodysplastic syndrome. *Annu. Rev. Med.*, **56**, 1–16.

135 Malcovati, L., Della Porta, M.G., Pascutto, C. *et al.* (2005) Prognostic factors and life expectancy in myelodysplastic syndromes according to WHO criteria: a basis for clinical decision making. *J. Clin. Oncol.*, **23** (30), 7594–7603.

136 Rollison, D.E., Howlader, N., Smith, M.T. *et al.* (2008) Epidemiology of myelodysplastic disorders and chronic myeloproliferative disorders in the United States, 2001–2004, using data from the NAACCR and SEER programs. *Blood*, **112**, 45–52.

137 Vannucchi, A.M., Guglielmelli, P., and Tefferi, A. (2009) Advances in the understanding and management of myeloproliferative neoplasms. *CA Cancer J. Clin.*, **59**, 171–191.

138 Osborne, W., Jones, G.L., Jackson, G.H. *et al.* (2012) Myeloproliferative disorders in older people. *Rev. Clin. Gerontol.*, **22**, 108–118.

139 Marx, J.A., Hockberger, R.S., Walls, R.M. *et al.* (eds) (2010) *Rosen's Emergency Medicine: Concepts and Clinical Practice*, Mosby/Elsevier, Philadelphia, PA.

140 McMullin, M.F., Bareford, D., Campbell, P. *et al.* (2005) Guidelines for the diagnosis, investigation and management of polycythaemia/erythrocytosis. *Br. J. Haematol.*, **130** (2), 174–195.

141 Siegel, R., Naishadham, D., and Jemal, A. (2013) Cancer statistics, 2013. *CA Cancer J. Clin.*, **63**, 11.

142 Eichhorst, B., Dreyling, M., Robak, T. *et al.* (2011) Chronic lymphocytic leukemia: ESMO Clinical Practice Guidelines for diagnosis, treatment and follow-up. *Ann. Oncol.-Engl. Ed.*, **22** (Suppl. 6), vi50.

143 Brenner, H., Gondos, A., and Pulte, D. (2008) Trends in long-term survival of patients with chronic lymphocytic leukemia from the 1980s to the early 21st century. *Blood*, **111** (10), 4916–4921.

144 Abrisqueta, P., Pereira, A., Rozman, C. *et al.* (2009) Improving survival in patients with chronic lymphocytic leukemia (1980–2008): the Hospital Clinic of Barcelona experience. *Blood*, **114**, 2044–2050.

145 Vion Pharmaceuticals, Inc. (2009) *OnriginTM (laromustine) Injection for Induction Therapy for Patients 60 Years or Older with De novo Poor-Risk Acute Myeloid Leukemia*, July 30th, 2009. http://www.fda.gov/downloads/advisorycommittees/committees meetingmaterials/drugs/oncologicdrugsadvisory committee/ucm180497.pdf (accessed 7 October 2013).

146 Chen, C.-Y., Tai, C.-H., Cheng, A. *et al.* (2012) Intracranial hemorrhage in adult patients with hematological malignancies. *BMC Med.*, **10** (1), 97.

147 Chen, C.-Y., Tai, C.H., Tsay, W. *et al.* (2009) Prediction of fatal intracranial hemorrhage in patients with acute myeloid leukemia. *Ann. Oncol.*, **20** (6), 1100–1104.

148 Baccarani, M. and Dreyling, M. (2010) Chronic myeloid leukaemia: ESMO Clinical Practice Guidelines for diagnosis, treatment and follow-up. *Ann. Oncol.*, **21** (Suppl. 5), v165–v167.

149 Faderl, S., Talpaz, M., Estrov, Z. *et al.* (1999) The biology of chronic myeloid leukemia. *N. Engl. J. Med.*, **341** (3), 164–172.

150 Calabretta, B. and Perrotti, D. (2004) The biology of CML blast crisis. *Blood*, **103** (11), 4010–4022.

151 Ganzel, C., Becker, J., Mintz, P.D. *et al.* (2012) Hyperleukocytosis, leukostasis and leukapheresis: practice management. *Blood Rev.*, **26** (3), 117–122.

152 Porcu, P., Cripe, L.D., Ng, E.W. *et al.* (2000) Hyperleukocytic leukemias and leukostasis: a review of pathophysiology, clinical presentation and management. *Leuk. Lymphoma*, **39** (1–2), 1–18.

153 Fox, M.J., Brody, J.S., and Weintraub, L.R. (1979) Leukocyte larceny: a cause of spurious hypoxemia. *Am. J. Med.*, **67**, 742–746.

23 Elder abuse and neglect

Michael C. Bond & Kenneth H. Butler
Department of Emergency Medicine, University of Maryland School of Medicine, Baltimore, MD, USA

Section I: Case presentation

An 83-year-old woman was brought to the emergency department (ED) via emergency medical services (EMSs) after being found wandering the streets in her nightgown at 3:00 in the afternoon. She was disheveled and confused. The paramedics reported that a bystander had called after seeing the patient wander out of a wooded area onto the street. The paramedics further stated that the patient had no complaints except being thirsty, and that she was not a patient known by them.

The patient was unable to give much information, other than her name. She was disoriented to date, time, and place, and did not know the name of the president. In review of the medical records from prior ED visits, she was determined to have a history of multi-infarct dementia, hypertension, chronic obstructive pulmonary disease, and diverticulitis. The medical record also recorded a history of frequent falls.

Upon examination, she was a thin, disheveled, unkempt, malodorous woman in no acute distress. The initial vital signs were as follows: temperature 36.6°C (97.8°F), heart rate 94 beats/min, blood pressure 154/84 mm Hg, respiratory rate 18 breaths/min, and O_2 saturation 94% on room air. The lungs were clear, the cardiovascular examination showed a regular rate and rhythm without murmurs, gallops, or rubs, and the abdomen was soft and nontender. Of note on skin examination there were multiple bruises in various stages of healing, multiple small bumps resembling hives with excoriation consistent with flea bites as well as what appeared to be dried feces.

Laboratory studies were unremarkable except for an elevated serum sodium of 152 meq/l. Computed tomography (CT scan) of her head showed multiple prior strokes as well as a small, left subdural hygroma. The family was contacted, and the woman's daughter and care giver arrived from work, declined further care, and desired to take the woman home.

Section II: Case discussion

Dr Peter Rosen (PR): How is elder abuse recognized?

Dr Jon Mark Hirshon (JMH): To recognize abuse in any patient, first there has to be recognition that abuse occurs and a willingness to consider the reasons behind the abuse. I think it's easy to overlook neglect and abuse in the busy ED. When the story doesn't quite fit the picture of the medical condition being presented, you have to be aware that abuse or neglect could be occurring.

PR: Do we have any information about the status of the daughter? Is she a court-appointed guardian, or is she merely an available relative?

Dr Michael Bond (MB): The daughter is the primary caregiver, whether or not she has legal documents, is not known.

PR: Is there any way to determine the social circumstances of the patient short of asking the daughter?

Dr Andrew Chang (AC): The daughter ideally would be helpful, but the fact that she wanted to abruptly

Geriatric Emergencies: A Discussion-Based Review, First Edition.
Edited by Amal Mattu, Shamai A. Grossman and Peter L. Rosen.
© 2016 John Wiley & Sons, Ltd. Published 2016 by John Wiley & Sons, Ltd.

take the patient away would make me suspicious of her history, and what she'll be able to report. Nevertheless, we do get many clues based on the description of the patient – the bruising, the flea bites, the disheveled appearance, even the laboratory work – the high sodium suggesting she's severely dehydrated and not getting adequate water – all of these findings combined suggest strongly that she is neglected or abused.

PR: Although these findings suggest abuse, on the other hand, there are certainly elderly patients who refuse assisted care, and try to live by themselves even though they really are not capable. These patients escape from their caretakers and then appear neglected and abused. This can be very difficult to sort out.

Dr Scott Wilber (SW): I would agree; when you first see this patient, you have information that she is disoriented, and that she has been found wandering. We really don't know if this is an acute change, or a progression of her chronic condition. First, we must try to determine the chronicity of her symptoms. A similar patient could present who was not a victim of abuse and neglect, and we could find that this patient has delirium. Therefore, the workup must be dependent on the history that we get, as is typical in emergency medicine (EM). With this patient's history, initially the baseline mental status is not very apparent. But when the daughter arrives, I assume she says that the patient's mental status is unchanged from her baseline, and that's why she wants to take her home abruptly. I would postpone doing a CT scan until I found out whether this was an acute change.

PR: These are very difficult points to work through in many of these patients. Frankly, if this is chronic, if she has been consistently and severely impaired by her dementia, she is really not capable of taking care of herself. You probably wouldn't try to do surgery on her even if she were found to have a surgically correctable lesion. On the other hand, if this is an acute change you want to correct it, if possible.

JMH: I would offer a different perspective. If I'm working in a busy ED, and someone comes in with altered mental status whose baseline status I don't know, I'm going to be relatively aggressive, at least initially in the evaluation and management. This workup includes a head CT scan.

PR: This presents a very clear-cut difference in philosophy. I wish I had the time to get all of the information I needed, but while we're trying to find out the circumstances, we can get ahead of the game by completing our workup. I often find that in many of these patients we never resolve what's chronic and what's acute, but because I find many of the workups we do and the therapies we give to be futile, I'm a little slower to initiate them. Nevertheless, I don't think there's anything wrong with the initiation of such workups, it probably represents a difference in style rather than standard.

Dr Shamai Grossman (SG): This case takes us somewhat out of the traditional role of the emergency physician in that we have to step back and look at whether there are medical issues here, or whether there are social issues here. When we begin to address some of the social issues, this pulls us away from actually curing her medical complaints. The problem is that we sometimes lose sight of the medical problems completely. I think part of the conflict we are having with those of us, who might want to do a head CT and those who don't, is a need to avoid losing sight of the medical issues while considering that this could be a social problem rather than a medical issue in the first place.

PR: Does daughter have the right to refuse care for the patient?

SG: This takes us back to my previous point. Even getting a medical history can be laden with social implications. In this case, we have to wonder whether we can actually trust the daughter to be the right person to both describe the patient's baseline and ultimately refuse health care. This is the patient's daughter, and, of course, she should be speaking for the patient. Yet, when we start thinking about the social issues and what the patient looks like, we have to wonder whether the daughter is really acting in the best interest of the patient. Before we actually release this patient to the daughter's care, I think we need to take a step back and (1) make sure she really is the healthcare proxy and (2) begin to investigate whether she's actually doing her job. Even if she legally is her healthcare proxy, our job may be to keep her from remaining in that capacity.

PR: What sort of social resources would help you to resolve some of these difficulties and do you have any available in your particular ED that we might recommend?

MB: In our ED, we have social workers who can come see the patient; unfortunately, at our hospital they are only on site between 8 a.m. and 5 p.m. There is somebody on call after hours; they will typically ask to admit the patient, whether it meets medical necessity or not, and then they can take care of the issues the next day. There is also an Adult Protection Services that can come and investigate a complaint. With this case, in my mind at least, we can definitely debate whether this is abuse or neglect. I would like to caution people about using the word abuse because it sounds like something you're doing on purpose and has a negative connotation. A lot of this seems like neglect, and a lot of time neglect is not a willful act. You're just too busy, just don't have the time, or just don't realize the resources that are out there for you.

PR: I think those are very strong points and I think part of the problem here is that we just simply don't have enough information.

MB: Unfortunately, I think we are going to see a lot more of these cases because of the aging of the population. There aren't enough nursing homes or assisted living facilities to take care of all the elderly; more and more are going to be living in their family's homes. Unfortunately, in the United States, nuclear families have become disjointed, and there are fewer people in the home to take care of grandma as we used to do 30 or 40 years ago. For this reason, we might see more and more of these cases – not reflecting willful acts of neglect, but just a lack of resources or people not knowing how to get resources that could help their family.

PR: I agree that much of the problem is ignorance about what is available and that we have fewer and fewer resources available to us. But the other side of the problem is that often elderly patients have the financial resources – they own the home, they own the bank account, while the relatives who are trying to take care of them in fact don't have resources of their own with which to do it. I think that one of the problems here is the suggestion that social services would make us automatically admit such a patient, and I think our inclination as physicians is not to admit such a patient. Perhaps a better idea would be to place her in an observation unit overnight, and give

ourselves a chance to see what sort of social resources are available, what the financial circumstances are, and how we can make a more rational disposition of this patient.

SW: I would agree that from the standpoint of reimbursement across the United States, placing this patient in observation would probably be acceptable, while admission would probably not be acceptable. I do have to say that in this particular case, we have electrolyte abnormalities that may allow us to admit the patient with the assumption that we have some medical reason for hypernatremia, or there are some untoward effects with a sodium of 150. There are also financial implications for the patient regarding charges and copayments for observation versus full admission status. At our hospital, we've moved many resources from the hospital setting to the ED setting. Even if the patient goes to observation, everything is started and we don't have to wait till the next morning to begin addressing these issues. I think we're going to find that hospitals stand to benefit financially by avoiding a wasted 24 h of observation before a social worker sees the patient.

PR: I think it behooves us to work with our administration, and see if we can gain 24-h access to case managers and social workers because it has become such a financial burden on the hospital. If you think a patient is abused, what would be your next step?

JMH: As has been highlighted already, the key is to obtain a history to try to understand the social circumstances. If I determine abuse or neglect, depending on the jurisdiction, I would be obligated to report the person for further investigation. But how I might respond to neglect or abuse would be different. Neglect may be a question of getting social services to help in finding resources, whereas abuse may require a stronger intervention including keeping the person in the hospital or in observation while we sort all the issues out. In Baltimore, we would report to Adult Protective Services.

PR: I'm sure that this varies from jurisdiction to jurisdiction, and we should all find out what is available in our own communities as well as what are the legal responsibilities in our own communities, particularly as elder abuse seems to be more and more common. Just like with child abuse, there are some legal ramifications if you detect elder abuse and fail to report it.

MB: Concerning decision-making capabilities, I've learned over the years, not to ask the family members to try to make decisions, but more to just express what their loved one's wishes would have been. I try to take that decision-making away from them, and put it back on the patient where it belongs. Clearly, they still have to make some decisions, but I think it helps the conversation a lot if you can let them, act as a proxy, a voice, to let us know what the patient's wishes would have been.

SW: I think that's a very important point that we talked about in the ethics chapter. As a principle of ethics, we need to ask the family members to use substituted judgment. To substitute their judgment for what the patient would have wanted rather than doing what's in the patient's best interest or their own best interest.

PR: Tell us some further information on how the case evolved.

JMH: With the family present, we then consulted with social services and felt it was unclear as to whether it was neglect or active abuse. Therefore, the patient was hospitalized for the medical management of dehydration and hypernatremia while the social and legal issues were fleshed out.

PR: I think that's often going to be the safest course for most of these patients. Again, we are used to making decisions in EM with time constraints and without much information, but we have to remember that sometimes the best decision is to not make a decision at all, but to get more information. How can we get more information? The relatives are likely to be defensive, hostile, and not terribly communicative, what more can we do in the ED?

JMH: Trying to understand the social circumstances of individuals, as with much of EM, is a kind of a puzzle. I usually start by doing a search of the medical records. We're fortunate enough in Maryland to be able to access medical records from other hospitals, though the system is still relatively limited, but a broad review of what's available from a medical records perspective comes first. At the same time, I would also try to talk to the family. If I have concerns about the primary caregiver, I would try to get in touch with other family members. If those steps are not adequate, I would broaden my search to look

for any legal issues that might be involved as well. Yet, I find that in general once I've done a thorough review of the medical records and had a chance to talk with family members present and perhaps by phone, I have a sense of my level of comfort or discomfort concerning the patient's current condition. As with any type of history taking, if there is a lot of disconnects or inconsistencies, it raises my concern and my level of desire to get additional information.

MB: We as physicians need to feel very comfortable that if there is any doubt at all that abuse or neglect is occurring that we need to make a phone call to social work or adult protective services – you're not casting blame, you're not making accusations, you're saying that there needs to be a more thorough assessment, and then they can go and do a home visit. On the visit, they can see what's going on and see what resources they might need.

MB: In summary, we need to be more aware that elder abuse and neglect occur and that there are many different facets from physical to sexual, to financial abuse, but most of it is actually neglect. They are not willful acts but more acts of omission, where people just don't know how to care for the elderly, or don't have the time or resources. We need to be very aggressive in trying to get other resources – social work, adult protective services – to investigate and be there to provide additional resources and to educate the general public. Yet, I don't think we will ever be able to build enough nursing homes or assisted living facilities to house all of our elderly people, so more and more of them will be moving in with their children and grandchildren. With the aging of society, we will unfortunately be seeing this more and more commonly.

Section III: Concepts

Background

The elderly are the fastest growing segment of the US population due largely to aging of baby boomers, but also due to advances in health care that has increased life expectancy. Members of the baby boomer generation currently account for 25% of the total US population, and this number will likely increase over the next decade [1]. According to the 2010 US census data, individuals older than 65 years constitute the fastest growing segment of our population [2, 3]. The population of individuals older than 65 increased 15.1% and those between 85 and 94 years (the old–old) increased 29.9% compared to the census in 2000. This is in comparison to the entire US census growing only 9.7% over the same decade [2]. A United Nations report predicts that by 2050, 22% of the world population will be 60 years or older, doubling the 2009 global population of older adults [4]. The number of elderly who are going to require some assistance with their care and daily needs is also going to increase. Some of these needs will be met by assisted living facilities and nursing homes, but many elderly individuals are going to rely on family and friends for assistance. This is extremely important, as most perpetrators of elder abuse and neglect are family and friends, and not employees of healthcare facilities [5].

The true incidence and prevalence of elder abuse may never be known. This is mostly due to the fact that many cases are not reported and others go unrecognized. The National Elder Mistreatment Study reports that approximately 11% of US elders have experienced some type of abuse or neglect over the previous year, and Lachs and Pillmer estimate the prevalence of elder abuse to be between 2% and 10% in 2004 [6, 7]. These estimates are thought to be low, as several authors suspect that as few as 1 in 5 to 1 in 14 cases of elder abuse are actually reported to authorities [5, 8, 9]. The best, most recent data that is available on the incidence of elder abuse is from the Adult Protective Services program that reports there were 381,430 cases of elder abuse and neglect in the United States in 2003 [10]. However, if abuse and neglect truly has an incidence of 11%, the 2010 census data would suggest that we could be seeing approximately 4.4 million cases of elder abuse and neglect per year. Clearly, this is a major public health problem that needs better recognition and resources.

Unfortunately, most of the "abuse" cases are not acts of commission but rather acts of omission, where the family neglects the patient and does not provide for the daily needs. This can be due to limited resources (i.e., food, money, heat, and shelter) or lack of knowledge of community resources that could assist the elderly and family. The neglect can also be due to the actions of the elderly person (i.e., self-neglect). Due to limited financial resources, many elderly may forego heat, water, medications, or other necessities in an attempt to make ends meet.

Key terms

Elder abuse and neglect can be divided into eight different types as defined by the National Center on Elder Abuse [11]. They are as follows:

- *Abandonment*: The desertion of an older person by an individual who has assumed responsibility for providing care for the older adult or by a person with physical custody.
- *Emotional or psychological abuse*: The infliction of anguish, pain, or distress through verbal or nonverbal acts. This is the second most common form of elder abuse, and can take on many forms (i.e., verbal harassment, belittling, threatening, and scolding). This type of abuse can be difficult to identify as the victim's reactions can range from withdrawal and apathy to worsening of cognitive function or new repetitive movements.
- *Financial or material exploitation*: The illegal or improper use of an older adult's funds, property, or assets. This form of abuse affects people of all socioeconomic statuses, and can be noted by sudden changes in the elder's bank account or will, bills not being paid, or lack of material goods (e.g., food and clothing) being provided to the victim.
- *Neglect*: The refusal or failure to fulfill any part of a person's obligations or duties to an older adult. Neglect is the most common type of harm, the hardest to prove, and can be intentional or unintentional [5, 12]. Intentional neglect would be the woeful failure to provide goods and services that are necessary for optimal health and safety of the victim, where unintentional neglect is often due to the inability to provide a resource or lack of knowledge on how to get a resource. Most neglect is unintentional, and the caregivers are providing the best care that they can, but might not have the knowledge, financial resources, or ability to meet all the needs of the victim.

Two specific forms of neglect are as follows:

- Psychological neglect includes the failure to provide social stimulation, imposed isolation, and restrictions on social interactions.
- Financial neglect includes the failure to use available funds for goods and services needed for an elder's health and safety.

- *Physical abuse*: The use of physical force that can result in bodily injury, physical pain, or impairment. Physical abuse can be the easiest to recognize, though several challenges can even make this form of abuse difficult to prove. These include the victim's reluctance or inability to report it, the difficulty in differentiating injuries sustained in a fall or accident from those that are intentionally done to the victim (e.g., thrown to ground). Patients with injuries should be interviewed separately from their care providers and asked about the infliction of abuse as both or either party may try to report an alternative explanation of how the injury occurred.

- *Sexual abuse*: Nonconsensual sexual contact of any kind with an older adult. This form of abuse is estimated to occur in only 1% of elderly patients making it the least common form of abuse, and often the most difficult to prove [13, 14]. Like most acts of abuse or neglect, the elderly are often reluctant to report that this has occurred. Be suspicious of any injuries to the genital or breast area. Sexual abuse can take many forms that include rape, sodomy, indecent exposure, or forced nudity. In some jurisdictions, suspicion of sexual abuse requires reporting to both law enforcement and social service officials. The most bothersome thing about sexual abuse is that the population that is least able to protect itself is also the least likely to see justice served. In 2001, Burgess and Hanrahan report the following [13]:
  - The older the victim, the less likely that the offender will be convicted.
  - Offenders are more likely to be charged with a crime if the victim has signs of physical trauma.
  - Victims in assisted living situations have a lower likelihood than those living independently that charges would be brought and the offender found guilty.

  Though the elderly are certainly entitled to engage in consensual sexual relations, patients with sexually transmitted diseases who lack the ability to consent to sexual relationships should have their case referred to the police or social services as a potential sexual abuse case.

- *Self-neglect*: A person's refusal or failure to provide him- or herself with adequate food, water, clothing, shelter, personal hygiene, medication, and safety precautions. Elder self-neglect is an important public health concern and is the most common form of elder abuse and neglect reported to social services, with the number of cases rising [10, 15]. Self-neglect can take on many different forms and includes everything from living without heat or water, to living in a home that is uninhabitable due to deterioration or infestation with insects or rodents, to not eating proper meals or having needed medications filled. Self-neglect is associated with increased rates of hospitalization (rate ratio 1.47, 95% CI 1.39–1.55 (CI = confidence interval)), mortality, and the severity of self-neglect is associated with the risk of death [16]. These patients also tend to use outpatient, emergency, and hospital services more, and are more likely to have an underlying mental disorder (e.g., dementia, depression, or substance abuse disorders) [16–18].

Elder abuse and neglect can be easily overlooked or forgotten, so it is imperative to remember that it exists and consider it as the underlying cause of an elderly person's condition. Oftentimes, the injuries or complaints can be attributed to falls, accidents, depression, or other causes, but an alert provider can pick up clues that suggest elder abuse or neglect. Some clues are inconsistencies in the history or on physical findings, vague complaints, frequent visits, lack of family presence, or an overbearing caregiver. A provider does not need definitive proof to report elder abuse but only needs to act in good faith when reporting to the appropriate authorities. It is up to the authorities to investigate the case and make a determination on whether abuse has occurred.

One of the biggest mistaken ideas about elder abuse is that it occurs predominately in nursing homes. Actually, less than 4% of elder abuse occurs in nursing homes, with most of it occurring in the patient's home by family members and friends [19, 20]. It is anticipated that the number of cases occurring in personal homes will increase with the aging of our population and an increased percentage of elderly being cared for by their families. Families that can afford paid care providers should know that they only account for 4.2% of abuse cases, where household members account for 89.7% of the cases (Table 23.1) [5].

Unfortunately, elder abuse does not fit a specific pattern, social or economic class, or a specific living situation that would make identifying it easier. Even though the elderly who are ill, mentally impaired, or depressed are at increased risk for elder abuse, any elderly person can be in an abusive situation, and no one is at

Table 23.1 Characteristics of perpetrators of elder abuse [5].

Men[a]	52.5%
Abandonment	83.4%
Physical abuse	62.6%
Emotional abuse	60.1%
Financial exploitation	59.0%
Neglect	48.6%
Age	
41–59 yr	38.4%
<40 yr	27.4%
>60 yr	34.3%
Race	
White	77.4%
Black	17.9%
Relationship	
Family member	89.7%
Adult child	47.3%
Spouse	19.3%
Other relatives	8.8%
Friend	6.2%
Home service provider	2.8%
Out-of-home service provider	1.4%

[a]Cases attributed to male perpetrators are listed by subcategory. Women had a lower incidence of abuse in all categories, except neglect, which was 52.4%.

zero risk. Everyone deals with the stress of caring for an elderly family member differently.

Section IV: Decision-making

The treatment of elder abuse and neglect is relatively straightforward. First, treat the presenting condition (e.g., trauma, dehydration, hypothermia, or medical illness) and then mobilize your support services (e.g., case management, social work, and adult protective services) to ensure that the elderly person will be cared for appropriately when discharged. The difficult part is recognizing that the elderly patient's condition is due to abuse or neglect.

Risk factors and recognition

One of the most important points in the recognition of elder abuse is that there is no stereotypical victim. Anybody can be a victim. Individuals from all races, cultures, and socioeconomic groups have

been victims, and the abuse can occur anywhere. People at increased risk include elderly women and the "old–old" (>85 years old) (Table 23.1) [18].

Risk factors for being a victim of elder abuse and neglect are presented in Box 23.1, and the risk factors for being a perpetrator are in Box 23.2. Some of the risk factors are not completely understood. It is unclear if poor health and cognitive impairment increase the risk of maltreatment by reducing the elderly person's ability to report the abuse or defend him- or herself from it, or is it the increased stress of the situation that causes the care provider to commit the abuse. Individuals who live alone are less likely to be abused though can still be the victim of self-neglect. Socially isolated elderly people are at increased risk as the abuse is less likely to be noticed by others. A history of violence, mental illness, alcohol, or drug abuse increases the risk of abuse [6, 21–26].

Box 23.1 Risk factors for elder abuse and neglect [27, 28].

- Decreased physical health (e.g., requiring more assistance with activities of daily living)
- Dementia or cognitive impairment
- Female
- History of violence
- Increased age
- Shared living arrangements
- Social isolation
- Alcohol or drug abuse
- Victim or caregiver with mental health or substance abuse issues.

Box 23.2 Risk factors for being a perpetrator [29].

- Alcohol and substance abuse
- Mental health problems (e.g., depression and personality disorders)
- Poor interpersonal relationships, premorbid relations
- Current marital, family conflict
- Lack of empathy, understanding of care needs and issues
- Financially dependent on victim.

Healthcare providers must be able to recognize the signs of elder abuse and neglect. Some red flags are highlighted in Box 23.3. Several screening tools have been designed to facilitate the detection of elder abuse. One that is easy to complete in the ED is the Elder Abuse Suspicion Index (EASI), which consists of the six questions presented in Box 23.4 [30]. Though this has not been validated in the ED setting, it has been validated in family practice offices and ambulatory care settings, demonstrating a sensitivity and specificity of 0.47 and 0.75, respectively. The EASI requires less than 2 min to complete. An answer of "yes" to one or more of questions 2–6 should prompt concern about abuse or neglect. Another screening tool created by the American Medical Association (AMA) consists of the nine questions presented in Box 23.5 [31]. An answer of "yes" to any one of these questions should raise concern and prompt a more thorough evaluation.

Box 23.3 Red flags of elder abuse and neglect [27, 32].

- *Signs of neglect*
  - Lack of medical aids (e.g., medication, walker, cane, and glasses)
  - Lack of adequate food, basic hygiene, heat, water, or appropriate clothing
  - Untreated medical issues (e.g., pressure sores, Foley catheters, or colostomy)
  - Confinement to a bed without assistance for long periods of time.
- *Signs of financial abuse*
  - Excessive financial gifts or reimbursements for care provided or companionship
  - Lack of amenities the patient should be able to afford (e.g., heat, water, and food)
- *Signs of psychological or emotional abuse*
  - Unexplained changes in behavior (e.g., depression, withdrawn, or altered mental status)
  - Isolation from family members and friends
  - A caregiver who appears to be controlling, demeaning, overly concerned about spending money, is verbally or physically aggressive toward the patient.
- *Signs of physical or sexual abuse*
  - Inadequately explained injuries (e.g., fractures, sores, lacerations, welts, or burns)

- Delay in seeking medical attention after an injury
- Unexplained sexually transmitted diseases.
- *General signs of abuse and neglect*
  - Incongruity between accounts given by the patient and caregiver
  - Vague or improbable explanations for injuries
  - Presentation of a mentally impaired patient without a care provider
  - Laboratory or radiology findings that are not consistent with the history provided.

Used with permission from Elsevier [3]. Originally adapted from Red Flags of Abuse 2012. Available at http://www.centeronelderabuse.org/docs/Red-Flags_2012.pdf.

Box 23.4 Elder abuse suspicion index (EASI) [30].

Questions 1–5 are answered by the patient. Question 6 is answered by the physician.

1 Have you relied on people for any of the following: bathing, dressing, shopping, banking, or meals?
2 Has anyone prevented you from getting food, clothes, medication, glasses, hearing aids, or medical care or from being with people you wanted to be with?
3 Have you been upset because someone talked to you in a way that made you feel ashamed or threatened?
4 Has anyone tried to force you to sign papers or to use your money against your will?
5 Has anyone made you afraid, touched you in ways that you did not want, or hurt you physically?
6 Doctor: Elder abuse may be associated with findings such as poor eye contact, withdrawn nature, malnourishment, hygiene issues, cuts, bruises, inappropriate clothing, or medication compliance issues. Did you notice any of these today or in the last 12 months?

The patient can answer "yes," "no," or "unsure." A response of "yes" on one or more of questions 2–6 should prompt concern for abuse or neglect.

Box 23.5 AMA screening questions for abuse [31].

1 Has anyone ever touched you without your consent?

2 Has anyone ever made you do things you didn't want to do?

3 Has anyone taken anything that was yours without asking?

4 Has anyone ever hurt you?

5 Has anyone ever scolded or threatened you?

6 Have you ever signed any documents you didn't understand?

7 Are you afraid of anyone at home?

8 Are you alone a lot?

9 Has anyone ever failed to help you take care of yourself when you needed help?

Book chapters and articles like this can educate the EM provider about elder abuse/neglect. However, education alone cannot increase the recognition of elder abuse, unless medical care providers actually have the time and resources to screen patients for this often occult problem. In the United States, the Joint Commission already requires that EDs screen all patients to ensure that they are not victims of abuse or neglect [33]. However, this typically just involves a nurse asking a simple question "Do you feel safe at home?", which is often not enough to identify all cases. Even worse, this is typically thought to be a domestic violence screen, but it is also meant to identify elder abuse. Moving forward, electronic medical records can be designed to prompt for elder abuse by incorporating one of the screening tools already discussed [34, 35].

Finally, in order to increase the chance of identifying elder abuse, a portion of the history should be conducted in private, without family members or care providers present, so that the EASI or AMA screening questions can be asked. A thorough physical examination should then be conducted. This includes completely disrobing the patient in order to visualize any signs of abuse. Bruises or lacerations in various stages of healing, burns, or injuries that are not consistent with the mechanism reported should alert the provider to potential abuse. Finally, decubitus ulcers, sores, dehydration, and poor hygiene should prompt concern for neglect or self-neglect.

Reporting of elder abuse

It is clear from the data that is available that elder abuse is a major public health concern that is underreported. Understanding why elder abuse is underreported and underrecognized can help providers develop tools and screening tests that can help overcome these hurdles. Some of the factors that are thought to contribute to the elderly not reporting or admitting to abuse are as follows [18, 36]:

• Fear of retaliation from the care provider

• Fear of being removed from their home and being placed in a nursing home

• Fear that their loved one, the care provider, will get in trouble with the law

• Embarrassment and shame over being abused

• Feeling that the abuse is deserved; poor self-esteem

• Inability to comprehend that the abuse has occurred or inability to communicate effectively due to cognitive or expressive dysphasia

• Denial.

A similar list can be made of factors that contribute to medical care providers not reporting elder abuse. They are as follows [18, 36]:

• Attributing a medical condition or accident as the cause of their injury resulting in failure to recognize the elder abuse

• Time constraints preventing asking the appropriate questions or making a report to the authorities

• Unfamiliarity with reporting laws

• Concern about one's own personal safety and fear of involvement

• Unfamiliarity with screening tools

• Unfamiliarity with available resources.

In order to help with the recognition of elder abuse, medical providers should be aware of the risk factors for elder abuse (Box 23.1) and the "red flags" of elder abuse (Box 23.2). In general, providers need to be suspicious of changes in personality, social isolation, and injuries that are not easily explained. Repeat ED visits should also prompt concern. Elder patients with mental health issues, dementia, or strokes that leave their ability to communicate impaired are at increased risk due to inability to comprehend their situation or inability to seek help. Medical providers should routinely ask about the elderly persons living situation. Some simple questions that can be asked to assess their living conditions are as follows:

- Do they live with anyone?
- Does anyone help them with their shopping?
- Are they having any trouble obtaining all of their medications?
- Are they able to maintain their home or apartment?
- Do they have all their basic necessities (i.e., heat and water)?
- Do they feel safe in their home?

Be aware of local reporting requirements and availability of resources that could assist the elderly. A provider does not need definitive proof in order to report a case but only needs to have a genuine suspicion. The authorities (e.g., adult protective services, social work, and police) will investigate the case, obtain additional information, and make a determination on whether abuse or neglect is occurring. Often, this simple intervention, even when there is no abuse present, is able to provide the elder person and the family a list of resources and programs that they would otherwise never learn about.

Legal implications

EM providers must be familiar with the laws in their state. Most states have mandatory reporting requirements for elder abuse and neglect. Physicians tend to be unfamiliar with these laws, and are *often* less effective than other professional groups in identifying elder abuse [37, 38, 27]. Most states that have mandatory reporting status grant immunity to providers who report their suspicions in good faith. State-specific information on reporting requirements is available on the National Center for Elder Abuse website: http://www.ncea.aoa.gov/ncearoot/Main_Site/Find_Help/State_Resources.aspx [39].

A 2004 survey of state Adult Protective Services programs shows that physicians make only 1.4% of the reports for elder abuse [10]. It is unclear if this is due to lack of recognition in general or if the reporting is delegated to other members of the healthcare team. In contrast, the most common reporters of elder abuse are family members (17.0%), social services representatives (10.6%), friends (8.0%), law enforcement officers (5.3%), and nurses/aides (38%) [10].

Even if an investigation does not reveal intentional abuse or neglect, it can be extremely helpful to the patient and family in identifying resources that they did not know existed through other channels (e.g., web search, social services, and physician referral).

As a final reminder, medical care providers who feel that a patient is at risk of continued harm, whether it is from neglect, self-neglect, or abuse, are obligated to protect the patient. This might necessitate hospital admission in order to sort out the social situation, and it could require assessment of the patient's decision-making capacity if he or she wants to leave against medical advice [40].

Conclusion

With the aging of our population, the prevalence of elder abuse and neglect will increase. We must improve on the underrecognition and underreporting of this condition. Increased educational efforts for healthcare providers, leading to increased awareness of this societal problem, are needed to protect our elderly patients. Physicians can make a huge impact on the quality of life of an elderly person by becoming familiar with the reporting requirements and the available assistance resources.

References

1 Report Elder Abuse (August 10, 2012) Nursing Home Neglect and Financial Exploitation. Elder Abuse Reporting. http://www.elder-abuseca.com (accessed 25 August 2015).
2 Werner, C.A. (2011) *The Older Population: 2010*, United States Census Bureau, Washington, DC.
3 Bond, M.C. and Butler, K.H. (2013) Elder abuse and neglect: definitions, epidemiology, and approaches to emergency department screening. *Clin. Geriatr. Med.*, 29 (1), 257–273.
4 United Nations, Department of Economic and Social Affairs PD (2009) *World Population Ageing 2009*, United Nations, New York, https://www.un.org/development/desa/publications/world-population-ageing-2009.html (accessed 10 September 2015).
5 US Department of Health and Human Services Administration on Aging and the Administration for Children and Families (1998) *The National Elder Abuse Incidence Study*, National Center for Elder Abuse, Washington, DC.
6 Lachs, M.S. and Pillemer, K. (2004) Elder abuse. *Lancet*, 364 (9441), 1263–1272.
7 Acierno, R., Hernandez, M.A., Amstadter, A.B. *et al.* (2010) Prevalence and correlates of emotional, physical, sexual, and financial abuse and potential neglect in the

United States: the National Elder Mistreatment Study. *Am. J. Public Health*, **100** (2), 292–297.

8 Davidson, J.L. (1979) Elder abuse, in *The Battered Elder Syndrome: An Exploratory Study* (eds M.R. Block and J.D. Sinnot), University of Maryland, College Park, MD, pp. 49–66.

9 Pillemer, K. and Finkelhor, D. (1988) The prevalence of elder abuse: a random sample survey. *Gerontologist*, **28** (1), 51–57.

10 Teaster, P.B., Dugar, T., and Mendiondo, M. (2012) *The 2004 Survey of State Adult Protective Services: Abuse of Adults 60 Years of Age and Older 2006 August 10, 2012*, http://www.apsnetwork.org/Resources/docs/AbuseAdults60.pdf (accessed 26 August 2015).

11 National Center on Elder Abuse (2012) *Major Types of Elder Abuse*, August 7, 2012, http://www.ncea.aoa.gov (accessed 24 August 2015).

12 Lachs, M.S., Williams, C., O'Brien, S. *et al.* (1997) Risk factors for reported elder abuse and neglect: a nine-year observational cohort study. *Gerontologist*, **37** (4), 469–474.

13 Burgess, A.W. and Hanrahan, N.P. (2001) *Identifying Forensic Markers in Elder Sexual Abuse*, National Institute of Justice.

14 Tatara, T. (1990) *Elder Abuse in the United States: An Issue Paper*, National Aging Resource Center on Elder Abuse, Washington, DC.

15 Dong, X., Simon, M., Mendes de Leon, C. *et al.* (2009) Elder self-neglect and abuse and mortality risk in a community-dwelling population. *J. Am. Med. Assoc.*, **302** (5), 517–526.

16 Dong, X., Simon, M.A., and Evans, D. (2012) Elder self-neglect and hospitalization: findings from the Chicago Health and Aging Project. *J. Am. Geriatr. Soc.*, **60** (2), 202–209.

17 Dyer, C.B., Goodwin, J.S., Pickens-Pace, S. *et al.* (2007) Self-neglect among the elderly: a model based on more than 500 patients seen by a geriatric medicine team. *Am. J. Public Health*, **97** (9), 1671–1676.

18 Abbey, L. (2009) Elder abuse and neglect: when home is not safe. *Clin. Geriatr. Med.*, **25** (1), 47–60.

19 Figart, J. (ed.) (2012) A Profile of Older Americans 2010, August 10, 2012, http://www.aoa.gov/aoaroot/aging_statistics/Profile/2010/docs/2010profile.pdf (accessed 10 September 2015).

20 Nasser, H.E. (2007) Fewer Seniors Live in Nursing Homes. USA Today (Sep 27).

21 Anetzberger, G. and Robbins, J.M. (1994) Podiatric medical considerations in dealing with elder abuse. *J. Am. Podiatr. Med. Assoc.*, **84** (7), 329–333.

22 Compton, S.A., Flanagan, P., and Gregg, W. (1997) Elder abuse in people with dementia in Northern Ireland: prevalence and predictors in cases referred to a psychiatry of old age service. *Int. J. Geriatr. Psychiatry*, **12** (6), 632–635.

23 Grafstrom, M., Nordberg, A., and Winblad, B. (1993) Abuse is in the eye of the beholder. Report by family members about abuse of demented persons in home care. A total population-based study. *Scand. J. Soc. Med.*, **21** (4), 247–255.

24 Homer, A.C. and Gilleard, C. (1990) Abuse of elderly people by their carers. *Br. Med. J.*, **301** (6765), 1359–1362.

25 Reay, A.M. and Browne, K.D. (2001) Risk factor characteristics in carers who physically abuse or neglect their elderly dependants. *Aging Ment. Health*, **5** (1), 56–62.

26 Williamson, G.M. and Shaffer, D.R. (2001) Relationship quality and potentially harmful behaviors by spousal caregivers: how we were then, how we are now. The Family Relationships in Late Life Project. *Psychol. Aging*, **16** (2), 217–226.

27 Lachs, M.S. and Pillemer, K. (1995) Abuse and neglect of elderly persons. *N. Engl. J. Med.*, **332** (7), 437–443.

28 Forum on Global Violence Prevention (2014) *Elder Abuse and Its Prevention*, National Academies Press, Washington, DC, http://www.ncbi.nlm.nih.gov/books/NBK189833/toc/?report=reader (accessed 10 September 2015).

29 Reis, M. and Nahmiash, D. (1998) Validation of the indicators of abuse (IOA) screen. *Gerontologist*, **38** (4), 471–480.

30 Yaffe, M.J., Wolfson, C., Lithwick, M., and Weiss, D. (2008) Development and validation of a tool to improve physician identification of elder abuse: the Elder Abuse Suspicion Index (EASI). *J. Elder Abuse Negl.*, **20** (3), 276–300.

31 Geroff, A.J. and Olshaker, J.S. (2006) Elder abuse. *Emerg. Med. Clin. North Am.*, **24** (2), 491–505.

32 National Center of Elder Abuse (2012) *Red Flags of Abuse*, http://www.centeronelderabuse.org/docs/Red_Flags_2012.pdf (accessed 25 August 2015).

33 Futures without Violence (2013) *Comply with the Joint Commission Standard PC.01.02.09 on Victims of Abuse*, http://www.futureswithoutviolence.org/section/our_work/health/_health_material/_jcaho (accessed 25 August 2015).

34 Bright, T.J., Wong, A., Dhurjati, R. *et al.* (2012) Effect of clinical decision-support systems: a systematic review. *Ann. Intern. Med.*, **157** (1), 29–43.

35 Kawamoto, K., Houlihan, C.A., Balas, E.A., and Lobach, D.F. (2005) Improving clinical practice using clinical decision support systems: a systematic review of trials to identify features critical to success. *Br. Med. J.*, **330** (7494), 765.

36 Kleinschmidt, K.C. (1997) Elder abuse: a review. *Ann. Emerg. Med.*, **30** (4), 463–472.

37 Blakely, B.E. and Dolon, R. (1991) The relative contributions of occupational groups in the discovery and treatment of elder abuse and neglect. *J. Gerontol. Soc. Work*, **17**, 183–199.

38 Clark-Daniels, C.L., Baumhover, L.A., and Daniels, R.S. (1990) To report or not to report: physicians' response to elder abuse. *J. Health Hum. Resour. Adm.*, **13** (**1**), 52–70.

39 National Center on Elder Abuse, Administration on Aging (2012) *State Directory of Helplines, Hotlines, and Elder Abuse Prevention Resources*, August 10, 2012, http://www.ncea.aoa.gov/Stop_Abuse/Get_Help/State/index.aspx.

40 Sessums, L.L., Zembrzuska, H., and Jackson, J.L. (2011) Does this patient have medical decision-making capacity? *J. Am. Med. Assoc.*, **306** (**4**), 420–427.

24 Geriatric emergency pain management case

Teresita M Hogan & Alexandra Wong

Section I: Case presentation

An 87-year-old woman presented to the emergency department (ED) after sustaining a fall. She reported that she lost her balance while getting out of the bathtub. She landed on her left shoulder, and now complains of severe pain in that shoulder. She did not strike her head. She denied loss of consciousness, headache, visual changes, nausea, vomiting, dizziness, weakness, or neck pain. She also denied chest or back pain. She was able to struggle to her feet, and called her daughter for help. Her daughter then drove her to the ED.

Her past medical history included hypertension, osteoporosis, gastroesophageal regurgitation disease, and bilateral cataract replacement surgery. Medications included bisoprolol fumarate, calcium and vitamin D, ranitidine, and Reclast injections annually. She lives alone in an apartment, manages activities of daily living (ADLs) and instrumental activities of daily living (IADLs) without assistance, and still drives but not at night or on expressways. She does note that she gets tired after doing laundry or carrying in her groceries. She does not smoke, and drinks occasional wine.

Physical examination was notable for a well-nourished woman, well-hydrated, nontoxic, and in obvious discomfort with left shoulder pain. She was oriented, coherent, and appropriate.

Her extremity examination is notable for left shoulder soft tissue swelling and ecchymosis; although there was no bony defect, she did have marked

tenderness to palpation of the shoulder diffusely. Any attempt to move the shoulder, and she would cry out and become diaphoretic. The remainder of her examination demonstrated no other focal tenderness or abnormalities. Neurologic examination was also normal, but she did not want to walk as it made her shoulder hurt too much.

Plain films revealed a nondisplaced fracture of the proximal humerus. Orthopedics recommended a sling and swath, pain control, and recheck with ortho clinic in 7–10 days. After application of sling and a total of 8 mg of morphine, the patient's pain was under control at rest, but she still complained of severe pain with attempts at ambulation.

The resident suggested prescribing hydrocodone applying the sling and discharging with follow-up as recommended by orthopedics.

Section II: Case discussion

Dr Peter Rosen (PR): Even though this appears to be a single organ injury in an elderly patient, how do you feel about the initial management of such a patient who herself appears to be focused on the target of the fall. As we all know, patients seem only able to complain about one bad pain at a time, but how far would you go with your workup of the rest of the patient?

Dr Scott Wilber (SW): The first thing to think about whenever we have a patient with a fall is the cause of

Geriatric Emergencies: A Discussion-Based Review, First Edition.
Edited by Amal Mattu, Shamai A. Grossman and Peter L. Rosen.
© 2016 John Wiley & Sons, Ltd. Published 2016 by John Wiley & Sons, Ltd.

the fall. From history and examination, it is important to evaluate why we think the patient fell. Frequently, we'll find other acute illnesses that precipitate a fall in the patient by causing weakness, and the one that always comes to mind the most is an acute infectious disease causing the patient to present with a fall, when in reality it is muscle weakness due to their infectious disease. I do think we need to consider other potential injuries. In this case, the resident discusses the idea of doing a head and neck computed tomography (CT) scan. I think we do need to think about whether it is necessary. We tend to have a low threshold for looking at other potential injuries in older patients especially if they have a distracting injury. In this situation, I don't see that there is evidence that the patient has any injury to the head. She says she did not strike it and there does not appear to be any evidence of head trauma or neck trauma. So in this patient, I probably would not immediately jump to evaluating and imaging the head and neck. I would probably try to achieve pain control, and do several repeat examinations to make sure that we are not missing something. In another patient who had evidence of more diffuse trauma, I would have a low threshold to image those areas.

PR: I think those are excellent points, as we have a patient whose history is very plausible. It is easy to lose your balance as you get older, and it is certainly easy to lose your balance in a bathtub; thus, the mechanism of injury here is quite compatible with what the patient says it is, as opposed to being induced by sepsis or cardiac dysrhythmia or some other problem. If this patient were taking an anticoagulant for some reason, given the same story, would you be more inclined to do a head CT?

Dr Maura Kennedy (MK): This depends on the situation. She is a great historian, and is very clear that she didn't hit her head; on the other hand, I am much more liberal with head CT scans when individuals are on anticoagulation so that if there was any hint that she might have hit her head, particularly in the setting of an anticoagulant, I would always do a head CT scan. It always raises the question, as well as whether you need to do a delayed head CT scan in patients taking warfarin, or if you need some additional discharge instructions because there is some concern for delayed intracranial hemorrhage. When I discharge a patient who is anticoagulated, who has had a head injury, I try to ensure that they have someone with them for the

first 24 h. Otherwise, I am obligated to watch them in the ED.

PR: I think you can put your brain in neutral and coast on a patient who is on an anticoagulant, and just go ahead and order the head CT scan. We also know that elderly patients frequently have no memory of the head blow that causes the subsequent subdural. Nevertheless, we have a patient here who is completely alert, who has no physical signs of head trauma, and who probably could be treated as a single organ trauma.

PR: Here is a patient who came to the ED with a chief complaint that her arm hurts. Could you tell me what your customary practice is, in regard to pain management in the patient while she is being worked up, and before you know the extent of the pathology?

Dr Ula Hwang (UH): The first important element of this patient's care is pain assessment. We want to, in some way, have her rate the pain, and give a description of the pain so that we have some baseline. This will enable us to evaluate whether this pain needs to be treated immediately. If we use a scale of 0–10 and the patient reports a 10, we may well conclude the patient needs treatment, whereas if someone else rates their pain a 2, we might be more inclined to hold off until the workup is complete. The next issue would be whether the patient desired treatment. It is always useful to ask the patient if they wish treatment, although some patients have to be encouraged not to be inappropriately stoic. The next important point in treating pain in the elderly is medication titration – "start low and go slow." I think this is particularly important in terms of analgesics that are chosen for patients. In our case under discussion, I would probably start the patient on a moderate-to-low dose of pain medication. You also need to assess dosage on the patient's size and underlying health status. Older adults have changes in their pharmacokinetics and pharmacodynamics, and this must be respected as you give analgesia. She is able to give a clear and convincing history of single organ trauma, and, therefore, I would start with 4 mg of morphine.

PR: Would you start pain medications before you obtained imaging?

UH: Yes, I would. I think in this case the pain treatment won't change anything in terms of imaging. The physical examination demonstrated a well-nourished, well-hydrated, nontoxic woman, who was in obvious discomfort with left shoulder pain.

PR: We are all familiar with the visual pain scale, and we all know that some patients will pick a level of pain that does not objectively appear to match the reason for the pain. Some patients do it because they want to get treated faster, and some patients do it because they don't think anyone will pay any attention if they don't have a major complaint, and some patients do it because they don't tolerate pain very well. On the other hand, there are patients who have what look like really painful injuries, who don't complain at all. Is there anything that you do to try to evaluate the patient's level of pain other than asking them what they perceive?

Dr Shamai Grossman (SG): I have not found pain scales to be particularly useful. They are reputed to be one of the few so-called objective methods that we have to actually evaluate patients for pain. Nevertheless, rather than being objective, I find that there is by necessity much subjectivity to them. I think that there are more and less stoic patients. If a patient appears to be in pain, I like to try to confirm this by speaking with them, by looking at the patient, by looking at their vital signs, and by examining them to determine if they are particularly tender. Although in our case, I really would not do too much manipulation to prove the pain, and certainly I would not try to make with her ambulate. If the patient is tachycardic or hypertensive, or tachypneic, it might imply that the patient is still in significant pain. That said, ultimately we rely on the patient's wishes since there are patients who simply won't want a lot of pain medication despite having a severe injury and an apparent great deal of pain.

PR: A lot of patients, especially older adults, may have underlying cognitive deficiencies, and they may not be able to report that they are having pain. We are going to have to assess them not necessarily just by numeric rating scales or their self-report. A lot of this may have to do with types of pain assessments that are specifically designed for patients who have cognitive impairment. I had a short hospitalization this weekend and there was a pain scale right in front of my bed. I was struck by how hard it was to distinguish between the levels of pain by the visual scale, and what was supposed to distinguish 9 from a 10 is that the patient

with a 10 was crying, and this degree of pain was rated as unbearable. I think that many elderly patients can't do that, and what they do present with is increased confusion, sometimes with erratic behavior because they are in pain, and they can't tell you about it.

PR: How would you feel about starting with a nonopiate for analgesia in this patient?

MK: I think that with the degree of pain that this patient appears to be in, a nonopioid analgesic alone is not going to be adequate. Certainly, in her discharge planning, I would encourage prescribing a nonopioid analgesic such as acetaminophen (APAP) around the clock rather than as an as-needed basis. I would schedule that analgesic so that she was routinely taking it, and then add on other analgesics as needed for pain. Specifically, as Dr Hwang noted, she will probably need analgesia prior to imaging. I suspect that a nonopioid analgesic is not going to provide adequate analgesia until she is immobilized. Once immobilized, it might be adequate, but I think she is going to need a more intensive analgesic, initially. But after imaging and immobilization, I would definitely implement a nonopioid analgesic, especially for her discharge planning.

PR: What do you like to start with?

MK: I would probably start with morphine at this stage. Fentanyl is also another good option given that it is short acting, but I would adjust the dose down generally choosing to give an older patient half the dose of what I would give a 30 year old. Also depending on weight, a frailer person definitely requires a lower dose.

PR: Would you prescribe it orally, intravenously (IV), or intramuscularly (IM)?

MK: Our patient already has an IV line in place. Given the need to get her comfortable quickly, and then obtain imaging quickly, I would start IV, but after imaging is done and we are looking toward discharge, my next step would be oral medications, both because they will provide a longer duration of pain relief, and importantly, to let us to know whether we can adequately control her pain in order to safely get her home.

PR: I don't disagree with any Drs Hwang, Grossman, and Kennedy's points, but what do we do with patients who have a reason for pain but need some kind of treatment besides pharmacology? In other words, you and I have both seen patients who have hip fractures or otherwise are very uncomfortable until some mild traction is placed on the fracture, and then they seem to be very comfortable. Do you ever take that into consideration before starting pharmacology or would you do both?

SW: My approach is to do both. I think that even when a patient has an injury that with reduction would have a reduction in pain, that patient still needs to have immediate pain relief. If I am worried about a patient's frailty, I might start with fentanyl. If I thought I was going to need moderate sedation later to put the patient to sleep, I could titrate fentanyl a lot better for pain control, and not worry about ongoing effects of a previously administered longer acting agent when I subsequently use, for instance, propofol or etomidate for a deep sedation procedure. I usually do these reduction procedures with a fairly significant sedation and treat them with analgesics as well as with a sedative agent, and here, fentanyl is my choice over one of the longer acting enteral opiates.

PR: I think those are good points. I was actually thinking of initial care as opposed to reduction or permanent casting, but let's say this patient came in with an obvious wrist fracture. I think it is very helpful to put a splint on the wrist and to put some ice on the wrist as well as to use pharmacology. I have seen many patients who came in complaining of a massive degree of pain, but after you get them splinted and iced, they don't need any medications.

SW: I think nonpharmacologic management of pain is great, and I do think that it is extremely important. It is always useful to relieve pain by splinting the fracture, placing the patient in a position of comfort, as well as by using elevation and icing. I would also consider doing a nerve block or an hematoma block to reduce the patient's pain. A femoral nerve block may be the best approach for that patient with a hip fracture whose analgesia is hard to control.

UH: The more ways we can directly block pain locally the better. If there is an option such as femoral nerve block we can provide analgesia without giving systemic medications. That is ideal in older patients, because they are often on multiple medications and

we cannot always easily predict how the analgesic medications.

PR: While I think that is often very useful, we also have to remember that the more we do to people, the more problems we have. For example, in this patient being discussed, you could do a very effective pain-relieving block with a brachial plexus block, but I think the complications of brachial block are so great that you really would not want to be dealing with any of them in this age patient, so I think that would preclude using it.

PR: Would you comment on inappropriate pain management? Although we've all agreed that we would want to start with low doses and reassess the patient often, but I see many physicians starting with much higher doses with different agents that are much stronger and much more long-lasting.

MK: With opioids, there are different degrees of strength; there are weaker opioids and stronger opioids. Codeine tends to be the next step in terms of strength of opioids, but often causes confusion, and generally doesn't provide good pain relief. Morphine and fentanyl are next up in terms of level of strength of pain relief, and after that hydromorphone. Thinking about IV pain medications, I think one of our common mistakes in the ED is dosing with 1 or 2 mg of hydromorphone because it sounds like a small number when actually it is a very large amount of narcotic medication. The equivalent is as much as 6 mg of morphine per milligram of hydromorphone.

PR: Would you also comment on nonopiates?

MK: APAP is a commonly used medication for geriatric patients with pain. It provides a mild degree of analgesia. Nonsteroidal anti-inflammatory drugs (NSAIDs), though we use them frequently in younger individuals, must often be avoided in older individuals because of the renal and gastrointestinal (GI) complications that they can produce. Nevertheless, in a situation, where you want plan to use them for a very short period of time, and where the anti-inflammatory effects are reasonable, you could consider using NSAIDs, but in general, I am less inclined to use ibuprofen for pain relief in older individuals. Some of the other medications that we use for pain relief, particularly for more neuropathic-type pain relief, such as tricyclic antidepressants (TCAs), have anticholinergic effects that older individuals often don't tolerate, so I don't typically prescribe those to my older patients.

PR: Many of my orthopedics colleagues don't like NSAIDs in any age group within the first 48 h post injury, because they think it increases bleeding at the site of the fracture. What do you do, if you have a patient who says : "a doctor gave me APAP, and I can't tolerate it, it doesn't do anything for me anyway. I've tried it for my arthritis and it never gives me any relief. The only thing that I get a relief from for my arthritis is Celebrex."

MK: In this particular patient presenting with a fracture, I would probably say that I don't think that is going to be the right choice for you right now. I would be concerned about the bleeding risk. I have frank conversation with patients at times when they request medications that I don't think are appropriate, or that I can't adequately monitor them for, and sometimes I say: "well, if that is something that your doctor prescribes you, I won't make a change to that, but I am not comfortable increasing the dose or prescribing that up-front," and I provide my explanation as to why.

PR: While I agree with you, I find that I don't have very many choices with which to help them other than opiates, and even opiates have severe complications.

PR: I was wondering whether you might consider using IV Tylenol, which was just approved by the FDA, and whether they have had any success with that particularly in the elderly as I have yet to use it.

SG: At our institution it is restricted, so we don't use it in the ED although I would say that the orthopedic surgeons find it particularly effective for postoperative pain

SW: I think IV Tylenol is a great idea, though I have no personal experience with it. I am laughing because yesterday I noticed a variety of articles about how doctors are advised not to use APAP anymore. This was not exactly what the FDA was saying, but it just tells me again, how hard our practice is when we have to deal with the Internet.

MK: I haven't had any direct experience in terms of doing a head-to-head comparison with pain relief, but I do know that IV APAP is very expensive, much more expensive than the oral or even rectal form. I think

that if cost weren't an issue, it is perhaps the safest drug we can use, I think that I would probably reach for it as a first-line pain medication, especially in older adults.

PR: We have a patient who responded pretty well to what is a modest amount of morphine. We know that the pathology is a humeral fracture, and we know that she is going to do pretty well with a splint and a sling, a swath and a sling. We also know that she is going to be uncomfortable as she starts moving about. Before we get into the issue of how she is to manage at home, would you consider admitting a patient like this to the observation (obs) unit for overnight care to make sure that you have the pain controlled, and to find out what in fact are the parameters of her mobility.

SG: That is an excellent suggestion. I think that this is a patient population that we often do admit to the obs unit for all those reasons, for pain control, for evaluation by our physical therapist for mobility and ability to care for themselves and as well as for case managers to get involved in the case to deal with some of the home care issues. The hours spent in the obs unit will give us a better idea of how well the patient can tolerate oral pain medication, and will also benefit the patient's ultimate disposition whether it is home, rehabilitation, or whether she will need full hospitalization for further pain control.

PR: How do you make it safe for the patient to be discharged? This is of particular concern when the patient lives alone.

UH: I think that of the key points mentioned here, the most pertinent one is having adequate pain control so that she is able to function. We have to remember this is a woman who lives alone, and prior to this ED visit, was pretty functional at home with regard to managing her own activities, the independent ADLs. I think the big concerns here are her ability to function at home, and now, the issue of her increased fall risk. She didn't have a prior history of falling, but she is going to be significantly at a greater risk now because she has the immobility of her left upper extremity. In this case, in addition to having a patient potentially to be put into observation, how are we going to manage her afterward? It is very easy to just say, ok, we are going to observe her, and then she is going to go home and have a 1-week follow-up with orthopedics, but how is she going to get from that day 2 to day 7 when she is supposed to follow up with orthopedics. In this particular case, the patient went to the obs unit, but then she was able to be transferred to a rehabilitation facility with social services assessment and assistance, and then from there, she went home with daily physical therapy and home assistance for her functional ADLs. Nevertheless, she still didn't have good pain control, despite having good follow-up, and despite having all of her care transitions managed. The patient continued to have a lot of pain that wasn't really managed that well thereafter.

PR: Those are all very important and useful points, and I would like to address two of them. First of all, this woman had a daughter, and in an institution where you don't have as much social services available to you, that this patient had, I would probably insist that the patient go to the daughter's home or that the daughter move in with the patient. I don't care what age you are, you cannot take care of your daily needs with one arm. It is just not possible and certainly not for a patient this age. I think a subsequent course is going to be mapped out by what kind of help you can arrange for her, and unfortunately this is the kind of patient where we frequently get into admission difficulties, because we don't have a relative who can move in with them or to whose home she could go, and there is no way to help a patient like this as an outpatient without getting 24-h assistance. Next, I would emphasize that orthopedics is often very stoic about a patient's agony, and they seem to think that just because they don't have to nail it, plate it, screw it, or cast it, therefore, it is a trivial injury, but while this wound would heal well in a sling and a swath, it is a particularly pain-inducing fracture. Every time the patient moves or turns during sleep, there is going to be an increase in discomfort. Therefore, this is one of those contentious injuries in which we may need to admit this patient for several days, just for pain control until we can get her to the point of function that she is in fact is comfortable without frequent doses of analgesia.

PR: What is your approach when you don't have major social service help?

SG: Unfortunately, it is more and more difficult to admit patients who don't have any clear indications, but in this patient, she clearly has pain that we cannot control in the ED. If I can't put that patient in the obs unit, then I will admit that patient for pain control, and that is still why we have inpatient beds. It is sometimes not safe to discharge a patient, and we all have to accept the responsibility for treating the patient until she can heal and resume autonomous living.

PR: What do you do about the issue of this patient deteriorating rapidly? She may have been functional at home, she may have in fact been taking care of herself quite well, but now we have removed her ability to do that. Dr Hwang mentioned that she has a great risk of falling again even if she doesn't take another bath, but what do you think about the other risks such as change in cognitive behavior, sundowning, and that sort of thing?

SW: Those are issues we do need to consider as well. Her medications could cause her to have delirium. It is possible we have missed some underlying reason for the fall that could cause her to become delirious, and I would really worry additionally when you place a patient like this into a sling and swath, giving them only one good arm, things like getting up from a chair are going to be extremely difficult for her. Moreover, it is going to affect her ability to ambulate, to transfer to toilet, and to get off of a toilet. When you are her age with one arm, every day activities may be very dangerous and difficult as well. There are many more issues here that are potentially problematic, and I think the best approach is, just what others have suggested at minimum, she is going to need some type of assistance with her ADLs. One way to test this, although a little more difficult with her shoulder, is have her do an informal up and go test where we have her seated, and see if she can get up out of a chair and walk with one arm.

PR: Would you like to summarize for us?

UH: This case presents an example of an older adult who comes in with severe pain secondary to a fracture. Not only do we have to deal acutely with the relief of her marked discomfort, but we have a lot to prepare for in regard to her decreased functional status, not just secondary to pain, but also due to the incapacitation of her injury.

PR: This is a tough case, she really needs some sort of rehabilitation or short-term nursing home placement just because she can't cook for herself, transfer to the toilet, or even get up and out of a chair, and is suddenly in need of 24-h assistance for probably a minimum of a week.

Section III: Concepts

Emergency pain management in older adults

Introduction

Pain is the most common chief complaint in Emergency Medicine (EM) [1]. Pain is also particularly common in the older adult population. About 40–50% of elderly patients presenting to the ED with pain are documented as having moderate-to-severe pain [2, 3]. The prompt relief of pain in the ED is important to patients, families, and regulatory agencies. In fact, all consider pain relief an important marker of quality of emergency care [4, 5]. Despite the prevalence and importance of quality pain treatment, little formal pain management education is provided in the training of emergency physicians (EPs).

Elder pain care is often quite complicated due to difficulties in pain assessment, medication management, side effects, and comorbidities, in addition to multiple elder-specific barriers. The complexity of elder patient care combined with lack of formal systematic education of providers causes ED elders to be at great risk for underassessment and poor pain treatment [2, 3, 6].

Poor pain treatment has many detrimental consequences. Unresolved pain has been linked with an overall decreased quality of life and is notable for its negative effects on elders' ADLs [7]. Furthermore, pain impedes the daily functioning of 25–50% of community-dwelling elders [8]. Decreased appetite, decreased socialization, depression, impaired ambulation, and impaired sleep have all been associated with the presence of pain [9]. Unresolved pain can precipitate a downward spiral resulting in sadness, illness, and even the untimely death of our elder patients. Recurring pain issues also result in increased healthcare utilization and costs [10].

To avoid these harmful consequences, quality pain management must be provided to ED elder patients. Quality ED pain management results from the smooth functioning of a multifactorial process that begins with the knowledge and skills of emergency healthcare providers and extends into coordinated processes, policies, monitoring, and reporting methods in ED operations. Many efforts to improve this multifactorial process exist. First, pain is often promoted as the "fifth vital sign" [11]. Toolkits have been developed facilitating the routine practice of ED pain score documentation [12]. In addition, organizations such as the American Pain Society (APS) [13], Agency for Healthcare Policy and Research (AHPR) [14], the Joint Commission on Accreditation of Healthcare Organizations (JCAHO), Institute of Medicine [15], and the American Geriatrics Society (AGS) [10] have published clinical guidelines for managing, treating, and controlling the pain of elderly patients.

As an example of one process, in 2005, the APS updated their clinical guidelines for pain management [13]. This includes the following:

1 Providers must recognize and treat pain promptly.
   a. This recognition is enabled through the performance of a comprehensive pain assessment.
   b. Providers must initiate preventive and prompt treatment.
2 Providers must involve patients and families in pain management plan.
   a. Customize care to the individual patient.
   b. Patients should participate in the development of the treatment plan.
3 Providers must improve their treatment patterns.
   a. Eliminate inappropriate practices.
   b. Patients should receive multimodal therapy.
4 Providers must reassess and adjust pain management plans as needed.
   a. Skilled providers respond not only to pain intensity but also to functional status and side effects.
5 Departments must monitor processes and outcomes of pain management.
   a. Quality indicators (QIs) and national performance indicators should be used in the evaluation of individual and department quality pain management.

Despite decades of the above educational and quality efforts to improve emergency elder pain care, over 40% of elderly patients receive analgesics at lower rates than younger adults and leave the ED with little or no pain relief [2, 3, 16–18]. This chapter is meant to enhance the competence of EPs in overcoming the many barriers to optimal emergent pain management of older adults.

369

Prevalence

Pain is prevalent among both nursing home and community-dwelling elders. Over one quarter of nursing home residents report or show signs of pain and over 30% of community-dwelling elderly report pain [19–21]. Abdominal pain and nonspecific pain are among the top 10 reasons older patients visit the ED [22]. Common ED presentations of pain include musculoskeletal pain, abdominal pain, and back pain, as well as fall-related pain [2]. The most common ED diagnoses of patients aged 65 and older include abdominal pain and fractures [22]. Fractures and falls are not only a frequent source of acute pain but are also problematic because of the subsequent loss of normal functioning [16].

Pain classification by duration

ED treatment of pain can be facilitated by classification of pain according to three duration-related categories and cancer pain [23]:

1 Acute
2 Acute exacerbation of a recurring condition
3 Chronic/persistent
4 Cancer pain.

Acute pain is defined as pain lasting from 0 to 7 days. Chronic pain typically lasts for months or years, or significantly longer than the expected time needed for resolution of pain due to an acute event [23]. Acute exacerbations of a painful recurring condition occur in diagnoses such as arthritis, gout, and migraine headaches. These exacerbations are defined by an increase from a baseline low-level pain or from a baseline pain-free state. Cancer pain is symptomatic of and related to a malignant disease. Cancer pain classically occurs until remission or death from the disease.

Barriers to elder pain care

The identification of barriers to care is often the first step in the improvement of care. The barriers to elder pain care are numerous and range from the individual person (provider/patient) to the system level. Providers must be aware of the classic barriers generally found in EDs as well as any site-specific barriers. Patient, caregiver, and provider misconceptions each pose barriers to pain management.

Ageism

One common misconception in all the groups above is that pain is a natural part of aging. This is false; pain occurs more often in elders because of its association with disease processes, but pain is not a necessary consequence of age alone.

Addiction

Misconceptions about addiction cause significant barriers to pain care. Elder patients commonly believe any opioid medication will cause them to become addicted; they prefer to bear pain than suffer addiction, and so avoid any narcotic use. Provider biases may also involve a fear of opioid abuse and prescribing opioids too broadly. Providers often hear of the rise in number of deaths resulting from prescription opioids, but less frequently consider the impact of untreated pain [24, 25].

Detection

Detection of pain in elders is difficult. Failure of detection means failure of treatment, and, therefore, this lack of detection must be understood and overcome. Providers may assume that a patient's lack of pain expression or failure to complain of pain indicates the absence of pain. Providers must therefore spend time and effort to elicit an appropriate pain history. This is difficult in a busy ED as it calls for providers to slow down, search for subtitle clues indicating pain and try varied approaches to communicate with these patients. Providers must know that elders are often afraid to express pain, fearing it represents serious illness they would rather deny. Stoicism is high in elder patients, as is the feeling that they do not want to trouble busy doctors and nurses or be a nuisance to anyone [26–28].

Subjective pain reporting versus objective pain observation

One of the most common barriers to appropriate pain management is the difficulty of communicating about a pain experience [29]. Pain is a subjective experience that to date escapes objective scientific measurement. Medical providers typically only know of the existence of pain because their patients report it. Therefore, in order to treat most pain, physicians must believe it exists as stated by the patient, as well as believe in the patient's self-reported pain intensity [14, 30, 31]. When providers do not trust this subjective report, or interpret objective patient behavior as contradictory to the self-report, patients receive less treatment and report less pain relief.

Although self-report is the gold standard for pain assessment [10], obtaining an accurate self-report from elderly patients can be a complex task [10, 28]. Many elders struggle to rate their pain on a numeric rating scale or have difficulty articulating the severity of their pain. These reporting difficulties often arise due to cognitive impairment, language barriers, other communication difficulties, or the many barriers described above [28].

Cognitive impairment

Another common barrier to elder pain care results from cognitive impairments. Patients with mild-to-moderate cognitive impairment are widely thought to be able to report a pain intensity level. Yet, no validated method exists to determine a cognitively impaired person's ability to self-report pain intensity [32]. Patients with cognitive impairment are at risk for underassessment and undertreatment. As a result, a number of tools have been developed to assess pain in cognitively impaired or nonverbal older adults [33, 34]. Based on a summary by Bjoro *et al.*, the most useful tools for ED evaluation of pain in the cognitively impaired include the Abbey Pain Scale, the Critical-Care Pain Observation Tool (CPOT), and the Algoplus [35–38]. All of these tools require an observation period of less than 1 min. The Checklist of Nonverbal Pain Indicators is appropriate for pain assessment in acute care settings and may be another useful pain assessment tool to use in the ED [39, 40]. Other pain scales that have been validated for use with cognitively impaired patients include the Assessment of Discomfort in Dementia Protocol, the Non-communicative Patient's Pain Assessment Instrument (NOPPAIN, the Pain Assessment Checklist for Seniors with Limited Ability to Communicate (PACSLAC), and the Pain Assessment in Advanced Dementia (PAINAD) Scale; however, many of these were validated in long-term care settings requiring too much time to be practical for use in the ED [35, 41–43].

In nonverbal or cognitively impaired patients, an attempt to obtain self-reported pain intensity should be supported by a search for potential causes of pain, observation of patient behavior, or surrogate reporting from a caregiver or relative [44]. The AGS has published a comprehensive list of cues indicating pain in cognitively impaired older adults [10]. Behavioral cues associated with pain in cognitively impaired older patients include facial expressions (i.e., grimacing and rapid blinking), body movements (i.e., guarding, changes in gait, and restricted movement), changes in interpersonal interactions (i.e., aggressive, withdrawn, and socially inappropriate actions), changes in activity patterns or routines (i.e., refusing food, changes to sleep/rest pattern, and sudden cessation of common routines), and mental status changes (i.e., crying, increased confusion, and distress). Verbal cues include grunting, groaning, noisy breathing, and being verbally abusive [10].

Medication side effects

Side effects are a concern with most pain medications, especially opioid preparations. Patients and providers alike fear effects such as respiratory depression, renal failure, injurious falls, constipation, vomiting, and delirium. Emergency providers often mistakenly believe that elderly patients cannot tolerate opioids. Many EPs are unaware of the many difficulties elders have with NSAIDs. These include congestive heart failure (CHF), renal failure, GI hemorrhage, risk of cardiovascular events, and multiple drug interactions. All these factors prevent relief from pain and suffering in vulnerable elder patients most in need of this care.

Provider knowledge gap

A lack of medical professional knowledge about specialized care for geriatric patients and a lack of standardized geriatric guidelines and protocols for pain management present other barriers impeding effective pain management [45]. Below are several areas that providers can quickly learn in order to enhance their skills in ED management of elder patients with pain. This begins with appropriate pain assessment, optimizing pharmacologic management of pain, and the standardized monitoring and reassessment of pain in the ED.

Pain assessment

Effective pain management is predicated on a comprehensive and thorough pain assessment. This comprehensive pain assessment enables the healthcare team to provide high-quality, individualized care [28].

1 *Establish existence of pain*: The goals of the comprehensive assessment are to first establish the existence of pain. Elder patients may not express symptoms at all or may not use the word "pain", and so their suffering may escape detection. Therefore, guidelines suggest using alternative words to describe pain such as "hurting," "aching," and "discomfort" [46, 47].

2 *Quantify the intensity of pain*: The second step is to quantify the intensity of the pain. Pain intensity is the most important component of the initial assessment because it guides the clinician's selection of pain treatment and establishes a baseline for measuring the progress of pain management. In most EDs, the triage nurse conducts the initial pain assessment and documentation. Intensity of pain is established through the use of pain scales as detailed in the section on Pain Scales.

3 *Document*: Documentation is critical to communication with the healthcare team, is often the essential step in the initiation of treatment, and is mandated by the Joint Commission. Documentation of pain existence and intensity facilitates high-quality delivery of pain relief. Multiple organizations such as AHCPR have established quality guidelines for documentation of pain assessment and the Department of Veterans Affairs has published a toolkit for implementing efficient methods of documenting pain scores in healthcare institutions [12, 14]. Establishment of pain intensity is a complex process often achieved through the use of scales as explained below.

4 *Complete the pain assessment*: After determination of the existence and intensity of pain, providers should determine the pain location, onset, duration, frequency, and exacerbating or relieving factors in addition to the consideration of preexisting conditions [48]. These are directly relevant to the history of present illness.Full pain assessment also includes past medical history, functional and psychosocial assessment, as well as physical examination. The past medical history and preexisting conditions are crucial for informing subsequent pain medication and treatment and avoiding any adverse drug–drug or drug–disease interactions.

A functional assessment should include assessment of the patient's cognition and physical function, particularly the patient's ability to perform ADLs, any sleep or appetite disturbances, and physical exercise habits. Psychosocial assessment should note depression, anxiety or issues the patient may have with lack of social support. It is in this assessment that goals of care and levels of tolerable pain for the patient can be established. Goals of pain are particularly important to help determine disposition and level of service needed upon discharge.

The physical examination should include musculoskeletal assessment as well as an assessment of mobility and balance. The timed "get up and go test" is a quick and easy way to gauge the elder patient's mobility and balance [49]. Assessing these factors is imperative because pain can lead to impaired mobility and falls in older adults [46, 48]. After a comprehensive pain assessment is documented, the next step is to attempt an analgesic trial to relieve the patient's pain [10, 32, 50].

Pain scales

The patient's self-report is the gold standard for pain assessment [10, 13]. A number of pain scales have been validated to enable the clinician to solicit a patient's self-reported pain intensity score that is useful for medication decision-making [10, 50, 51]. One-dimensional pain intensity scales, which include numeric rating scales, visual analog scales, verbal descriptor scales, and pictorial scales, are most practical for use in the ED [32, 52]. Although many scales have not been validated specifically for use with geriatric ED patients, the numeric rating scale and the verbal descriptor scale are the most commonly used in the ED setting. Multidimensional scales, such as the McGill Pain Questionnaire, take longer to complete and may not be practical for use in the ED when rapid pain assessment is necessary [32].

Numeric rating scale

The gold standard for patient self-report of pain intensity is verbal administration of the numeric rating scale [10]. Patients are asked to rate the severity of their pain from 0 to 10, 0 being no pain and 10 being the worst pain possible [10].

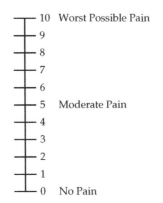

1. Do you have any pain or discomfort today?

2. Can you tell me about your pain, aches, soreness or discomfort?

3. Please point to the number that best represents the intensity of your pain or discomfort NOW.

Used with permission Keela Herr, PhD, RN, The University of Lowa, College of Nursing. December 2013

Visual analog scale

The visual analog pain scale is a 10-cm line with "no pain" marked at the left end and "worst pain possible" marked at the right end. Patients are asked to use a pen or pencil to mark the point on the line that best represents the intensity of their pain. The scale can be presented to the patient horizontally or vertically; however, studies found that patients prefer the horizontal orientation [28]. The visual analog scale has been shown to be a highly sensitive scale; however, it is not suggested for use with older adults because it is a relatively abstract tool and with a higher error rate than other pain assessment instruments [50].

Pictorial scales

We will discuss the two most commonly used pictorial pain scales, The Iowa Pain Thermometer and the Wong–Baker Scale. The Iowa Pain Thermometer uses a modified version of the verbal descriptor scale alongside a visual aid of a "pain thermometer." The pain thermometer indicates pain as cool to hot using seven different pain descriptors (most intense pain imaginable, very severe pain, severe pain, moderate pain, mild pain, slight pain, and no pain) that are presented on the right side of the image of a thermometer [50]. This thermometer scale has been validated for use with both younger and older adults [50]. The Wong–Baker faces scale is a popular example of a pictorial scale. This scale was originally developed for pediatric patients and consists of six images of faces expressing different degrees of distress. The faces are labeled as no hurt, hurts little bit, hurts little more,

hurts even more, hurts whole lot, and hurts worst [51]. Although some believe the Wong–Baker faces scale will be more easily understood by cognitively impaired adults, further evaluation of the scale for use with cognitively impaired older patients is needed [28].

Multidimensional scales

These scales assess qualities of pain other than intensity, such as sensory, affective, and temporal factors. The McGill Pain Questionnaire is a popular tool for pain assessment; however, it takes about 30–45 min to administer, making it impractical for use in the ED [32].

The Brief Pain Inventory is another multidimensional scale that was originally developed for cancer pain assessment and has been translated into over 10 languages. It has also been validated for use with patients who have chronic nonmalignant pain and may be a viable option for use in the ED when it is necessary to evaluate the impact of pain on a patient's overall quality of life [28, 32, 53].

Pharmacologic pain management for elderly patients

Geriatric considerations

The rate and intensity of adverse drug events (ADEs) is astounding; 700,000 ED visits and 120,000 hospitalizations annually are due to ADE, with elders affected twice as often as younger persons [54].

Well-meaning practitioners must become knowledgeable in aging pharmacokinetics and pharmacodynamics, so a drug they prescribe to help a patient does not cause that patient needless suffering or premature death.

Physiologic changes

The physiological changes that accompany aging and the potential for adverse drug–disease and drug–drug interactions must all be accounted for before prescribing pain medication. Drug absorption from the large intestine is largely unaltered in older patients, leaving them susceptible to harm from physiologic changes in drug distribution, metabolism, and elimination. Drug distribution is affected by changes in water, lean and fat mass composition. In general, older patients have more body fat and less water, causing a longer half-life and delayed distribution, especially for water-soluble drugs, such as morphine [29].

It is critical to understand that acute illness superimposed on an aging physiology can rapidly reduce renal clearance; this is especially true of any event causing acute dehydration. Dosage of medications must be further reduced for any elder with acute illness and dehydration.

The central nervous system (CNS) in elders is especially vulnerable to dangerous drug effects. Anesthetic, opioid, psychotropic, or anticonvulsant drugs may impede intellectual function causing anything from confusion, to agitation, to frank delirium; these agents also impair motor coordination causing accidents and falls with injuries that range from trivial to fatal. Reduced hepatic functioning is common with aging resulting in a higher risk for drug intoxication. Reduced renal excretion necessitates dose adjustment for many analgesics. Older patients often have decreased blood flow to the GI tract, which increases the risk of GI side effects, such as bleeding, constipation, and ulcerations, from common pain medications [45].

Frail patients are at great risk for decline in mobility and ADLs, as well as hospitalization and death [55]. Frailty is determined using the following characteristics: weight loss, loss of muscle mass, weakness (measured by grip strength), poor endurance, slowness (measured by a timed walk test), and low physical activity. If patients exhibit three or more of these criteria, they are categorized as frail [55]. ADEs occur more often and can be more devastating in frail elders.

Drug–disease interactions

Drug–disease interactions are common due to the prevalence of multiple comorbidities among older patients. Two thirds of American elders suffer from multiple chronic conditions [56]. Many of these preexisting conditions, such as CHF, peptic ulcer disease (PUD), and chronic kidney disease, may be exacerbated by pain medications and contraindicate the prescription of certain pain medications.

Drug–drug interactions

Polypharmacy causes enormous injury and even death in elder patients. Up to 30% of elderly patients presenting to the ED have been found to have potential adverse drug interactions on their medication lists, and prescriptions added during ED visits also create the possibility of adverse drug interactions [57–59]. The potential for adverse drug–drug interactions is common for older patients in need of pain relief. On average, older patients are taking from four to eight daily medications [57, 60, 61]. A thorough review of a patient's medications is necessary to avoid adverse effects of polypharmacy.

Strategies to decrease adverse drug reactions include the following:

1 *Use of the Beers Criteria*: The Beers Criteria for potentially inappropriate medication use in older adults compiled by the AGS is a listing of medications that should be avoided in elder patients. This is a straightforward and effective way to check medications that generally should not be used in elders and doses that may be inappropriate.

2 *Use of registered pharmacy consultants*: Review by experts of either individual patient prescriptions or ED-specific medication protocols commonly used by a group of emergency providers can prevent common ADEs by alerting providers to potential interactions.

3 *Computer-generated review*: Specific programs exist that may be utilized in clinical settings that automatically check for drug–drug interactions. These programs can automatically generate renal dosing guidelines.

Pharmacologic guidelines

Several organizations have developed standardized methods to address the pharmacologic treatment of pain. The most familiar of these is the World

Health Organization (WHO) pain ladder, which was originally developed for cancer pain, and has been adapted with recommendations for opioid use in elderly patients with noncancer pain. To guide appropriate pain medication selection, the WHO ladder groups pain intensity into three levels: mild, moderate, and severe [62]. It then suggests classes of drugs best suited to relieve pain for each intensity level. The AGS also published clinical practice guidelines for managing persistent pain in older patients [10]. Another useful tool takes the opposite approach, instead of suggesting the most appropriate drug the Beers Criteria provides a list of analgesics and adjuvant drugs to avoid in older adults, this list includes the level of quality of evidence and strength of recommendation for each drug. The Beers list was updated in 2012 by the AGS [63].

Pain medications can be broadly grouped into nonopioid analgesics, opioid analgesics, and adjuvants. Nonopioid and opioid analgesics are most effective in relieving nociceptive pain, whereas adjuvant medications are frequently prescribed for neuropathic pain. Nociceptive pain is signaled through the neural pathways, resulting from tissue damage or stimuli that are potentially tissue-damaging, whereas neuropathic pain results from a pathophysiologic abnormality in the peripheral or CNS and is caused by lesion or disease in the nervous system [10]. This clinical classification differentiates between pain resulting from a normal or abnormally functioning nervous system. Patients with nociceptive pain tend to respond well to conventional analgesics and nonpharmacologic interventions, whereas patients with neuropathic pain have been shown to respond to unconventional analgesia, particularly, adjuvant drugs.

Nonopioid analgesics

Acetaminophen (APAP)

APAP is the first line of medication for mild and moderate pain in elders. It is most appropriate for musculoskeletal pain, headache, earache, and low back pain. Patients must refrain from taking doses greater than 4 g every 24 h and must be careful to reduce the dose of APAP if they are consuming combination agents that may contain additional APAP. Dose reductions should also occur if a patient has acute hepatic failure or is taking large doses of APAP for a prolonged period [29]. Decreased hepatic phase II metabolism in elders increases risk of hepatotoxicity. Patients simultaneously taking anticonvulsants and oral anticoagulants, such as warfarin [64, 65], are at increased risk for adverse drug interactions.

Nonsteroidal anti-inflammatory drugs (NSAIDs)

NSAIDs are more appropriate for localized nonneuropathic pain, including acute headache, renal and biliary colic, and gout [8, 65]. Unfortunately, there are a number of contraindications and side effects for NSAIDs that are specifically severe in elders. Therefore, many physicians do not consider NSAIDs as the first line of medication for mild-to-moderate pain in older patients [66]. The prevalence of serious GI ADE in elders is twice that of younger patients. The AGS strongly recommends against prescribing NSAIDs for pain in the Beers Criteria for potentially inappropriate medication in older adults [63]. NSAIDs can have adverse interactions with angiotensin-converting enzyme (ACE) inhibitors, angiotensin II receptor blockers, diuretics, warfarin, corticosteroids, and other NSAIDs [65]. The potential side effects for NSAIDs include renal or liver toxicity, dehydration, cardiovascular complications, CHF, GI bleeding, and PUD [64–66]. NSAIDs are contraindicated in patients with these preexisting conditions. Because of the adverse GI side effects of NSAIDs, if the provider decides to prescribe an NSAID, proton pump inhibitors (PPIs) should always be added to decrease the risk of GI bleeding. PPIs, such as omeprazole, lansoprazole, or pantoprazole [67, 68], should be added even if the NSAID is in the form of COX2-specific agents (such as celecoxib or valdecoxib) [67–70]. Although PPIs decrease the risk of GI problems due to NSAID use, PPIs can have adverse interactions themselves. PPI are contraindicated in combination with oral anticoagulants, ACE inhibitors, diuretics, and glucocorticoids [65]. In addition, COX2-specific agents have similar side effects to nonspecific NSAIDs, such as cardiovascular complications and renal dysfunction [65]. There is strong evidence to avoid prescribing ketorolac in at least some older patients. Ketorolac increases the risk of PUD and GI bleeding in patients who are at high risk of developing these GI issues [63].

Opioid analgesics

Opioids are the recommended treatment for moderate and severe pain [29]. Studies comparing pain relief with opioids in older and younger cohorts reveal that elders respond just as well if not better to opioid treatment [71]. Short- and intermediate-acting opioids are ideal for acute pain relief. The most common opioids prescribed in the ED are vicodin, morphine, hydromorphone, and percocet [22]. Many opioids, including codeine, hydrocodone, and hydromorphone, are prodrugs that are metabolized in the liver to morphine, the active agent.

Morphine

Morphine is an effective pain reliever for moderate and severe acute pain that has been the mainstay of pain treatment for decades. The duration of morphine is about 4 h. Morphine is conjugated in the liver and the kidneys excrete its metabolites. Dosing adjustment should be made in patients with renal impairment as accumulation of morphine metabolites can cause CNS toxicity, manifested by jerks, delirium, or tremors. Cognitive function may be impaired for up to 7 days after a new dose, but after a few days of stable and moderate doses cognitive function is well maintained in elders [72]. Morphine is also a histamine releaser and may cause pruritus and hives; however, this is often a transient reaction and should not be considered an allergic reaction [65]. Other adverse effects include nausea and vomiting that can be decreased in oral agents by ingestion of food. Constipation can be a severe side effect and a bowel regimen is essential in all patients discharged with opioids. Although morphine is historically considered the opioid gold standard, its histamine and GI side effects indicate that it may not be the best option for older patients [64, 65, 73].

Dosage in elderly or frail patients is suggested to begin at 5 mg every 4 h to reduce drowsiness confusion or balance issues. The dose should be increased gradually by 33–50% with frequent reassessment of pain until the patient deems satisfactory relief. Total analgesia is not always possible or desired.

Codeine

Weak opioids are ideal first-line treatment for patients with moderate pain. Codeine is one of the weak opioids commonly prescribed for mild-to-moderate pain. Codeine's therapeutic effect is limited by its adverse GI side effects, making it impractical to administer codeine in doses greater than 60 mg [74]. Codeine's side effects include pruritus, nausea,

constipation, and dizziness. Studies have found that codeine works additively with APAP for analgesic effect, making oral codeine-APAP the prototypical form of opioids administered for moderate pain. Common oral formulations use codeine doses of 30 and 60 mg, which are combined with 300 mg of APAP. Limitations due to maximum recommended daily amount of APAP should be considered when prescribing codeine combination agents to avoid potential adverse effects of exceeding an intake of 4 g of APAP in 24 h.

Hydrocodone

Hydrocodone is a prodrug that is metabolized first to hydromorphone, then to its active agent morphine. Hydrocodone has also been found to have an additive analgesic effect with APAP and is commonly administered in the form of an oral combination agent. Common formulations include Vicodin (5 mg hydrocodone and 500 mg APAP), Norco (10 mg hydrocodone and 325 mg APAP), and Lorcet (10 mg hydrocodone and 650 mg APAP).

Hydromorphone

Hydromorphone is a prodrug that is ideal for moderate-to-severe acute pain. Side effects include nausea, drowsiness, and pruritus. Hydromorphone has been found to have few GI adverse side effects and may be more ideal for severe pain relief in older patients.

Oxycodone

Oxycodone is an opioid agonist suitable for moderate and severe pain. Its side effects include nausea, headache, drowsiness, and dizziness. Percocet, an oral combination agent, is formulated by 5 mg oxycodone and 325 mg APAP.

Tramadol

Tramadol is another weak opioid that can be prescribed for moderate pain; however, it can lower the seizure threshold and should be avoided in patients with past medical history of seizures. If severe pain is present or an attempt at pain relief using weaker opioids does not control the pain, strong opioids such as morphine are advisable. Morphine, oxycodone, and hydromorphone are recommended for breakthrough or acute recurrent pain although very few studies have focused on their use specifically in older patients [10, 29].

Meperidine

Meperidine should be avoided in geriatric patients because it may cause neurotoxicity, and there are many safer, more effective options [4, 10, 63].

Fentanyl

Fentanyl is a synthetic, lipid-soluble drug, which is most commonly administered in the form of an extended-release (q72 h) transdermal patch [65]. It is appropriate for both musculoskeletal and neuropathic pain. Due to its high potency, it should not be prescribed in opioid naïve patients [29].

Opioid dose adjustment in elders

Experts debate the most appropriate types of opioids for geriatric physiology and their specific dosages that should be used [64, 75]. Many advocate a "start low, go slow" procedure, lowering the dosage for a normal adult by 25–50% [64, 76]. Physiological differences in geriatric patients make timely reassessment after pain medication administration imperative. Pain should be reassessed 15–30 min after administration of IV opioids and 60 min after administration of oral medications. During reassessment and prior to discharge home, clinicians should document that there have been no adverse side effects from the analgesia.

Route of administration

When selecting the route of medication administration, the ideal choice is the least invasive method. In most cases, oral administration is the most convenient route of administration, making it preferable for older patients. Opioids can be administered orally, IM, IV, and intranasally. IV administration will provide the most rapid delivery of pain relief and is the preferable route of opioid delivery. IM administration should be avoided in geriatric patients because of prevalent muscle-wasting and loss of fatty tissue, which make the absorption time longer and delays the time it will take relieve a patient's pain [10, 29, 64].

Side effects of opioid medications

A number of side effects and risk factors accompany the prescription of opioids to older patients. Geriatric patients who are prescribed opioids are at risk for respiratory depression, delirium, sedation, nausea, and vomiting [75, 77]. Respiratory depression is of special concern in patients taking other CNS depressants and in those patients with underlying pulmonary diseases. Renal dysfunction, frailty, and the possibility of falling must be taken into consideration during pain management for geriatric patients. In these conditions consider both lower dose and longer dosage intervals [75, 78]. In older adults, constipation is one of the most common side effects of using opioids. A stool softener or laxative should be prescribed in conjunction with narcotics in any discharged patient.

Topical medications

It is important to understand the difference between transdermal and topical pain medication delivery. Transdermal medications are placed on the skin but are effective via systemic absorption to the general circulation and have systemic effects. Topical analgesia medications, however, do not depend on systemic absorption but act through diffusion to local peripheral nerves preventing pain transmission by suppressing sodium channels. Topical analgesia may only be effective if the site of pain is superficial. As no systemic absorption is found with the use of these topical analgesics, they can be useful in a wide range of patients who do not respond to other methods or in whom systemic medications may be contraindicated or targeted local therapy sufficient to control pain. Clinicians may consider topical agents in conjunction with other agents as part of a multimodal pain treatment protocol [79].

Topical NSAIDs

Many NSAIDs are available in a topical form and have been proved to reduce pain with the potential to reduce side effects. As a class, these topical NSAIDs are underutilized considering their effectiveness and lack of ADEs. Compared with APAP, topical NSAIDs yield three times the pain relief, in addition to providing improved function and decreased stiffness of the affected joints [80].

In the US, diclofenac sodium topical solution 1.5% and diclofenac sodium 1% gel are approved for osteoarthritis (OA) of the knee, ankle, foot, elbow, wrist, and hand. The American College of Rheumatology (ACR) 2012 guidelines recommends topical NSAIDs as a first-line treatment for OA among patients aged 75 years or older. In 2007, the diclofenac epolamine 1.3% topical patch (DETP) was FDA approved for acute pain due to sprains, strains, and contusions [81].

377

These topical preparations decreased the incidence of GI, cardiovascular, and renal events from those of oral preparations. Topical NSAID limitations include cost, creams and gels are associated with inaccurate dosing and need for frequent applications; this can be avoided by using a patch. However, patch use is limited in the hands [82].

Lidocaine

The second most common local pain medication delivered topically is lidocaine. It can be administered in a 5% plaster or patch. However, variable drug absorption, body mass issues, and delay in analgesic effects have been reported. Therefore, a microneedle-integrated transdermal patch was recently developed to overcome these issues [83]. Topical lidocaine has been found effective in the treatment of rib fractures, vertebral body fractures, OA, and chronic low back pain as well as in shoulder impingement syndromes [84, 85]. Lidocaine has also been suggested to treat postherpetic neuralgia; however, a recent Cochrane review casts doubt on the efficacy of this treatment [86].

Other topical agents

Topical rubefacients containing salicylate or nicotinate esters are not supported for acute conditions as they may predispose to salicylate toxicity and cause skin breakdown [87].

Capsaicin is available in a topical cream to provide relief for osteoarthritic and neuropathic pain. A single 60 min application of an 8% capsaicin patch produced significant relief in postherpetic neuralgia pain that was sustained for up to 12 weeks [88]. However, many patients experience an uncomfortable burning sensation after applying the cream.

Adjuvant agents

Adjuvant drugs were originally developed for a purpose other than relieving pain. Medications such as antidepressants, antiepileptics, and muscle relaxants are categorized as adjuvant drugs. TCAs are first-line drugs for treating neuropathic pain and should be considered even in older adults. Anticholinergic side effects can be limited by using secondary amines (nortriptyline and desipramine) [89]. TCAs can also be used in combination with nonopioid and opioid analgesics [10]. Antiepileptics, such as gabapentin

and pregabalin, are also good choices for relieving neuropathic pain [10, 45].

Nonpharmacologic interventions

Application of superficial cold or heat (ice or hot packs) is a potential source of pain alleviation. In addition, repositioning or applying a sling or wrap can be used as nondrug interventions in appropriate situations. Cognitive or psychological treatments, such as distraction and relaxation techniques, are also viable options for care post discharge from the ED. Although they are not appropriate for acute pain relief in the ED, many cognitive-behavioral therapies have been shown to be effective for older patients with chronic pain [90–92]. Studies have shown the benefits of physical activity on maintaining independent functioning and quality of life for elderly patients. The Arthritis Foundation provides recommendations for physical activity programs, such as water exercise, to alleviate the symptoms of OA [10]. Arthrocentesis is an option for patients who present with inflammatory knee pain. During arthrocentesis, the joint is punctured and synovial fluid is aspirated to provide therapeutic relief and occasionally is used for analysis. The risk of infection is low and significant adverse effects are rare. Medications, such as anesthetics, can also be injected into the joint space to provide pain relief for a more extended period [93].

Femoral nerve blocks have been shown to be an effective intervention for pain relief in elderly patients with hip fractures. Ultrasound-guided nerve blocks are a feasible option in the ED for pain relief [94, 95].

Discharge pain management

Discharge instructions

Good quality discharge instructions ensuring patient comprehension of ED diagnosis and directions for future care are essential to avoid unnecessary adverse health complications after an ED visit [4]. Studies have shown low patient comprehension of discharge instructions is common and even more problematic in elders [96]. In addition, only 20% of the patients who did not understand their discharge instructions were aware of this failure. Other studies have found a trend between patients who did not understand the diagnosis or did not understand the course of illness and their increased risk of return visit to ED or hospitalization within 90 days from discharge [97]. Patients' dissatisfaction with discharge instructions has also been correlated with patients not filling discharge prescriptions and missing follow-up appointments [98]. The Society for American Academic Emergency Medicine (SAEM) has recognized the need to improve physician–patient communication. A Task Force was established to develop guidelines for physician–patient communication in the ED. The Task Force recognized discharge instructions as an area for improvement in communication and developed recommendations for discharge planning [99]. More recently, the SAEM Geriatric Task Force also developed guidelines for ED discharge planning, specifically for geriatric patients [4]. A summary of clinical information from the ED visit should be sent to the patient's primary care provider (PCP), home care provider, or other downstream providers involved in transfer of care. Before discharge, medication reconciliation should ensure that the patient knows which medications to stop, start, or continue. A written list of medications and written discharge instructions should be provided to the patient; the provider should assume that the patient will not remember verbal instructions [99].

Providers must consider clinical, epidemiological, social, cultural, and economic factors that can impact an elder patient's adherence to discharge medications. Understanding barriers to adherence is necessary to ensure adequate treatment. Patients should know the relationship of the medication to pain relief. Either the patient or a caregiver should be able to verbalize time from taking the medication to expectation of pain relief, dosage schedule, and duration of pain relief. Extra caution is needed if patients are to self-adjust dosage according to the severity of pain. The typical prescription for combination opioids, which states "one to two pills every 3–4h as needed for pain," has much potential for error. Any drug dosage should be titrated to a clear clinical response. A careful practitioner will ensure follow-up discussion with a healthcare provider in 1–2 days after ED discharge to check on quality of pain relief and provide further instructions as appropriate.

Transitions of care

Each year, over 2 million residents from nursing homes or other institutions visit the ED. In many cases, the ED does not receive complete information from the nursing home regarding the patient's health, and conversely, nursing homes do not receive complete documentation of the care provided to the patient in the ED. The SAEM Geriatric Task Force identified QIs for the transition of care between nursing homes and EDs. When a patient arrives at the ED from a nursing home, the following written information should accompany the patient: (1) reason for ED visit, (2) code status, (3) medication list and allergies, and (4) contact information for the nursing home, the PCP or on-call physician, and legal relative or healthcare representative. When a patient is transferred to a nursing home from the ED, the EP should document communication with a provider at the nursing home or the on-call physician. The patient's paperwork should include an ED diagnosis and list of tests performed in the ED with all of the accompanying results.

Pain management monitoring and quality assurance

Only modest gains in ED pain management have been made despite two decades of efforts, leading many organizations and institutions to advocate for different tactics including the application of quality improvement methods to this area [15, 100]. ED providers must rapidly assess and treat a broad range of health issues in a high-stress, high-acuity environment [5, 101], while striving to make care safe, efficacious, patient-centered, timely, efficient, and equitable [101]. Therefore, quality efforts are best removed from the individual patient encounter and should center on staff education and monitoring of compliance with what has been taught.

Education is required because EPs are variably trained in how to best achieve appropriate initial pain control and how to ensure continued optimal pain relief upon ED discharge; this variability frequently leads to sustained pain and worsened physical function after discharge [102]. Although significant improvement in pain evaluation and treatment has been seen after institution of an EM resident and nursing pain education programs [103, 104],

379

education alone fails to achieve sustained behavior change in medical staff [105–107].

Enhancing staff skills in pain assessment by using pain scales increases the likelihood of analgesic administration in the ED [107]. Simple and easily applicable protocols for pain management permit satisfactory pain relief during a patient's ED stay [108]. These types of protocols have the potential to substantially improve pain management in diverse ED settings [109]. However, just as with educational change, adherence to these protocols must be monitored regularly in order to sustain optimal pain management [110].

It is clear; staff education and institutional protocols must be partnered with department operations via process and outcome measures. Process measures are considered more useful because they are more easily measured and sensitive to the quality of care, do not require substantial adjustment in their analysis, and can be addressed directly through provider action [4].

The question of what needs to be measured to ensure optimal ED elder pain management is paramount. Measurable targets include improved care through earlier and repeated pain assessment, optimizing medical management and enhanced disposition. Professional organizations have determined what markers best ensure the quality of elderly pain care in the ED. The SAEM Geriatric Task Force developed the following QIs for pain management of geriatric patients in the ED:

1 A formal pain assessment should be documented within 1 h of arrival.
2 If the patient remains in the ED for over 6 h, a second pain assessment should be documented within 6 h of arrival.
3 If the patient receives pain treatment in the ED, a pain reassessment should be documented prior to discharge home.
4 For patients with moderate-to-severe pain, pain treatment should be initiated or a reason why treatment was not initiated should be documented.
5 Meperidine should be avoided.
6 If a patient receives an opioid analgesic upon discharge, a bowel regimen should also be provided (or a reason documented as to why one was not).

In 2005, the APS also published six QIs for pain management [13]:

1 Intensity of pain documented with numeric or descriptive (mild, moderate, or severe) scale

2 Pain intensity documented in frequent intervals
3 Pain treated by route other than intramuscular
4 Pain treated with regularly administered analgesics; multimodal approach used when possible
5 Pain prevention and control to degree that facilitates function and quality of life
6 Patients are adequately informed and knowledgeable about pain management.

The QIs proposed by the SAEM Geriatric Task Force and APS highlight the need for pain assessment and reassessment documentation, as well as specialized treatment. SAEM focuses on timely initial pain documentation, whereas the APS emphasizes the use of a validated pain scale (numeric or descriptive). Tightly linking geriatric-specific pain education to routine monitoring of the above quality markers should achieve sustained clinical practice impact that will promote optimal, goal-directed, quality analgesia management for older adults in the ED.

Summary

ED providers must take action to improve the quality of pain relief delivered to older adults. Quality elder pain management requires specific knowledge and skills. However, despite enhanced education, efforts by professional organizations, and the generation of multiple care guidelines; failures in ED pain care are common and have serious adverse consequences. Improvements can be achieved through staff education, the early systematic use of patient self-report scales and the understanding of common barriers to care. Pain is a personal, subjective experience. Therefore, providers must find a way to meld the patient's self-reported pain intensity with their own observations and biases. Patients and caregivers should be involved in the selection of pain interventions and assist in the goals of care, so all have realistic expectations of what can and cannot be accomplished in the ED encounter.

Pharmacologic management should focus on the physiologic changes of aging, drug–drug, and drug–disease interactions in order to prevent adverse drug reactions and maximize pain relief through appropriate choice and dosage of analgesic agents. Topical and adjuvant agents should be considered along with nonpharmacologic interventions.

Thorough documentation from initial evaluation throughout the ED course to and including ED discharge and transitions of care are essential for ensuring patient safety and continued pain relief after departure from the ED.

Quality assurance programs must be used in conjunction with staff education in order to sustain improvements. SAEM and the APS have identified the performance measures most likely to improve quality of pain management in elder adults. These can be implemented in any ED to ensure maximal quality improvement. Training providers to provide specialized care for older patients, accompanied by ongoing monitoring of ED pain management processes, will enable healthcare systems to achieve and sustain high-quality standards of care for the aging population.

Section III: Decision making

- The delivery of good quality pain management requires providers to tailor pain assessment, treatment, and ED discharge to the needs of geriatric patients.
- Pain Assessment is key! Determine the existence and intensity of pain, establish pain location, onset, duration, frequency, and exacerbating or relieving factors in addition to what the patient has done to treat the pain so far.
- Determine the functional impact of pain and then titrate pain control to enable optimal function.
- Drug treatment in elders means providers must select the optimal age and disease-compatible drug and the lower age appropriate dose.
- When giving pain medications in elders, "Start Low (dose) Go Slow!"
- Departments should utilize QIs and benchmark national performance indicators to evaluate individual and departmental performance in quality pain management.
- Strategies to decrease adverse drug reactions include the use of (a) the Beers list, (b) registered pharmacy consultants, and (c) computer-generated review.
- Educate on discharge, ensure understanding and ability to adhere to recommendations.
- Coordinate a smooth transition of care and maintain pain control until the next provider contact.

References

1 Cordell, W., Keene, K., Giles, B. *et al.* (2002) The high prevalence of pain in emergency medical care. *Am. J. Emerg. Med.*, 20 (3), 165–169.

2 Hwang, U., Richardson, L.D., Harris, B., and Morrison, R.S. (2010) The quality of emergency department pain care for older adults. *J. Am. Geriatr. Soc.*, 58 (11), 2122–2128.

3 Platts-Mills, T., Esserman, D., Brown, L. *et al.* (2012) Older US emergency department patients are less likely to receive pain medication than younger patients: results from a national survey. *Ann. Emerg. Med.*, 60, 199–206.

4 Terrell, K., Hustey, F.M., Hwang, U. *et al.* (2009) Quality indicators for geriatric emergency care. *Acad. Emerg. Med.*, 16, 441–449.

5 Adams, J. and Biros, M. (2002) The elusive nature of quality. *Ann. Emerg. Med.*, 9 (11), 1067–1070.

6 Rupp, T. and Delaney, K.A. (2004) Inadequate analgesia in emergency medicine. *Ann. Emerg. Med.*, 43 (4), 494–503.

7 Cooper, J. and Kohlmann, T. (2001) Factors associated with health status of older Americans. *Age Ageing*, 30, 495–501.

8 Gloth, F. (2011) Pharmacological management of persistent pain in older persons: focus on opioids and nonopioids. *J. Pain*, 12 (3), S14–S20.

9 Bosley, B., Weiner, D., Rudy, T., and Granieri, E. (2004) Is chronic nonmalignant pain associated with decreased appetite in older adults? Preliminary evidence. *J. Am. Geriatr. Soc.*, 52 (2), 247–251.

10 American Geriatrics Society (AGS) (2002) The management of persistent pain in older persons. *J. Am. Geriatr. Soc.*, 50 (6), S205–S224.

11 Lanser, P. and Gesell, S. (2001) Pain management: the fifth vital sign. *Healthc. Benchmarks*, 8 (6), 68–70, 62.

12 Geriatrics and Extended Care Strategic Healthcare Group NPMCC (2000) *Pain as the 5th Vital Sign Toolkit*, October 2000.

13 Gordon, D., Dahl, J.L., Miaskowski, C. *et al.* (2005) American pain society recommendations for improving the quality of acute and cancer pain management. *Arch. Int. Med.*, 165 (14), 1574–1580.

14 Agency for Health Care Policy and Research APMGP (1992) *Acute Pain Management: Operative or Medical Procedures and Trauma*, U.S. Department of Health and Human Services editor, Rockville, MD.

15 Institute of Medicine (2001) *Crossing the Quality Chasm: A New Health System for the 21st Century*, National Academy Press, Washington, DC.

16 Hwang, U., Richardson, L.D., Sonuyi, T.O., and Morrison, R.S. (2006) The effect of emergency department crowding on the management of pain in

older adults with hip fracture. *J. Am. Geriatr. Soc.*, **54**, 270–275.

17 Jones, J., Johnson, K., and McNinch, M. (1996) Age as a risk factor for inadequate emergency department analgesia. *Am. J. Emerg. Med.*, **14** (2), 157–160.

18 Iyer, R. (2011) Pain documentation and predictors of analgesic prescribing for elderly patients during emergency department visits. *J. Pain Symptom Manage.*, **41** (2), 367–373.

19 Sengupta, M., Bercovitz, A., and Harris-Kjoetin, L. (2010) *Prevalence and Management of Pain, by Race and Dementia Among Nursing Home Residents: United States, 2004*, NCHS editor, Hyattsville, MD.

20 Reyes-Gibby, C., Aday, L., and Cleeland, C. (2002) Impact of pain on self-rated health in the community-dwelling older adults. *Pain*, **95**, 75–82.

21 Bernabei, R., Gambassi, G., Lapane, K. *et al.* (1998) Management of pain in elderly patients with cancer. *J. Am. Med. Assoc.*, **279** (23), 1877–1882.

22 National Center for Health Statistics (2010) *National Hospital Ambulatory Medical Care Survey: 2010 Emergency Department Summary Tables*, Hyatsville, MD.

23 Joint statement from American Society of Pain Management Nursing tENA, the American College of Emergency Physicians and the American Pain Society (2010) *Optimizing the Treatment of Pain in Patients with Acute Presentations*. Approved January 2010.

24 Centers for Disease Control and Prevention (CDC) (2011) *Vital Signs: Overdose of Prescription Opioid Pain Relievers–United States 1999–2008*.

25 Substance Abuse and Mental Health Services Administration (SAMHSA) (2010) *The DAWN Report: Trends in Emergency Department Visits Involving Nonmedical Use of Narcotic Pain Relievers*, US Department of Health and Human Services, Rockville, MD, June 18, 2010.

26 AGS Panel (2009) Pharmacological management of persistent pain in older persons. *J. Am. Geriatr. Soc.*, **57** (8), 1331–1346.

27 Hadjistavropoulos, T., Herr, K., Turk, D. *et al.* (2007) An interdisciplinary expert consensus statement on assessment of pain in older persons. *Clin. J. Pain*, **23** (1), S1–S43.

28 Herr, K. and Garand, L. (2001) Assessment and measurement of pain in older adults. *Clin. Geriatr. Med.*, **17** (3), 457–478, vi.

29 American Geriatrics Society (AGS) (2013) Guidance on the management of pain in older people. *Age Ageing*, **42**, i1–i57.

30 American Pain Society (APS) (1990) Standards for monitoring quality of analgesic treatment of acute pain and cancer pain. *Oncol. Nurs. Forum*, **17**, 952.

31 Pasero, C. and McCaffery, M. (2001) Pain control: the patient's report of pain. *Am. J. Nurs.*, **101** (12), 73–74.

32 Richards, C. (2005) Establishing an emergency department pain management system. *Emerg. Med. Clin. North Am.*, **23** (2), 519–527.

33 Husebo, B., Strand, L., Moe-Nilssen, R. *et al.* (2008) Who suffers most? Dementia and pain in nursing home patients: a cross-sectional study. *J. Am. Med. Dir. Assoc.*, **9** (6), 427–433.

34 Herr, K. (2010) Pain in the older adult: an imperative across all healthcare settings. *Pain Manag. Nurs.*, **11** (2), S1–S10.

35 Bjoro, M. and Herr, K. (2009) Chapter 5-assessment of pain in the nonverbal and/or cognitively impaired older adults, in *Current Therapy in Pain* (ed H.S. Smith), Saunders Elsevier, Philadelphia, PA, pp. 24–37.

36 Abbey, J., Piller, N., De Bellis, A. *et al.* (2004) The Abbey pain scale: a 1-minute numerical indicator for people with end-stage dementia. *Int. J. Palliat. Nurs.*, **10** (1), 6–13.

37 Gelinas, C., Fillion, L., Puntillo, K. *et al.* (2006) Validation of the critical-care pain observation tool in adult patients. *Am. J. Crit. Care*, **15** (4), 420–427.

38 Rat, P., Jouve, E., and Pickering, G. (2011) Validation of an acute pain-behavior scale for older persons with inability to communicate verbally: Algoplus. *Eur. J. Pain*, **15** (2), 198.e1–198.e10.

39 Bjoro, K. and Herr, K. (2008) Assessment of pain in the nonverbal or cognitively impaired older adult. *Clin. Geriatr. Med.*, **24** (2), 237–262.

40 Feldt, K. (2000) The checklist of nonverbal pain indicators (CNPI). *Pain Manag. Nurs.*, **1** (1), 13–21.

41 Snow, A., Weber, J., O'Malley, K. *et al.* (2004) NOPPAIN: a nursing assistant-administered pain assessment instrument for use in dementia. *Dement. Geriatr. Cogn. Disord.*, **17** (3), 240–246.

42 Fuchs-Lacelle, S. and Hadjistavropoulos, T. (2004) Development and preliminary validation of the pain assessment checklist for seniors with limited ability to communicate (PACSLAC). *Pain Manag. Nurs.*, **5** (1), 37–49.

43 Warden, V., Hurley, A., and Volicer, L. (2003) Development and psychometric evaluation of the pain assessment in advanced dementia (PAINAD) scale. *J. Am. Med. Dir. Assoc.*, **4** (1), 9–15.

44 Herr, K., Coyne, P.J., Manworren, R. *et al.* (2006) Pain assessment in the nonverbal patient: position statement with clinical practice recommendations. *Pain Manag. Nurs.*, **7** (2), 44–52.

45 Rastogi, R. and Meek, B. (2013) Management of chronic pain in elderly, frail patients: finding a suitable, personalized method of control. *Clin. Interv. Aging*, **8**, 37–46.

46 Royal College of Physicians BGSaBPS (2007) *The Assessment of Pain in Older People*, RCP, London.

47 Hadjistavropoulos, T. and Craig, K.D. (2002) A theoretical framework for understanding self-report and observational measures of pain: a communications model. *Behav. Res. Ther.*, **40** (5), 551–570.

48 Bruchenthal, P. (2008) Assessment of pain in the older adult. *Clin. Geriatr. Med.*, **24** (2), 213–236, vi-vi.

49 Podsiadlo, D. and Richardson, S. (1991) The timed "Up & Go": a test of basic functional mobility for frail elderly persons. *J. Am. Geriatr. Soc.*, **39** (2), 142–148.

50 Herr, K., Spratt, K., Garand, L., and Li, L. (2007) Evaluation of the Iowa pain thermometer and other selected pain intensity scales in younger and older adult cohorts using controlled clinical pain: a preliminary study. *Pain Med.*, **8** (7), 585–600.

51 Wong, D. and Baker, C. (1988) Pain in children: comparison of assessment scales. *Pediatr. Nurs.*, **14**, 9–17.

52 Bijur, P., Latimer, C., and Gallagher, E. (2003) Validation of a verbally administered numerical rating scale of acute pain for use in the emergency department. *Acad. Emerg. Med.*, **10** (4), 390–392.

53 Tan, G., Jensen, M., Thornby, J., and Shanti, B. (2004) Validation of the brief pain inventory for chronic nonmalignant pain. *J. Pain*, **5** (2), 133–137.

54 Budnitz, D., Pollock, D., Weidenbach, K. *et al.* (2006) National surveillance of emergency department visits for outpatient adverse drug events. *J. Am. Med. Assoc.*, **296**, 1858–1866.

55 Fried, L., Tangen, C., Walston, J. *et al.* (2001) Frailty in older adults: evidence for a phenotype. *J. Gerontol.*, **56A** (3), M146–M156.

56 2013 *Health, United States, 2012: With Special Feature on Emergency Care*, National Center for Health Statistics, Hyattsville, MD.

57 Hohl, C., Dankoff, J., Colacone, S., and Afilalo, M. (2001) Polypharmacy, adverse drug-related events, and potential adverse drug interactions in elderly patients presenting to an emergency department. *Ann. Emerg. Med.*, **38** (6), 666–671.

58 Chin, M., Wang, L., Jin, L. *et al.* (1999) Appropriateness of medication selection for older persons in an urban academic emergency department. *Acad. Emerg. Med.*, **6** (12), 1232–1242.

59 Beers, M., Storrie, M., and Lee, G. (1990) Potential adverse drug interactions in the emergency room: an issue in the quality of care. *Ann. Intern. Med.*, **112** (1), 61–64.

60 Nixdorff, N., Hustey, F., Brady, A. *et al.* (2008) Potentially inappropriate medications and adverse drug effects in elders in the ED. *Am. J. Emerg. Med.*, **26**, 697–700.

61 Stromski, C., Popavetsky, G., and DeFranco, B. (2004) The prevalence and accuracy of medication lists in en elderly population. *Am. J. Emerg. Med.*, **22**, 497–498.

62 Pergolizzi, J., Boger, R.H., Budd, K. *et al.* (2008) Opioids and the management of chronic severe pain in the elderly: consensus statement of an International Expert Panel with focus on the six clinically most often used World Health Organization step III opioids (buprenorphine, fentanyl, hydromorphone, methadone, morphine, oxycodone). *Pain Pract.*, **8** (4), 287–313.

63 American Geriatrics Society (AGS) (2012) American Geriatrics Society updated Beers Criteria for potentially inappropriate medication use in older adults. *J. Am. Geriatr. Soc.*

64 Ardery, G., Herr, K.A., Titler, M.G. *et al.* (2003) Assessing and managing acute pain in older adults: a research base to guide practice. *Medsurg Nurs.*, **12** (1), 1–18.

65 Innes, G. and Zed, P.J. (2005) Basic pharmacology and advances in emergency medicine. *Emerg. Clin. North Am.*, **23**, 433–465.

66 Barkin, R., Beckerman, M., Blum, S.L. *et al.* (2010) Should nonsteroidal anti-inflammatory drugs (NSAIDs) be prescribed to the older adult? *Drugs Aging*, **27** (10), 775–789.

67 Goldstein, J. (2004) Challenges in managing NSAID-associated gastrointestinal tract injury. *Digestion*, **69** (**Suppl. 1**), 25–33.

68 Rostom, A., Dube, C., Wells, G.A. *et al.* (2010) Prevention of NSAID-induced gastroduodenal ulcers. *Cochrane Lib.*, **16** (6), 1–68.

69 Chan, K. (2010) Celecoxib versus omeprazole and diclofenac in patients with osteoarthritis and rheumatoid arthritis (CONDOR): a randomised trial. *Lancet*, **376** (9736), 173–179.

70 Lovell, S., Taira, T., Rodriguez, E. *et al.* (2004) Comparison of valdecoxib and an oxycodone-acetaminophen combination for acute musculoskeletal pain in the emergency department: a randomized controlled trial. *Acad. Emerg. Med.*, **11** (12), 1278–1282.

71 Likar, R., Vadlae, E., Breschan, C. *et al.* (2008) Comparable analgesic efficacy of transdermal buprenorphine in patients over and under 65 years of age. *Clin. J. Pain*, **24** (6), 536–543.

72 Ballantyne, J. and Mao, J. (2003) Opioid therapy for chronic pain. *N. Engl. J. Med.*, **349** (20), 1943–1953.

73 Linklater, D., Pemberton, L., Taylor, S., and Zeger, W. (2005) Painful dilemmas: an evidence-based look at challenging clinical scenarios. *Emerg. Clin. North Am.*, **23**, 367–392.

74 Moore, A., Collins, S., Carroll, D., and McQuay, H. (1997) Paracetamol with and without codeine in acute pain: a quantitative systematic review. *Pain*, **70** (2–3), 193–201.

75 McLachlan, A., Bath, S., Naganathan, V. *et al.* (2011) Clinical pharmacology of analgesic medicines in older people: impact of frailty and cognitive impairment. *Br. J. Clin. Pharmacol.*, **71** (3), 351–364.

76 Lynch, T. (2011) Management of drug–drug interactions: considerations for special populations–focus on opioid use in the elderly and long term care. *Am. J. Manag. Care*, **17** (**Suppl. 11**), S293–S298.

77 Morrison, R.S., Magaziner, J., Gilbert, M. *et al.* (2003) Relationship between pain and opioid analgesics on the development of delirium following hip fracture. *J. Gerontol.*, **58A** (**1**), 76–81.

78 Miller, M., Sturmer, T., Azrael, D. *et al.* (2011) Opioid analgesics and the risk of fractures in older adults with arthritis. *J. Am. Geriatr. Soc.*, **59**, 430–438.

79 Pasero, C. (2013) Lidocaine patch 5% for acute pain management. *J. Perianesth. Nurs.*, **28** (3), 169–173.

80 Zhang, W., Nuki, R., Moskowitz, S. *et al.* (2010) OARSI recommendations for the management of hip and knee osteoarthritis part III: changes in evidence following systematic cumulative update of research published through January 2009. *Osteoarthr. Cartil.*, **18** (4), 476–499.

81 Lionberger, D., Lanzarotti, A., Piercahala, L. *et al.* (2010) Analgesic efficacy and safety of diclofenac epolamine topical patch (Flector Patch) by location of injury in trials of acute pain: a pooled analysis of five trials. *J. Appl. Res.*, **10** (3), 97–107.

82 Durand, C., Alhammad, A., and Willett, K. (2012) Practical considerations for optimal transdermal drug delivery. *Am. J. Health-Syst. Pharm.*, **69** (2), 116–124.

83 Kochhar, J., Lim, W., Zou, S. *et al.* (2013) Microneedle integrated transdermal patch for fast onset and sustained delivery of lidocaine. *Mol. Pharmaceutics*, **10** (11), 4272–4280.

84 Farr, B. (2013) Unclear study methods still confusing readers despite CONSORT guidelines (e.g., lidocaine patch does relieve pain of covered rib fractures). *J. Clin. Epidemiol.*

85 Radnovich, R. and Marriott, T. (2013) Utility of the heated lidocaine/tetracaine patch in the treatment of pain associated with shoulder impingement syndrome: a pilot study. *Int. J. Gen. Med.*, **6**, 641–646.

86 Khaliq, W., Alam, S., and Puri, N. (2013) WITH-DRAWN: topical lidocaine for the treatment of postherpetic neuralgia. *Cochrane Database Syst. Rev.*, **18**(Art. No.: CD004846), DOI: 10.1002/14651858 .CD004846.pub3

87 Hochberg, M., Altman, R., April, K. *et al.* (2012) American college of rheumatology 2012 recommendations for the use of nonpharmacologic and pharmacologic therapies in osteoarthritis of the hand, hip, and knee. *Arthritis Care Res.*, **64** (4), 465–474.

88 Irving, G., Backonja, M., Dunteman, E. *et al.* (2011) A multicenter, randomized, double-blind, controlled study of NGX-4010, a high-concentration capsaicin patch, for the treatment of postherpetic neuralgia. *Pain Med.*, **12** (1), 99–109.

89 Chai, E. and Horton, J. (2010) Managing pain in the elderly population: pearls and pitfalls. *Curr. Pain Headache Rep.*, **14** (6), 409–417.

90 Morley, S., Eccleston, C., and Williams, A. (1999) Systematic review and meta-analysis of randomized controlled trials of cognitive behaviour therapy and behaviour therapy for chronic pain in adults, excluding headache. *Pain*, **80** (1–2), 1–13.

91 Waters, S., Woodward, J., and Keefe, F. (2005) Cognitive-behavioral therapy for pain in older adults, in *Pain in Older Persons, Progress in Pain Research and Management* (eds S. Gibson and D. Weiner), IASP Press, Seattle, WA, pp. 239–261.

92 Morone, N., Greco, C., and Weiner, D. (2008) Mindfulness meditation for the treatment of chronic low back pain in older adults: a randomized controlled pilot study. *Pain*, **134** (3), 310–319.

93 Voll, S. (2013) Arthrocentesis: the latest on joint pain relief. *Nurs. Pract.*, **38** (9), 37–39.

94 Beaudoin, F., Nagdev, A., Merchant, R., and Becker, B. (2010) Ultrasound-guided femoral nerve blocks in elderly patients with hip fractures. *Am. J. Emerg. Med.*, **28**, 76–81.

95 Fletcher, A., Rigby, A., and Heyes, F. (2003) Three-in-one femoral nerve block as analgesia for fractured neck of femur in the emergency department: a randomized, controlled trial. *Ann. Emerg. Med.*, **41**, 227–233.

96 Engel, K., Heisler, M., Smith, D. *et al.* (2009) Patient comprehension of emergency department care and instructions: are patients aware of when they do not understand? *Ann. Emerg. Med.*, **53** (4), 454–461.e15.

97 Hastings, S., Barrett, A., Weinberger, M. *et al.* (2011) Older patients' understanding of emergency department discharge information and its relationship with adverse outcomes. *J. Patient Saf.*, **7** (1), 19–25.

98 Thomas, E., Burstin, H., O'Neil, A. *et al.* (1996) Patient noncompliance with medical advice after the emergency department visit. *Ann. Emerg. Med.*, **27** (1), 49–55.

99 Rosenzweig, S., Knpp, R., and Fereas, G. (1997) Physician–patient communication in the emergency department, part 3: clinical and educational issues. *Acad. Emerg. Med.*, **4**, 72–77.

100 Gordon, D., Dahl, J.L., Miaskowski, C. *et al.* (2002) A 10-year review of quality improvement in pain management: recommendations for standardized outcome measures. *Pain Manag. Nurs.*, **3**, 116–130.

101 Burstin, H. (2002) "Crossing the quality chasm" in emergency medicine. *Ann. Emerg. Med.*, **9** (**11**), 1074–1077.

102 Heins, A., Grammas, M., Heins, J. *et al.* (2006) Determinants of variation in analgesic and opioid prescribing practice in an emergency department. *J. Opioid Manag.*, **2** (**6**), 335–340.

103 Jones, J. (1999) Assessment of pain management skills in emergency medicine residents: the role of a pain education program. *J. Emerg. Med.*, **17** (**2**), 349–354.

104 Linkewich, B., Sevean, P., Habjan, S. *et al.* (2007) Educating for tomorrow: enhancing nurses' pain management knowledge. *Can. Nurse*, **103** (**4**), 24–28.

105 Davis, D., O'Brien, M., Freemantle, N. *et al.* (1999) Impact of formal continuing medical education: do conferences, workshops, rounds, and other traditional continuing education activities change physician behavior or health care outcomes? *J. Am. Med. Assoc.*, **282** (**9**), 867–874.

106 Leach, D. (2001) Changing education to improve patient care. *Qual. Health Care*, **10** (**Suppl.** 2), ii54–ii58.

107 Silka, P., Roth, M., Moreno, G. *et al.* (2004) Pain scores improve analgesic administration patterns for trauma patients in the emergency department. *Acad. Emerg. Med.*, **11** (**3**), 264–270.

108 Viallon, A., Marjollet, O., Guyomarch, P. *et al.* (2007) Analgesic efficacy of orodispersible paracetamol in patients admitted to the emergency department with an osteoarticular injury. *Eur. J. Emerg. Med.*, **14** (**6**), 337–342.

109 Yanuka, M., Soffer, D., and Halpern, P. (2008) An interventional study to improve the quality of analgesia in the emergency department. *Can. J. Emerg. Med.*, **10** (**5**), 435–439.

110 Stephan, F., Nicke, C., Martin, J. *et al.* (2010) Pain in the emergency department: adherence to an implemented treatment protocol. *Swiss Med. Wkly.*, **140** (**23–24**), 341–347.

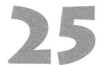

Ethical issues and end-of-life care

Phillip D. Magidson[1] & Jon Mark Hirshon[2]

[1]*Departments of Emergency Medicine and Internal Medicine, University of Maryland Medical Center, Baltimore, MD, USA*
[2]*Department of Emergency Medicine, National Study Center for Trauma and EMS, University of Maryland, Baltimore, MD, USA*

Section I: Case presentation

An 84-year-old woman presented to the emergency department (ED) at 2 a.m. via emergency medical service (EMS) transport with a complaint of shortness of breath and fever. The patient, who suffered from dementia and severe osteoarthritis, was a resident of a local nursing home. Per EMS report, the patient was found to be febrile to 38.6 °C (101.4°F) with increased work of breathing and worsening confusion by nursing home staff who called 911. EMS brought a packet of paper from the nursing home that included basic demographic information, an out-of-state niece's emergency contact information, and a list of medications, which included lisinopril, simvastatin, iron, ibuprofen, and docusate. There were no advance directives (ADs).

Evaluation of the patient revealed an elderly, frail-appearing woman who appeared sleepy, dyspneic, and in mild discomfort. Upon questioning, the patient knew her name only, and that her back and right knee were hurting. She was otherwise unable to tell you the date, her location, or any other medical history. She asked that you contact her daughter whose name she didn't remember. The vital signs were as follows: temperature of 39.1°C (102.3°F), blood pressure of 94/56 mmHg, pulse of 116 beats/min, respiratory rate of 24 breaths/min with accessory muscle use, and oxygen saturation of 87% on room air. Physical examination was notable for left lower lobe rales on pulmonary examination, and pain with passive movement of her right knee.

A quick call to the nursing home revealed the patient was confused at baseline, but able to answer basic questions. According to the staff, she normally would remember her daughter's name as the daughter visited twice a week and lived locally. No do not resuscitate (DNR)/do not intubate (DNI), AD or goals of care were known to the nursing home. They provided the daughter's phone number.

Section II: Case discussion

Dr Peter Rosen (PR): What's interesting to me about this case is how often we have to act in the ED with a paucity of information. Is it your custom to obtain an AD from every patient, or to find out about an AD before beginning to care for any patient? If not, in which ones do you do so and why?

Dr Jon Mark Hirshon (JMH): In Maryland, there is a relatively rigorous AD law, so people should come in with their ADs, particularly if they're coming from a skilled nursing facility. But, when do I access their directives? This depends on the clinical situation. I need to understand what the wishes of the patient and of the family are. These will be critically important in the decisions I'm going to make, the type of management we're going to offer, and how aggressive we're going to be with her care.

PR: When we have patients like this, it's easy to conclude that they are demented and that the quality

Geriatric Emergencies: A Discussion-Based Review, First Edition.
Edited by Amal Mattu, Shamai A. Grossman and Peter L. Rosen.
© 2016 John Wiley & Sons, Ltd. Published 2016 by John Wiley & Sons, Ltd.

of their life is terrible. This can inhibit what we try to attain for the patient. But, do you make an effort to distinguish between chronic problems that have an acute exacerbation or problems that have a quick reversal, without worrying about the underlying status of the patient's quality of life?

Dr Shamai Grossman (SG): Quality of life is truly a relative term. What one person might deem a poor quality of life for another might serve as something quite meaningful. It's a judgment that must be individually based. In the ideal situation, the patient has already set up a healthcare proxy or signed some sort of DNR/DNI form prior to resuscitation, enabling you to have some idea where the patient stands as far as quality of life goes. That said, when this doesn't exist, and a patient presents with symptoms that are readily reversible as opposed to say someone who has a terminal malignancy presenting in their end stages, I would be more inclined to aggressively attempt resuscitation.

PR: I think that those are very important points. We tend to confuse our personal attitudes toward quality of life with patient desires, and here's a patient who is not going to be able to express her desires even though she might have when she was well. In your institution, does a DNR order preclude your admitting a patient to the intensive care unit (ICU) or to the OR?

Dr Andrew Chang (AC): Yes, however, if the patient is DNR/DNI, we still have our critical care team come down to assess the patient, but generally we will not send that patient to the ICU, mainly for resource issues. They still will be admitted to a general medical ward on a ventilator if they're intubated. In terms of the OR, that is situation dependent, but, in general, after discussions the surgeon has with any family members or surrogates who are there, they will not go to the operating room.

AC: I think it becomes much more problematic when there's no conversation with family, when you're trying to do something with limited knowledge. In the case presented, until you reach the family, you have no idea what this person's wishes are, and you have to be relatively aggressive. But even in the setting of an executed DNR/DNI, depending on the quality of that document, it can be very confusing. Perhaps it's no measures at all. Perhaps it's antibiotics. Perhaps it's just no cardiopulmonary resuscitation (CPR). With the complexities of modern medicine, it becomes very

important to understand the person's wishes. Without that information, it becomes a more difficult process to try and decide the level of care and the amount of care that's appropriate for the patient.

PR: How do you feel about a patient who may be a little confused, but who is febrile and may well be septic as the source of the confusion? The patient seems to indicate to you that she wants help, but there is a relative there who says that the patient didn't want that and was going to fill out an AD, but never got around to it.

Dr Rob Anderson (RA): I think in that situation, my goal is to relieve suffering immediately when the patient comes in, regardless of what's going on. My second role is to try and educate the family as to what the patient's outcome might be. I feel like we're straddling the roles between paternalism and autonomy with these individuals, and trying to help the patient and the family understand what the disease course might be. In the case that you described, it might be reasonable to say: "Boy, I hear what you're saying, but I think that in this case we can really do some good for your loved one with some simple interventions."

JMH: One thing is important from an educational perspective. Advance directives are very nice, but you, as a patient, really need to have a healthcare advocate particularly if you're having significant interactions with the healthcare system. The healthcare system is very complex and the decisions are very complex, and so having someone to accompany you if you're making essentially lifesaving or life-denying types of decisions is very important. I think educating family to make sure that they have adequate support for their loved ones and for themselves is something that we as physician educators should be doing.

PR: I couldn't agree with you more that it really isn't done very well in our ICUs and in our private doctor's offices, and we see a large number of patients in the ED whose family doesn't understand what's happening, and are not in consonance with the patient, and trying to sort that out in the acute situation with the patient like this one, who is febrile and probably septic is very, very difficult. Have you experienced patients who you are told are either delusional or demented, but when you've treated the various diseases and they cleared up, they turned out not to be demented at all but actually had been having a chronic episode of disease that wasn't well managed?

SG: Absolutely. It's often very difficult to know what the patient's true mental status is and what the patient's true quality of life in the setting of acute disease. What we have found as well is that when you explain to a patient or family that resuscitating or intubating this patient in the ED will not necessarily cause undo distress but might bring this patient and her quality of life back to some prior baseline, they will often reverse a prior DNR order.

PR: I think that those are really critical issues that we can almost never define in the ED, and it certainly makes the case for ignoring some ADs, at least until you have a patient stabilized and treated acutely reversible conditions sufficiently.

PR: We have the opposite experience as well, families that continue to want everything done for a patient, who is either already dead or already so close to dying that it's a matter of just a short wait – do you have any suggestions for when you depart from family wishes from doing more to doing less?

JMH: Again, it's important to minister to the family as well as to the patient in that instance, and I try to educate the family to the best of my ability. There are times that you end up admitting people who you feel have a very unlikely chance of survival in the short term, but they're not there yet.

PR: What about patients who need an acute reversal as opposed to patients who have, say, metastatic prostatic disease or breast cancer in whom death might be a welcome end point – if you know that the patient has a DNR order, does it limit your diagnostic efforts on behalf of that patient even when you feel that you have an acute reversible condition?

Dr Scott Wilbur (SW): I think in those situations, I would still try to determine what the patient would have wanted, typically with a family member, and try to tailor the workup to what they would consider an acceptable evaluation. In my experience, most patients or proxies would say that doing blood work and a urinalysis, a chest X-ray study, and administration of antibiotics would be acceptable. I do think that even a patient in whom we think things are readily reversible though, the patient, through themselves or through the family, has the right to

say that he or she would not want to have a workup or treatment for pneumonia. We used to refer to pneumonia as "the old man's friend." I think that in a patient, for instance, who has dementia and continually aspirates, it may be reasonable to forgo even what we may consider simple treatments, so I think it does depend on the patient's wishes.

PR: Would you like to summarize the ethical position that we have dissected on this case? I think we are close to being done here.

SG: I think that all of us are faced with situations that are very similar to the case that we presented today on a daily basis. Each of us, when that patient arrives in our ED, has tried our best to follow the wishes of the patient. Sometimes, it's very challenging if the patient can't talk, or a family member can't be found, and they haven't documented what they would want in this situation or any situation. We have to use our best judgment to determine what the patient would have wanted and try to act in the best interest of the patient. We can try to reach family to figure out what the patient really wants in this situation, and if not, then to try and do our best to do what should be done for that patient, which usually means to resuscitate them until more information or until the patient is able to tell us thank you or I really didn't want that. This is what happens when you don't have a health-care proxy.

Section III: Concepts

Prognosis

Medical prognostication is very challenging, even under ideal conditions, when a physician and patient have had a long established relationship. Emergency medicine presents an additional challenge in that emergency physicians (EPs) frequently have no preexisting relationship with the patient and are unfamiliar with patient's medical history and baseline level of health. Furthermore, the time in which ED clinicians first interact with their patients, during a medical emergency with time urgency and limited data sources, makes it even more challenging to gather enough historical data to form a clear picture of a patient's overall health.

It is well established in the literature that a provider's estimation of overall prognosis is generally very poor. Some have suggested that as few as 20% of prognostic estimations are accurate with nearly 70% representing overestimates in that patients are predicated to live longer than they eventually do [1, 2]. Use of prognostication tools may help providers to better estimate overall prognosis. One instrument, the Palliative Performance Scale (Table 25.1), which looks at a total of five domains, is relatively easy to use, and scores from this scale have been correlated with overall survival [3]. Although prognostic instruments can provide some estimation of survival, their use in a busy ED may be impractical [4].

Understanding of four basic "death trajectories" can aid the EP in the provision of meaningful prognostic information to patients and families (Figure 25.1). First described by Lunney *et al.* in 2002 after review of Medicare data, these trajectories may allow an ED clinician to begin to better recognize what and when these patients may benefit from palliative or hospice care [5, 6]. In addition, broad guidelines, provided by the Centers for Medicare and Medicaid Services, do exist in helping determine which patients may be eligible for hospice care. Although these guidelines help to determine specific insurance coverage for patients, they may assist providers in determining the most appropriate disposition.

Sudden death only accounts for 7% of all deaths, meaning most geriatric patients follow some predictable trajectory with time between an identifiable onset of disease and their eventual death. The EP should, however, be able to identify specific geriatrics patients seen in the ED as those whose prognosis is overall poor, who may be appropriate for either hospice or more palliative, rather than curative, interventions. Use of prognostic instruments and an understanding of various death trajectories and recognition of patients who meet hospice criteria may aid providers in this identification. For these patients, this is likely to lead to better control of end-of-life symptoms, decreased medical care costs, and overall improvement in patient satisfaction and perceived quality of life [7, 8].

Table 25.1 Palliative Performance Scale.

PPS Level	Ambulation	Activity & Evidence of Disease	Self-Care	Intake	Conscious Level
100%	Full	Normal activity & work No evidence of disease	Full	Normal	Full
90%	Full	Normal activity & work Some evidence of disease	Full	Normal	Full
80%	Full	Normal activity *with* Effort Some evidence of disease	Full	Normal or reduced	Full
70%	Reduced	Unable Normal Job/Work Significant disease	Full	Normal or reduced	Full
60%	Reduced	Unable hobby/house work Significant disease	Occasional assistance necessary	Normal or reduced	Full or Confusion
50%	Mainly Sit/Lie	Unable to do any work Extensive disease	Considerable assistance required	Normal or reduced	Full or Confusion
40%	Mainly in Bed	Unable to do most activity Extensive disease	Mainly assistance	Normal or reduced	Full or Drowsy +/- Confusion
30%	Totally Bed Bound	Unable to do any activity Extensive disease	Total Care	Normal or reduced	Full or Drowsy +/- Confusion
20%	Totally Bed Bound	Unable to do any activity Extensive disease	Total Care	Minimal to sips	Full or Drowsy +/- Confusion
10%	Totally Bed Bound	Unable to do any activity Extensive disease	Total Care	Mouth care only	Drowsy or Coma +/- Confusion
0%	Death	–	–	–	–

From Ref. [3]. Copyright Victoria Hospice Society, BC, Canada (2001) www.victoriahospice.org

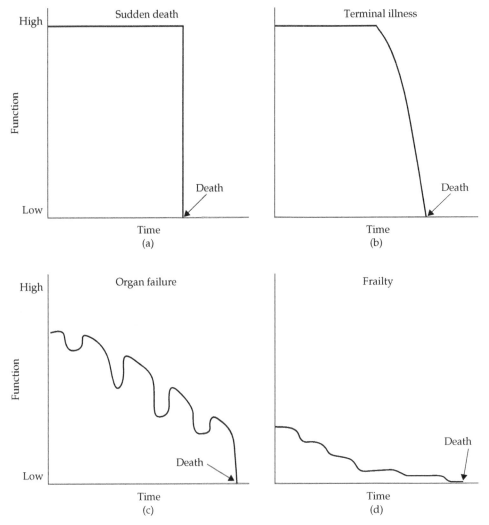

Figure 25.1 (a–d) Theoretical trajectories of dying. Lunney *et al.* [6]. Reproduced with permission from American Medical Association.

Goals of care and advance directives

Traditionally, the EP has focused on identification and management of acute and life-threatening illnesses with the primary goal of prolonging life. This default model is perhaps a reasonable approach for many patients seen in the ED. However, in ill geriatric patients who likely have multiple medical problems, this approach may not be ideal, and perhaps will be inconsistent with the patient's wishes [9].

Geriatric patients may initially present to the ED for acute injury or illness. However, these patients will also frequently present for progressive physical or mental decline secondary to long-standing and multiple chronic diseases. Numerous studies have shown some impairment, from problems with vision to mental status, in patients over the age of 65 presenting to the ED [10–12]. Miller and colleagues find that nearly 70% of patients aged 65 and older presenting to the ED are dependent in at least one activity of daily living [10]. Chief complaints related to chronic functional decline can be frustrating to the EP as a clear intervention to "cure" the patient and resolve the complaint is often not possible.

Furthermore, for geriatric patients who present with an acute illness, the patient and family may not desire aggressive intervention or any intervention. For example, an 85-year-old man with metastatic lung cancer and large pleural effusions causing significant dyspnea may not be an appropriate candidate for the placement of a chest tube. The challenge for the EP is being able to balance acute illness management where timely decisions must be made and the overall goals of the patient who may wish no care.

Goals of care can be defined as curing a disease, extending life, maintaining independence and functionality, and alleviation of pain or some combination thereof [13]. The need for and specifics revolving around diagnostic and treatment interventions should always be discussed with the patient as well as with his or her family member or legally authorized representative. In this way, the EP may be able to determine the patient's true wishes concerning goals of care. The challenge frequently faced with this approach in the acute setting as well as with geriatric patients is the potential inability for these patients, either as a result of their acute illness or chronic decline, to communicate their true wishes or make an informed decision. Moreover, determination of decisional capacity of geriatric patients by EPs, discussed in more detail later, has been shown to frequently be inaccurate [14–17]. These facts often leave ED clinicians with one of three options in determining a patient's goals of care.

As the first option, ED clinicians may have access to the patient's written ADs. The use of AD, particularly in the ED in geriatric patients, is one method of ensuring all providers, especially those unfamiliar with a patient's medical history, have some understanding of a patient's goals of care, whether curative or palliative.

Although the Federal Patient Self-Determination Act of 1991 requires many healthcare institutions such as hospitals and nursing homes to provide information on ADs to patients, historically most patients presenting to the ED, by some estimates as many as three quarters, do not have an AD [9, 18, 19]. One study finds that although ADs are more common among older patients, overall, only 27% of patients presenting to the ED have any form of AD [20].

However, the lack of AD can be turned into an opportunity for interventions. Preparation of some form of AD in the ED or in the hospital by providers, likely with the assistance of a departmental social worker, can expedite future ED visits and ensure that the patient's wishes are respected. Time constraints in the ED are often the primary impediment to creating an AD in the ED setting. Although overall success of an ED-based AD initiative, for geriatric patients, has not been studied, to our knowledge, success in community-based initiatives has been studied. Hammes and Rooney have published work that suggests an extensive AD education program can increase the number of patients with AD. In this study completed in the La Crosse, Wisconsin area, 85% of decedents (median age of 82 years) over an 11-month period have an AD. Prior to the initiative of the community AD education program, only 15% of individuals sampled from that same area had an AD. Marco and colleagues find that although 94% of EPs feel "legal concerns" influence decisions regarding resuscitations, 80% would still honor an AD on resuscitation including withholding care [21].

The second option is relying on surrogate decision-makers, most likely family members and ideally with some written healthcare power of attorney. EPs utilize this resource on a daily basis when clarifying past medical history, medications, and so on, when treating patients who are unable to report such information themselves. Two complications arise when this method is used to determine goals of care. One complication stems from potential disagreement among family members as well as the patient's true wishes. The second complication relates to how successful surrogates are able to use substitute judgment in determining goals of care for a family member. In a 2006 article published in the *Journal of the American Geriatric Society*, Vig and colleagues find that many surrogate decision-makers rely on factors such as their own personal interests, when making decisions about end-of-life care [22]. To that end, written ADs are clearly preferential to this second option.

The final option, when addressing goals of care in geriatric patients in the ED, is to simply provide aggressive resuscitation in an attempt to preserve the patient while determination of goals of care is made [9]. This is generally the default approach in the ED. Although this approach may be the most straightforward and easiest from a provider's perspective, it is the one approach that allows for no patient input to be considered, and should be undertaken when patients or their next of kin cannot express the goals of care.

Assumptions about goals of care of patients presenting to the ED are frequently made by providers, and, in many circumstances that may be appropriate. Geriatric patients, particularly those nearing the end of life, however, may have goals of care quite different from a default, aggressive resuscitation approach. EPs should attempt when possible to determine these goals in order to provide all patients with the most appropriate care.

Decision-making capacity and refusal of care

Legally, there is clear precedent that allows competent adult patients to make informed decisions about their medical care. This includes refusing care, even lifesaving care. The United States Supreme Court decision in Cruzan v. Director, Missouri Department of Health as well as the California Court of Appeal's decision in Bouvia v. Superior Court upheld the right of patients to refuse care. At issue in these cases was the question as to whether a patient, or his/her representative, has the right to refuse care, even if refusal may result in death. The Courts find that the Due Process Clause of the Fourteenth Amendment, which prohibits government deprivation of life, liberty or property, protects competent adult patients against forced medical interventions [23].

The challenge, of course, is determining which patients have decision-making capacity and which patients do not. There are numerous approaches to making this determination, objective cognitive evaluation scales and institutional standards an ED clinician can use to determine if a patient has decisional capacity. We would advise the following four-step approach in determining if a geriatric patient in the ED has decision-making capacity:

Step 1: It is imperative to ensure that general medical stability is achieved. That is to say, patients who are significantly hypoxic, hypotensive, intoxicated, or otherwise unstable medically should not be making decisions about their medical care, especially a decision against medical advice or standard of care. These derangements should be corrected. Special attention to iatrogenic causes of impairment, such as medication administration, should be examined.

Step 2: The physician's assessment of patients' competence has been called into question in the past [24]. For this reason, objective cognitive scales and standardized questionnaires that are evidence based and validated should be used to help guide an EP in determining if any and to what degree, cognitive impairment may exist. This includes

the Mini-Mental Status Examination, Montreal Cognitive Assessment Scale, and Quick Confusion Scale among others. Mild cognitive impairment is by no means an absolute contraindication in allowing a patient to make decisions about his or her medical care. However, severe impairment, confusion, and advanced dementia may require that others be involved in helping make informed decisions on behalf of the patient.

Step 3: Perhaps the most important step is ensuring that patients are able to communicate and explain their understanding of options, alternatives, and the potential consequences of various choices. Although more time intensive, ED clinicians must allow patients the chance to explain options in their own words, and not simply ask for confirmation of understanding with a simple yes or no. Patients unable to understand the consequences of their actions, specifically refusal of lifesaving care, may not have decisional capacity.

Step 4: Documentation of end-of-life goals, especially refusal of care, is essential. This is not only essential for being able to communicate with other providers, but also prudent from a legal standpoint. Although the frequently repeated expression "if it wasn't documented, it wasn't done" is perhaps overly simplistic, having proper documentation certainly makes it easier for the provider to defend his or her decisions. Furthermore, continued reassessment is necessary. Although perhaps not as germane to the ED setting, patients' medical conditions continually change, as do their goals of care, and this should be monitored and reassessed over time.

Patient-centered goals and patient-directed decision-making should be a key focus whenever caring for a geriatric patient in the ED. However, given geriatric patients high burden of disease and potential cognitive impairment, especially near the end of life, EPs should, if possible, complete proper evaluation of a patient's decisional capacity.

Section IV: Decision-making

- Although prognosis is challenging in general, ED clinicians should always attempt to identify geriatric patients who may be reaching the end of life and who are unlikely to benefit from aggressive interventions.

- Goals of care of ill geriatric patients may be determined by spending time with the patient and his or her family, the best initial approach. Written ADs, prepared prior to an emergency situation in the ED, is another method in which patients may be able to communicate their goals of care. For patients without ADs, the ED may be an opportunity to begin this conversation with utilization of social workers to assist in this process.
- Geriatric patients nearing the end of life may be referred to both inpatient and outpatient hospice from the ED directly. Consultation with hospice and palliative care providers should be made when these dispositions would most benefit the patient.

References

1 Higginson, I.J. and Costantini, M. (2002) Accuracy of prognosis estimates by four palliative care teams: a prospective cohort study. *BMC Palliat. Care*, **1**, 1.

2 Christakis, N.A. and Lamont, E.B. (2000) Extent and determinants of error in doctors' prognoses in terminally ill patients: prospective cohort study. *Br. Med. J.*, **320**, 469–473.

3 Head, B., Ritchie, C., and Smoot, T.M. (2005) Prognostication in hospice care: can palliative performance scale help? *J. Palliat. Med.*, **8**, 492–502.

4 Willner, L.S. and Arnold, R.M. (2006) The palliative prognostic score #62. *J. Palliat. Med.*, **9**, 993.

5 Lunney, J.R., Lynn, J., and Hogan, C. (2002) Profiles of older Medicare decedents. *J. Am. Geriatr. Soc.*, **50**, 1109–1112.

6 Lunney, J.R., Lynn, J., Foley, D.J. *et al.* (2003) Patterns of functional decline at the end of life. *J. Am. Med. Assoc.*, **289**, 2387–2392.

7 Bailey, C., Murphy, R., and Porock, D. (2011) Trajectories of end-of-life care in the emergency department. *Ann. Emerg. Med.*, **57**, 362–369.

8 Grudzen, C.R., Hwang, U., Cohen, J. *et al.* (2012) Characteristics of emergency department patients who receive a palliative care consultation. *J. Palliat. Med.*, **15**, 369–399.

9 Cobbs, E.L. and Lynn, J. (2000) Ethics in emergency care of critically ill patients, in *Acute Emergencies and Critical Care of the Geriatric Patient* (eds T.T. Yoshikawa and D.C. Norman), Marcel Dekker, Inc., New York, pp. 11–30.

10 Miller, D.K., Lewis, L.M., Nork, M.J., and Morley, J.E. (1996) Controlled trial of geriatric case-finding and liaison service in an emergency department. *J. Am. Geriatr. Soc.*, **44**, 513–520.

11 Gerson, L.W., Rousseau, E.T., Hogan, T.M. *et al.* (1995) Multicenter study of case finding in elderly emergency department patients. *Acad. Emerg. Med.*, **2**, 729–734.

12 Peter, D.J. and Gerson, L.W. (2000) Functional assessment and decline, in *Geriatric Emergency Medicine* (eds S.W. Meldon, O.J. Ma, and R. Woolard), McGraw-Hill, New York.

13 Von Gunten, C.F., Ferris, F.D., and Emanuel, L.L. (2000) Ensuring competency in end-of-life care: communication and relational skills. *J. Am. Med. Assoc.*, **23**, 3051–3057.

14 Rodriguez-Molinero, A., Lopez-Dieguez, M., Tabuenca, A.I. *et al.* (2010) Physicians' impression on the elder's functionality influences decision making for emergency care. *Am. J. Emerg. Med.*, **28**, 757–765.

15 Hustey, F.M. and Meldon, S.W. (2002) The prevalence and documentation of impaired mental status in elderly emergency department patients. *Ann. Emerg. Med.*, **39**, 248–253.

16 Husty, F.M., Meldon, S.W., Smith, M.D., and Lex, C.K. (2003) The effect of mental status screening on the care of elderly emergency department patients. *Ann. Emerg. Med.*, **41**, 678–684.

17 Rodriguez-Molinero, A., Lopez-Dieguez, M., Tabuenca, A.I. *et al.* (2006) Functional assessment of older patients in the emergency department: comparison between standard instruments, medical records and physicians' perceptions. *BMC Geriatr.*, **6**, 13.

18 Marco, C.A. (2000) Ethical issues in geriatric emergency medicine, in *Geriatric Emergency Medicine* (eds S.W. Meldon, O.J. Ma, and R. Woolard), McGraw-Hill, New York, pp. 40–50.

19 Llovera, I., Ward, M.F., Ryan, J.G. *et al.* (1999) Why don't emergency department patients have advance directives. *Acad. Emerg. Med.*, **6**, 1054–1060.

20 Llovera, I., Mandel, F.S., Ryan, J.G. *et al.* (1997) Are emergency department patients thinking about advanced directives? *Acad. Emerg. Med.*, **4**, 976–980.

21 Marco, C.A., Bessman, E.S., Schoenfeld, C.N., and Kelen, G.D. (1997) Ethical issues of cardiopulmonary resuscitation: current practice among emergency physicians. *Acad. Emerg. Med.*, **4**, 898–902.

22 Vig, E.K., Taylor, J.S., Starks, H. *et al.* (2006) Beyond substituted judgment: how surrogates navigate end-of-life decision-making. *J. Am. Geriatr. Soc.*, **54**, 1688–1693.

23 Furrow, B.R., Greaney, T.L., Johnson, S.H. *et al.* (2001) *Bioethics: Health Care Law and Ethics*, West Group, St. Paul, MN.

24 Markson, L.J., Kern, D.C., Annas, G.J., and Glantz, L.H. (1994) Physician assessment of patient competence. *J. Am. Geriatr. Soc.*, **42**, 1074–1080.

26

Geriatric dispositions and transitions of care

Barbara Morano[1], Carmen Morano[2], Kevin Biese[3], Eric A. Coleman[4] & Ula Hwang[5]

[1] *Brookdale Department of Geriatrics and Palliative Medicine, Icahn School of Medicine at Mount Sinai, New York, NY, USA*
[2] *Hunter College of the City University of New York, New York, NY, USA*
[3] *Division of Geriatrics, Department of Emergency Medicine and Internal Medicine, University of North Carolina School of Medicine, Chapel Hill, NC, USA*
[4] *Division of Health Care Policy and Research, University of Colorado Anschutz Medical Campus, Aurora, CO, USA*
[5] *Department of Emergency Medicine, Icahn School of Medicine at Mount Sinai, New York, NY, USA*

Section I: Case presentation

Chief complaint: shortness of breath

HPI (History of Presenting Illness): This was a 67-year-old woman who had increasing number of emergency department (ED) visits for shortness of breath. She was the primary caregiver for her husband who had dementia. Her priorities in life were to be able to breathe better without having to use oxygen, but wanted to continue to care for her husband. As far as social supports were concerned, she had a son who did not live nearby. He was a very busy executive. Mrs M was a 67-year-old married woman with a high school education and no advance directives. She was the primary caregiver for her 73-year-old husband, who was diagnosed with early stage dementia approximately 3 years prior. Mr M was on medications for agitation that was believed to be related to his dementia. Mrs M. was a librarian, and Mr M. was a teacher at the local high school. They have been in the community for a very long time. Their son was an executive in a biotech company, and had a very demanding job and work schedule. When asked about her self-rated health

status (scale = excellent, very good, good, fair, poor) she reported fair.

Past Medical History: Congestive heart failure (CHF), chronic obstructive pulmonary disease (COPD), diabetes, coronary artery disease, hypertension, low blood count, acid reflux, depression, cholecystectomy, elevated cholesterol, heart attack, decreased kidney function, tubal ligation, and carpel tunnel syndrome.

Allergies: penicillin, tetracycline, and augmentin.

Pre-ED visit medications: Insulin Humulin N 35 plus 10 regular in AM; Insulin Humulin N 25 plus 10 regular in PM; Glyburide 2.5 meq. twice per day; Ecotrin 81 mg once per day; Furosemide 80 mg once per day; Allopurinol 100 mg once per day; Potassium 750 mg once per day; Amitriptyline 25 mg at bedtime; Vicodin 5/500 every 3–4 h as needed; Fluoxetine 20 mg once per day; Ranitidine 300 mg once per day; Oxygen 2.5 l; Nitroglycerine as needed.

Social History: Patient had kept the extent of her caregiving from her son, and was now extremely anxious about what to do about her husband. Although the son had a good relationship with his mother and

---

Geriatric Emergencies: A Discussion-Based Review, First Edition.
Edited by Amal Mattu, Shamai A. Grossman and Peter L. Rosen.
© 2016 John Wiley & Sons, Ltd. Published 2016 by John Wiley & Sons, Ltd.

called frequently, he had little contact with his father because as the patient indicated, "my husband was never one for talking." The patient had been a fairly independent person, but was now faced with having to care for herself, and not being able to care for her husband. She had lived in her home for 45 years, and refused to move closer to the son. She repeatedly visited the ED due to shortness of breath (SOB), but did not inform her son when the situation escalated. In discussion with the son, he voices a goal of encouraging his parents to move out of their home and into assisted living, while the patient voices goals of being able to breathe without oxygen, and to continue caring for her husband.

Section II: Case discussion

Dr Peter Rose (PR): It is my understanding that this is a patient who is presently in the ED who is not terribly sick, but is a frequent visitor, probably for her COPD exacerbations. Is that correct?

Dr Ula Hwang (UH): Yes, that's correct.

PR: Before we go down this path, I just want to make sure that everyone is clear where we are. We are in the ED, we have a patient who is a frequent visitor and that always irritates us, and we try to figure out how to stop that with no success. Where would you commence your care on a patient like this?

Dr Andrew Chang (AC): Obviously, there are a lot of social issues. In busy EDs, we have some difficulty teasing that out. Clearly this is a complicated case. The patient has a goal. The son has a goal. In my own ED, we are particularly lucky because in addition to social workers, we also have a patient navigator who can help us to deal with issues, and to try to keep patients from being readmitted to the ED. In addition to doing my examination and getting whatever basic screening tests I would need, I would also involve both the social worker and our patient navigator with this case. Even on repeated ED visits, with an elderly patient with shortness of breath, I think there's a tendency to be conservative and admit these patients.

PR: We frequently see patients like this in whom the issues seem to be more social than actually acutely medical. At what point is it the responsibility of the ED to become involved in decisions such as "Is this patient ready for assisted living? Is this patient no longer capable of autonomous living? Is this patient someone who really needs a different social structure than they have available?" These are the questions we never really used to ask in emergency medicine, and while we are happy when we have social workers to pose these to, I think we're becoming more and more involved with patients who have problems like this.

Dr Scott Wilber (SW): When I started in emergency medicine in the early 1990s, we focused on the medical objectives, and never paid any attention to the social issues. I think increasingly as we see more and more patients with a lot of medical complexities, many of whom are geriatric patients, and in addition with changes in health care, where we have moved a lot more of healthcare delivery to the outpatient setting, it has become a reasonable role for emergency physicians to have greater knowledge of, and be involved in outpatient care. I think the days are gone, where you can basically state in your discharge instruction, "See your doctor in 48 h and everything will be ok," or else admit the patient to the hospital. I think we must start thinking about things like: How do we understand the role of assisted living or nursing facilities or rehabilitation facilities? How do we help this person with home care? Could we get her home on oxygen if she were to need home oxygen? In this case, she's already on home oxygen, but wants to function without it, but in the case of a patient who wasn't yet on it, would we be able to arrange home oxygen for the patient? – can we become part of care management teams? What we don't want to have happen to us is to have care management teams say, "This is how the patient will be managed when they come to the ED," and not have involvement in that care management team.

PR: This patient is 67, which I personally don't think is very old. At what point do you think geriatric concerns kick in? After all, we see many younger patients who have complex medical histories, and we don't seem to worry about their sociology quite as much as we do with the older patient.

Dr Donald Melady (DM): I think "old" is often used as a proxy for a bunch of other issues that are not always related to chronological age. The fact that she is 67 doesn't really tell us anything. All the other factors that travel with increasing age do – multimorbidity, polypharmacy, cognitive status and mental health, functional capacity, or social support system. No one really knows exactly what "old" means. For example, anyone working in a place that deals with a large street-dependent population knows that if you're living on the street, by the time you're 40 or 45, you are the equivalent of a 90-year-old living in stable housing. When we say "old," we probably mean the mix of physiological, pathological, and social instability or decline. So is this woman "old?" Whether we use that term or not, we can see what she is. She is a woman with complex medical problems, pharmacological problems, psychological issues, as well as a challenging social situation. So as Dr Wilber already said, we have to include all of these issues when assessing her immediate medical presentation.

PR: When we see younger patients with complex problems, we tend to focus more on their medical problems than on their sociology. At one point, do we start considering the sociology of the patients?

DM: One of the problems about being old is that it is very difficult to just say that there is one "active problem." The care of all older patients is complex. I think we can usually make the assumption (*usually* correctly) that a 35 year old with abdominal pain only has one problem. The emergency paradigm has always been to determine what that one active problem is, and to act on it. That's why we simple-minded people have always gravitated toward emergency medicine: because we like our problems simple! With this woman, it's impossible at any point in her trajectory to say there is only one active problem. All of her problems are interacting. Her social situation is *part* of her problem. Likely the reason she keeps getting so short of breath is that, because of the complex care she needs to provide to her husband, she may forget to take her furosemide, and her CHF gets a little worse. So, how do you separate out the pathology (the CHF) and its pharmacology from her social situation? I think, whenever we decide to start calling someone "old," that's when you have to start considering their social situation as part of their medical problem.

PR: We have a patient who, like many patients, wishes fulfillment of fantasies that are not going to come true. She is dependent on oxygen, but does not want to be. Clearly, we deal all the time with patients whose

compliance is sometimes a matter of lack of intelligence. How do we ensure that her life becomes somewhat easier if she were to become more compliant? Or, is that one more indication that the patient needs some sort of assistance in her living?

Dr Maura Kennedy (MK): The first part of the question is encouraging her to be compliant. I think focusing on what her goals are, and tying in her compliance with her goals are going to be very useful. She wants to be able to care for her husband; I presume she wants to be able to be active, and to be at her home, if that is a safe possibility for her. She might have to allow herself to be on oxygen to improve her general well-being, and to allow her to continue to care for her husband. I think that may be part of it – getting her to have a change in mindset, where she may have to accept some limitations on her ideal life circumstances (allowing herself to be on oxygen) to improve the other aspects in her life.

PR: We don't seem to allow older patients the freedom to be stupid or noncompliant the way we do with younger patients. We tend to be more protective and in fact more paternalistic. Do you think this is necessary or just our unwillingness to allow independence to older patients when we disapprove of their decision-making?

MK: I think, in part, it is reflective of concern for safety. Certainly, with young children when they come in with falls and injuries that seem atypical we worry about their safety and act paternalistic with them. As individuals age, sometimes for cognitive reasons, they are not aware of their limitations, or they are not aware of safety issues. In those situations, there is some responsibility to think of their safety and to address it. With our patient, the issue is complicated as she appears cognitively intact, and she is caring for someone who isn't. I am not quite clear as to whether there are any immediate issues of safety at home. Obviously, there are issues of transitions of care from the ED to home and back to the PCP. Perhaps with this discharge, there will be opportunities to address that, to try to improve her care at home for her COPD and CHF. But the big question I have, because the son is encouraging them to move out of their home into an assisted living facility, is whether there is an immediate safety issue that we need to address, or can this be done on a more gradual basis. If there is a safety issue, we need to look at it now. Otherwise, I think it is a longer-term process to identify the best living situation for them.

PR: We frequently overestimate the amount of family support that is available, simply because there is a younger relative somewhere. But I find that in families there is often dissonance between what they would want for their parent, and that sometimes the issues are being decided on a financial basis instead of what is best for the patients. How do you attack that problem in a patient like this who has a son who appears to be remote, but is looking for a way to perhaps make his family safe, while also enhancing his own convenience in how much he has to visit and take care of them?

Dr Vaishal Toila (VT): I think this is an important challenge that not only has to be fixed in the ED, but also on the inpatient side. One of the most important actions we can accomplish in the ED is to communicate. First, of course with the patient, then perhaps with the family members, if available. But one resource we often underutilize is the actual PCP. Oftentimes, the PCP has seen this patient several times in clinic, and has tried to face these issues, and has had communication with several family members, and has seen the trajectory of the needs that this patient might have as well as the safety issues that might be starting to arise at home. Particularly in this case, if Mrs M is well enough to be discharged home from the ED, it might be worthwhile in the ED spending extra time and using any resources we have available to us, like the social worker or case manager to help arrange the most appropriate transition for her.

Dr Shamai Grossman (SG): I would add that conversation with the PCP may be critical as that physician may have a rapport with the patient that is very difficult to replicate in a short time in the ED. That rapport may be more useful than any cure or any attempted cure we can try to implement in the ED.

PR: While I agree with that, one of the problems in the patients who are frequent ED users is either that they don't have good primary care, or that they don't have access to it at the times that they need it, so that they keep on bouncing back to the ED.

PR: I was wondering if you would comment on what you could do when you have someone who ostensibly has a PCP, but does not use that person, or doesn't have access to them in a timely manner. We've seen a wide range of variability in trying to reach a PCP in less than 48 h. Do you think that's part of the transition problem here? Or do you think we're dealing with the kind of patient who is so worn out by caregiving responsibilities that what she really needs is for someone to relieve her from that responsibility, so that she could concentrate on her own health a little more?

UH: I think the patient in question here is somewhat more in the middle. The points to be emphasized here are as follows: We don't really have (at least with what's presented here) a lot of information as to what her relationship is with her PCP. Perhaps the follow-up hasn't been as rigorous as it could be. That points to an opportunity to look at the reasons. Is it simply that her PCP is not available? Is it that she is not able to get to her appointments in a timely manner? The other question is "What is timely from an ED perspective." Is it that the patient needs to be seen within 24 h, or 5 days, or a week? Perhaps this is why the ED now needs to utilize an interdisciplinary force: case managers and social workers to help investigate further what's going on. Why is the patient coming back? Maybe it is for medical reasons. On the other end of the extreme, I think what this case also demonstrates is that there are other things going on at her home and in her life that may very well be exacerbating or causing her health to decline leading to an increasing number of these shortness of breath visits. Using other resources to help us figure these things out is going to be important. It will also be time-consuming. But it is a direction we will probably have to take in emergency medicine, especially when we are caring for complex patients like this.

DM: This woman's problems are not going to be solved or even well addressed by any *solo* physician, neither the emergency physician nor her family doctor. To believe that this amount of complexity can be solved by one person is just magical thinking. I agree that having an interdisciplinary team involved in her care, where she lives, which in this case is in her own house in the community, is the best way to tease out and address all the multifaceted components of her care. While we can get some of that started in the ED, I don't know what other EDs have, but if she were seen in our place, she would be assessed by an ED-based interdisciplinary team offering clear direction back to the emergency physician (EP) and to community-based care. *Part* of that team is the EP, me, dealing with the medical issues, and probably some medication debridement. But I'm just one part because I don't know that much about her fall prevention, about physiotherapy, whether she would be getting along better with a walker, how to readjust her home environment, how to get her medication into a blister pack so that she's actually taking them on a regular basis. We need to stop whining about her frequent ED visits, and start doing something *in the ED* to allow her to live better so that she doesn't need to come to the ED. I think that is in part the responsibility of the EP and the ED to develop strong links with community-based care so that there can be a transition in both directions: when she needs to come to the ED, and when she returns to the community.

PR: I guess that we've quickly concluded the problems in this case are more sociologic, and more related to what happens in her home than medical. I think this is a habit that we get into when we see frequent visitors to the ED. We sometimes forget that chronic diseases have a natural history of getting worse, and that sometimes we need to do yet another workup on a patient in order to find out if that chronic disease is, in fact, worsening. What do you use as clues to help you decide to do yet another workup before you turn to the interdisciplinary team to help you manage the patient as an outpatient? – not that I'm objecting to what I think is a terrific resource if you have it, but I also think we have a responsibility as physicians not to underestimate chronicity and exacerbation of those diseases.

SG: I think that any time a patient comes into the ED, you always have to look at them fresh like this is their first visit. That said, medical records are often invaluable. Looking at patients' similar complaints, similar vital signs, similar examinations, and similar test results can often be priceless clues. Nevertheless, it's really difficult to decide that this time the patient is definitely coming back because she can't deal with the problems at home, and what we really need is a social solution. The best we can do is do a basic evaluation, do the physical examination, and do the electrocardiogram (EKG), in her case it might be obtaining a BNP (B-type natriuretic peptide) level, and checking a chest X-ray study, and putting the data together and saying this really doesn't look different from the way she was when she was discharged from the hospital just a few weeks prior. If that's the case, all the patient really needs is outpatient care or social care. I think that's the best surrogate we have for knowing exactly what's going on in each acute situation.

PR: Let's assume you don't have access to one of these interdisciplinary teams. How would you solve the situation for a patient like this? Would you consider admitting her to the hospital to get her some relief from her caretaking duties, as well as to get more focus on straightening out her medical problems and to get better access to social work?

DM: Who is going to be providing care to her husband while she is in hospital?

SW: It has to be taken into consideration that, we come from fairly large health systems that may have more resources than smaller institutions have. I sometimes practice in a smaller rural hospital, and while we do have the availability of a care manager, she is shared with the entire hospital. When that occurs, sometimes the resources have to be delivered in the hospital rather than being done purely in the ED. Also it is fairly easy for me to get someone connected with our outpatient geriatrics clinic, and yet in the rural area where I practice, there are no geriatricians in the town. It does suggest that there are going to be many different ways to care for the patient. One thing to keep in mind though is that in general, the hospital is not a kind place to someone who is older. A few days of not getting up and moving around the way they should is probably going to make them weak, and necessitate some rehabilitation. Also, there is the possibility of nosocomial infection. So whenever possible, I think, trying to deliver outpatient care is probably safer for the patient, and will allow her to care for her husband. The one resource that I didn't hear mentioned was trying to consider a palliative care consultation as well. In an oxygen-dependent COPD patient, hospice care is a possibility, but even prior to hospice, palliative care for symptom management of her dyspnea is what she really needs.

DM: I do some consulting with small hospitals around geriatric emergency medicine and my question is this: If we are admitting this person to get access to services, and the services are available in the hospital, why are the services not available in the ED? The ED is also part of the hospital. It is certainly not going to be good for this patient to admit her to the hospital.

It is going to be bad for her because of the hazards of hospitalization. It is going to be bad for her husband to have no one at home looking after him. But it is also bad for the hospital. Surely, it must be more expensive to have to admit her to the hospital for 3 or 4 days than to make these services available to her in the ED. I do think we need to start rethinking the system that we are working in, and to realize that the ED is not only part of the hospital but also part of the community.

PR: I think that unfortunately many of our hospitals are not rationally administered, and that as well, many of our Medicare mandates are not rational, and sometimes we have to do what is bad for a patient in order to get the kind of care we are trying to give.

SG: This involves some very simple, practical issues here in 2015. If you're at a community hospital, and even if you're at an academic center, it is unlikely that you're going to have all those services available 24 h a day. If you don't have an observation unit, then often your only other alternative is to admit this patient to the hospital. Also, you may not only have to admit her, but may need to have an ambulance go and pick up her husband and bring him to the hospital because that's the only way he will be safe until services he needs can be arranged.

DM: Contrarily, you might rethink the system you have and say, "That's the way things are now, and we can change it." If we're thinking of a senior-friendly ED in a society that has more and more old people around, we may have to start rethinking the way we do things. For example, at our place we now have a protocol for holding people overnight in the ED to get a more comprehensive discharge-specific assessment. It has been our hospital's opinion that this is better for everybody. We don't put the internists in the hospital through the unnecessary work process of admitting somebody who is only going to be in the hospital for 12–16 h. It is better for the emergency physicians and the ED because we actually get the patient out with their problems addressed, and they're not back a week later. It's certainly better for the patient who doesn't have to go through the process of a hospital admission that's not necessary.

PR: We've made an issue of the dependent husband at home, and yet we see patients all the time at any age group for whom their care is going to compromise

their nonillness responsibilities. At what point would you call the son and say, "Go take care of your father for a few days," as opposed to trying to create two admissions instead of one because of her outpatient responsibilities.

VT: Having those conversations is difficult, especially from the ED. But if this patient is ill enough then she would require admission or care coordination from an admission standpoint, and if that infrastructure is not there already, the son is going to have to discuss and have communications with his mom and the PCP, if available, and with us as to what would be the plan. Presumably, this patient has been admitted to the hospital multiple times in addition to her frequent ED visits, so there is some outpatient failure of her management, and that may only get worse in terms of the care plan for her husband. She is probably spending hours in the ED, so what is going on with her husband during those frequent ED visits? Does one admission solve the problem and help? Perhaps that's a possibility. If we can arrange a home nurse visit, which can often be done directly from the ED if the infrastructure is available, that would be the best alternative. But I would have that conversation with the son and say, "Look, this is the situation with your mom. She may be noncompliant, or may not have access. She may have some issue with her medication. Her illness may be getting progressively worse. We will have to make arrangements. Do you or some family member want to come to the hospital now and have that conversation? And what is your plan for moving forward?" I think you have to have that conversation.

DM: Building care around the availability of family members is rarely going to be a successful strategy. If we got this phone call saying we had to drive 4 h or to fly across the continent to suddenly take care of our aging parent, how many of us right now would be able to go? This son is an executive in a biotech company likely in a different state, if not country. I don't think it is likely that he is going to be able to step up and assume those responsibilities.

VT: I don't think he is going to be able to do so either, but I think you have to start that conversation. "This is the situation your parents are in." If he's really kind of hands off about this, "Look I'm busy, I live in another country, and I can't participate in their care," then so be it. Then, it's really our responsibility. Then, we again look at the best interest of our patient and try to mobilize as many resources as we have available. However, having that conversation with that family member is still imperative; we may discover another family member who is local who the patient hasn't really talked about. Those resources are also likely to fail, but there are certain instances when there are some family members, cousins, friends, or even neighbors who are willing to help and check on the husband, and care for him while our patient is actually admitted to the hospital.

PR: I think you make a good point, and while I agree that families are often not very helpful, I've been impressed by how many resources there are within a family structure that we don't often call upon that can be implemented in cases of crisis. They may be friends, they may be relatives, they may be church members, but there are resources that we can call upon other than just pure family. But as Dr Toila says, we have to start somewhere.

PR: Dr Hwang can you summarize for us?

UH: Much of the discussion we've had here focused on care transitions. This is probably relatively new to most EPs. This is not what we're typically taught. This is now the time for emergency medicine to think, "What can we do, or what should we be doing in terms of care transitions?" and "What are the definitions of care transitions from the ED setting?" Eric Coleman is a national expert on care transitions from a broader perspective, from the hospital to the home setting. He describes what are called the four pillars of care transitions. These focus on the patient's understanding of medication/self-management, an understanding of and access to their own health record, the ability to get follow-up and timely follow-up (usually/hopefully with their PCP), and knowing what the red flags of their conditions are, and when they may be in situations or have symptoms that may put them at greater risk. These care transition tenets do not just apply to older adults, but should be considered for all patients once they leave the ED. It is to ensure the safe and efficient transition of ED patients to the appropriate care setting consistent with their care needs and preferences. High-quality care transitions should include these elements: assessment of the patient's care needs, understanding of the patient's and the families' care

preferences, linking the patient to appropriate care settings, identifying (hopefully) a single care coordinator, delivering effective education to the patient, family and caregiver, and facilitating their timely disposition from the ED. We have discussed some of these ideas here and the question remains: when are we officially able to "hand off" our responsibility as emergency clinicians in terms of the patient's transition?

DM: From a system's point of view, our healthcare system and its units (specifically our EDs), really need to understand that doing things the way we used to is not going to work in the future, and that addressing solutions that work for older people is part of having a successful ED. In cases such as the one we have been discussing, I do think that implementing social care is feasible in most EDs in larger centers, cost-effective, and good for the patient. Yet, often these three things do not come together. I think it is the responsibility of EPs (and those of us training future EPs), as well as administrators to start putting some of those things in place. The key components are access to an interdisciplinary team in the ED and establishing robust and easy communications with the community of which we are a part.

PR: Dr Rob Anderson has described another solution to us in the past – making house calls on patients like this – unfortunately, this is probably a solution that isn't available to most of us.

DM: Our department has developed a close liaison with a home-based primary care service, a real family practice that operates only in people's homes. So we refer our most complicated patients to that service, and they're able to ensure medical follow-up in that patient's home within 2 days.

PR: I think that's a terrific plan. There was a service in San Diego called "Call Doc" that basically made house calls on Medicare patients, and showed that they were able to reduce the number of admissions for those patients by about 50% as well as to give much more effective and cheaper care because they weren't being admitted. That would enable probably some of this woman's repeat visits to be cut back. Perhaps we can summarize by saying that we have a community responsibility, we have a sociologic responsibility, that is not particularly in the forefront of emergency medicine discussions but is going to be more and more essential as we have more and more patients like this.

Case resolution

The patient was provided a pharmacy consult which allowed her to get a better understanding of her own medication management. Post-ED visit medications were as follows: Insulin Humulin N 30 mg plus 10 Regular in AM; Furosemide twice per day; Oxygen 4 l; Lovastatin 2 tablets with dinner; Flovent 88 mcg oral inhalation twice daily; Losartan 100 mg once per day; multivitamin.

She was seen by a social worker who was able to link her up to community resources and support groups. Discussion with these services allowed the patient to have a better understanding of her diseases (COPD, CHF, and depression), which in turn allowed her to have a better understanding of her own condition, and talk to others about what was going on. The social worker was also able to help with care for her husband by facilitating his going to an adult day care for parts of the day. This gave the patient some respite from the continuous and increasing needs of her husband's caretaking as well as her own deteriorating health. Finally, a family meeting was convened that allowed for the discussion with the patient and her son about advanced directives, her own goals of care, and what would happen if she were to pass away before her spouse.

Section III: Concepts

Introduction

There is a growing body of literature that suggests older adults transfer between settings, sites, and systems of care more often than their younger counterparts [1, 2]. The safe transition between these settings is a priority in healthcare reform (i.e., Affordable Care Act (ACA) and a growing focus in the healthcare literature). Although the ED has been recognized as the most common entry system into the healthcare system for older adults, little attention has been given to transitional care from ED to home. Older patients discharged to home from the ED are at

high risk of experiencing adverse outcomes, including receiving inappropriate medications, return to the ED, and death [2]. A greater understanding of the risks associated with an ED visit for older adults as they transition back to home can contribute to improved health outcomes and satisfaction, and a decrease in return visits and hospitalization. This chapter elucidates these risks and explores how to tailor optimal care transition interventions for this vulnerable population when they transition from ED to home.

In their review of the healthcare system, Wagner and colleagues at the Group Health Research Institute acknowledge that inadequate care for chronic illnesses stems from the "culture and structure of medical practice," [3] which results in patients' lack of knowledge regarding their own disease, poor medical care, and dissatisfaction with the care received [4]. Similarly, as stated by the American Geriatrics Society, poorly executed care transitions lead to poor health outcomes, patient dissatisfaction, unnecessary tests, and inappropriate use of hospital and emergency services [5]. The onset of an acute incident requiring a visit to the ED not only exacerbates any preexisting stress on the patient or family caregiver, but also frequently triggers a sequence of new transitions. The stress of the acute episode combined with the lack of communication between providers and patients is compounded by the additional stress of navigating a fragmented system of health care [3]. Thus, it should not be surprising that what follows is a series of failures such as poor patient comprehension of the medical condition, medication errors, inaccurate or incomplete transmittal of patient medical records, and costly hospital readmissions [6, 7]. Transitional care interventions are an effective way to manage these adverse events and organize our fragmented healthcare system. In turn, this will improve outcomes for older adults.

There are a number of evidence-based transitional care programs designated to reduce hospital readmissions such as the Care Transitions Intervention (Coleman) [5, 8], Project RED (Boston University Medical Center) [9], and Project BOOST (Society of Hospital Medicine) [10, 11]. However, their applicability in the ED is variable, and still being determined. As hospital systems face the challenge of meeting the Triple Aim of the ACA to (1) improve patient health care, (2) improve patient healthcare access, and (3) reduce total healthcare costs (including unnecessary hospitalizations and costly return visits to the ED), focused attention on transitional care programs implemented in the ED may be an effective solution. There is robust evidence that transitional care programs implemented from an inpatient setting reduce total costs of care and improve patient outcomes [11–15]. Earlier upstream implementation of such programs in the ED is a logical place to begin in a patient's health care continuum. It is important to recognize that unlike younger persons or patients free of chronic conditions at baseline for whom an ED visit likely represents a new acute problem, ED utilization by chronically ill older adults often represents an important sentinel event signifying a breakdown in care coordination for an already existing condition or conditions. This may result in a decline in functional status, increased healthcare utilization, nursing home admission, and even mortality [14].

Transitioning patients from the ED

Though the focus of this chapter is on enhancing care transitions for older adults being transitioned to home from the ED, it is worth touching briefly upon best practices for receiving older adults into the ED. Given the complexity of these patients and the fact that many of them may not be able to give an adequate history, it is critical to do the following things upon an older adult's arrival to the ED.

- If the patient is sent from a skilled nursing or other facility, a mechanism needs to be in place to ensure the facility is responsibly sending timely and accurate information including the history of present illness and reason for visit.
- Obtain as accurate a medication list as possible. If not readily available from the patient or family, this may be best obtained through the primary physician, pharmacy, or skilled nursing facility.
- In those cases where the patient is unable to communicate (i.e., cognitively impaired, even temporarily, or cannot speak on behalf of him-/herself), the healthcare power of attorney or proxy should be contacted if not present.
- Attempt to discover or elucidate the patient's goals of care and any advanced directives as soon as possible.

Transitioning patients to home from the ED

Improving transitions between sites of care require that the sending site, in this case the ED, where patients are transferred to another level of care, prepare and educate the patient, conduct medication reconciliation with the current regimen, and make arrangements for the next level of care, whether returning to an identified primary care physician (PCP), or subacute care facility [8]. Optimally, the sending and receiving clinicians are in communication during this transition. It is the recommendation of the Geriatric Task Force of the Society for Academic Emergency Medicine that this be verbal communication [16].

When considering a model of transitional care from ED to home, consider the fast-paced nature of the ED encounter. Such brief encounters do not afford the luxury of working with a patient on numerous occasions, over multiple days, prior to the patient's discharge. Nonetheless, the ED provides a unique opportunity to initiate transitional care as part of the patient's care continuum. This will require the ED to utilize appropriate screenings and assessments to identify quickly those older adults who have the potential for safe discharge to home by the early initiating of a transitional care intervention during the ED visit. In addition to the ED medical evaluation that would assess for health conditions, engagement by a social worker to assess for any psychosocial barriers to appropriate discharge to the patient's home is recommended. While not every ED may have access to social workers, case managers, or designated clinical care coordinators such as NPs or nurses, it is recommended that such individuals become critical members of the team to ensure successful transitional care, and all attempts should be made by hospitals to incorporate such personnel in the ED setting. Early engagement by a member of the transitional care team will facilitate referrals for a more in-depth assessment by the transitional care team that may also consist of other members, such as pharmacists, physical therapists, and social workers. As a result of the ACA, there are an increasing number of care coordination initiatives (i.e., accountable care organization (ACO) and community-based care transitions program (CCTP)), which provide care coordination and transitional care. Determining if the patient is already engaged in one of these initiatives is recommended early in the ED visit to prevent a duplication of services and to ensure continuity of care and timeliness of the intervention.

Determining the best use of the limited time with the patient while in the ED needs to be considered when developing any transition intervention. The literature suggests that patient education related to medication compliance and knowledge of signs and symptoms of a worsening condition is fundamental [8–10]. It is important that a patient understand the significance of follow-up with one's PCP soon after the ED visit. However, the transitional care professional, whether a nurse, nurse practitioner (NP), or social worker, must understand the patient and family caregiver's ability to grasp the necessary information and to follow through independently. Although a thorough psychosocial assessment is ideal, it may not be feasible in the fast-paced and resource-limited ED environment. Screening tools for dementia, activities of daily living and instrumental activities of daily living status, depression, or similar are useful and should be considered when available and feasible. At a minimum, the ED provider is encouraged to get some basic insights into the patient's physical and cognitive functioning through electronic medical record (EMR) review and by patient/family interview.

When engaging the patient in preliminary education to prepare for discharge, the "teach-back" method (also known as the "show-me" or "closing the loop" method) is a way to confirm that the patient understands what has been explained [17]. This may also reveal deficits in the patient's comprehension of discharge instructions as well as the potential for an unsafe transition to home [18]. The patient's inability to focus and be attentive to discharge instructions while in crisis during an ED visit is another factor that complicates working with patients and their families or caregivers in the ED. Several studies have found that comprehension of discharge instructions is a significant barrier to care compliance [19–22]. A visit to the ED can be viewed as a situational crisis that results in patients (of all ages) function at a lower level than before the ED visit [23]. When available, involving the patient's support system (family caregivers) in preparation for discharge is recommended, even if telephonically.

A common theme in the majority of the various transitional care models is the focus on empowering patients with information and disease-specific knowledge to better self-manage their medical condition(s) and medications. It has been well established that regardless of the setting of care, compliance with medication regimes is problematic. One follow-up study reveals that 65% of patients contacted after discharge from the ED have at least one medication problem and 53% need some corrective action [24, 25]. Consequently, when the older patient arrives at the ED during an acute crisis, it is critical that accurate information about current medications is immediately available to first responders and ED personnel. Unfortunately, access to and reconciliation of the patient's medication regime during an acute crisis in the ED is problematic if not impossible. Not only is it time-intensive to contact outside pharmacies to confirm medication lists, it is not always accurate as patients often receive medications from multiple sources. When possible, utilizing the skills of a pharmacist to consult with the patient and family members or caregivers in the ED to obtain an accurate medication history, and to provide the patient with a medication self-management tool is recommended. It is recognized that not every ED has a pharmacist as an available resource. It is recommended that at a minimum, if any of the patient's usual medications has been changed, it is conveyed both verbally and in writing to the patient and the usual source of care.

Recommended elements in transitional care to home

When developing a specific transitional care model, the following elements must be considered: early engagement and assessment; in-person or telephonic follow-up; schedule of follow-up; duration of intervention; staffing; and outcomes desired. Whether utilizing a nurse, NP, or social worker-driven model of transitional care, there is a consensus on how to improve outcomes as patients transition between settings of care. Limpahan and colleagues [26] through a review of the literature developed ED best practice guidelines to improve communication during transitions of care. These include the following:

1 Record the name of the primary care provider who provides regular source of care.
2 Record the name of the home care community-based medical, nursing, or social service provider.
3 Send summary clinical information to PCP.
4 Send summary clinical information to home care provider/s.

403

5 Send summary clinical information to downstream receiving physicians.

6 Perform medication reconciliation.

7 Provide patient education.

8 Provide written discharge instructions.

Another example of goals and elements necessary in ED to home transitional care are those of a transitional care initiative currently being implemented and launched as part of an innovative model of care with Geriatric Emergency Department Innovations in care through Workforce, Informatics, and Structural Enhancements (GEDI WISE) [27]. The group has proposed the following preliminary definition and necessary elements of transitional care from the ED to home: *To ensure the safe and efficient transition of ED patients to the appropriate care setting consistent with their care needs and preferences.*

High-quality ED care transitions should include the following elements:

1 Assessment of care needs

2 Understanding the patient's/family's care preferences

3 Linkage to appropriate care setting

4 Identification of single care coordinator

5 Delivering effective patient/family/caregiver education

6 Facilitating a timely disposition from the ED setting.

We suggest, if possible, a follow-up appointment be made for the patient before discharge from the ED. It is during this "no-care zone" – between discharge from the ED and reconnection to a PCP – that undesirable outcomes occur [28]. Assuring that this reconnection is successful in a timely manner may prevent ED revisits or hospital admissions.

Specific steps that can be taken when planning to discharge a patient to home from the ED so that the above elements can be accomplished include the following:

• Engage any help available to you (pharmacist, social worker, etc.) early in the course of ED care.

• Review the discharge plans in detail with the patient and family caregiver if possible, using the "teach-back" method.

• Send summary information to the PCP and other physicians caring for the patient, as well as the home health, skilled nursing facility, social workers, or other individuals caring for the patient.

• Perform medication reconciliation with existing medications to ensure that none of the medications the patient is being prescribed from the ED interfere with the current regimen. (A classic example includes the interaction of many antibiotics and warfarin.)

• Provide clear, concise written instructions printed in large font.

• Make follow-up appointments for patients when possible.

• When possible, arrange for phone call or other follow-up of at-risk patients within 24–72 h of discharge from the ED to review discharge plans and to help patients with any obstacles in completing these plans they may encounter.

Follow-ups performed in the patient's home are optimal, but they are not always feasible. Time limitations, financial burden, staffing, or liability issues make home visits a challenge. It is for this reason that telephonic models of transitional care are more feasible and are becoming more widely utilized. Patients who receive follow-up calls have lower readmission rates, higher rates of follow-up visits, and fewer undesirable outcomes [29]. In one study of patients aged 65 and older discharged to home from the ED, the patients who receive a call by a trained nurse within 72 h of discharge from the ED are nearly twice as likely to see a doctor within 5 days as those patients who have not been called, and are less likely to return to the ED, or to be admitted to the hospital within 35 days [30]. When considering a telephonic model, Johnson *et al.* delineate three decision points to consider: (1) who should make the call, (2) what information is essential, and (3) when calls are made and for what period of time [29]. Calls should be made within 24–72 h after discharge and should continue periodically until the patient is reconnected to the PCP. We recommend a follow-up call within 24 h after discharge from the ED, considering the added risk of the shortened time available while in the ED to implement a transitional care plan. Reviewing medications and red flags through the teach-back method is optimal during the call as well as assessment of other social issues (caregiving, transportation, etc.) that may have arisen since discharge. The culture of the healthcare organization and local environment and its resources will dictate the appropriate person to make these follow-up calls, but usually these can be completed by NPs, nurses, or social workers.

Summary

Transitions in care for older patients in the ED setting will increasingly become a critical element of emergency care. Understanding the risks associated with an ED visit for an older adult during the transition back to home and addressing the challenges to be faced after discharge from the ED may lead to improved health outcomes and satisfaction, and a decrease in return visits and hospitalization. The goal should be safe transition from ED back to the community. Key elements to accomplish this include assessing the patient's care needs, assessing the patient's or care giver's understanding of medical conditions and medications, clear and concise discharge instructions that have been reviewed and comprehended by the patient or care giver, connection of the patient with the PCP, early follow-up with the patient about the medical condition, and whether the transition home has been successful.

Section IV: Decision-making

- Older adults transfer between settings, sites, and systems of care more often than their younger counterparts.
- Older patients discharged to home from the ED are at high risk of experiencing adverse outcomes, including receiving inappropriate medications, return to the ED, and death.
- ED utilization by chronically ill older adults often represents an important sentinel event signifying a breakdown in care coordination for an already existing condition or conditions.
- Transitional care interventions are an effective way to manage adverse events and organize our fragmented healthcare system.
- There are a number of evidence-based transitional care programs designated to reduce hospital readmissions; however, their applicability in the ED is variable and still being determined.
- Insight into the patient's physical, social, and cognitive functioning through EMR review and by patient/family interview, either in person or telephonically, is needed to safely discharge older adults from the ED.
- Follow-up calls to patients result in lower readmission rates, higher rates of follow-up visits, and fewer undesirable outcomes.

References

1 Roberts, D.C., McKay, M.P., and Shaffer, A. (2008) Increasing rates of emergency department visits for elderly patients in the United States, 1993 to 2003. *Ann. Emerg. Med.*, 51 (6), 769–774.

2 McCusker, J., Roberge, D., Vadeboncoeur, A., and Verdon, J. (2009) Safety of discharge of seniors from the emergency department to the community. *Healthc. Q.*, 12, 24–32.

3 Wagner, E.H., Austin, B.T., and Von Korff, M. (1996) Organizing care for patients with chronic illness. *Milbank Q.*, 74 (4), 511–544.

4 Rothman, A.A. and Wagner, E.H. (2003) Chronic Illness management: what is the role of primary care? *Ann. Intern. Med.*, 138 (3), 256–261.

5 Coleman, E.A., Boult, C., and American Geriatrics Society Health Care Systems Committee (2003) Improving the quality of transitional care for persons with complex care needs. *J. Am. Geriatr. Soc.*, 51 (4), 556–557.

6 Aminzadeh, F. and Dalziel, W.B. (2002) Older adults in the emergency department: a systematic review of patterns of use, adverse outcomes, and effectiveness of interventions. *Ann. Emerg. Med.*, 39 (3), 238–247.

7 Friedmann, P.D., Jin, L., Karrison, T.G. *et al.* (2001) Early revisit, hospitalization, or death among older persons discharged from the ED. *Am. J. Emerg. Med.*, 19 (2), 125–129.

8 Coleman, E.A. (2003) Falling through the cracks: challenges and opportunities for improving transitional care for persons with continuous complex care needs. *J. Am. Geriatr. Soc.*, 51 (4), 549–555.

9 Project RED (Re-Engineered Discharge) http://www.bu.edu/fammed/projectred/ (accessed 29 August 2015).

10 Society of Hospital Medicine *Project Boost (Better Outcomes by Optimizing Safe Transitions)*, http://www.hospitalmedicine.org/AM/Template.cfm?Section=Home&TEMPLATE=/CM/HTMLDisplay.cfm&CONTENTID=27659 (accessed 29 August 2015).

11 Hansen, L.O., Greenwald, J.L., Budnitz, T. *et al.* (2013) Project BOOST: effectiveness of a multihospital effort to reduce rehospitalization. *J. Hosp. Med.*, 8 (8), 421–427.

12 Parry, C., Min, S.J., Chugh, A. *et al.* (2009) Further application of the care transitions intervention: results of a randomized controlled trial conducted in a fee-for-service setting. *Home Health Care Serv. Q.*, 28 (2–3), 84–99.

13 Bennett, H.D., Coleman, E.A., Parry, C. *et al.* (2010) Health coaching for patients with chronic illness. *Fam. Pract. Manag.*, 17 (5), 24–29.

14 Coleman, E.A., Eilertsen, T.B., Kramer, A.M. *et al.* (2001) Reducing emergency visits in older adults with

chronic illness. A randomized, controlled trial of group visits. *Eff. Clin. Pract.*, 4 (2), 49–57.

15 Coleman, E.A., Parry, C., Chalmers, S., and Min, S.J. (2006) The care transitions intervention: results of a randomized controlled trial. *Arch. Intern. Med.*, 166 (17), 1822–1828.

16 Terrell, K.T., Hustey, F.M., Hwang, U. *et al.* (2009) Quality indicators for geriatric emergency care. *Acad. Emerg. Med.*, 16, 441–450.

17 Schillinger, D., Piette, J., and Grumbach, K. (2003) Closing the loop: physician communication with diabetic patients who have low health literacy. *Arch. Intern. Med.*, 163 (1), 83–90.

18 White, M., Garbez, R., Carroll, M. *et al.* (2013) Is "Teach-Back" associated with knowledge retention and hospital readmission in hospitalized heart failure patients? *J. Cardiovasc. Nurs.*, 28 (2), 137–146.

19 Clark, C., Friedman, S., Arenovich, T. *et al.* (2005) Emergency discharge instruction comprehension and compliance study. *Can. J. Emerg. Med.*, 7, 5–11.

20 Engel, K.G., Heisler, M., Smith, D.M. *et al.* (2009) Patient comprehension of emergency department care and instructions: are patients aware of when they do not understand? *Ann. Emerg. Med.*, 53, 454–461.

21 Hastings, S.N., Barrett, A., Weinberger, M. *et al.* (2011) Older patients' understanding of emergency department discharge information and its relationship with adverse outcomes. *J. Patient Saf.*, 7, 19–25.

22 Engel, K.G., Buckley, B.A., Forth, V.E. *et al.* (2012) Patient understanding of emergency department discharge instructions: where are knowledge deficits greatest? *Acad. Emerg. Med.*, 19, 1035–1044.

23 Kanel, K. (2012) *A Guide to Crisis Intervention*, 4th edn, Linda Schreiber-Ganster, http://crisis9.com/download/201 (accessed 29 August 2015).

24 Pincus, K. (2013) Transitional care management services: optimizing medication reconciliation to improve the care of older adults. *J. Gerontol. Nurs.*, 39 (10), 10–15.

25 Cesarz, J.L., Steffenhagen, A.L., Svenson, J., and Hamedani, A.G. (2013) Emergency department discharge prescription interventions by emergency medicine pharmacists. *Ann. Emerg. Med.*, 61 (2), 209–214 e201.

26 Limpahan, L.P., Baier, R.R., Gravenstein, S. *et al.* (2013) Closing the loop: best practices for cross-setting communication at ED discharge. *Am. J. Emerg. Med.*, 31 (9), 1297–1301.

27 Centers for Medicare and Medicaid Innovation (2012) *Health Care Innovation Award Project Profiles*, http://innovation.cms.gov/Files/x/HCIA-Project-Profiles.pdf (accessed 27 May 2014).

28 Tarkan, L. (2008) E.R. Patients Often Left Confused After Visits. New York Times (Sep 16).

29 Johnson, M.B., Laderman, M., and Coleman, E.A. (2013) Enhancing the effectiveness of follow-up phone calls to improve transitions in care: three decision points. *Jt. Comm. J. Qual. Patient Saf.*, 39 (5), 221–227.

30 Biese, K., LaMantia, M., Shofer, F.S. *et al.* (2014) A randomized trial exploring the impact of a phone call follow-up on care plan compliance among older adults discharged home from the emergency department. *Acad. Emerg. Med.*, 21, 188–195.

The geriatric ED

*Phillip D. Magidson[1], John G. Schumacher[2], &
Elizabeth A. Couser[3]*

[1] *Departments of Emergency and Internal Medicine, University of Maryland Medical Center, Baltimore, MD, USA*
[2] *Department of Sociology and Anthropology, University of Maryland, Baltimore, Baltimore County (UMBC), MD, USA*
[3] *Department of Sociology and Anthropology, University of Maryland, Baltimore, Baltimore County (UMBC), MD, USA*

Section I: Case presentation

A 76-year-old woman was brought to the emergency department (ED) via Emergency Medicine Section (EMS) from the local airport on a Saturday evening. The patient, traveling alone from out of state, to visit family, had tripped and fallen while rushing to make a connecting flight. Reports from paramedics indicated she had struck her head with a brief loss of consciousness, and was complaining of right shoulder and wrist pain. The paramedics reported that the wrist was broken, and the shoulder was dislocated.

The patient was in mild pain on initial examination. The patient further gave a medical history consistent with chronic back pain, type II diabetes, and hypertension. Her medications, which remain at the airport in her checked baggage, included ibuprofen as needed for pain, 25 units of glargine taken each morning, hydrochlorothiazide, and lisinopril. The vital signs were notable for a heart rate of 104 beats/min and blood pressure of 142/84 mmHg. The patient's physical examination revealed an area of ecchymosis over the right superior orbit, swelling and tenderness on the dorsal aspect of the right forearm, and a humerus that appeared to be anteriorly dislocated. She was neurovascularly intact.

The patient was triaged as a middle-level priority patient, and her workup began. Over the next 8–10 h (the department was very busy), as the patient waited

on an interior hallway stretcher, she had plain film X-ray studies, a noncontrast head computerized tomography (CT) scan, IV opiate pain medication, and q6 hour vital sign checks. A fracture of her right wrist, which might require surgery, was confirmed. The orthopedic surgeon, current in the operating room (OR), asked that you keep the patient nil per os (NPO) until they can fully assess her injuries, and determine whether to operate. Your department has no weekend evening social worker or case manager coverage.

Nearly 10 h after her arrival, the nurse alerts you that the patient is tachycardiac to 130 beats/min, diaphoretic, mildly hypotensive to 102/58 mmHg, appears confused, somnolent and now complains of vague chest pain. The blood glucose level is 56 mg/dl, and the only notable finding on her repeat physical examination are pupils of 2 cm bilaterally.

Section II: Case discussion

Dr Peter Rosen (PR): Would you like to start off the discussion on the recent publication of guidelines for geriatric EDs and the utility of geriatric EDs in general?

Dr Shamai Grossman (SG): Guidelines have been published in many different forms and by many different organizations. The American College of

Geriatric Emergencies: A Discussion-Based Review, First Edition.
Edited by Amal Mattu, Shamai A. Grossman and Peter L. Rosen.
© 2016 John Wiley & Sons, Ltd. Published 2016 by John Wiley & Sons, Ltd.

Emergency Physician (ACEP) has tried to publish guidelines in many different parts of emergency medicine over the years, and the issue that I have is when guidelines are published, they have historically lacked evidence behind them. Moreover, people tend to use these guidelines as dogma. Yet, that isn't what they are intended for; they are simply guidelines that are based on, often, a group of physicians who feel this is the correct management because this is the way we do it. Once guidelines are published, however, the medical legal community stamps them as a standard of care using the ACEP as the authority rather than any evidence that might have been gleaned that would refute the guideline.

Dr Ula Hwang (UH): I wanted to make a couple of clarifications concerning the recent geriatric ED guidelines. These are not just ACEP guidelines or policy. This is actually a joint effort by the Society for Academic Emergency Medicine (SAEM), ACEP, the American Geriatrics Society (AGS), and the Emergency Nurses Association (ENA). The geriatric guidelines were not intended as a standard of care, but rather more as recommendations; as a place to commence special attention for geriatric patients. We think the situation is analogous to the need for special care for pediatric populations, or psychiatric patients, perhaps even a need for a geriatric-oriented ED. The case can be made that we need to somehow change how we approach patients, especially older adults, and it is not one size fits all. Geriatric EDs did not exist 10 years ago, but now there are self-proclaimed geriatric EDs being developed in many places throughout the country. Just as the American College of Surgeons thought there should be some criteria met in order to be designated a as trauma center, the Geriatric Task Force with members from ACEP, AGS, SAEM, and ENA convened to say that we need to lay forth some specific criteria, and some set of recommendations. So even though there is no evidence upon which to base the recommendations, at least some thoughtful people have tried to recommend what might improve care for geriatric patients. A finalized set of recommendations of the task force was presented to ACEP's board of directors, to SAEM's board of directors, and also to AGS's board of directors who all supported and endorsed it. It has been published in the three journals of these societies: Annals of Emergency Medicine, Journal of American Geriatric Society, and Academic Emergency Medicine. Hopefully, with these recommendations as a place to start from, we will be able to study what parameters are useful, and how best to improve geriatric care. The textbook that we are working on is also making recommendations that we hope are based on good practice, and we think that the publication of the guidelines will affirm the work that we are doing.

PR: The problems that I have with guidelines were pretty well summarized by Dr Grossman. I would not have any problem referring to this as considerations and goals, and I think that is what the point of the text is. We try to present a style of management that is based on experience and consideration and safety, while we may not have prospective, randomized evidence for every piece of recommendation; what we are trying to do is to say, well, you ought to think of these things, and here is a safe management style that you can try on your own practices. The problem that I have with societal guidelines is that they aren't guidelines, they are mandates, and I think it does exactly what we are trying to get away from: a group of people around a room give expert-based opinions, some of whom are very confident and experienced, and some of whom are there for political reasons who don't have any more experience than those of us who are on the front lines managing these cases. Frequently, they harm us rather than help us.

My second objection is I am theoretically and philosophically vehemently opposed to geriatric EDs. Yes, our society is aging, yes we are going to have to learn to take care of these patients in a better manner, but if we try to split off the pediatrics on one end and the geriatrics on the other end, the trauma along the way, how are we going to support the care of all the rest of the emergency patients that don't have an easy label for their own particular ED. I think we will have done an enormous disservice to our specialty because the reality is not everybody can afford to have a pediatric ED, or a geriatric ED, and we have to take care of both ends of the spectrum as part of our general responsibilities. I have a big problem if we are using the guidelines to suggest that we proceed with the development of geriatric patient only, EDs.

UH: I think that that is a very good point, and I don't think that the intention is to say that self-standing or distinct geriatric EDs should exist. I think that in many ways, the guidelines are put out there as a modality through which, hopefully, we can shift the needle in terms of what and how overall care is delivered. I think many of the tenets that are brought up within the guidelines have come through in the discussion of many of the cases in this book. Some of the models that we are recommending, or that are proposed in the Geriatric ED Guidelines, are applicable in regard to universal care, so most patients should have consideration in terms of what does the patient want and need. That is not just for older adults. I would like this consideration, too, when I am being seen, and I am sure that my children would like that in terms of their preferences. So, I think this is a first step, because for many, many years, there has been very little interest in the geriatric patient population. Now there is a growing interest, there is a growing need. The guidelines are not to say that all places need to create geriatric EDs. This was never the intention of this. Unfortunately, I think you are right, I think some people will use this for political reasons or policy purposes and make this a mandate, but that was not the intention.

Section III: Concepts

Background

The US population continues to age with the increasing proportion of older Americans. The most recent US Census data from 2010 shows the total US population increased 9.7% between 2000 and 2010. Over the same decade, the number of individuals over the age of 62 increased by more than 21% [1]. With an increasing population comes an increasing number of ED visits, especially for geriatric patients. The Centers for Disease Control and Prevention's most recent National Ambulatory Medical Care Survey shows a nearly 10% increase in total ED visits in the United States between 2006 and 2010. Patients over the age of 65 represent the age group with the largest increase in visits over that same time period, more than 11%, for a total of nearly 20 million visits [2, 3]. Nearly 2.5 million alone are from patients coming directly from a nursing home facility [4]. By some estimates, these numbers will continue to rise so that by 2030, 35,000,000 ED visits will be by patients over the age of 65 [5]. These demographic changes present new challenges to the healthcare system, including the ED, where resources must be best allocated to care

for an aging population. Geriatric patients seen in the ED are not simply "older adults." Emerging data suggests they present with distinct needs, are treated differently, and their dispositions from the ED, be that admission or discharge, may be more complex than that of younger patients.

First, geriatric patients are more likely to arrive via ambulance than any other age group. In fact, 38% of all patients over 65, and nearly half of those over 75, arrive in the ED in this way [3]. By contrast, the next closest age group to have these many patients arrive via ambulance are those aged 45–64 at only 20%. Arrival via ambulance may suggest these patients are less likely to come with family and friends, and have already begun to be less in control of their ED visit, before they even arrive. These patients are also likely to arrive already taking prescription medications; 90% of those over 65 seen in the ED are taking at least one medication, which obscures the diagnostic picture, and creates the potential for polypharmacy [6]. This is especially true given that up to 50% of these patients will be prescribed additional medication upon discharge from the ED [5].

Older adult patients are, not surprisingly, more complex than younger patients, and their workup less straightforward. These patients are more likely to exhibit nonspecific symptoms or atypical presentations, and this can further complicate an evaluation. This patient population is generally less healthy, and presents with numerous complicating conditions. One third of all patients over the age of 75 arrive in the ED with "severely high" initial blood pressure measurements [3]. In one study, 67% of geriatric patients seen in the ED were dependent on at least one activity of daily living [7]. Hustey and Meldon further find that over 15% of geriatric patients seen in the ED are cognitively impaired; what is more, 81% of these patients do not carry this diagnosis prior to being seen in the ED [8]. This suggests an underdiagnosis of cognitive impairment in this population, and these patients are less likely to have specialized services such as home health care compared to those with a history of cognitive impairment. This can make a discharge to home from the ED significantly more challenging [8].

Furthermore, geriatric patients seen in the ED generally need more diagnostic tests, utilize more resources, have longer ED stays, are more likely to be admitted to the hospital, and are more likely to be admitted to the intensive care unit (ICU) [3, 9–11]. This increase in stays and rates of admission are not without risk. Up to 20% of older patients develop delirium during hospitalization [12, 13]. Furthermore, Horwitz and colleagues find that over half of ED providers have reported an adverse event or near miss during the transfer of patients from the ED to the inpatient units [14].

With the increasing number of geriatrics patients being seen and the unique needs of these patients, an increase in specialized ED resource centers, broadly identified as Geriatric Emergency Departments (GEDs), have emerged across the country with the first one developed in 2008. This new organization of ED care is designed to respond to the unique needs and challenges that older adult patients can bring to the traditional ED settings with improved patient outcomes and lower total costs.

Development of the geriatric emergency department model

The GED concept is an emerging model of care that broadly focuses on the care of older adults in the ED setting. The model itself is relatively new with the first two GEDs appearing in 2008. GEDs are currently proliferating rapidly with over 50 hospitals self-identifying as providing some level of GED care as of 2013 [15]. At present, hospitals simply self-identify and promote their ED care as a GED, Senior Emergency Center, Senior Emergency Room, or Senior-Friendly ED among several related terms. As is common in an emerging area, there is not yet an established criterion for what constitutes a GED, and the model remains heterogeneous. For example, at one end of the spectrum are some relatively comprehensive GEDs with separate, dedicated geriatric ED space and beds, staffed with geriatric trained advanced practice nurses and ED physicians utilizing assessments, policies, and procedures modified for geriatric patients, and ED case management staff do patient follow-up calls 24 h later. In contrast, other EDs marketed as GEDs may have simply increased their mattress thickness in several ED gurneys, provided magnifiers, lowered the lighting and market themselves aggressively as GEDs. In light of the current GED heterogeneity, several major professional associations including the ACEPs, the SAEM, the AGS, and the ENA, have recently engaged in 2 years of consensus-based work and offer an initial set of

guidelines for GEDs [16]. For this chapter, the term Geriatric Emergency Department will be used to refer to all of the self-identified EDs that explicitly describe modifications to their care of older adult patients in order to capture the broadest range of ED activities related to caring for older ED patients.

In the context of emergency medicine, it should be acknowledged that the absence of a GED does not imply that emergency physicians (EPs) do not know how to treat older adult patients. A characteristic of EDs is their ability to respond to and care for any patient who may present regardless of age, condition, or ability to pay. EDs provide universal care to all patients; however, GEDs are designed to begin to optimize care for the growing population of older ED patients. This is similar to the concept of pediatric emergency medicine and the emergence of specific departments and centers aimed at providing emergency care to younger populations.

Historically, the concept of dedicated care of the geriatric emergency patient stretches back to at least the mid-1980s and beyond, with the publication of articles as well as Wilson *et al.*'s [17] book title Handbook of Geriatric Emergency Medicine. In the early 1990s, there was publication of a series of articles in the Annals of Emergency Medicine by the Geriatric Emergency Medicine Task Force of SAEM funded by the John A. Hartford Foundation [18–20] that helped to focus attention on older adults in the ED. This project culminated in the creation of an instructor's manual, curriculum, video, and textbook edited by Sanders [21] entitled "Emergency Care of the Elder Person." Following this period, interest in geriatric emergency medicine remained modest; however, several professional associations began to organize sections on geriatric issues including SAEM's Academy of Geriatric Emergency Medicine (AGEM), ACEP's Geriatric Emergency Medicine Section (GEMS), and the ENA's Geriatric Committee. Building on the work to date, Hwang and Morrison's [22] article "The GED" first described the general features of a dedicated GED including staffing patterns, physical environment, policies, and procedures. The following year, in 2008, the first GEDs opened in Maryland and New Jersey, and GEDs began rapidly growing across the county [15]. The area of geriatric emergency medicine has received more attention with Hogan *et al.*'s [23] publication of the "Competencies for Emergency Medicine Resident's in Geriatric Care," which identifies eight domains and 26 key competencies for emergency medicine residents in the care of older adults. The recent joint dissemination of the guidelines on GEDs by the major emergency medicine professional associations will further advance the field.

GED staffing patterns

The goal of a GED is to optimize the care provided to older adult patients presenting to the ED. In general, fundamental principles of geriatric medicine help to guide the application and modification of principles of emergency medicine to the older adult population. Compared to other patient populations, the geriatric patient population represents the very highest level of heterogeneity of patient characteristics on key dimensions in the ED. Older adult patients' age range runs from age 65 to over 110 years, a span of over 50 years. With a 50-year age span comes heterogeneity in factors such as comorbidities, medication history, functional reserve, organ system function and drug metabolism, hearing, pain, cognitive function, communication, basic presentation of disease, and social situation. For these reasons, older adult patients may represent some of the most challenging cases for ED providers.

Staffing in the GED typically includes a combination of geriatric-trained ED nurses, Emergency Medicine–trained physicians, and case managers for enhanced discharge planning. Nurse–patient ratios are generally lower than in the average adult ED. Some GEDs have dedicated geriatric nurse practitioners, ED pharmacists, and may have on-call specialists (e.g., cardiology, surgery, radiology, and psychiatry), who have received some level of geriatric training related to emergency medicine. Beyond these staff, Carpenter et al. [24] report the innovative use of "geriatric technicians" to screen for geriatric syndromes in the ED. GED use of volunteers and sitters has also been described. In contrast to the 24-h operation of the main ED, GEDs are typically open and staffed with more limited hours, and some staff, such as specialists and case managers, may not be available on nights or weekends.

Most GEDs include some level of case management through the use of a geriatric social worker or a geriatric case manager who assesses the individual's living environment, and social supports in relation to the person's medical requirements. Such staff members have been shown to greatly sustain treatment efficacy received in the GED and decrease readmission rate [25]. The geriatric case manager typically meets with and counsels the patient and his or her family on discharge plans and enlists community supports if necessary.

After discharge, the geriatric case manager or another designated GED provider routinely places a follow-up call to the patient within 24–48 h of discharge to address concerns and assess treatment efficacy and needs. If any types of services are recommended (e.g., visiting nurse, physical therapy, home care, and meals on wheels), the GED provider calls to assess compliance, and to assist with any challenges in obtaining services. Follow-up calls through the GED are also designed to reduce avoidable readmissions to the ED.

GED education and training

Appropriately training and educating GED staff is an important issue for GEDs. Some EDs have opted to train all of their nursing staff in elements of geriatric emergency medicine, which permits flexibility in nurse staffing of the GED and the rest of the ED. Other GEDs have trained specific nurses designated to work in the GED. ED physician training is more variable. Significant educational opportunities for geriatric ED care have developed over the past decade. The eight domains of Hogan et al.'s [23] "Minimum Geriatric Competencies for Emergency Medicine Residents" provide a useful range of key educational domains including (1) atypical presentation of disease, (2) trauma including falls, (3) cognitive and behavioral disorders, (4) emergent intervention modifications, (5) medication management, (6) transitions of care, (7) pain management/palliative care, and (8) effect of comorbid conditions. These topics are covered in greater details in other chapters of this book. Specific online geriatric ED education resources include the Portal of Geriatrics Online Education (POGOE), which lists over 100 geriatric emergency medicine-specific resources ranging from an introduction to geriatric emergency medicine to palliative ED care [26]. Also, the ENA offers the online Geriatric Emergency Nurses Education (GENE) course with 17 modules from geriatric assessment to care coordination [27]. Beyond these resources, the

411

scientific meetings of SAEM and ACEP increasingly include geriatric emergency medicine symposia, presentations, posters, workshops, seminars, and continuing medical education credits. Fellowship training in geriatric emergency medicine is now available at more than five sites. These organized educational programs on geriatric emergency medicine provide the opportunity for training ED physicians, nurses, staff, and volunteers.

GED environmental modifications

Turning to the GED environment, GEDs typically make some degree of modification to their physical environment related to optimizing care for older adult patients. A range of environmental modifications currently in use are listed in Table 27.1. Modifications may focus on the physical space and architectural features (e.g., separate GED space, interior design, and railings), furnishings (e.g., thicker mattresses), availability of adaptive equipment (e.g., magnifiers and amplification systems), or comfort items (e.g., food availability/kitchen access), among other innovations (e.g., harpist) [28]. Environmental modification also includes planning space to accommodate family members in ED rooms, and for GED case managers involved in enhanced discharge planning [28].

GED procedures and policy modifications

GEDs make a range of modifications to their ED procedures and policies with the goal of optimizing care

Table 27.1 Potential environmental modifications for geriatric emergency departments.

Environmental Modifications	
Separate GED space/rooms	Thicker mattresses
Space for family members in room	Recliner chairs for patients
Lighting flexibility and natural light	Blanket warmers and pillows
Nonglare and nonskid flooring	Orientation devices: large numbered clocks and calendars
Wall color selection	Magnifiers and amplification systems
Noise reduction: ceiling, curtains, and no overhead paging	Food availability/kitchen access
Improved signage	Music and aroma therapy

for their older adult patients. The following section describes some of the common procedural and policy modifications made in GEDs.

Screening and assessment

To begin, GEDs may have criteria for initial triage/admission to the GED including age, cardiac stability, vital sign parameters, nursing level required, and other factors. Triage assessment for older patients may include screening tests developed and modified for a geriatric ED patient population tests including the Triage Risk Screening Tool (TRIST) and the Identifying Seniors at Risk (ISAR) tool. In addition, GEDs report using screening tests for cognitive impairment and dementia, functional decline, fall risk and mobility, medication history or polypharmacy, and pain as described in more detail in the following sections. However, there continues to be a need for validation of many of these instruments for older adults in the ED environment [29] (Table 27.2).

Cognition

In the acute setting, many older adults may present with cognitive impairment, which may be due to underlying dementia, delirium, depression, pain, sensory deficits, including visual and hearing impairment among other factors. Typical screening tests may include the Cognitive Assessment Method (CAM), the Montreal Cognitive Assessment (MoCA), the Short Blessed Test, and the Brief Alzheimer's Screen. In addition, the patient's mood and emotional status should be assessed as depression and anxiety may impact cognitive functioning [30, 31].

Function

Many of the older adult patients who are seen in the GED may have a decreased level of physical functioning, especially during an acute medical emergency or after an injury [22]. Poor physical functioning may lead to falls and an increased risk of additional injury [32]. It is essential to assess an individual's functional ability upon entrance to the GED. Fall risk is a multifactorial entity. Poor nutrition, dehydration, hypotension, cognitive impairment, delirium, and injury are all factors that heighten an individuals' risk for falling in the GED environment. They should be assessed simultaneously with general functional capacity. Assessing ability to perform activities of daily living (ADLs) and instrumental ADL are good

Table 27.2 Potential patient screening and assessment tests for geriatric emergency departments.

Summary of Range of GED Screening and Assessment Tests			
Cognition	Function	Medication	Pain
Mini mental status examination	Timed get up and go	BEERS criteria	Brief pain inventory
The brief Alzheimer's screen	ADL/IADL	–	Pain assessment in advanced dementia scale
Montreal cognitive assessment	Performance-oriented assessment of balance and gait	–	–
Short Blessed test	–	–	–
Ottawa 3DY	–	–	–
Geriatric depression scale	–	–	–

starting points for assessing baseline functional ability prior to their admittance to the GED. The GED professional can interview the individual or the caregiver about the individual's ability to perform such tasks. Additional measures of function include the Timed Get Up and Go Test and the Performance-Oriented Assessment of Balance and Gait. Once in the acute setting, ED providers should consider strategies to minimize iatrogenic fall risk in the acute unit including the use of wireless monitoring and in-room commodes.

Medication

Ninety percent of geriatric patients entering the GED will be taking at least one prescribed medication, and most are prescribed additional medications upon discharge [33]. Polypharmacy is a clear risk for all GED patients (see Chapter 4). Due to the complexity of the medications in the ED, the availability of a dedicated ED pharmacist with training in geriatrics is an important resource. To the extent possible, all medications should be reviewed, not only for correct dosage, but also for expiration date, prescription compliance, interactions with other medications, and possible side effects of each medication. Misuse of both prescription and over-the-counter medications may impact functional ability and cognitive status [34]. The GED provider should attempt to follow the most recent BEERS Criteria (2012) identifying potentially inappropriate medications for older adults when reviewing medications for potential risk in older adults.

Risks and benefits to the patient should be considered when administering a known high-risk BEERS medication. Appropriate monitoring actions should be taken in such an event, based on potential side effects. For example, benzodiazepines, while effective in the younger population, are known to cause cognitive impairment, delirium, falls, and risk of motor vehicle accidents in the older adult population, due in part to a slower metabolism of the medications. Some high-risk drugs may be ineffective in the older adult population and should not be used. Upon discharge, the patient and caregivers should receive medication counseling by ED providers on the appropriate use, compliance, possible side effects, and interactions of all newly prescribed medications. In addition, the ED provider should review all previous and current medications with patients to ensure prescriptions are current, necessary, and will not interact with new medications.

Pain

Pain is an additional area of concern when assessing older adult patients in the ED. Pain may hinder physical functioning as well as distort cognitive status, depending on the severity. Acute pain should be assessed in conjunction with chronic pain. One method of pain assessment in the ED is the Brief Pain Inventory (BPI), which is available in a short form to assess pain intensity and severity. Some patients may be unable to communicate the severity of their pain, especially individuals who are cognitively impaired or whose clinical condition has rendered them unable to communicate. The Pain Assessment in Advanced Dementia Scale is useful in such patients as it assesses pain based on facial grimacing and vocalizations. The individual may be reluctant to discuss the severity of pain or ask for pain management, due to social or emotional reasons [35]. The GED provider should be aware of this concern and offer pain management appropriately as pain is often reported to be inadequately managed in the ED setting.

Additional procedural and policy considerations in the GED

End-of-life preferences should be integrated, when appropriate, into the initial ED triage and screening to avoid potential ethical and legal dilemmas. Any relevant advance directives should be documented and included in the medical record, particularly those involving the patient preferences for resuscitation or life support. In some cases, soliciting information from designated proxies may be necessary. Assessing patients for signs of elder abuse in all forms (physical, verbal, sexual, financial, and emotional) should be routine in this population and investigated further if suspected (see Chapter 23). Older adults are a vulnerable population and highly susceptible to abuse, especially when they are cognitively or physically impaired [36]. Finally, in terms of discharge planning, inquiries regarding social supports and living environment should be conducted during the ED stay. A strong social support system is optimal in discharge planning and recovery process. The GED professional should assess the safety of the individual's environment upon discharge and the patient's ability to live independently including potential challenges that he or she may face.

Section IV: Decision-making

GED integration with larger hospital

Ideally, the GED will initiate standing relationships and training with various departments (admissions, imaging, pharmacy, lab, transportation, food service, and social work) in the main hospital. Working collaboratively with the range of hospital service departments outside the ED can contribute significantly to the provision of care in an optimal manner for the older adult patient population. For example, in some hospitals, GED patients may have priority admission status to the larger hospital to address their medical needs. The same may be true of pharmacy services, imaging, lab, transportation, and food

services depending on how services are currently delivered. At minimum, it is important to bring the voices of these departments to the table to discuss the GED setting.

Conclusions

GEDs represent an emerging model of care designed to optimize the care of older adults in the emergency medicine setting. Current GEDs settings range from relatively comprehensive, purpose built, dedicated GED settings to "senior-friendly" EDs with relatively limited modifications and represent an ongoing trend in both community and academic emergency settings. Overall, there remains a lack of systematic information and peer-reviewed evidence regarding the GED model including its structure, operation, and outcomes. Anecdotal evidence from the early GEDs suggests high levels of patient and ED staff satisfaction with the GED environment; however, such findings need to be rigorously researched and verified. As with other new models of care, GEDs would benefit from research studies focused on key patient care outcomes such as mortality, readmission rates, patient satisfaction, ED provider satisfaction, and costs. Furthermore, due to the rapidly growing size of the older adult population and ongoing ED crowding, research identifying the specific types of older patients who would optimally benefit from GED care represents another important goal. To address these research and policy issues, leadership by emergency medicine professional organizations will be required to argue for resources to further develop and assess the efficacy of GEDs nationwide.

References

1 Howden, L. and Meyer, J. (2010) *Age and Sex Compositions: 2010*, http://censusgov/prod/cen2010/briefs/c2010br-03pdf (accessed 25 August 2015).

2 Pitts, S., Niska, R., Xu, J., and Burt, C. (2006) *National Hospital Ambulatory Medical Care Survey: 2006 Emergency Department Summary*, http://wwwcdcgov/nchs/achd/web_tableshtm#namcs.

3 CDC (2010) *National Hospital Ambulatory Medical Care Survey: 2010 Emergency Department Summary Tables*, http://wwwcdcgov/nchs/achd/web_tableshtm#namcs.

4 Wang, H.E., Shah, M.N., Allman, R.M., and Kilgore, M. (2011) Emergency department visits by nursing home residents in the United States. *J. Am. Geriatr. Soc.*, **59** (**10**), 1864–1872.

5 Wilber, S.T., Gerson, L.W., Terrell, K.M. *et al.* (2006) Geriatric emergency medicine and the 2006 Institute of Medicine reports from the Committee on the Future of Emergency Care in the U.S. Health System. *Acad. Emerg. Med.*, **13** (**12**), 1345–1351.

6 Hohl, C.M., Dankoff, J., Colacone, A., and Afilalo, M. (2001) Polypharmacy, adverse drug-related events, and potential adverse drug interactions in elderly patients presenting to an emergency department. *Ann. Emerg. Med.*, **38** (**6**), 666–671.

7 Miller, D.K., Lewis, L.M., Nork, M.J., and Morley, J.E. (1996) Controlled trial of a geriatric case-finding and liaison service in an emergency department. *J. Am. Geriatr. Soc.*, **44** (**5**), 513–520.

8 Hustey, F.M., Meldon, S.W., Smith, M.D., and Lex, C.K. (2003) The effect of mental status screening on the care of elderly emergency department patients. *Ann. Emerg. Med.*, **41** (**5**), 678–684.

9 Grief, C.I. (2003) Patterns of ED use and perceptions of the elderly regarding their emergency care: a synthesis of recent research. *J. Emerg. Nurs.*, **29** (**2**), 122–126.

10 Roberts, D.C., McKay, M.P., and Shaffer, A. (2008) Increasing rates of emergency department visits for elderly patients in the United States, 1993 to 2003. *Ann. Emerg. Med.*, **51** (**6**), 769–774.

11 Strange, G.R. and Chen, E.H. (1998) Use of emergency departments by elder patients: a five-year follow-up study. *Acad. Emerg. Med.*, **5** (**12**), 1157–1162.

12 Inouye, S.K. (2006) Delirium in older persons. *N. Engl. J. Med.*, **354** (**11**), 1157–1165.

13 Fernandez, H.M., Callahan, K.E., Likourezos, A., and Leipzig, R.M. (2008) House staff member awareness of older inpatients' risks for hazards of hospitalization. *Arch. Intern. Med.*, **168** (**4**), 390–396.

14 Horwitz, L.I., Meredith, T., Schuur, J.D. *et al.* (2009) Dropping the baton: a qualitative analysis of failures during the transition from emergency department to inpatient care. *Ann. Emerg. Med.*, **53** (**6**), 701–710.e4.

15 Schumacher, J.G. and Couser, E. (2012) *Emergency Departments and Older Adults: Analysis of the Emerging Trend of Senior Emergency Centers*, Gerontological Society of America Scientific Meetings, San Diego, CA.

16 Carpenter, C.R., Bromley, M., Caterino, J.M. *et al.* (2014) Optimal older adult emergency care: introducing multidisciplinary geriatric emergency department guidelines from the American College of Emergency Physicians, American Geriatrics Society, Emergency Nurses Association, and Society for Academic Emergency Medicine. *Ann. Emerg. Med.*, **63** (**5**), e1–e3.

17 Wilson, L. (1984) *Handbook of Geriatric Emergency Care*, University Park Press, Baltimore, MD, p. xix, 275 pp.

18 Strange, G.R., Chen, E.H., and Sanders, A.B. (1992) Use of emergency departments by elderly patients: projections from a multicenter data base. *Ann. Emerg. Med.*, **21** (**7**), 819–824.

19 McNamara, R.M., Rousseau, E., and Sanders, A.B. (1992) Geriatric emergency medicine: a survey of practicing emergency physicians. *Ann. Emerg. Med.*, **21** (**7**), 796–801.

20 Singal, B.M., Hedges, J.R., Rousseau, E.W. *et al.* (1992) Geriatric patient emergency visits part I: comparison of visits by geriatric and younger patients. *Ann. Emerg. Med.*, **21** (**7**), 802–807.

21 Sanders, A.B. (1996) *Emergency Care of the Elder Person*, Beverly Cracom Publications, St. Louis, MO, p. xiii, 305 pp.

22 Hwang, U. and Morrison, S. (2007) The geriatric emergency department. *J. Am. Geriatr. Soc.*, **55** (**11**), 1873–1876.

23 Hogan, T.M., Losman, E.D., Carpenter, C.R. *et al.* (2010) Development of geriatric competencies for emergency medicine residents using an expert consensus process. *Acad. Emerg. Med.*, **17** (**3**), 316–324.

24 Carpenter, C.R., Griffey, R.T., Stark, S. *et al.* (2011) Physician and nurse acceptance of technicians to screen for geriatric syndromes in the emergency department. *West. J. Emerg. Med.*, **12** (**4**), 489–495.

25 Mion, L., Palmer, R., Anetzberger, G., and Meldon, S. (2001) Establishing a case-finding and referral system for at-risk older individuals in the emergency department setting: the SIGNET model. *J. Am. Geriatr. Soc.*, **49** (**10**), 1379–1386.

26 Portal of Geriatrics Online Education (2014) [cited 2014 January 13], http://www.pogoe.org/ (accessed 3 September 2015).

27 Emergency Nurses Association. (n.d.) *Geriatric Emergency Nurses Education Online Course* Des Plaines, IL, [cited 2014 January 15], http://www.ena.org/education/education/GENE/Pages/default.aspx (accessed 25 August 2015).

28 Carpenter, C.R. and Platts-Mills, T.F. (2013) Evolving prehospital, emergency department, and "inpatient" management models for geriatric emergencies. *Clin. Geriatr. Med.*, **29** (**1**), 31–47.

29 Carpenter, C.R., Heard, K., Wilber, S. *et al.* (2011) Research priorities for high-quality geriatric emergency care: medication management, screening, and prevention and functional assessment. *Acad. Emerg. Med.*, **18** (**6**), 644–654.

30 Crocco, E.A., Castro, K., and Loewenstein, D.A. (2010) How late-life depression affects cognition: neural mechanisms. *Curr. Psychiatry Rep.*, **12** (**1**), 34–38.

31 Baune, B.T., Miller, R., McAfoose, J. *et al.* (2010) The role of cognitive impairment in general functioning in major depression. *Psychiatry Res.*, **176** (2–3), 183–189.

32 Kearney, F.C., Harwood, R.H., Gladman, J.R.F. *et al.* (2013) The relationship between executive function and falls and gait abnormalities in older adults: a systematic review. *Dement. Geriatr. Cogn. Disord.*, **36** (1–2), 20–35.

33 Hohl, C., Robitaille, C., Lord, V. *et al.* (2005) Emergency physician recognition of adverse drug-related events in elder patients presenting to an emergency department. *Acad. Emerg. Med.*, **12** (3), 197–205.

34 Huang, A.R., Mallet, L., Rochefort, C.M. *et al.* (2012) Medication-related falls in the elderly: causative factors and preventive strategies. *Drugs Aging*, **29** (5), 359–376.

35 Platts-Mills, T.F., Hunold, K.M., Weaver, M.A. *et al.* (2013) Pain treatment for older adults during prehospital emergency care: variations by patient gender and pain severity. *J. Pain*, **14** (9), 966–974.

36 Widera, E., Steenpass, V., Marson, D., and Sudore, R. (2011) Finances in the older patient with cognitive impairment: "he didn't want me to take over". *J. Am. Med. Assoc.*, **305** (7), 698–706.

Index

Page numbers in *italic* refer to figures; those in **bold** to tables; those <u>underlined</u> to definitions

Printed and bound by CPI Group (UK) Ltd, Croydon, CR0 4YY

16/04/2025

14658535-0005